HEALTH
The Basics

Rebecca J. Donatelle

Custom Edition for Pasadena City College

Taken from:

Health:The Basics, Seventh Edition
by Rebecca J. Donatelle

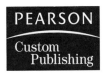

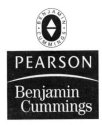

PEARSON

Custom
Publishing

PEARSON

Benjamin
Cummings

Cover images by Richshell Allen

Taken from:

Health:The Basics, Seventh Edition
by Rebecca J. Donatelle
Copyright © 2007 by Pearson Education, Inc.
Publishing as Benjamin Cummings
Sansome St., San Francisco, California 94111

This special edition published in cooperation with Pearson Custom Publishing.

Printed in the United States of America

10 9 8 7 6 5 4 3 2 1

ISBN 0-536-27444-4

2006280039

AL

Please visit our web site at *www.pearsoncustom.com*

PEARSON CUSTOM PUBLISHING
75 Arlington Street, Suite 300, Boston, MA 02116
A Pearson Education Company

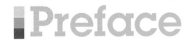
Preface

It is difficult to imagine a time when concerns over health were not headline news. Fears over pandemic flu and new strains of infectious diseases, concerns about the safety of our drinking water and the air we breathe, worries over global warming and catastrophic environmental events such as hurricanes and winter storms, threats from sexually transmitted infections, and reports of epidemic increases in obesity and chronic disease seem to permeate our lives and cause concern for our future.

We are forced on a daily basis to make decisions that may impact our own health or the health of others based on a media blitz of information that is confusing to even the most savvy consumers. Will the foods we eat make us sick or clog our arteries? Is that person who sneezes two seats over in the airplane going to be responsible for our own illnesses? Should we eat more flaxseed to avoid risks from inflammatory diseases? What can we do to protect ourselves, prevent disease and promote our own health and the health of others? Can changing our health behaviors really make a difference? In order to better understand the infinite health possibilities of our actions, it's necessary to look back and see how far we've advanced when it comes to health.

The challenges to our health we face today could not have been imagined by our ancestors. While pandemic disease has always been part of the human experience, threats from pollution and environmental degradation, harmful drugs that drain our potential, threats of bioterrorism, and other modern day issues were unthinkable just a generation or two ago. Disease and illness were seen as phenomena people had little power over — people who became sick from an infectious disease either weathered the illness and recovered or, in all too many cases, died. Few choices were available in foods, medicines, and services; consequently, health care decisions usually focused on cleanliness, avoiding known hazards, and staying away from others who were sick. Over the decades, our list of options for improved health has steadily grown. Technological advances, improvements in vaccines and antibiotics, new treatments for a wide range of illnesses, and new scientific knowledge about risks and hazards have helped us sift through the information overload and begin to make some sense of things.

Today's health-conscious individuals have an abundance of choices when making health decisions: pharmacies loaded with prescription and over-the-counter drugs, health food stores with thousands of products that claim to promote wellness and prevent illness, Yellow Pages filled with doctors and alternative practitioners to choose from, grocery stores and fast-food restaurants packed with every imaginable food, and transportation moving people to and from far-flung continents in a matter of hours. Books, television, the Internet, and other media-driven sources are constantly luring consumers into buying miracle products. Talk show hosts offer formulas for relationship success, sexual prowess, and a slew of other behaviors and products that promise happier and healthier living.

Juxtaposed against the threats to health are advances in medical research, recognition that we need to do more to remove barriers and reduce disparities for some groups when it comes to health, new attention to policies designed to preserve health and protect against harm, and improved strategies for promoting health and preventing premature disease and disability. Technologies continue to be developed, with concomitant improvements in diagnosis of disease and treatment occuring daily. Daily, newspapers and scientific journals report evidence that dietary choices, exercise behaviors, and improvements in interpersonal relationships really matter. At no time in history has it been more evident that by taking action, an individual can prevent illness and prolong a productive, fully functional life. Regardless of whether changes in public policy and community and corporate behavior are necessary to help improve health status, this much is true: the better individuals prepare themselves to make wise decisions, and the more community leaders and representatives of the health care system work together to help achieve and maintain excellent health status, the more likely that everyone's quality of life will improve. In the last year, major changes in food labeling, national nutritional guidelines, policies covering smoking in public places, changes in child protection, auto safety, and numerous other aspects of life have made it easier for people to be healthy even as they face numerous challenges.

Each new class of college students represents a more savvy group of health consumers, complete with its own unique perspectives on health. An astounding, often contradictory and confusing, array of health information is available through the simple click of a mouse, the routine turn on of the television, cell phone, or other media device, or the casual perusal of a magazine. Because there is no single recipe for achieving health, it is important to consider the various opinions and options available to determine what information is the most scientifically defensible and which poses the least amount of risk to wellness.

After more than 30 years of teaching public health students from a wide range of health and other disciplines and after working on several editions of this book, I continue to be excited about the tremendous opportunities that students today have to make a difference to their health, the health of their loved ones, and the health of others. Part of my goal in writing this book is to help students be better "agents of change" as they view the health controversies of today and those that will shape their future—not just in the arena of personal health behaviors, but also in the larger realm of policy changes and community behaviors, which ultimately can assist the global population in living smarter, longer, and better. In short, this book is designed not just to teach health facts but to present health as a much broader concept, something that everyone desires and deserves. By understanding the factors that contribute to health risk, exploring concepts provided in this text, contemplating action plans that might serve to reduce risk, and using the technological tools provided, students can take the first steps in accessing better health.

New to the Seventh Edition

Every year as I face a new class of students, I am struck by the fact that these students will face a new set of health challenges surpassing anything that their parents or I could imagine at their age. These students must be able to find and assess accurate information about health, understand basic foundational material, and choose from a myriad of alternatives as they seek to maintain or improve their health. Each page of this text is designed to provide the latest information, engage students in active thinking and learning, and guide students to make health decisions based on the best science, rather than pop mythology.

As with previous editions of this text, I have been committed to ensuring that this new edition provides students with the latest in cutting-edge research as well as describing the latest discoveries, controversies, and realities that today's students face on a daily basis. Page by page, *Health: The Basics* is designed to pack maximum information into a smaller and relatively moderately priced text. It is designed to be engaging and to move students from just thinking about health improvements to being actively involved in their own health behavior changes. In keeping with my philosophy of leading the market in covering the "hottest" health topics for each new group of students, this edition of *Health: The Basics* includes the following major enhancements and additions.

- **Assess Yourself! boxes** now incorporate the **Make It Happen!** feature, previously located at the end of each chapter. The redesign of this feature will strengthen the connection between assessment and action in making a positive behavior change. We hope to give students the tools that they need to make real and lasting behavior changes and to see these changes as something that can continue long after they have completed their health class.

- **New chapter opener questions** touch on topics students are interested in and help to capture students' attention and engage them in what they will be learning later in the chapter. Questions are repeated within the chapter, where answers can be found.

- **New Try It Now features** highlight simple actions that students can do immediately to improve their overall health and encourage positive lifestyle changes. These new activities, found in each chapter, further emphasize the overall course goal of behavior change and the impact small, daily changes have on overall wellness.

- **New Multiple Choice Review questions** appear in the Take Charge! end-of-chapter material and help students immediately review what they have learned. Answers appear at the back of the text for easy chapter review.

- **A brand new design and enhanced photo program** includes new chapter opener photographs, vibrant colors, redesigned boxes that key students into the importance of each type of box, and approximately five new photographs per chapter to enhance the visual appeal of the text. The redesign of the text provides the same pedagogical standards as in previous editions of *Health: The Basics,* with a modern and bold look aimed at engaging the student.

- **New Behavior Change Contracts** are found at the front of the book and in the Health Resources section; contracts may be filled out as part of the students' Make It Happen! behavior change plans. An example of a completed contract is also included.

- **References** for numbered endnotes now appear at the end of each chapter. This change will make it easier for professors and students to locate additional sources for information and research. The references have also undergone a thorough review for currency.

- **Updates on the status of our nation's health.** We cover the latest trends and threats to health, including tobacco and obesity, the concept of healthy life expectancy, and improving overall quality of life, and provide key information about risk reduction for major areas that are within individual control.

- **New information on health disparities.** We are not created equal when it comes to health. Health problems vary considerably by gender, race, education, ethnicity, age, socioeconomic status, sexual orientation, relationship status, culture, country of origin, and other factors. We provide current information about key disparities and their effects on health and about programs and policies to reduce disparities.

- **Increased coverage of global health issues.** In an era of constant travel and instant communication, we would be remiss in not addressing the interaction of individual, community, and global health. Textbooks that only focus on the individual concerns leave out an important factor: we all live and work in a broader community and are increasingly affected by factors that evolve in our external world. Knowing how to cope and how to reduce risks at all levels is crucial to overall health.

- **Updated information on the role our psychosocial health plays in overall wellness.** Information covers the spiritual resurgence taking place across America, how certain personality traits such as resiliency enhance our ability to cope with threats to psychosocial health, and how to evaluate your own level of happiness or satisfaction with life and improve upon it.

- **New information on mental illness on campus.** Coverage includes how to recognize depression and ways campuses and universities are recognizing and addressing mental illness in college students. This coverage supplies students with the knowledge that they are not alone if they struggle with depression and will help them to better understand how to recognize and cope with a deterioration in psychosocial health.

- **New information on how to evaluate stress levels and techniques that can help students cope with stressful circumstances.** This information will give students valuable coping skills at a time when they are experiencing many changes and new pressures associated with college life. Also featured is new information on alternative stress management techniques (such as deep breathing and Qigong) and tips for controlling anger.

- **Updated coverage on violence, crime on campus, terrorism, and bioterrorism.** These topics are intended to increase student awareness of the tremendous toll that violence takes. New facts and figures include trends in crime, economic implications of crime, and the emotional and physical burden of violent crime among selected populations, particularly college students. Date rape, stranger rape, and marital rape are all discussed in terms of factors that contribute to these crimes, the impact on those affected by rape, and related societal issues.

- **Greatly updated coverage of nutrition covers the USDA's new MyPyramid Plan.** Key goals and features of the plan, detailed information on serving sizes and caloric needs, and the role of physical activity in the new plan are included. Information on portion distortion, how to eat healthfully when dining out, and healthy eating tips for college students are discussed.

- **Major expansion of information on the global epidemic of obesity and the unique risks for people with weight problems.** Risk factors for obesity, new methods for assessing body composition, strategies for risk reduction, and other weight management trends are discussed.

- **Update of the fitness chapter reflecting ever-growing interest in this area.** Coverage has been increased on the role of strength training in weight control and increased metabolic activity, distinctions between physical activity and physical fitness, and how to develop the best exercise program for you. We also cover a unique, often ignored, area: exercise programs for overweight, obese, and very out-of-shape individuals. Information on factors to consider when buying exercise equipment and fitness club memberships should be of interest to students of all ages.

- **New and expanded coverage of infectious and chronic diseases and conditions.** Topics include diabetes, meningitis, SARS, avian influenza, antibiotic resistance, pathogens related to bioterrorism threats, hepatitis A, B, and C, tuberculosis, sleep apnea, and asthma.

- **New statistics on cancer and heart disease** and the most current guidelines for blood pressure and cholesterol monitoring are included.

- **New discussion on the facts and myths surrounding marriage** from the National Marriage Project at Rutgers University, and information on how to determine if your own relationship is a healthy one, or needs some work.

- **Expanded coverage of environmental issues and concerns.** Included are discussions of our roles and responsibilities for environmental health, conservation, and protection of the environment. We added new information on potential risks from prolonged exposure to cell phones and dangers from molds and other environmental health risks at home and outdoors. Comparisons in consumption patterns between Americans and persons in other nations are designed to stimulate discussion and critical thinking.

- **New coverage of widely publicized drugs** including methamphetamine, GHB, Ecstasy, and other substances that are widely discussed in the media but whose risks are often misunderstood are described.

- **New information on recent steps the FDA has taken to ensure prescription drug safety** in light of health problems associated with the popular class of COX-2 inhibitor medications.

- **Updated information on the newest contraceptive methods available to students today,** including their relative effectiveness, issues with use, and other key aspects of effective use. Lea's Shield, Ortho Evra, Seasonale, and Mirena are among the products described and assessed. Also included is information on ECPs, their safety, effectiveness, and controversy surrounding the availability.

- **Updated and expanded coverage on the dual epidemic of diabetes and obesity,** including the relationship between the two and the importance of diet and exercise in risk reduction

Maintaining a Standard of Excellence

With every edition of *Health: The Basics,* the challenge has been to make the book better than before and to provide information and material that surpass the competition at every level. We have painstakingly considered our reviewer feedback from the previous edition and strengthened and improved pedagogical standards.

Chapter 1 establishes both the individual and social context of health and disease and the importance of health to society as a whole, a dual approach used throughout the text. In order to assist students in their efforts to achieve health, we provide a foundation for sound decision making based on well-established theories of health behavior.

Decision making through critical thinking and awareness continues to form the cornerstone of each chapter. Pedagogical aids such as the What Do You Think? questions throughout the chapter encourage students to apply information acquired from the chapter to their own lives.

The roles of the community, health policies, and health services in disease prevention and health promotion are integrated throughout the text. The public health approach is often ignored in health texts in favor of individual action only. I believe that optimum health changes will occur only in environments that are con-

ducive to change, in which individuals can maximize resources to make long-term behavior changes.

Within a strong pedagogical framework, the importance of building health skills is emphasized and integrated consistently throughout the text. Readers will learn specific applications in every chapter through the Assess Yourself, Skills for Behavior Change, Reality Check boxes, and Try it Now feature throughout the text.

Special Features

Each chapter of *Health: The Basics* includes several of the following special features in various combinations. These features are designed to help students think about healthy behavior skills and how to apply concepts found in the boxes to their everyday lives.

- **Assess Yourself** boxes provide quick, general indicators of personal health status in various areas, which students may consider when initiating behavior change. The Make It Happen feature provides students with the opportunity to use the results of the self-assessment, and create a plan for healthy behavior change.

- **Skills for Behavior Change** boxes focus on practical strategies that students can use to improve their personal health and reduce their risks from harmful health behaviors.

- **Reality Check** boxes focus attention on potential risks and safety issues, often as they relate to college-age students. Statistical information and trends help students recognize risks as they relate to particular behaviors and outcomes.

- **Health in a Diverse World** boxes increase awareness and appreciation for individual and cultural differences. They promote acceptance of diversity on college campuses and help students thrive in an increasingly diverse world. In particular, these boxes focus on health implications and issues for diverse populations.

- **Consumer Health** boxes promote consumer skills by increasing awareness about the health market and focusing on particular consumer issues.

- **New Horizons in Health** boxes report on late-breaking health news and topics of recent concern. They show students that health is a dynamic and constantly changing field.

- **Women's Health/Men's Health** boxes, which discussed the unique aspects of men's and women's health and the challenges faced by each group have now been incorporated into the text and the coverage integrated where appropriate.

Learning Aids

- Each chapter is introduced with **chapter objectives** to alert students to the key concepts to be covered in upcoming material.

- Groups of **What Do You Think? questions** that encourage students to think critically are highlighted and strategically placed throughout each chapter.

- To emphasize and support understanding of material, pertinent health terms are boldfaced in the text and defined in the **running glossary** located at the bottom of text pages.

- At the end of each chapter, the **Taking Charge** section wraps up the chapter content with a focus on application by the student. The summary, multiple choice review questions, questions for discussion and reflection, Accessing Your Health on the Internet, and further reading sections offer more opportunities to explore areas of interest.

- **Health Resources** provides practical information in a convenient format at the end of the book. The Injury Prevention and Emergency Care section describes procedures that may prevent injury and save lives. This section also includes a Behavior Change Contract and a sample of a completed contract.

Student Supplements

Available with *Health: The Basics,* seventh edition, is a comprehensive set of ancillary materials designed to enhance learning:

- **MyHealthLab (www.myhealthlab.com).** This online resource lets students access a wide range of print and media supplements that make studying convenient and fun. Contents include the Behavior Change Log Book and Wellness Journal; Tutor Center, ABC Lecture Launcher Video Clips, and the text's Companion Website (all described further below). The instructor resources on the site are described later in this preface.

- **Companion Website (www.aw-bc.com/donatelle).** This easy-to-navigate site offers complete articles from the *New York Times* relevant to the text content, interactive self-assessment activities, practice quizzes, open-ended critical-thinking questions, hypothetical case studies, journal and log activities, and web links for the Accessing Your Health on the Internet section found at the end of each chapter. The website also includes the Flashcard program, with the entire list of terms and their definitions from the textbook available for study.

- **Take Charge of Your Health! Worksheets (ISBN 0-8053-6037-9).** This pad of 38 self-assessment activities (selected from the Take Charge Workbook) is available separately from the workbook.

- **Behavior Change Log Book and Wellness Journal (ISBN 0-8053-7844-8).** This assessment tool helps students track daily exercise and nutritional intake and create a long-term nutrition and fitness prescription plan. It also includes a Behavior Change Contract and topics for journal-based activities.

- **MyDietAnalysis ISBN 0-8053-7387-X (stand-alone CD); 0-8053-7386-1 (student access kit); 0-8053-7839-1 (website virtual ISBN).** Powered by ESHA Research, Inc., MyDietAnalysis features a database of nearly 20,000 foods and multiple reports. This easy-to-use program, on CD or online, allows students to track their diet and activity and generate and submit reports electronically. It is available at a discount when packaged with our Nutrition, Personal Health, and Fitness and Wellness titles.

Instructor Supplements

A full resource package accompanies *Health: The Basics* to assist the instructor with classroom preparation and presentation.

- **MyHealthLab.** This online resource provides everything in one convenient location that instructors need to teach health. MyHealthLabs' course management system is loaded with valuable free teaching resources that make giving assignments and tracking student progress easy. Powered by CourseCompass™, the preloaded content in MyHealthLab includes PowerPoint slides, Test Bank questions, Instructor's Manual material, and more.

- **ABC News Health and Wellness Lecture Launcher Videos, VHS vol. 1 0-8053-0438-X; vol. 2 0-8053-0174-7**

- **Teaching Tool Box (ISBN 0-8053-3859-4).** Developed to support adjunct and part-time faculty teaching the personal health course, this kit will offer all the tools necessary to guide an instructor through the course. Requiring little to no preparation, this adjunct pack will provide detailed information on the resources available for each chapter, including visual lecture outlines, class assignments, and discussion topics. The box includes the IM, TB, Media Manager with ABC News Lecture Launcher videos, Course-at-a-Glance Grid, First-Time Teaching Tips Manual, MyHealthLab Instructor Access Kit, Great Ideas: Active Ways to Teach Health and Wellness,

The Behavior Change Logbook and Wellness Journal, Take Charge! of Your Health Worksheets, and Transparencies.

- **Instructor's Resource Manual (0-8053-7468-X).** This teaching tool provides student and classroom activities, chapter objectives, lecture outlines, and Companion Website resources to reinforce chapter concepts and develop effective student learning. It also includes ideas for incorporating the ABC News video clips into your course and discussion questions for the e-themes articles.

- **Printed Test Bank (0-8053-7843-X)** and **Computerized Test Bank (0-8053-8095-7).** The questions in the comprehensively revised test bank were reviewed by a panel of instructors for relevance and accuracy. The Test Bank includes approximately 1,500 multiple-choice, short-answer, true/false, matching, and essay questions, all with answers and page references. The cross-platform TestGen CD-ROM enables you to create tests, edit questions, and add your own material to existing exams.

- **Media Manager CD-ROM (0-8053-7927-4).** This cross-platform CD-ROM includes figures and tables from the book and lecture outlines that may be customized for lecture presentation. Links to media and appropriate questions for discussion have been added within each chapter lecture. Also included is the two-volume CD-ROM with ABC News video clips.

- **Transparency Acetates (0-8053-8108-2).** The figures and tables from the text are also available as full-color transparencies.

- **Great Ideas: Active Ways to Teach Health and Wellness (0-8053-2857-2).** This new publication provides instructors with effective, proactive strategies contributed by health educators from around the country for teaching health topics in a variety of classroom settings.

- **Course Management.** In addition to MyHealthLab, WebCT, and Blackboard are also available. Contact your Benjamin Cummings sales representative for details.

- **Clickers in the Classroom (0-8053-8728-5).** This handbook provides detailed guidance in enhancing lectures using clicker (Classroom Response Systems) technology.

Acknowledgments

After writing seven editions of *Health: The Basics*, I can only marvel at the dedication and professionalism of the many fine publishing experts who have helped make such a text successful. With each subsequent edition of *Basics*, their skills in dealing with the complexities and considerations of the publication process have become more apparent. I have been extremely fortunate in having a steady stream of fine publishing teams to help me create the foundations of a text that was responsive to students, creative in approach, and reflective of the most important health trends of the times.

Since the acquisition of *Health: The Basics* by the Benjamin Cummings group, I have been extremely pleased by the professionalism, dedication, and attention to detail that this publication team has displayed as we've progressed through several editions of the text. They are truly outstanding and a pleasure to work with. From the highly skilled and enthusiastic Acquisitions Editor, Deirdre Espinoza, to the outstanding editorial staff, I have been uniformly amazed at their consistent efforts to produce a great finished product. Although I wouldn't have thought it was possible to beat past publishing efforts, I must honestly say that my experiences with Benjamin Cummings have been the best of my publishing years; and, remarkably, it just keeps getting better! They personify key aspects of what it takes to be successful in the publishing world, from this author's perspective: (1) drive and motivation for hard work and efficient process, (2) commitment to excellence, (3) a vibrant, youthful, and enthusiastic approach that is in tune with college student needs, and (4) personalities that motivate an author to continually strive to produce market-leading texts. In previous editions of *Health: The Basics,* I was extremely impressed by the superb effort, expertise, level-headed perspective, and guidance of Susan Malloy. With this edition, Alison Rodal proved to be an outstanding addition to the writing team and provided the necessary skill, attention to detail, and creative flair that helped make this edition come alive. Like her predecessors, Alison is a wonderful project editor, and it is largely through her efforts that this book was completed in a timely and efficient manner. I feel fortunate that BC invests in their staff and picks outstanding professionals dedicated to producing high quality texts. While authors provide the "bones" of the book, the editorial staff provides the flesh, life, and heart that entice students to step inside and enjoy the visual and pedagogical enhancements that make a book unique. Without her efforts, in particular, these texts would not have come to fruition or enjoyed the successes that they have achieved. Thank you, Alison!

In addition, I would like to acknowledge the wonderful editorial assistance provided by Developmental Editor Alice E. Fugate, who did an outstanding job in a short time frame to merge some of the newest features of *Health: The Basics* with content from *Access to Health* and in suggesting revisions and modifications based on reviewer comments and market demands. This was a huge and complicated task, and Alice did a remarkable job.

Although these women were key contributors to the finished work, there were many other people who worked on this revision of *Health: The Basics*. In particular, I would like to thank Production Supervisor Beth Masse and The Left Coast Group for their invaluable assistance in final book development and refinement. I would also like to thank Marketing Manager Sandra Lindelof, who spent countless hours making sure that *Health: The Basics* got into instructors' hands, and the rest of the outstanding BC sales staff. Part of the success of any book depends on the efforts of those who work diligently to make sure that the strengths of the book are outlined and that instructors are able to make good decisions about what their students will be reading. In keeping with my overall experiences with Benjamin Cummings, the sales staff and editorial staff are among the best of the best. I am very lucky to have them working with me on this project and want to extend a special thanks to all of them!

Contributors to the Seventh Edition

Many colleagues, students, and staff members have provided the feedback, reviews, extra time and assistance, and encouragement that have helped me meet the demands of rigorous publishing deadlines over the years. With each edition of the book, your assistance has made the vision for *Health: The Basics* a reality. Rather than just creating an upscale version of a high school text, we have worked diligently to provide a text that is alive for readers. With each edition, we would not have developed a book like this one without the outstanding contributions of several key people. Whether acting as reviewers, generating new ideas, providing expert commentary, or writing chapters, each of these professionals has added his or her skills to our collective endeavor.

I would like to thank specific contributors to chapters in this edition. Dr. Christopher Eisenbarth (University of Idaho) did an outstanding job of updating and revising Chapter 3: Managing Stress to reflect his many years of study and work in this area. Thanks to Dr. Patricia Ketcham (Oregon State University) for her work on Chapter 6: Birth Control, Pregnancy, and Childbirth; Chapter 7: Licit and Illicit Drugs;

Chapter 8: Alcohol, Tobacco, and Caffeine; and Chapter 17: Consumerism, and for the insight she brings into the problems faced by students on today's campuses. Dr. Peggy Pederson's (Department of Health at Western Oregon State University) expertise and outstanding writing style greatly enhanced the quality and presentation of Chapter 5: Healthy Relationships and Sexuality. Dr. Amy Eyler (St. Louis University) provided significant expertise and a wealth of teaching and research knowledge to prepare Chapter 11: Personal Fitness. Last but not least, Karen Elliott, a doctoral student in Public Health at Oregon State University, contributed significant time and energy in providing updated information in the area of weight control, with particular emphasis in eating disorders. Each of these professionals provided expertise that went above and beyond my own and which contributed to a well-referenced, scientifically accurate overview of key topics relevant to today's students.

Reviewers for the Seventh Edition

The expertise of many professionals is necessary to create a finished work that represents the best available health information source for college level students. Clearly, *Health: The Basics* continues to be an evolving work in progress incorporating the help of many fine minds in ensuring a quality product. Each new edition builds on the combined expertise of many colleagues throughout the country who are dedicated to the education and positive behavioral change of students and the health of the population as a whole. My thanks go to the following reviewers who have helped us with this admirable tradition: Susan MacLaury, Kean University; Brent Hardin, University of Alabama–Tuscaloosa; Elisha Nixon-Cobb, Kean University; Troy Adams, Arizona State University; Christopher Eisenbarth, University of Idaho; Carolyn Clancy, Phillips Community College; Robert Dollinger, Florida International University; Tanya Morgan, West Chester University of Pennsylvania; Justin Laird, State University of New York–Brockport; Donald Tickle, Radford University; Wanda Taylor, South Carolina State University; Kerry Morgan, Oklahoma State University; McKinley Thomas, Augusta State University; and Susan Moore, Western Illinois University.

Rebecca J. Donatelle
Health & Kinesiology
Benjamin Cummings
1301 Sansome Street
San Francisco, California 94111

Brief Contents

Contents

Part Six
Facing Life's Challenges

Taking Charge

Feature Boxes

Do my friends and family influence my health choices?

How can I differentiate between a bogus health claim and a real one?

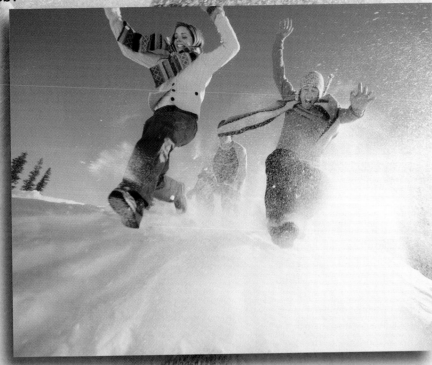

What can I do to change an unhealthy habit?

How can I set a realistic health goal?

1 Promoting Healthy Behavior Change

Objectives

- *Discuss* health in terms of historical perspectives and its multidimensional elements.
- *Explain* the importance of a healthy lifestyle in preventing premature disease and in promoting wellness.
- *Discuss* the health status of Americans and the importance of *Healthy People 2010* and other national initiatives to promote health.

- *Evaluate* the role of gender and health disparities in health status, research, and risk.
- *Focus* on current risk behaviors and how they influence current and future health.
- *Examine* how beliefs, attitudes, and significant others affect a person's health behavior.
- *Assess* behavior-change techniques and apply them to your own lifestyle.

Interested in improving your health? Concerned about the health of a loved one or family member and not sure what to do about it? If so, you are not alone. At no time in our history have so many individuals, government agencies, community groups, businesses, policymakers, and health organizations focused so intently on a growing list of health concerns. Epidemic rates of obesity and diabetes, a growing list of infectious and chronic diseases, a wide range of environmental threats, and other health problems are highlighted daily in the popular media. This widespread focus on health problems makes even the most healthy among us wonder if there is anything we can do to "get it right" and avoid risks to health.

The good news is that the list of actions that we might take to prevent premature disease and disability grows daily. Millions of us are working hard to change our lifestyles, protect our environment, have healthier relationships, and be smarter health consumers. So, why isn't the good news even better?

Let's face it: Getting healthy and maintaining health is a challenge for most of us and requires knowledge and willpower. We know that we should eat right, exercise more, and manage stress—but when a pizza with "the works" is placed in front of us, we can't resist or eat in moderation, or if it's rainy outside, we skip our daily walk and watch TV instead. We are creatures of habit and comfortable habits are often hard to break.

The ability to make wise health choices is complicated by conflicting health claims, faulty research, and scientific reports written in technical language. For example, just when we think our pain medications are safe and helping people live productively, we face major recalls and reports of serious health consequences. Even the best scientists struggle to determine which research is valid and which provides only a preliminary indicator of harm or benefit. The average person is often left wondering how to wade through the information available on the Internet and in the media and to determine the best course of action.

Not only must we negotiate the variety of information sources available to us, but we must also have an awareness of how the media often exploits our weaknesses and how businesses profit by catering to our fears and desires through clever ad campaigns. Food advertisements encourage us to consume enormous portions of high-fat foods and influence us to eat when we aren't hungry, are overstressed, or feeling blue.

The struggle to make personal health choices is not just a matter of willpower and knowledge. For some people, positive lifestyle choices are even more difficult because they lack necessary resources to purchase healthy foods or don't have adequate insurance to have preventive screenings. Social and environmental conditions play an important role in the health choices we make and the options we have. Real disparities exist, and not all have equal access to health opportunities.

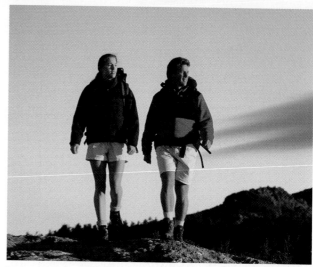

Today, health and wellness mean taking a positive, proactive attitude toward life and living it to the fullest.

These inequities in health care and information access can make our choices easier or much more difficult.

In spite of the many factors and challenges influencing our health, many people have made real strides in reducing risks to health. They have become smart and savvy health consumers by successfully negotiating the information available and have taken action to improve their health. Most importantly, these individuals have found their own unique ways to make small changes to sustain long-term, positive behavior change. They have identified an unhealthy behavior, planned a course of action, and changed their lifestyle for the better. Have you ever wondered, for example, how one of your friends was able to lose weight and now walks up four flights of stairs to class, while you dash to the nearest elevator? Or, why another friend seems to thrive under pressure, while you break down into a crying fit? Why do so many good health intentions remain only intentions?

This text cannot provide a foolproof recipe for achieving health or answer all of your questions. It is designed to provide fundamental knowledge about health topics, to help you use personal and community resources to create your own health profile, and to challenge you to think more carefully before making decisions that affect your health or the health of others. It shows how policies, programs, media, culture, ethnicity, gender, and socioeconomic status directly and indirectly influence health in the United States and around the world.

It is our hope that you will gain appreciation for the many achievements that we have made in health and the many challenges that lie ahead. In addition, we hope that you will look at health not in an ethnocentric way, in which you only appreciate those who look and talk like you and have habits and customs like yours, but rather in a more inclusive way.

Health decisions should be based on the best available research and should be consistent with who you are, your values and beliefs, and who you want to become. Although health is not always totally within your control, certain behavior choices will affect you positively today and reduce future health risks. For those risk factors beyond your control, you can learn to react, adapt, respond appropriately, and use a reasoned rather than purely emotional rationale for your choices. By making informed, rational decisions, you will improve the quality and the length of your own life and have a positive influence on those around you.

PUTTING YOUR HEALTH IN PERSPECTIVE

Although we use the term *health* almost unconsciously, few people understand the broad scope of the word. For some, health simply means the antithesis of sickness. To others, it means being in good physical shape and able to resist illness. Still others use terms such as *wellness* or *well-being* to include a wide array of factors that lead to positive health status. Why all of these variations? In part, the differences in perception are due to an increasingly enlightened way of viewing health that has taken shape over time. As our understanding of illness has improved, so has our ability to understand the many nuances of health. Although our current understanding about health has evolved over centuries, we have a long way to go in achieving a truly comprehensive view of this complex subject.

Health: Yesterday and Today

Prior to the 1800s, if you weren't sick, you were not only regarded as lucky, but also healthy. When deadly epidemics such as bubonic plague, influenza, and cholera killed millions of people, survivors were believed to be of hearty stock, and they congratulated themselves on their good fortune. Poor health was often associated with poor hygiene and unsanitary conditions, and a stigma was attached to households that harbored illnesses. Not until the late 1800s did researchers discover that victims of epidemics were not simply dirty or unhealthy. Rather, they were victims of environmental factors (microorganisms found in contaminated water, air, and human waste) over which they had little control. Public health officials moved swiftly to address these problems, and as a result, *health* became synonymous with *good hygiene*. Colleges offered courses in health and hygiene, the predecessors of the course you are taking today.

Investigation into the environment as the primary cause of disease continued into the twentieth century as outbreaks of tuberculosis, pneumonia, and influenza

surged in many regions of the world. People who made it through the first few years of life without succumbing to an infectious disease usually were able to survive to old age. (Keep in mind, however, that the average life expectancy in 1900 was only 47 years.) Continued improvements in sanitation brought dramatic changes in life expectancy. The development of vaccines and antibiotics added even more years to the average life.

By the 1940s, progressive thinkers began to note that there was more to health than hygiene or disease. At an international conference in 1947, the World Health Organization took the landmark step of trying to clarify what health truly meant: "Health is the state of complete physical, mental, and social well-being, not just the absence of disease or infirmity."[1] For the first time, the concept of health came to mean more than just not being ill.

It wasn't until the 1960s and 1970s that the definition of health begin to mirror the comprehensive model that public health professionals had advocated for decades. Scientists argued that **health** was much more than the absence of disease; it includes the physical, social, and mental elements of life, as well as environmental, spiritual, emotional, and intellectual dimensions of life. To be truly healthy, a person must be capable of functioning at an optimal level in each of these areas, as well as interacting with others and the greater environment. In addition, public health leaders argued that it wasn't just length of life or the number of disease-free years that mattered, but rather achieving your potential for a happy, healthy, and productive life. Today, *quality of life* is considered as important as years of life.

Morbidity (illness) rates indicate that people less frequently contract common infectious diseases that devastated previous generations. Yet, longer life and less frequent disease are not proof that people are indeed healthier. Since most childhood diseases are preventable or curable and massive public health efforts are aimed at reducing the spread of infectious diseases, many people are living well into their 70s and 80s. Today, life expectancy at birth in the United States is 77.6 years. According to **mortality** (death) rate statistics, people are now living longer than at any time in our history, but this trend may not continue.[2] A recent study projects that today's newborns will be the first generation to have a lower life expectancy than that of their parents. Largely attributable to the consequences of

---

Health The ever-changing process of achieving individual potential in the physical, social, intellectual, emotional, environmental, mental, and spiritual dimensions.

Morbidity The relative incidence of disease.

Mortality The proportion of deaths to population death.

obesity, researchers report that life expectancy could decline by as much as five years over the course of the next few decades.[3] This dire prediction is not inevitable if we take steps to become healthier as a nation.

The Evolution toward Wellness

René Dubos, biologist and philosopher, aptly summarized the thinking of his contemporaries by defining health as "a quality of life, involving social, emotional, mental, spiritual, and biological fitness on the part of the individual, which results from adaptations to the environment."[4] The concept of adaptability, or the ability to successfully cope with life's ups and downs, became a key element of the overall health definition. Eventually the term *wellness* became popular. It included the previously mentioned elements, and also implied that there were levels of health in each category. To achieve high-level wellness, a person would move progressively higher on a continuum of positive health indicators. Those who fail to achieve these levels may move to the illness side of the continuum. Today, the terms *health* and *wellness* are often used interchangeably to mean the dynamic, ever-changing process of achieving one's potential in each of several interrelated dimensions. These dimensions typically include those presented in Figure 1.1 and described below.

- *Physical health.* This dimension includes characteristics such as body size and shape, sensory acuity and responsiveness, susceptibility to disease and disorders, body functioning, physical fitness, and recuperative abilities. Newer definitions of physical health also include our ability to perform normal **activities of daily living (ADLs),** or those tasks necessary to normal existence in today's society. Being able to get out of bed in the morning, bend over to tie your shoes, and other usual daily tasks are examples of ADLs.

- *Social health.* This dimension refers to the ability to have satisfying interpersonal relationships, including interactions with others, adaptation to social situations, and appropriate daily behaviors.

Wellness   The achievement of the highest level of health possible in each of several dimensions.

Activities of daily living (ADLs)   Performance of tasks of everyday living, such as bathing and walking up the stairs.

Mental health   The thinking part of psychosocial health; includes your values, attitudes, and beliefs.

- *Intellectual health.* This dimension refers to the ability to think clearly, reason objectively, analyze critically, and use brain power effectively to meet life's challenges. It means learning from successes and mistakes and making responsible decisions that take into consideration all aspects of a situation.

- *Emotional health.* This dimension refers to the ability to express emotions when they are appropriate, controlling them when they are not, and avoiding expressing them inappropriately. Self-esteem, self-confidence, self-efficacy, trust, love, and many other emotional reactions and responses are all part of emotional health.

- *Environmental health.* This dimension refers to an appreciation of the external environment and the role individuals play in preserving, protecting, and improving environmental conditions.

- *Spiritual health.* This dimension may involve a belief in a supreme being or a way of life prescribed by a particular religion. Spiritual health also includes the feeling of unity with the environment—a feeling of oneness with others and with nature—and a guiding sense of meaning or value in life. It also may include the ability to understand and express one's purpose in life; to feel a part of a greater spectrum of existence; to experience love, joy, pain, sorrow, peace, contentment, and wonder over life's experiences; and to respect all living things.

Although typically not considered a dimension in most wellness continuums, **mental health** is an important concept. Often confused with emotional, social, spiritual, or intellectual health, it is a broader concept that encompasses all of these dimensions. According to the U.S. Surgeon General, this umbrella term refers to the "successful performance of mental function, resulting in productive activities, fulfilling relationships with others, and the ability to adapt to change and cope with adversity. From early childhood until late life, mental health is the springboard of thinking and communication skills, learning, emotional growth, resilience, and self-esteem."[5] Mental health is a critical public and community health priority.

A *well* individual might display the following characteristics:

- A realistic sense of self, including personal capabilities and limitations

- An appreciation of all living things, no matter how ugly or beautiful, how unique, or how great or small

- A willingness to understand imperfection, forgive others' mistakes, and grow from personal mistakes or shortcomings

- The ability to laugh, cry, and genuinely feel emotions without getting lost in emotional upsets

- The ability to function at a reasonable level physiologically
- The ability to maintain healthy relationships with family, friends, and intimate partners, and to interact appropriately with strangers
- An appreciation for one's role in preserving and protecting the environment
- A sense of satisfaction with life and an appreciation for the stages of the life experience
- A zest for living, coupled with a curiosity about what each new day will bring
- A respect for self and for others
- A realistic perspective about life's challenges and stressors and the skills to cope with them
- A balance in all things

Many people believe that wellness can best be achieved by adopting a *holistic* approach, which emphasizes the integration of and balance among mind, body, and spirit. Achieving wellness means attaining the optimum level of wellness for a person's unique limitations and strengths. A physically disabled person may function at his or her optimum level of performance; enjoy satisfying interpersonal relationships; maintain emotional, spiritual, and intellectual health; and have a strong interest in environmental concerns. In contrast, those who spend hours lifting weights to perfect the size and shape of each muscle but pay little attention to nutrition may *look* healthy but not have a good balance in all areas of health. Although we often consider physical attractiveness and other external trappings in measuring overall health, appearance is actually only one sign of wellness and indicates little about the other dimensions.

How healthy are you? Complete the Assess Yourself box on page 8 to gain perspective on your own level of wellness in each dimension.

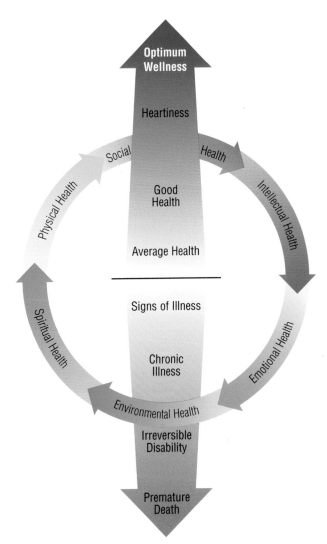

Figure 1.1 ■ The Dimensions of Health and the Wellness Continuum

What Do You Think? Based on the wellness dimensions discussed, what are your key strengths in each dimension? ■ What are your key deficiencies? ■ What one or two things can you do to enhance your strong areas? ■ To improve your weaknesses?

NEW DIRECTIONS FOR HEALTH

In 1990, in response to the indications that Americans were not as healthy as they should be, the U.S. Surgeon General proposed a national plan for promoting health among individuals and groups. Known as *Healthy People 2000*, the plan outlined a series of long-term objectives. Despite many communities working toward

achieving these goals, as a nation we still had a long way to go by the new millennium.

Healthy People 2010

Healthy People 2010 takes the original initiative to the next level. It is a nationwide program with two broad goals: (1) eliminate health disparities, and (2) increase the life span and quality of life. The plan includes 28 focus areas, each representing a public health priority such as nutrition, tobacco use, substance abuse, access to quality health services, and common health conditions (such as heart disease and diabetes). Also included is a list of leading health indicators (LHIs) that spell out specific health issues (Table 1.1).

For each focus area, the plan presents specific objectives for the nation to achieve during the next decade. For instance, nutrition data show that only 42 percent of Americans aged 20 and older are at their healthy weight; the goal is to raise that number to

Table 1.1

What Is *Healthy People 2010*?

Overarching Goals

1. Increase quality and years of healthy life
2. Eliminate health disparities

Focus Areas

1. Access to quality health services
2. Arthritis, osteoporosis, and chronic back conditions
3. Cancer
4. Chronic kidney disease
5. Diabetes
6. Disability and secondary conditions
7. Educational and community-based programs
8. Environmental health
9. Family planning
10. Food safety
11. Health communication
12. Heart disease and stroke
13. Human immunodeficiency virus (HIV)
14. Immunization and infectious diseases
15. Injury and violence prevention
16. Maternal, infant, and child health
17. Medical product safety
18. Mental health and mental disorders
19. Nutrition and overweight
20. Occupational safety and health
21. Oral health
22. Physical activity and fitness
23. Public health infrastructure
24. Respiratory disease
25. Sexually transmitted disease
26. Substance abuse
27. Tobacco use
28. Vision and hearing

Leading Health Indicators

1. Physical activity
2. Overweight and obesity
3. Tobacco use
4. Substance abuse
5. Responsible sexual behavior
6. Mental health
7. Injury and violence
8. Environmental quality
9. Immunization
10. Access to health care

Source: Office of Disease Prevention and Health Promotion, U.S. Department of Health and Human Services, "Healthy People 2010," 2000, www.health.gov/healthypeople/About/hpfact.htm.

60 percent. In the focus area of physical activity and fitness, 40 percent of Americans aged 18 and older do not engage in any leisure-time physical activity. The objective is to reduce this number to 20 percent by 2010.[6] As part of the goal to eliminate **health disparities,** *Healthy People 2010* also must address issues of social justice. Disparities in health care among various groups are often the result of disadvantages faced by minority groups, women, and children, whose health care suffers due to their race, ethnicity, gender, and/or socioeconomic status. The attention to social justice issues in the *Healthy People 2010* program is designed to address these disparities.

National Changes: Improving Health and Reducing Disparities

Are we making progress? From all indicators, national priorities are shifting and health professionals and public and private organizations are beginning to work together to help people make better health decisions.

Health disparities   Differences in the incidence, prevalence, mortality, and burden of diseases and other health conditions among specific population groups.

For example, in early 2005, after years of work and considerable research, a new, more readily adaptable Food Guide Pyramid and major changes in food labeling were completed to assist individuals in dietary choices. In addition, major changes in recommended exercise levels for fitness, weight loss, and other objectives were established.[7] These landmark actions are designed to improve one's life span and quality of life. On the flip side, we do still see evidence of disparities in health care, especially evident during the Hurricane Katrina disaster.

To help reduce disparities in costs, quality of care, and access to health care services, national groups have called for actions or goals including improvements in health insurance for the uninsured and underinsured, better access to low-cost, high-quality health care, improvements in education about health risks, creation of policies to protect health, and enhancement of environments to help reduce risk. Importantly, each of us must also act responsibly, take appropriate action, and do what we can to improve our own health status.

A New Focus on Health Promotion

The objectives of *Healthy People 2010* have prompted action to promote health and prevent premature disability through social, environmental, policy-related, and community-based programming. There is also a new emphasis on assisting individuals in changing unhealthy behaviors—which is not easy without an arsenal of resources and a supportive environment.

The term *health promotion* describes the educational, organizational, procedural, environmental, social, and financial supports that help individuals and groups reduce negative health behaviors and promote positive change. Health promotion programs identify healthy people who are engaging in **risk behaviors,** or actions that increase susceptibility to negative health outcomes, and motivate them to change their actions. Effective stop-smoking programs, for instance, don't simply say, "Just do it." Instead, they provide information about possible consequences to smokers and their secondhand smoke victims (educational support); encourage smokers to participate in smoking cessation classes and allow time off for worker attendance or set up buddy systems to help them (organizational support); establish policies governing smokers' behaviors and supporting their decisions to change, such as banning smoking in the workplace and removing cigarettes from vending machines (environmental support); and provide monetary incentives to motivate people to participate (financial support).[8]

Health promotion programs also encourage those with sound health habits to maintain them. By attempting to modify behaviors, increase skills, change attitudes, increase knowledge, influence values, and improve health decision making, health promotion goes well beyond the simple information campaign. By basing programs and services in communities, organizations, schools, and other places where most people spend their time, health promotion increases the likelihood of long-term success on the road to health and wellness.

Whether we use the term *health* or *wellness*, we are talking about a person's overall responses to the challenges of living. Occasional dips into the ice cream bucket and other dietary indulgences, failures to exercise every day, flare-ups of anger, and other deviations from optimal behavior should not be viewed as major failures. Actually, the ability to recognize that each of us is an imperfect being attempting to adapt in an imperfect world signals individual well-being.

We must also remember to be tolerant of others. Rather than be warriors against pleasure in our zeal to change the health behaviors of others, we need to be supportive, nonjudgmental, and helpful to those trying to achieve their own health goals.

Disease Prevention

Most health promotion initiatives include **disease prevention**. Historically, the health literature describes three types of prevention: primary, secondary, and tertiary.

In a general sense, *prevention* means taking positive actions *now* to avoid becoming sick *later*. Getting immunized against diseases such as polio, deciding not

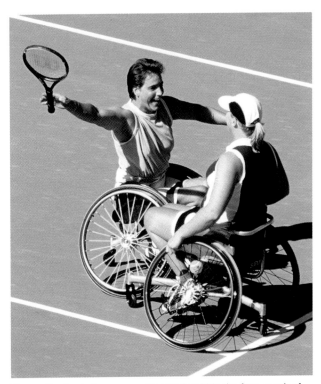

The motivation to improve quality of life within the framework of one's own unique capabilities is crucial to achieving health and wellness.

to smoke cigarettes, and practicing safer sex constitute **primary prevention**—actions designed to reduce risk and avoid health problems before they start. **Secondary prevention** (also referred to as **intervention**) involves recognizing health risks or early problems and taking action (intervening) to stop them before they lead to actual illness. Getting a young smoker to quit is an example of secondary prevention. The third type, **tertiary prevention,** involves treatment and/or rehabilitation after a person is already ill. Typically, health care professionals practice tertiary prevention.

Health promotion Combined educational, organizational, policy, financial, and environmental supports to help people reduce negative health behaviors and promote positive change.

Risk behaviors Behaviors that increase susceptibility to negative health outcomes.

Disease prevention Actions or behaviors designed to keep people from getting sick.

Primary prevention Actions designed to stop problems before they start.

Secondary prevention (intervention) Intervention early in the development of a health problem.

Tertiary prevention Treatment and/or rehabilitation efforts.

How Healthy Are You?

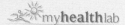

Fill out this assessment online at
www.aw-bc.com/MyHealthLab or www.aw-bc.com/donatelle.

Although we all recognize the importance of being healthy, it can be a challenge to sort out which behaviors are most likely to cause problems or which ones pose the greatest risk. Even when we recognize our unique risks and know what to do, it isn't always easy to stay motivated enough to maintain a specific set of health behaviors. Before you decide where to start, it is important to take a careful look at your health status right now. Think carefully about where you believe that you are today in each of the dimensions of health. Circle the number in each category that you think best describes you. Rate your health status in each of the following dimensions by circling the number on the line that comes closest to describing the way you are most of the time.

	Poor Health		Average Health		Excellent Health
Physical health	1	2	3	4	5
Social health	1	2	3	4	5
Emotional health	1	2	3	4	5
Environmental health	1	2	3	4	5
Spiritual health	1	2	3	4	5
Intellectual health	1	2	3	4	5

After completing the above section, how would you rate your *overall* health? _____

Which area(s), if any, do you think you should work on improving? _____

If we were to ask your closest friends how healthy they think you are, which area(s) do you think they would say you need to work on and improve? _____

By completing the following assessment, you will have a clearer picture of health areas in which you excel and those that could use varying degrees of work. Taking this assessment will also help you to reflect on various components of health that you may not have thought much about.

Use the results from this assessment as a guide and as a way to begin analyzing potential areas for improvement and/or maintenance. Answer each question, then total your score for each section and fill it in on the Personal Checklist at the end of the assessment for a general sense of your health profile. Think about the behaviors that influenced your score in each category. Would you like to change any of them? Choose the area that you'd like to improve, then complete the Behavior Change Contract at the front of your book. Use the contract to think through and implement a behavior change over the course of this class.

Each of the categories in this questionnaire is an important aspect of the total dimensions of health, but this is not a substitute for the advice of a qualified health care provider. Consider scheduling a thorough physical examination by a licensed physician or setting up an appointment with a mental health counselor at your school if you think you need help making a behavior change.

For each of the following, indicate how often you think the statements describe you.

Physical Health

	Never	Rarely	Some of the Time	Usually or Always
1. I am happy with my body size and weight.	1	2	3	4
2. I engage in vigorous exercises such as brisk walking, jogging, swimming, or running for at least 30 minutes per day, 3–4 times per week.	1	2	3	4
3. I do exercises designed to strengthen my muscles and increase endurance at least 2 times per week.	1	2	3	4
4. I do stretching, limbering up, and balance exercises such as yoga, pilates, or tai chi to increase my body awareness and control and increase my overall physical health.	1	2	3	4
5. I feel good about the condition of my body and would be able to respond to most demands placed upon it.	1	2	3	4
6. I get at least 7–8 hours of sleep each night.	1	2	3	4

	Never	Rarely	Some of the Time	Usually or Always
7. I try to add moderate activity to each day, such as taking the stairs instead of the elevator and walking whenever I can instead of riding.	1	2	3	4
8. My immune system is strong, and my body heals itself quickly when I get sick or injured.	1	2	3	4
9. I have lots of energy and can get through the day without being overly tired.	1	2	3	4
10. I listen to my body; when there is something wrong, I try to make adjustments to heal it or seek professional advice.	1	2	3	4

Total score for this section: ———

Social Health

	Never	Rarely	Some of the Time	Usually or Always
1. When I meet people, I feel good about the impression I make on them.	1	2	3	4
2. I am open, honest, and get along well with other people.	1	2	3	4
3. I participate in a wide variety of social activities and enjoy being with people who are different than I.	1	2	3	4
4. I try to be a "better person" and work on behaviors that have caused problems in my interactions with others.	1	2	3	4
5. I get along well with the members of my family.	1	2	3	4
6. I am a good listener.	1	2	3	4
7. I am open and accessible to a loving and responsible relationship.	1	2	3	4
8. I have someone I can talk to about my private feelings.	1	2	3	4
9. I consider the feelings of others and do not act in hurtful or selfish ways.	1	2	3	4
10. I try to see the good in my friends and do whatever I can to support them and help them feel good about themselves.	1	2	3	4

Total score for this section: ———

Emotional Health

	Never	Rarely	Some of the Time	Usually or Always
1. I find it easy to laugh, cry, and show emotions like love, fear, and anger and try to express these in positive, constructive ways.	1	2	3	4
2. I avoid using alcohol or other drugs as a means of helping me forget my problems.	1	2	3	4
3. When viewing a particularly challenging situation, I tend to view the glass as "half full" rather than "half empty" and perceive problems as opportunities for growth.	1	2	3	4
4. When I am angry, I try to let others know in nonconfrontational and nonhurtful ways and try to resolve issues rather than stewing about them.	1	2	3	4
5. I try not to worry unnecessarily and try to talk about my feelings, fears, and concerns rather than letting them become chronic issues.	1	2	3	4
6. I recognize when I am stressed and take steps to relax through exercise, quiet time, or other calming activities.	1	2	3	4
7. I feel good about myself and believe others like me for who I am.	1	2	3	4
8. I try not to be too critical and/or judgmental of others and to understand differences or quirks that I may note in others.	1	2	3	4

(continues)

(continued)

	Never	Rarely	Some of the Time	Usually or Always
9. I am flexible and adapt or adjust to change in a positive way.	1	2	3	4
10. My friends regard me as a stable, emotionally well-adjusted person whom they trust and rely on for support.	1	2	3	4

Total score for this section: _____

Environmental Health

	Never	Rarely	Some of the Time	Usually or Always
1. I am concerned about environmental pollution and actively try to preserve and protect natural resources.	1	2	3	4
2. I buy recycled paper and purchase biodegradable detergents and cleaning agents whenever possible.	1	2	3	4
3. I recycle my garbage, purchase refillable containers when possible, and try to minimize the amount of paper and plastics that I use.	1	2	3	4
4. I try to wear my clothes for longer periods between washing to reduce water consumption and the amount of detergents in our water sources.	1	2	3	4
5. I vote for pro-environment candidates in elections.	1	2	3	4
6. I write my elected leaders about environmental concerns.	1	2	3	4
7. I turn down the heat and wear warmer clothes at home in winter and use the air conditioner only when necessary or at higher temperatures in summer.	1	2	3	4
8. I am aware of lead pipes in my living area, chemicals in my carpet, and other potential hazards and try to reduce my exposure whenever possible.	1	2	3	4
9. I use both sides of the paper when taking class notes or doing assignments.	1	2	3	4
10. I try not to leave the faucet running too long when I brush my teeth, shave, or shower.	1	2	3	4

Total score for this section: _____

Spiritual Health

	Never	Rarely	Some of the Time	Usually or Always
1. I believe life is a precious gift that should be nurtured.	1	2	3	4
2. I take time to enjoy nature and the beauty around me.	1	2	3	4
3. I take time alone to think about what's important in life—who I am, what I value, where I fit in, and where I'm going.	1	2	3	4
4. I have faith in a greater power, be it a God-like force, nature, or the connectedness of all living things.	1	2	3	4
5. I engage in acts of caring and goodwill without expecting something in return.	1	2	3	4
6. I feel sorrow for those who are suffering and try to help them through difficult times.	1	2	3	4
7. I look forward to each day as an opportunity for further growth and challenge.	1	2	3	4
8. I work for peace in my interpersonal relationships, in my community, and in the world at large.	1	2	3	4
9. I have a great love and respect for all living things, and regard animals, etc., as important links in a vital living chain.	1	2	3	4
10. I go for the gusto and experience life to the fullest.	1	2	3	4

Total score for this section: _____

Intellectual Health

	Never	Rarely	Some of the Time	Usually or Always
1. I carefully consider my options and possible consequences as I make choices in life.	1	2	3	4
2. I learn from my mistakes and try to act differently the next time.	1	2	3	4
3. I follow directions or recommended guidelines, avoid risks, and act in ways likely to keep myself and others safe.	1	2	3	4
4. I consider myself to be a wise health consumer and check reliable information sources before making decisions.	1	2	3	4
5. I am alert and ready to respond to life's challenges in ways that reflect thought and sound judgment.	1	2	3	4
6. I have at least one hobby, learning activity, or personal growth activity that I make time for each week; something that improves me as a person.	1	2	3	4
7. I actively learn all I can about products and services before making decisions.	1	2	3	4
8. I manage my time well rather than let time manage me.	1	2	3	4
9. My friends and family trust my judgment.	1	2	3	4
10. I think about my self-talk (the things I tell myself) and then examine the evidence to see if my perceptions and feelings are sound.	1	2	3	4

Total score for this section: _____

Although each of these six dimensions of health is important, there are some factors that don't readily fit one dimension. As college students, you face some unique risks that others may not have. For this reason, we have added an additional section to this self-assessment that focuses on personal health promotion and disease prevention. Answer these questions and add your results to the Personal Checklist in the following section.

Personal Health Promotion/ Disease Prevention

	Never	Rarely	Some of the Time	Usually or Always
1. I know the warning signs of common sexually transmitted infections, such as genital warts (HPV), chlamydia, and herpes, and read new information about these diseases as a way of protecting myself.	1	2	3	4
2. If I were to be sexually active, I would use protection such as latex condoms, dental dams, and other means of reducing my risk of sexually transmitted infections.	1	2	3	4
3. I find ways other than binge drinking when at parties or during happy hours to loosen up and have a good time.	1	2	3	4
4. When I have more than 1 or 2 drinks, I ask someone who is not drinking to drive me and my friends home.	1	2	3	4
5. I have eaten too much in the last month and have forced myself to vomit to avoid gaining weight.	4	3	2	1
6. I have several piercings and have found that I enjoy the rush that comes with each piercing event.	4	3	2	1

(continues)

(continued)

	Never	Rarely	Some of the Time	Usually or Always
7. If I were to have a tattoo or piercing, I would go to a reputable person who follows strict standards of sterilization and precautions against bloodborne disease transmission.	1	2	3	4
8. I engage in extreme sports and find that I enjoy the highs that come with risking bodily harm through physical performance.	4	3	2	1
9. I am careful not to mix alcohol or other drugs with prescription and over-the-counter drugs.	1	2	3	4
10. I practice monthly breast/testicle self-examinations.	1	2	3	4

Total score for this section: _____

Personal Checklist

Now, total your scores in each of the health dimensions and compare them to what would be considered optimal scores. Which areas do you need to work on? How does your score compare with how you rated yourself in the first part of the questionnaire?

	Ideal Score	Your Score
Physical health	40	_____
Social health	40	_____
Emotional health	40	_____
Environmental health	40	_____
Spiritual health	40	_____
Intellectual health	40	_____
Personal health promotion/ disease prevention	40	_____

WHAT YOUR SCORES IN EACH CATEGORY MEAN

Scores of 35–40: Outstanding! Your answers show that you are aware of the importance of these behaviors in your overall health. More important, you are putting your knowledge to work for you by practicing good health habits that should reduce your overall risks. Although you received a very high score on this part of the test, you may want to consider areas where your scores could be improved.

Scores of 30–34: Your health practices in these areas are very good, but there is room for improvement. Look again at the items you answered that scored one or two points. What changes could you make to improve your score? Even a small change in behavior can help you achieve better health.

Scores of 20–29: Your health risks are showing! Find information about the risks you are facing and why it is important to change these behaviors. Perhaps you need help in deciding how to make the changes you desire. Assistance is available from this book, your professor, and student health services at your school.

Health Status Report: How Well Are We Doing?

In the United States, chronic diseases account for seven of the ten leading causes of death, and are linked to preventable lifestyle behaviors such as tobacco use, poor nutrition and lack of physical activity leading to obesity, alcohol use, car crashes, risky sexual behavior, and drug use.[9] These preventable risk behaviors not only kill us, but they affect quality of life for nearly 100 million Americans and account for 70 percent of total medical expenditures.[10]

Primary and secondary prevention offer our best hope for reducing the **incidence** (number of new cases), and **prevalence** (number of existing cases) of disease and disability. Community intervention programs have proven effective, and certain ones have become model programs for public health.[11]

Incidence The number of new cases.

Prevalence The number of existing cases.

Scores below 20: You may be taking unnecessary risks with your health. Perhaps you are not aware of the risks and what to do about them. Identify each risk area and make a mental note as you read the associated chapter in the book. Whenever possible, seek additional resources, either on your campus or through your local community health resources, and make a serious commitment to behavior change. If any area is causing you to be less than functional in your class work or personal life, seek professional help. In this book you will find the information you need to help you improve your scores and your health. Remember that these scores are only indicators, not diagnostic tools.

■■■ Make It Happen!

Assessment: The Assess Yourself activity gave you the chance to look at the status of your health in several dimensions. Now that you have considered these results, you can begin to take steps toward changing certain behaviors that may be detrimental to your health.

Making a Change: In order to change your behavior, you need to develop a plan. Follow these steps below and complete your Behavior Change Contract to take action.

1. Evaluate your behavior, and identify patterns and specific things you are doing. What can you change now? What can you change in the near future?
2. Select one pattern of behavior that you want to change.
3. Fill out the Behavior Change Contract found at the front of your book. It should include your long-term goals for change, your short-term goals, the rewards you'll give yourself for reaching these goals, potential obstacles along the way, and strategies for overcoming these obstacles. For each goal, list the small steps and specific actions that you will take.
4. Chart your progress in a journal. At the end of a week, consider how successful you were in following your plan. What helped you be successful? What made change more difficult? What will you do differently next week?
5. Revise your plan as needed: Are the short-term goals attainable? Are the rewards satisfying?

Example: Felipe assessed his health and discovered that his score in the Personal Health promotion section was low—25 points—because of some risky behaviors in which he was engaging. In particular, he realized that he had driven several times after drinking and that he was not performing monthly testicle self-examinations. Felipe decided to tackle one of these issues at a time. He completed a Behavior Change Contract to drive only when he had had fewer than two drinks. Steps in his contract included finding out about designated driver programs, moderating his drinking so that he was sober and competent to drive at the end of a night out with friends, and finding concerts and other events to attend that did not involve drinking. The rewards he chose for these steps included tickets to a concert and a new computer game. After a few months Felipe realized that he had been in several situations in which he might previously have driven under the influence. Instead, he had given himself alternatives such as designated drivers, budgeting for a taxi, and moderating his drinking, and thus had avoided unsafe situations.

Next month, Felipe will get a pamphlet from the health center on testicular self-exams and choose a day of the month to be his self-examination day. Every month that he does the exam, he'll sleep in an extra hour that weekend as a reward.

A focus on prevention and early intervention rather than tertiary prevention can create a significant decrease in preventing chronic diseases and the tolls they take on U.S. citizens. Health educators in our schools and communities offer an effective delivery mechanism for prevention and intervention programs. **Certified Health Education Specialists (CHES)** make up a trained cadre of public health educators with special credentials and competencies in planning, implementing, and evaluating prevention programs that offer scientifically and behaviorally sound methods to help individuals and communities increase the likelihood of success in achieving optimal health. Trained exercise science and nutrition specialists can provide excellent advice on specific dietary and exercise behaviors which can support specific aspects of health promotion activities. Together, these specialists have the skills and experience

> **Certified Health Education Specialists (CHES)**
> Academically trained health educators who have passed a national competency examination for prevention and intervention programming.

Ten Greatest Public Health Achievements of the Twentieth Century

1. Vaccinations
2. Motor vehicle safety
3. Workplace safety
4. Control of infectious diseases
5. Cardiovascular disease (CVD) and stroke deaths
6. Safe and healthy foods
7. Maternal and infant care
8. Family planning
9. Fluoridated drinking water
10. Recognition of tobacco as a health hazard

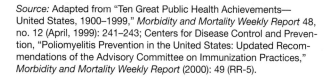

Source: Adapted from "Ten Great Public Health Achievements—United States, 1900–1999," *Morbidity and Mortality Weekly Report* 48, no. 12 (April, 1999): 241–243; Centers for Disease Control and Prevention, "Poliomyelitis Prevention in the United States: Updated Recommendations of the Advisory Committee on Immunization Practices," *Morbidity and Mortality Weekly Report* (2000): 49 (RR-5).

to greatly enhance the nation's health. A major shift in focus from treatment to prevention is necessary to achieve our national goals.

Improving Quality of Life

In the last decade, a shift in the way we look at health has been quietly emerging. This new view will have a profound impact on how we perceive our nation's health status. For decades we have looked at steadily increasing life expectancy rates and proudly proclaimed that the health of Americans has never been better. However, in the late 1990s health organizations and international groups attempted to quantify the number of years a person lives with a disability or illness, compared to the number of healthy years. In a 2002 report, the World Health Organization summarized the concept of **healthy life expectancy.**[12] Simply stated, *healthy life expectancy* refers to the number of years a newborn can expect to live in full health, based on current rates of illness and mortality. For example, if you could delay the onset of diabetes so that a person didn't develop the disease until she was 60 years old, rather than developing it at 30, there would be a dramatic increase in the number of healthy years the individual could except to live. A focus on disease prevention could vastly improve quality of life and create huge cost reductions in the amount spent on premature disease.

This concept of healthy life expectancy can have tremendous implications for your health and motivation to

Healthy life expectancy The equivalent number of years a newborn can expect to live, based on current rates of illness and mortality.

change behaviors now. For example, you know that you should exercise, maintain a healthy weight, and not drink and drive; however, the threat of heart disease, cancer, or accident-related injuries seems decades away. Recognizing how your present actions will play a role in your future health and overall quality of life can motivate you to make behavior changes now to ensure the maximum number of years you can live happily and healthfully.

What Do You Think?

Think about your own health right now. ■ On a scale from 1 to 10, with 1 being the lowest and 10 the highest, rate your fitness level (going for a run; hiking up a hill), your ability to form and maintain healthy relationships, and your ability to cope with daily stressors.

Achievements in Public Health

Shortcomings aside, for those of us in the field of public health, the saying "We've come a long way, baby" accurately reflects the health achievements of the past 100 years. Table 1.2 lists the ten greatest public health achievements of the past century according to the Centers for Disease Control and Prevention (CDC).

While past achievements are indeed remarkable, the possibilities for health and well-being in the future defy the imagination. Living longer, living more disease-free years, and injecting more quality into the extra years of life will be major goals. The more we learn about the remarkable resilience of the human body and spirit, and the more that technology stretches our imagination and enlarges our possibilities, the more likely that the twenty-first century will surpass the twentieth in health-related breakthroughs.

What Do You Think?

What do you consider the greatest achievements in public health in your lifetime? ■ What do you think would be the most important achievement that public health could make in the next 50 years?

PREPARING FOR BETTER HEALTH IN THE TWENTY-FIRST CENTURY

Many health challenges still lie ahead. While it is important that each of us work to preserve and protect our own health, it is also important to become actively engaged in the health of our communities, our nation, and the global population.

Global Health Issues

Everyone's health is profoundly affected by economic, social, behavioral, scientific, and technological factors. The world economy has become increasingly interconnected and globalized; every day, 2 million people worldwide move across national borders. Globalization has benefited people in virtually every country while creating a remarkable degree of mutual interdependence.[13] In addition to the advantages, these changes also bring health risks that cannot be addressed by one country alone. The SARS outbreak in 2003, and the current concern over pandemic flu serve as grim reminders of the need for a proactive international response to disease prevention. Health risks are not limited to disease; contaminants to our food, air, and water supplies, bioterrorists, and chemical toxins, are modern health threats to the global community.[14]

Global health in the twenty-first century will require each of us to do our part to protect our own health and the health of others, whether at home or abroad. We will need time to understand the vast differences in health status across various social groups and to promote community action that addresses the unique needs of each population.

Gender Differences and Health

When it comes to health-related differences, men and women really do seem to be from Mars and Venus. Though much of the male and female anatomy is identical, researchers are discovering that the same diseases and treatments can affect men and women very differently. Many illnesses—for example, osteoporosis, multiple sclerosis, diabetes, and Alzheimer's disease—are much more common in women, even though rates for these diseases seem to be increasing in men. Why these differences? Is it simply a matter of lifestyle? Clearly, it is much more complicated than that. Consider the following:[15]

- The size, structure, and function of the brain differs in women and men, particularly in areas that affect mood and behavior and areas of the brain used to perform the same tasks. Reaction time is slower in women, but accuracy is higher.
- Bone mass in women peaks in their twenties; in men, it peaks gradually until age 30. At menopause, women lose bone at an accelerated rate, and 80 percent of osteoporosis cases are women.
- Women's cardiovascular systems are different in size, shape, and nervous system impulses, and women have faster heart rates.
- Women's immune systems are stronger than men's, but women are more prone to autoimmune disease

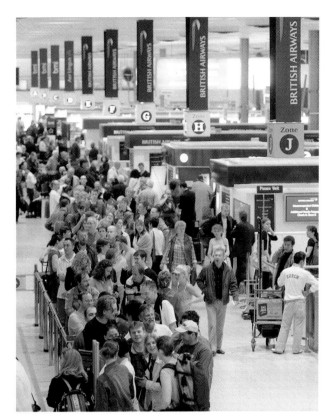

Modern travel has made health and the spread of disease a global issue. The deadly flu pandemic of 1918 took over one year to travel around the globe. Today, modern air travel could spread illness globally in a matter of weeks.

(diseases in which the body attacks its own tissues, such as multiple sclerosis, lupus, and rheumatoid arthritis) than men. Women experience pain in different ways than men and may react to pain medications differently.

Differences do not stop there; according to a report by the Society for Women's Health Research:[16]

- When consuming the same amount of alcohol, women have a higher blood alcohol content then men, even allowing for size differences.
- Women who smoke are 20 to 70 percent more likely to develop lung cancer than men who smoke the same amount of cigarettes.
- Women are more likely than men to suffer a second heart attack within one year of their first heart attack.
- The same drugs—even common drugs like antihistamines and antibiotics—can cause different reactions and different side effects in women and men.
- Women are two times more likely than men to contract a sexually transmitted infection and ten times more likely to contract HIV when having unprotected intercourse.
- Depression is two to three times more common in women than in men.

Table 1.3

Leading Causes of Death in the United States by Age (Years), 2002

All Ages		15–24	
Diseases of the heart	696,947	Unintentional injuries	15,412
Malignant neoplasms	557,271	Homicide	5,219
Cerebrovascular diseases	162,672	Suicide	4,010
Chronic lower respiratory diseases	124,816	Malignant neoplasms	1,730
Unintentional injuries	106,742	Diseases of the heart	1,022
Under 1 Year		**25–44**	
Congenital anomalies	5,623	Unintentional injuries	29,279
Short gestation or low birth weight	4,637	Malignant neoplasms	19,957
Sudden infant death syndrome	2,295	Diseases of the heart	16,853
Maternal complications	1,708	Suicide	11,897
Complications of placenta, cord, membranes	1,028	Homicide	7,728
1–4		**45–64**	
Unintentional injuries	1,641	Malignant neoplasms	143,028
Congenital anomalies	530	Diseases of the heart	101,804
Homicide	423	Unintentional injuries	23,020
Malignant neoplasms	402	Cerebrovascular diseases	15,952
Diseases of the heart	165	Diabetes mellitus	15,518
5–14		**65+**	
Unintentional injuries	2,718	Diseases of the heart	576,301
Malignant neoplasms	1,072	Malignant neoplasms	391,001
Congenital anomalies	417	Cerebrovascular diseases	143,293
Homicide	356	Chronic lower respiratory diseases	108,313
Suicide	260	Influenza and pneumonia	58,826

Source: R. N. Anderson and B. L. Smith, "Deaths: Leading Causes for 2002," in *National Vital Statistics Reports* 53 (Hyattsville, MD: National Center for Health Statistics, 2005).

Surprisingly, although these and countless other disparities in health have long been recognized, researchers largely ignored the unique aspects of women's health until the 1990s, when a highly publicized 15-year, $625 million dollar government study was funded by the National Institutes of Health (NIH). Known as the **Women's Health Initiative (WHI),** this study was designed to focus research on the uniqueness of women when it came to drug trials, development of surgical instruments, and other health issues rather than just assuming that women were just like the males previously studied. This and follow-up studies are providing invaluable information about women's risks and potential strategies for prevention, intervention, and treatment.

Women's Health Initiative (WHI) National study of postmenopausal women; in conjunction with the NIH mandate for equal research priorities for women's health issues.

What Do You Think? Why do you think there are differences between men and women in their risks for certain diseases? ■ Which of the differences highlighted in the previous section could be modified through changes in health behavior?

IMPROVING YOUR HEALTH

Factors That Influence Your Health Status

Table 1.3 summarizes the leading causes of death in the United States. Note that Americans aged 15 to 24 and 25 to 44 are most likely to die from unintentional injuries, followed by homicide and suicide.[17] In 2005, cancer replaced cardiovascular disease as the number one cause of death for all persons under the age of 85, for the first time in U.S history.[18]

Individual behavior is a major determinant of good health, but heredity, access to health care, the environment, and many other factors can also influence health status (Figure 1.2). When these factors are considered together and form the basis of a person's lifestyle choices, the net effect on health can be great.

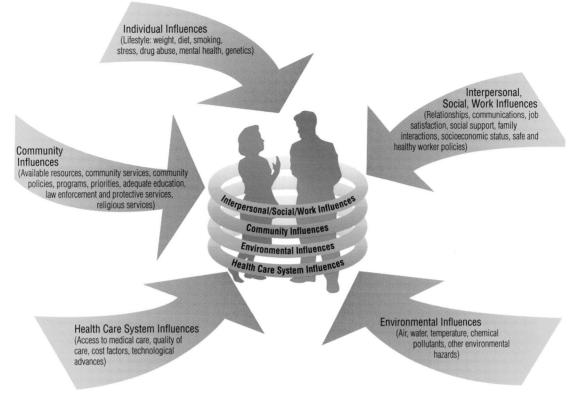

Figure 1.2 ■ Factors That Influence Health Status

Healthy Behaviors

Most experts believe that several key behaviors will help people live longer, such as

- Getting a good night's sleep (minimum of seven hours)
- Maintaining healthy eating habits and managing weight
- Participating in physical recreational activities
- Practicing safer sex
- Limiting intake of alcohol and avoiding tobacco products
- Scheduling regular self-exams and medical checkups

Several other actions may not add years to your life, but they can add significant life to your years. They include:

- Controlling real and imaginary stressors
- Maintaining meaningful relationships with family and friends
- Making time for yourself and being as kind to yourself as you are to others
- Participating in at least one fun activity each day
- Respecting the environment and the people in it
- Considering alternatives when making decisions and assessing how actions affect others

- Valuing each day and making the best of opportunities
- Viewing mistakes as opportunities to learn and grow
- Understanding the health care system and using it wisely

All of us, no matter where we are on the health and wellness continuum, have to start somewhere.

PREPARING FOR BEHAVIOR CHANGE

As Mark Twain said, "Habit is habit, and not to be flung out the window by anyone, but coaxed downstairs a step at a time." The chances of successfully changing negative habits improve when you identify a key behavior that you want to change and develop a plan for gradual modification that allows you time to unlearn negative patterns and substitute positive ones.

Factors That Influence Behavior Change

Figure 1.3 identifies major factors that influence behavior and behavior-change decisions. They can be divided into three general categories: predisposing, enabling, and reinforcing factors.

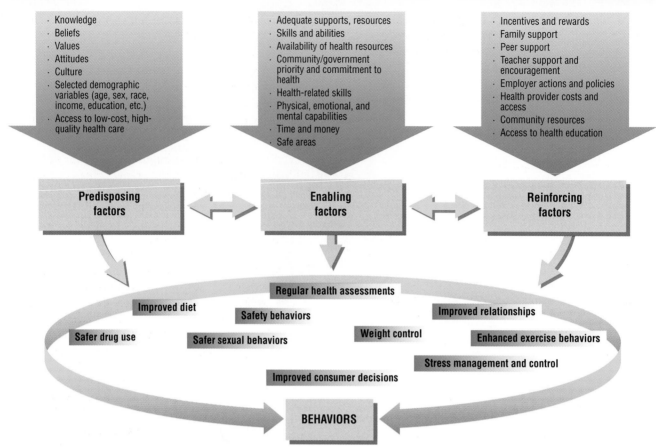

Figure 1.3 ■ Factors That Influence Behavior-Change Decisions

Predisposing Factors Our life experiences, knowledge, cultural and ethnic heritage, and current beliefs and values are all *predisposing factors* that influence behavior. Factors that may predispose us to certain conditions include age, sex, race, income, family background, educational background, and access to health care. For example, if your parents smoked, you are 90 percent more likely to start smoking than someone whose parents didn't smoke. If your peers smoke, you are 80 percent more likely to smoke than someone whose friends don't smoke.

Enabling Factors Skills and abilities; physical, emotional, and mental capabilities; community and government priorities and commitment to health; and safe and convenient resources and facilities that make health decisions easy or difficult are *enabling factors.* Positive enablers encourage you to carry through on your intentions to change. Negative enablers work against your intentions to change. For example, if you would like to join a local fitness center but discover that the closest one is four miles away and the membership fee is $500, those negative enablers may convince you to stay home. On the other hand, if your school's fitness center is two blocks away, stays open until midnight, and offers a special student membership, those positive

enablers will probably convince you to join. Identifying positive and negative enabling factors and devising alternative plans when the negative factors outweigh the positive are part of planning for behavior change.

Reinforcing Factors *Reinforcing factors* include the presence or absence of support, encouragement, or discouragement that significant people in your life bring to a situation; employer actions and policies; health provider costs and access; community resources; and access to health education. For example, if you decide to stop smoking and your family and friends continue smoking in your presence, you may be tempted to start smoking again. In other words, your smoking behavior is reinforced. If, however, you are overweight and you lose a few pounds and all your friends tell you how terrific you look, your positive behavior is reinforced and you will likely continue your weight-loss plan.

The manner in which you reward or punish yourself in the process of change also plays a role. Accepting small failures and concentrating on your successes can foster further achievements. Berating yourself because you binged on ice cream or argued with a friend may create an internal environment in which failure becomes almost inevitable. Telling yourself that you're worth the extra effort and giving yourself a pat on the back for small accomplishments are often overlooked factors in positive behavior change. It is also important to invest time in your friendships. Not only is it rewarding to spend time with your friends, but when you need help making a change, you'll have the social support you need.

Motivation and Readiness

Wanting to change is a prerequisite of the change process, but there is much more to the process than motivation. *Motivation* must be combined with common sense, commitment, and a realistic understanding of how best to move from point A to point B.[19] *Readiness* is the state of being that precedes behavior change. People who are ready to change possess the attitudes, knowledge, skills, and internal and external resources that make change possible.

Beliefs and Attitudes

We often assume that when rational people realize their actions put them at risk, they will act to reduce that risk—but this is not necessarily true. Consider the number of health professionals who smoke, consume junk food, and act in other unhealthy ways. They surely know better, but their "knowing" is disconnected from their "doing." Why is this so? Two strong influences on behavior are beliefs and attitudes.

A **belief** is an appraisal of the relationship between some object, action, or idea (for example, smoking) and some attribute of that object, action, or idea (for example, smoking is expensive, dirty, and causes cancer—or, it is relaxing). An **attitude** is a relatively stable set of beliefs, feelings, and behavioral tendencies in relation to something or someone.

Psychologists studying the relationship between beliefs and health habits have determined that although beliefs can subtly influence behavior, they may not actually cause people to behave differently. In 1966, psychologist I. Rosenstock developed a classic theory, the **Health Belief Model (HBM),** to show when beliefs affect behavior change.[20] Although many other models attempt to explain the influence of beliefs on behaviors, the HBM remains one of the most widely accepted. It holds that several factors must support a belief before change is likely:

- *Perceived seriousness of the health problem.* How severe would the medical and social consequences be if the health problem were to develop or to be left untreated? The more serious the perceived effects, the more likely that the person will take action.

- *Perceived susceptibility to the health problem.* What is the likelihood of developing the health problem?

People who perceive themselves at high risk are more likely to take preventive action.

- *Cues to action.* Those who are reminded or alerted about a potential health problem are more likely to take action. For example, having your doctor tell you that your blood sugar levels indicate a prediabetic state may be the cue that pushes you to lose weight and exercise.

Three other factors are linked to perceived risk for health problems: *demographic variables*, including age, gender, race, and ethnic background; *sociopsychological variables*, including personality traits, social class, and social pressure; and *structural variables*, including knowledge about or prior contact with the health problem.

People follow the HBM many times every day. Take, for example, smokers. Older smokers are likely to know other smokers who have developed serious heart or lung problems. They are thus more likely to perceive tobacco as a threat to their health than is a teenager who has just begun smoking. The greater the perceived threat of health problems caused by smoking, the greater the chance a person will quit.

However, many chronic smokers know the risks yet continue to smoke. Why do they miss these cues to action? According to Rosenstock, some people do not believe that they will be affected by a problem—they act as if they have some kind of immunity to it—and are unlikely to change their behavior.[21] In some cases, they may think that even if they get cancer or have a heart attack, the health care system will cure them. They also may feel that the immediate pleasure outweighs the long-range cost.

Intentions to Change

Our attitudes reflect our emotional responses to situations and follow from our beliefs. According to the **Theory of Reasoned Action,** our behaviors result from our intentions to perform actions. An intention is a product of our attitude toward an action and our beliefs about what others may want us to do.[22] A *behavioral in-*

Belief   Appraisal of the relationship between some object, action, or idea and some attribute of that object, action, or idea.

Attitude   Relatively stable set of beliefs, feelings, and behavioral tendencies in relation to something or someone.

Health Belief Model (HBM)   Model for explaining how beliefs may influence behaviors.

Theory of Reasoned Action   Model for explaining the importance of our intentions in determining behaviors.

Many of us resolve to change a given behavior only to return to the behavior after a short time.

Why do so many good intentions fail? According to Drs. James Prochaska and Carlos DiClemente, it's because we are going about things in the wrong way, and fewer than 20 percent of us are really prepared to take action. Yet, health professionals continue to exhort us to "Just do it! And do it now!" After considerable research, Prochaska and DiClemente believe that behavior changes usually fail if they start with the change itself. Instead, we must go through a series of stages to prepare ourselves for that change.

1. *Precontemplation.* People in the precontemplation stage have no current intention of changing. They may have tried to change a behavior before and given up, or they may be in denial and unaware of any problem.
Strategies for Change: Sometimes a few frank yet kind words from friends may be enough to make precontemplators take a

closer look at themselves. This is not to say that you should become a "warrior against pleasure" or tell people what to do when they haven't asked for advice. Recommending readings or making tactful suggestions, however, can help precontemplators consider making a change.

2. *Contemplation.* In this phase, people recognize that they have a problem and begin to contemplate the need to change. Acknowledgment usually results from increased awareness, often due to feedback from family and friends or access to information. Despite this acknowledgment, people can languish in this stage for years, realizing that they have a problem but lacking the time or energy to make the change.
Strategies for Change: Often, contemplators need a little push to get them started. This may come in the form of helping them set up a change plan (for example, an exercise routine), buying a helpful gift (such as a low-fat

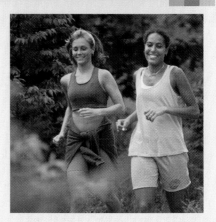

cookbook), sharing articles about a particular problem, or inviting them to go with you to hear a speaker on a related topic. People often need time to think about a course of action or to build skill. Your assistance can help them move off the point of indecision.

3. *Preparation.* Most people at this point are close to taking action. They've thought about what they might do and may even have come up with a plan. Rather than

---

tention, then, is a written or stated commitment to perform an action.

In brief, the more consistent and powerful your attitudes about an action and the more you are influenced by others to take that action, the greater will be your stated intention to do so. The more you verbalize your commitment to change, the more likely you are to succeed. The more you have social support from family and friends to encourage you, the more your intentions will be bolstered.

Significant Others as Change Agents

Many of us are highly influenced by the approval or disapproval (real or imagined) of close friends, loved ones, and the social and cultural groups to which they belong. Such influences can support healthy behavior, or they can interfere with even the best intentions.

Your Family From the time of your birth, your parents or other family members have given you strong cues about which actions are and are not socially acceptable. Brushing your teeth, bathing, wearing deodorant, and chewing food with your mouth closed are behaviors that your family probably instilled in you long ago. Your family culture influenced your food choices, religious and political beliefs, and all your other values and actions. If you deviated from your family's norms, a family member probably let you know fairly quickly. Good family units share unconditional trust, dedication to the healthful development of all family members, and commitment to work out difficulties.

Do my friends and family influence my health choices?

When a loving family unit does not exist, when it does not provide for basic human needs, or when dysfunctional, irresponsible individuals try to build a family under the influence of drugs or alcohol, it becomes difficult for a child to learn positive health behaviors.

thinking about why they can't begin, they have started to focus on what they can do.

Strategies for Change: People in the preparation stage can benefit from following a few simple guidelines. Set realistic goals (large and small), take small steps toward change, change only a couple of things at once, reward small milestones, and seek support from friends. Identify factors that have enabled success or served as a barrier to success in the past, and modify them where possible. Fill out the Behavior Change Contract in the front of this book to help you commit to making these changes.

4. *Action.* In this stage, people begin to follow their action plans. Those who have prepared for change, thought about alternatives, engaged social support, and made a realistic plan of action are more ready than those who have given it little thought. Unfortunately, too many people start behavior change here rather than going through the first three stages. Without a plan, without enlisting the help of others, or without a realistic goal, failure is likely.

Strategies for Change: Publicly stating the desire to change helps ensure success. Encourage friends who are making a change to share their plans with you. Offer to help, and try to remove potential obstacles from the person's intended action plan. Social support and the buddy system can motivate even the most reluctant person.

5. *Maintenance.* Maintenance requires vigilance, attention to detail, and long-term commitment. Many people reach a goal, only to relax and slip back into the undesired behavior. In this stage, it is important to be aware of the potential for relapses and develop strategies for dealing with such challenges. Common causes of relapse include overconfidence, daily temptations, stress or emotional distractions, and self-deprecation.

Strategies for Change: During maintenance, continue taking the same actions that led to success in the first place. Find fun and creative ways to maintain positive behaviors. This is where a willing and caring support group can be vital. Knowing where on campus to turn for help when you don't have a close support network is also helpful.

6. *Termination.* By this point, the behavior is so ingrained that the current level of vigilance may be unnecessary. The new behavior has become an essential part of daily living. Can you think of someone you know who has made a major behavior change that has now become an essential part of that person's life?

Source: J. O. Prochaska, and C. C. DiClemente, "Stages and Processes of Self-Change of Smoking: Toward an Integrative Model of Change," *Journal of Consulting and Clinical Psychology* 51 (1983): 390–395.

Healthy behaviors get their start in healthy homes; unhealthy homes breed unhealthy habits. Healthy families provide the foundation for a clear and necessary understanding of what is right and wrong, what is positive and negative. Without this fundamental grounding, many young people have great difficulties.[23]

The Influences of Others Just as your family influences your actions during your childhood, your friends and significant others influence your behaviors as you grow older. Most of us desire to fit the "norm" and avoid hassles in our daily interactions with others. If you deviate from the actions expected in your hometown, or among your friends, you may suffer ostracism, strange looks, and other negative social consequences. Understanding the subtle and not-so-subtle ways in which other people influence our actions is an important step toward changing our behaviors.

The behavior choices we make can be explained by the *Theory of Planned Behavior*.[24] This theory outlines three reasons for how we choose to behave:

1. *Our attitudes toward the behavior;* for example, what we think about the positive or negative effects of our actions and the importance of each of those

2. *Our level of perceived behavioral control,* or our beliefs about the constraints and/or opportunities we might have concerning the behavior

3. *Our subjective norms,* or whether or not we think our actions will meet the approval or disapproval of people important to us.

For example, if you want to lose weight because you believe it will make you more desirable, you'll have strong intentions to begin a weight loss program (attitudes toward the behavior*). Intentions* are powerful indicators of successful behavior change. If there is a convenient, affordable fitness center near you, and if the schedule works for you, you'll be even more motivated and believe you can make the change (control beliefs). Finally, if friends offer encouragement (subjective norms), we are more likely to remain motivated to change our behaviors. On the other hand, if we perceive

Finding Reliable Health Information on the Internet

Looking for reliable health information on the Internet? Wondering if that e-mail warning of a deadly pathogen in your hamburger is fact or fiction? Dazed by searching for a topic, only to be confronted with 300,000 websites in your search results? Each year more than 100 million people seek health information on the Internet. Many of them end up frazzled, confused, and—worst of all—misinformed.

The Internet can be a wonderful resource for rapid answers. However, some of the answers you'll find are better than others. How can you maximize your chances of locating high-quality information? Follow these tips:

How can I differentiate between a bogus health claim and a real one?

■ Look for websites sponsored by an official government agency, a university or college, or a hospital/medical center. These typically offer accurate, up-to-date information about a wide range of health topics. Government sites are easily identified by their .gov extensions (for example, the National Institute of Mental Health is www.nimh.nih.gov); college and university sites typically have .edu extensions (Johns Hopkins University is www.jhu.edu). Hospitals often have an .org extension (Mayo Clinic is www.mayoclinic.org). Major philanthropic foundations, such as the Robert Wood Johnson Foundation, the Legacy Foundation, the Kellogg Foundation, and others, often provide information about selected health topics.

■ Search for well-established, professionally peer-reviewed journals such as *The New England Journal of Medicine* (www.nejm.org) or *The Journal of the American Medical Association (JAMA)* (http://jama.amaassn.org). While some of these sites require a fee for access, often you can locate concise abstracts and information, such as a weekly table of contents, that can help you conduct a search. Other times, you can pay a basic fee for a certain number of hours of unlimited searching. You may also find that your college or university library receives an online subscription to a number of these journals.

■ Consult the Centers for Disease Control and Prevention (www.cdc.gov) or consumer news and updates. The CDC also provides consumer alerts on topics such as buying antibiotics online and e-mail health hoaxes.

■ There are many government and education-based sites that are independently sponsored and reliable. The following is just a sample. We'll provide more in each chapter as we cover specific topics:

- Aetna Intelihealth: www.intelihealth.com
- Dr. Koop.com: www.drkoop.com
- Drug Infonet: www.druginfonet.com
- Health AtoZ.com: www.healthatoz.com
- WebMD health: http://my.webmd.com

The American Accreditation Healthcare Commission (www.urac.org), has devised over 50 criteria that health sites must satisfy to display its seal. Look for the "URAC Accredited Health WebSite seal" on websites you visit. In addition to policing the accuracy of health claims, URAC evaluates health information and provides a forum for reporting misinformation, privacy violations, and other complaints.

■ Finally, don't believe everything you read. Cross-check information against reliable sources to see if facts and figures are consistent. Be especially wary of websites that try to sell you something. Just because a source claims to be a physician or an expert does not mean that this is true. When in doubt, check with your own physician, health education professor, or state health division website.

Sources: L. Landro, "Health Journal: Online Groups Step Up Attempts to Enforce Standards," *The Wall Street Journal,* July 20, 2001, B1. URAC, "URAC's Health Web Site Standards," 2005, www.urac.org/consumer_standards.asp.

that our friends will think we are "nerds" for going to the gym, or if the gym is inconvenient or expensive, we may quickly lose our motivation. The opinions of key people play a powerful role in our motivation to change behaviors.

The influence of others serves as a powerful *social support* for positive change. If you are engaged in an abusive relationship, having friends you trust and can confide in can give you the strength to walk away from the situation. Someone who will accept you unconditionally and be there for you can be a wonderful asset and give you the support to deal with life's challenges. The more *social support* options you have, and the closer the relationship or *social bonds,* the greater the chances that you will be able to deal with crises in healthy ways. If you expand your social support network to include counselors, ministers/pastors/rabbis, and others, you will further increase your likelihood of success. Who would you call if you were stranded in the middle of a cold, snowy night on a remote road? Who would get out of bed and, without question, come and get you? Surprisingly, many people have no one to call under any circumstances, let alone when they are in crisis. The importance of cultivating and maintaining close social ties with others is an important part of overall health.

CHOOSING A BEHAVIOR-CHANGE TECHNIQUE

What can I do to change an unhealthy habit?

Once you have analyzed all the factors that influence your behaviors, you must consider what actions you can take to change the negative ones. Behavior-change techniques include shaping, visualization, modeling, controlling the situation, reinforcement, and changing self-talk. The options don't stop here, but these are the most common strategies.

Shaping

Regardless of how motivated you are, some behaviors are almost impossible to change immediately. To reach your goal, you may need to take a number of individual steps, each designed to change one small piece of the larger behavior. This process is known as **shaping.** For example, suppose that you have not exercised for a while. You decide that you want to get into shape, and your goal is to jog three miles every other day. But you realize that you'd face a near-death experience if you tried to run even a few blocks in your current condition. So you decide to build up to your desired fitness level gradually. During week 1, you will walk for one hour every other day at a slow, relaxed pace. During week 2, you will walk for the same amount of time but speed up your pace and cover slightly more ground. During week 3, you will speed up even more and try to go even farther. You will continue taking such steps until you reach your goal.

Whatever the desired behavior change, all shaping involves the following actions:

- *Start slowly,* and try not to cause undue stress during the early stages of the program.
- *Keep the steps small* and achievable.
- *Be flexible.* If the original plan proves uncomfortable or you deviate from it, don't give up! Start again, and move forward.
- *Don't skip steps* or move to the next step until you have mastered the previous one.
- *Reward yourself* for meeting regular, pre-set goals.

Remember, behaviors don't develop overnight, so they won't change overnight.

Visualization

Mental practice can transform unhealthy behaviors into healthy ones. Athletes and others use a technique known as **imagined rehearsal** to reach their goals. By visualizing their planned action ahead of time, they are better prepared when they put themselves to the test.

For example, suppose you want to ask someone out on a date. Imagine the setting (walking together to class). Then practice exactly what you want to say ("There's a great concert this Sunday, and I was wondering if. . . . ") in your mind and aloud. Mentally anticipate different responses ("Oh, I'd love to, but I'm busy that evening. . . . ") and what you will say in reaction ("How about if I call you sometime this week?"). Careful mental and verbal rehearsal—you could even try out your scenario on a friend—will greatly improve the likelihood of success.

Try it ▸NOW

Stay connected. **Having a broad base of social support is an important part of insuring overall health. Make an effort to strengthen social bonds. Call a friend right now and make a date for coffee, lunch or "fun time," to catch up on each other's lives and show you care.**

Modeling

Modeling, or learning behaviors by watching others perform them, is one of the most effective strategies for changing behavior. For example, suppose that you have trouble talking to people you don't know very well. One of the easiest ways to improve your communication skills is to select friends whose social skills you envy. Observe them. Do they talk more or listen more? How do people respond to them? Why are they such good communicators? If you observe behaviors you admire and isolate their components, you can model the steps of your behavior-change technique on a proven success.

Controlling the Situation

Sometimes, the right setting or the right group of people will positively influence your behaviors. Many situations and occasions trigger certain actions. For example, in libraries, houses of worship, and museums, most people talk softly. Few people laugh at funerals.

Shaping Using a series of small steps to get to a particular goal gradually.

Imagined rehearsal Practicing through mental imagery to become better able to perform an event in actuality.

Modeling Learning specific behaviors by watching others perform them.

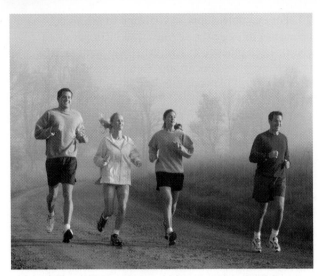

The support and encouragement of friends who have similar goals and interests will strengthen your commitment to develop and maintain positive health behaviors.

The term *situational inducement* refers to an attempt to influence a behavior by using occasions and social settings to control it.

For example, you may be more apt to stop smoking if you work in a smoke-free office, a positive situational inducement. Additionally, policies such as those to prevent sales of cigarettes and alcohol to minors can provide real inducements to resist temptation. But a smoke-filled bar, a negative situational inducement, may tempt you to resume or to keep smoking. Careful consideration of which settings will help and which will hurt your effort to change, and your decision to seek the first and avoid the second, will improve your chances for change.

Reinforcement

A **positive reinforcement** seeks to increase the likelihood that a behavior will occur by presenting a reward for it. Each of us is motivated by different reinforcers. Although a special T-shirt may be a positive reinforcer for young adults entering a race, for example, it would not be for a 40-year-old runner who dislikes message-bearing T-shirts.

> **Situational inducement** Attempt to influence a behavior through situations and occasions that are structured to exert control over that behavior.
>
> **Positive reinforcement** Presenting something positive following a behavior that is being reinforced.

Most positive reinforcers can be classified into five categories: consumable, activity, manipulative, possessional, and social.

- *Consumable reinforcers* are delicious edibles, such as candy, cookies, or gourmet meals.
- *Activity reinforcers* are opportunities to do something enjoyable, such as watching TV or going on a vacation.
- *Manipulative reinforcers* are incentives, such as getting a lower rent in exchange for mowing the lawn or the promise of a better grade for doing an extra-credit project.
- *Possessional reinforcers* are tangible rewards, such as a new TV or a sports car.
- *Social reinforcers* are signs of appreciation, approval, or love, such as loving looks, affectionate hugs, and praise.

When choosing reinforcers, determine what would motivate you to act in a particular way. Research has shown that people can be motivated to change their behaviors, such as not smoking during pregnancy or abstaining from cocaine, if they set up a *token economy* system whereby they earn tokens or points that can be exchanged for meaningful rewards, such as financial incentives.[25] The difficulty often lies in determining *which* incentive will be most effective. Your reinforcers may initially come from others (extrinsic rewards), but as you see positive changes in yourself, you will begin to reward and reinforce yourself (intrinsic rewards). Although reinforcers should immediately follow a behavior, beware of overkill. If you reward yourself with a movie every time you go jogging, this reinforcer will soon lose its power. It would be better to give yourself this reward after, say, a full week of adhering to your jogging program.

What Do You Think? What consumable reinforcers would be a healthy reward for your new behavior? ■ If you could choose one activity reinforcer with which to reward yourself after one week of success in your new behavior, what would it be? ■ If you could obtain something (possessional reinforcer) after you reach your goal, what would it be? ■ If you maintain your behavior for one week, what type of social reinforcer would you like to receive from your friends?

Changing Self-Talk

Self-talk, or the way you think and talk to yourself, can also play a role in modifying health-related behaviors. Here are some suggested strategies for changing self-talk.

Rational-Emotive Therapy This form of cognitive therapy or self-directed behavior change is based on the premise that there is a close connection between what people say to themselves and how they feel. According to psychologist Albert Ellis, most emotional problems and related behaviors stem from irrational statements that people make to themselves when events in their lives are different from what they would like them to be.[26]

For example, suppose that after doing poorly on a test, you say to yourself, "I can't believe I flunked that easy exam. I'm so stupid." By changing this irrational, "catastrophic" self-talk into rational, positive statements about what is really going on, you increase the likelihood that positive behaviors will occur. Positive self-talk might be phrased as follows: "I really didn't study enough for that exam, and I'm not surprised I didn't do very well. I'm certainly not stupid. I just need to prepare better for the next test." Such self-talk will help you to recover quickly and take positive steps to correct the situation.

Problem Solving: The Art of Self-Instruction

Some people seem to naturally take on challenges and deal with stressful life events in positive ways. However, most of us aren't skilled at tackling and overcoming problems in our lives, but we can learn to do a better job. According to psychologist Donald Meichenbaum, we can learn to inoculate ourselves against stressful events or control our anger over certain situations. Before a stressful event (for example, going to the doctor for sexually transmitted infection tests), Meichenbaum encourages his patients to practice coping skills, such as deep breathing or progressive muscle relaxation, or to practice self-instruction ("I'll feel better once I know what is going on here"). He provides a list of strategies that are designed to help each of us cope with stressors and modify anger reactions or other negative behaviors:[27]

- Define your stressor or stress reactions as problems to be solved.
- Set concrete, realistic goals and specific behaviors you can do to reach goals.
- Try out the most acceptable and practical solution, and generate a wide range of possible alternative courses of action.
- Imagine and consider how others might respond if asked to deal with similar problems.
- Evaluate the pros and cons of each proposed solution and organize the solutions from least to most practical and desirable.

- Rehearse strategies and behaviors by means such as imagery or role playing the behavior in advance.
- Expect some failures, but reward yourself for having tried.
- Reconsider the original problem in light of the attempt at problem-solving.

Blocking/Thought Stopping By purposefully blocking or stopping negative thoughts, a person can concentrate on taking positive steps. For example, suppose you are preoccupied with your ex-partner, who has recently deserted you for someone else. You consciously stop dwelling on the situation and force yourself to think about something more pleasant (such as dinner tomorrow with your best friend). By refusing to dwell on negative images and forcing yourself to focus elsewhere, you can save wasted energy, time, and emotional resources and move on to positive change.

CHANGING YOUR BEHAVIOR

Self-Assessment: Antecedents and Consequences

Behaviors, thoughts, and feelings always occur in a context, that is, in a situation. Situations can be divided into two components: the events that come before and after. *Antecedents* are the setting events for a behavior; they stimulate a person to act in certain ways. Antecedents can be physical events, thoughts, emotions, or the actions of other people. *Consequences*—the results of behavior—affect whether a person will repeat that action.[28] Consequences also can consist of physical events, thoughts, emotions, or the actions of other people.

Suppose you are shy and must give a speech in front of a large class. The antecedents include walking into the class, feeling frightened, wondering whether you are capable of doing a good job, and being unable to remember a word of your speech. If the consequences are negative—if your classmates laugh or you get a low grade—your terror about speaking in public will be reinforced, and you will continue to dread this kind of event. In contrast, if you receive positive feedback from the class or instructor, you may actually learn to like speaking in public.

Learning to recognize the antecedents of a behavior and acting to modify them is one method of changing behavior. A diary noting your undesirable behaviors and identifying the settings in which they occur can be a useful tool. Figure 1.4 identifies factors that can make behavior change more difficult.

COMMON BARRIERS	STRATEGY
Not enough time	Prioritize your time. Categorize your activities as: (1) Must Do's; (2) Should Do's; and (3) Free Time.
Stress	Identify your sources of external stress. Use the "self-instructional" methods in this chapter to develop methods for reducing your stress levels.
Habits	Identify bad habits and the social pressures that encourage them. Think about how you might handle these pressures differently. Let your friends know your behavior change goal, and ask for their support.
Self-blame or criticism	Acknowledge that no one, including you, is perfect. Examine what you think you did wrong and think about what you would do differently. Think of mistakes as learning opportunities.
Low self-efficacy	Break large, difficult tasks into smaller, manageable parts. Develop new skills, ask for help, and focus on successes.
Lack of motivation	Make an effort and set goals. Reward yourself for achievements.

Figure 1.4 ■ Overcoming Barriers to Healthy Behaviors

There are a number of obstacles that might make it difficult to change your behavior. Each strategy can help you overcome these obstacles.

Source: From *Self-Directed Behavior: Self-Modification for Personal Adjustment,* 8th edition by D. L. Watson and R. G. Tharp. 2002 by Wadsworth Publishing, a division of Thomson Publishing Inc. Reprinted by permission of the publisher.

Analyzing Personal Behavior

Successful behavior change requires determining what you want to change. All too often we berate ourselves by using generalities: "I'm lousy to my friends; I need to be a better person." Determining the specific behavior you would like to modify—in contrast to the general problem—will allow you to set clear goals. What are you doing that makes you a lousy friend? Are you gossiping or lying about your friends? Have you been a taker rather than a giver? Or are you really a good friend most of the time?

Let's say the problem is gossiping. You can analyze this behavior by examining the following components.

- *Frequency.* How often do you gossip—all the time or only once in a while?
- *Duration.* How long have you been doing this?
- *Seriousness.* Is your gossiping just idle chatter, or are you really trying to injure other people? What are the consequences for you? For your friends? For your relationships?
- *Basis for problem behavior.* Is your gossip based on facts, perceptions of facts, or deliberate embellishment of the truth?
- *Antecedents.* What kinds of situations trigger your gossiping? Do some settings or people bring it out in

you more than others do? What triggers your feelings of dislike or irritation toward your friends? Why are you talking behind their backs?

Once you assess your actions and determine what motivates you, consider what you can do to change your behavior.

Decision Making: Choices for Change

Now it is time to make a decision that will lead to positive health outcomes. Try to anticipate what might occur in a given setting and think through all possible safe alternatives. For example, knowing that you are likely to be offered a drink when you go to a party, what response could you make that would be okay in your social group? If someone is flirting with you and the conversation takes on a distinct sexual overtone, what might you do to prevent the situation from turning bad? Advance preparation will help you stick to your behavior plan.

Fill out the Behavior Change Contract at the beginning of this book to help you set a goal, anticipate obstacles, and create strategies to overcome those obstacles. Remember that things typically don't "just happen." Making a commitment by completing a contract helps you stay alert to potential problems, be aware of your alternatives, maintain a good sense of your own values, and stick to your beliefs under pressure.

Setting Realistic Goals

How can I set a realistic health goal?

Changing behavior is not easy, but sometimes we make it even harder by setting unrealistic and unattainable goals. To start making positive changes, ask yourself these questions.

1. *What do I want?* What is your ultimate goal—to lose weight? Exercise more? Reduce stress? Have a lasting relationship? Whatever it is, you need a clear picture of the target outcome.

2. *Which change is the greatest priority at this time?* Often people decide to change several things all at once. Suppose that you are gaining unwanted weight. Rather than saying "I need to eat less, start jogging, and really get in shape," be specific about the current behavior you need to change. Are you eating too many sweets? Too many high-fat foods? Perhaps a realistic goal would be, "I am going to try to eat less fat during dinner every day." Choose the behavior that constitutes your greatest problem, and tackle that first. You can always work on something else later. Take small steps, experiment with alternatives, and find the best way to meet your goals.

3. *Why is this important to me?* Think through why you want to change. Are you doing it because of your health? To look better? To win someone else's approval? Usually, doing something because it's right for you rather than to win others' approval is a sound strategy. If you are changing for someone else, what happens when that other person isn't around?

4. *What are the potential positive outcomes?* What do you hope to accomplish?

5. *What health-promoting programs and services can help me get started?* Nearly all campuses offer helpful resources. You might buy a self-help book at the campus bookstore, speak to a counselor, or enroll in an aerobics class at the local fitness center.

6. *Are there family or friends whose help I can enlist?* Social support is one of your most powerful allies. Getting a friend to exercise with you, asking your partner to help you stop smoking by quitting at the same time you do, and making a commitment with a friend to never let each other drive if you've been drinking alcohol—these are all examples of how people can help each other make positive changes.

What Do You Think? Why is it sometimes hard to make decisions? ■ What factors influence your decision making? ■ Select one behavior that you want to change and refer to the Behavior Change Contract. Using the goal-setting strategies discussed here, outline a plan for change.

■ Taking Charge

Summary

- Health encompasses the entire dynamic process of fulfilling one's potential in the physical, social, emotional, spiritual, intellectual, and environmental dimensions of life. Wellness means achieving the highest level of health possible in several dimensions.

- Although the average American life expectancy has increased over the past century, we also need to increase the quality of life. Programs such as *Healthy People 2010* have established national objectives for improving life span and quality of life for all Americans through health promotion and disease prevention.

- Gender continues to play a major role in health status and care. Women have longer lives but more medical problems than do men. To close the gender gap in health care, researchers have begun to include more women in medical research and training.

- For the U.S. population as a whole, the leading causes of death are cancer, heart disease, and stroke. But in the 15- to 24-year-old age group, the leading causes are unintentional injuries, homicide, and suicide. Many of the risks associated with cancer, heart disease, and stroke can be reduced through lifestyle changes. Many of the risks associated with accidents, homicide, and suicide can be reduced through preventive measures.

- Several factors contribute to a person's health status, and a number of them are within our control. Beliefs and attitudes, intentions to change, support from significant others, and readiness to change are factors over which individuals have some degree of control. Access to health care, genetic predisposition, health policies that support positive choices, and other factors are all potential reinforcing, predisposing, and enabling factors that may influence health decisions.

- Behavior-change techniques, such as shaping, visualization, modeling, controlling the situation, reinforcement, and changing self-talk, help people succeed in making behavior changes.

- Decision making has several key components. Each person must explore his or her own problems, the reasons for change, and the expected outcomes. The next step is to plan a course of action best suited to the individual's needs.

Chapter Review

1. Our ability to perform everyday tasks, such as walking up the stairs, is an example of
   a. improved quality of life.
   b. physical health.
   c. health promotion.
   d. activities of daily living.

2. Janice describes herself as confident and trusting and she displays both high self-esteem and self-efficacy. The dimension of health this relates to is
   a. social.
   b. emotional.
   c. spiritual.
   d. intellectual.

3. After Jill was hospitalized for dehydration and was diagnosed with anorexia nervosa, she began an inpatient treatment program designed to treat individuals with eating disorders. The type of disease prevention she is receiving is called
   a. primary prevention.
   b. secondary prevention.
   c. tertiary prevention.
   d. disease prevention.

4. What statistic is used to describe the number of new cases of AIDS in 2005?
   a. morbidity
   b. mortality
   c. incidence
   d. prevalence

5. Because Craig's parents smoked, he is 90 percent more likely to start smoking than someone whose parents didn't. This is an example of what factor influencing behavior change?
   a. circumstantial factor
   b. enabling factor
   c. reinforcing factor
   d. predisposing factor

6. According to the Health Belief Model, all of the following factors must support a belief before change is likely, *except*
   a. cues to action.
   b. our subjective norms.
   c. perceived seriousness of the health problem.
   d. perceived susceptibility to the health problem.

7. Suppose you want to lose 20 pounds. To reach your goal, you take small steps to gradually lose weight. You start by joining a support group and count calories. After two weeks, you begin an exercise program and gradually build up to your desired fitness level. What behavior-change strategy are you using?
   a. shaping
   b. visualization
   c. modeling
   d. reinforcement

8. After Kirk and Tammy pay their bills they reward themselves by watching TV together. The type of positive reinforcement that motivates them to pay their bills is
   a. activity reinforcer.
   b. consumable reinforcer.
   c. manipulative reinforcer.
   d. possessional reinforcer.

9. The setting events for a behavior that cue or stimulate a person to act in certain ways are called
   a. antecedents.
   b. frequency of events.
   c. consequences.
   d. cues to action.

10. What strategy for change is advised for an individual in the *preparation* stage of change?
    a. recommended readings
    b. find creative ways to maintain positive behaviors
    c. set realistic goals
    d. publicly state the desire for change

Answers to these questions can be found on page A-1.

Questions for Discussion and Reflection

1. How are the terms *health* and *wellness* similar? What, if any, are important distinctions between these terms? What is health promotion? Disease prevention? What does it really mean to be healthy?

2. How healthy are Americans today? How will health promotion and illness/accident prevention both increase life expectancy and improve quality of life right now? In the future?

3. What are some of the major differences in the way men and women are treated in the health care system? Why do you think these differences exist?

4. What are the leading causes of death across different ages? What are the leading causes of death for Americans aged 15 to 24? Why are these statistics

so different? Explain why it is important to look at these statistics by age rather than just looking at them in total. What lifestyle changes can you make to lower your risks for contracting major diseases?

5. What is the HBM? What is the Theory of Reasoned Action? How may each of these models operate when a young woman decides to smoke her first cigarette? Her last cigarette?

6. Explain the predisposing, reinforcing, and enabling factors that might influence a young mother on welfare as she decides whether to sell drugs to support her children.

7. Using the Stages of Change model found in the Skills for Behavior Change box on page 20, discuss what you might do (in stages) to help a friend stop smoking. Why is it important that a person be ready to change before trying to change?

Accessing Your Health on the Internet

The following websites explore further topics and issues related to personal health. For links to the websites below, visit the Companion Website for *Health: The Basics,* Seventh Edition at www.aw-bc.com/donatelle.

1. *CDC Wonder.* Outstanding reference for comprehensive information from the CDC, including special reports, guidelines, and access to national health data.

2. *Mayo Clinic.* Reputable resource for specific information about health topics, diseases, and treatment options. Easy to navigate and consumer friendly.

3. *National Center for Health Statistics.* Outstanding place to start for information about health status in the United States. Links to key documents such as *Health United States* (published yearly); national survey information; and information on mortality by age, race, gender, geographic location, and other important data. Includes comprehensive information provided by the CDC, as well as easy links to at least ten of the major health resources currently being used for policy and decision making about health in the United States.

4. *National Health Information Center.* Excellent resource for consumer information about health.

5. *WebMD.* Reputable and comprehensive overview of various diseases and conditions. Written for the public in an easy-to-understand format with links to more in-depth information.

Further Reading

Robins, A. and A. Wilner. *Quarterlife Crisis: The Unique Challenges of Life in Your 20s.* New York: JP Tarcher Paperbacks, 2001.

Overview of challenges facing young adults in America today.

Institute of Medicine. *Who Will Keep the Public Healthy? Educating Public Health Professionals for the 21st Century.* Washington, DC: National Academies Press, 2003.

An edited text featuring experts from throughout the country discussing the role of health professionals in health change. It outlines an ecological approach to improving the nation's health and has served as a catalyst for initiatives focused on current health issues and future plans to improve health and prevent premature death and disability.

Institute of Medicine. *The Future of Public Health in the 21st Century.* Washington, DC: National Academies Press, 2003.

The summary of a national effort to examine the nation's health status and describe how key individuals and organizations can work as a public health system to create conditions in which people can be healthy. In addition, this text recommends the evidence-based actions necessary to make the U.S. health system work effectively.

Lee, P. and C. Estes. *The Nation's Health,* 7th ed. Sudbury, MA: Jones and Bartlett, 2003.

An overview of key writings on public health and issues affecting individuals and populations. Special emphasis on health determinants, emerging threats to health, the health of diverse populations, and issues of health care quality, costs, and access.

U.S. Department of Health and Human Services. *Healthy People 2010: National Health Promotion and Disease Prevention Objectives for the Year 2010.* Washington, DC: Government Printing Office, 1998.

This plan contains the U.S. Surgeon General's long-range goals for improving the life span for all Americans by three years and improving access to health for all Americans, regardless of sex, race, socioeconomic status, and other variables.

U.S. Department of Health and Human Services. *Health, United States: 2004.* Centers for Disease Control and Prevention. Washington, DC: Government Printing Office, 2004.

Provides an up-to-date overview of U.S. health statistics, risk factors, and trends.

References

1. World Health Organization (WHO), "Constitution of the World Health Organization," *Chronicles of the World Health Organization* (Geneva, Switzerland: WHO, 1947).
2. National Center for Health Statistics, Table 12 from "United States Life Tables, 2002." *National Vital Statistics Reports* 53, no. 6 (November 2004).
3. S. J. Olshansky et al., "A Potential Decline in Life Expectancy in the United States in the 21st Century," *New England Journal of Medicine* 352, no. 11 (March 2005): 1138–1145.
4. R. Dubos, *So Human the Animal* (New York: Scribners, 1968), 15.
5. D. Satcher, *Keynote Address* (Washington, DC: National Association of School Psychologists, Government and Professional Relations Committee, Public Policy Institute, February 2001), 10–12.
6. National Center for Health Statistics, "About *Healthy People 2010,*" www.cdc.gov/nchs.
7. U.S. Department of Agriculture and U.S. Department of Health and Human Services, "Dietary Guidelines for Americans 2005," www.health.gov/dietaryguidelines/dga2005/recommendations.htm; U.S. Department of Agriculture, "My Pyramid Food Guidance System, 2005," www.mypyramid.gov.

8. R. Donatelle et al., "Incentives in Smoking Cessation: Status of the Field and Implications for Research and Practice with Pregnant Smokers," *Nicotine and Tobacco Research* 6, Supplement 2 (April 2004): S163–S179.

9. Centers for Disease Control and Prevention, "Chronic Disease Prevention, 2004" (Atlanta, GA: U.S. Department of Health and Human Services, 2004), www.cdc.gov/nccdphp.

10. Centers for Disease Control and Prevention, "The Burden of Chronic Diseases and Their Risk Factors: National and State Perspectives 2004," February 2004, www.cdc.gov/nccdphp/burdenbook2004.

11. Examples of organizations: American Cancer Society, Association for Healthcare Quality Research, Centers of Disease Control and Prevention, National Cancer Institute, Substance Abuse and Mental Health Services Administration, 2005. See also Cancer Control Planet which provides links to resources for comprehensive cancer control at http://cancercontrolplanet.cancer.gov; and the Task Force on Community Preventive Services' site "Guide to Community Preventive Services" at www.thecommunityguide.org.

12. World Health Organization (WHO), "The World Health Report 2002." *Reducing Risks, Promoting Health Life* (Geneva, Switzerland: WHO, 2002) www.who.int/whr/2002/en.

13. Institute of Medicine. *Who Will Keep the Public Healthy? Educating the Public Health Professionals for the 21st Century* (Washington DC: National Academies Press, 2003).

14. U.S. Department of Health and Human Services, "The Fifty-Eighth World Health Assembly, Geneva, Switzerland, 2005," www.who.int/mediacentre/events/2005/wha58/en/index.html.

15. C. Garnet, "What's Next for Women's Health Research? NIH Word on Health. Women's Health Research." April 2003, www.nih.gov/news/WordonHealth/apr 2003/womenshealth.htm.

16. Institute of Medicine, Committee on Understanding the Biology of Sex and Gender Differences, *Exploring the Biological Contributions to Human Health: Does Sex Matter?* (Washington, DC: National Academies Press, 2001).

17. R. N. Anderson. "Deaths: Leading Causes for 2000," *National Vital Statistics Reports* 50, no. 16 (Hyattsville, MD: National Center for Health Statistics, 2004.)

18. A. Jemal et al., "Cancer Statistics," *A Cancer Journal for Clinicians* 55 (January/February 2005): 10–30; E. Ward, News Conference, American Cancer Society, ACS (19 January 2005).

19. K. Glanz, F. Lewis, and B. Rimer, *Health Behavior and Health Education: Theory, Research and Practice,* 3rd ed. (San Francisco: Jossey-Bass, 2002), Chapter 4.

20. I. M. Rosenstock, "Historical Origins of the Health Belief Model," *Health Education Monographs* 2 (1974): 328–335.

21. Ibid.

22. G. D. Bishop, *Health Psychology* (Boston: Allyn and Bacon, 1994), 84–86.

23. K. Glanz et al., *Health Behavior and Health Education,* Chapters 8 and 9.

24. I. Ajzen, "The Theory of Planned Behavior." *Organizational Behavior and Human Decision Processes* 50 (1991): 179–211.

25. Ibid.

26. A. Ellis, *The Essence of Rational Emotive Behavior Therapy* (New York: The Albert Ellis Institute, 1994).

27. D. Meichenbaum, *Treatment of Patients with Anger Control Problems* (Toronto: Pergamon Press, 2003); D. Meichenbaum, *Stress Inoculation Training* (Toronto: Pergamon Press, 2004).

28. P. Watson and R. Tharp, *Self-Directed Behavior: Self-Modification for Personal Adjustment* (Pacific Grove, CA: Brooks/Cole, 1993), 13.

Do I have to be religious to be spiritual?

How do I know if I've had a panic attack?

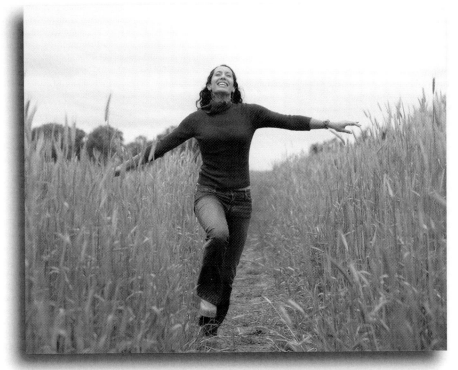

Can negative emotions make me sick?

How can I choose the right therapist for me?

2

Psychosocial Health
Being Mentally, Emotionally, Socially, and Spiritually Well

Objectives

- **Define** each of the four components of psychosocial health, and identify the basic traits shared by psychosocially healthy people.
- **Consider** how each internal and external factor that influences psychosocial health may affect you and the positive steps you can take to enhance your psychosocial health.

- **Discuss** the mind–body connection and how emotions influence health status.
- **Identify** common psychosocial problems of adulthood, including suicide, and explain their causes, methods of prevention, and treatments.
- **Explain** the goals and methods of different types of health professionals and therapies.

One of the great ironies of life is that children may long for adulthood—a time of life they believe will give them the power and control necessary to be happy—while adults young and old tend to pine for their youth, wishing for a carefree, less complicated time in their lives. In truth, all age groups, races, and cultures face unique challenges, threats, and periods of great health and happiness. As we transition between ages and stages of life, the real challenge is to recognize the complexities of life and to learn to adapt, cope, or simply "go with the flow." College students, in particular, face challenges as they move from the security of their hometowns, friends, and family into foreign environments where they are virtual unknowns and must quickly establish themselves as intelligent, socially adept, and worthy of friendship and acceptance.

Although the vast majority of college students describe their college years as among the best of their lives, many find the pressure of grades, financial concerns, relationship problems, and the struggle to find themselves to be extraordinarily difficult. Steven Hyman, provost of Harvard University and former director of the National Institutes of Mental Health states, "The mental state of many students is so precarious that it is interfering with the core mission of the university."[1] According to an annual survey of counseling center directors, the severity of the problems that students experience has been increasing since 1988.[2] Psychological distress caused by relationship issues, family issues, academic competition, and adjusting to life as a college student is rampant on college campuses today. Experts believe that the anxiety-prone campus environment is a major contributor to poor health decisions such as high alcohol consumption and, in turn, to health problems. "Much of collegiate social activity is centered on alcohol consumption because it's an anxiety reducer and demands no social skills . . . it provides an instant identity; it lets people know that you are willing to belong."[3] Increasingly, student health professionals recognize the importance of a solid social network, emotional and mental health, and developing spiritual capacity to not only academic success, but success in life.

DEFINING PSYCHOSOCIAL HEALTH

What Is Psychosocial Health?

While the college years can be fraught with struggles, the good news is that most young adults are resilient, have solid networks of support, and are able to cope,

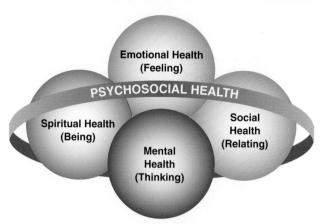

Figure 2.1 ■ Psychosocial Health
Psychosocial health is a complex interaction of mental, emotional, social, and spiritual health.

adapt, and thrive, regardless of life's challenges. They develop into well-adjusted, psychosocially healthy individuals and learn from the ups-and-downs of their early years, recognizing that they have remarkable reserves. The term *psychosocial health* encompasses the mental, emotional, social, and spiritual dimensions of what it means to be healthy (Figure 2.1). It is the result of a complex interaction between a person's history and his or her thoughts about and interpretations of the past and what it means to the present. Psychosocially healthy people are emotionally, mentally, socially, intellectually, and spiritually resilient. They respond to challenges and frustrations in appropriate ways most of the time, despite occasional slips (Figure 2.2). When they do slip, they recognize it and take action to rectify the situation. Most authorities identify several basic characteristics shared by psychosocially healthy people.[4]

■ *They feel good about themselves.* They are not typically overwhelmed by fear, love, anger, jealousy, guilt, or worry. They know who they are, have a realistic sense of their capabilities, and respect themselves even though they realize they aren't perfect.

■ *They feel comfortable with other people.* They enjoy satisfying and lasting personal relationships and do not take advantage of others or allow others to take advantage of them. They recognize that there are others whose needs are greater than their own. They can give love, consider others' interests, take time to help others, respect personal differences, and feel responsible for their fellow human beings.

■ *They control tension and anxiety.* They recognize the underlying causes and symptoms of stress in their lives and consciously avoid irrational thoughts, hostility, excessive excuse making, and blaming others for their problems. They use resources and learn skills to control reactions to stressful situations.

■ *They meet the demands of life.* They try to solve problems as they arise, accept responsibility, and plan

---

Psychosocial health The mental, emotional, social, and spiritual dimensions of health.

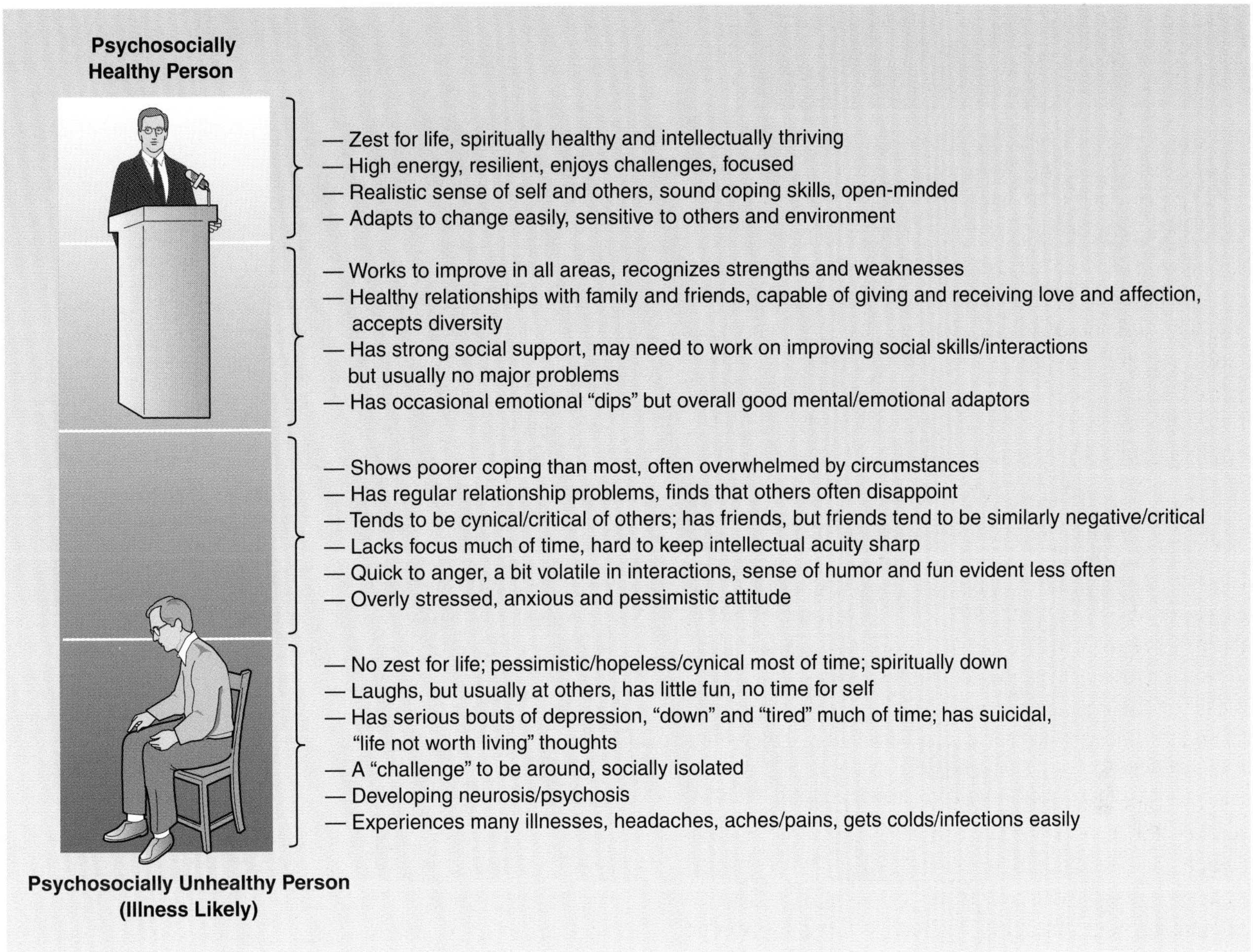

Psychosocially Healthy Person

— Zest for life, spiritually healthy and intellectually thriving
— High energy, resilient, enjoys challenges, focused
— Realistic sense of self and others, sound coping skills, open-minded
— Adapts to change easily, sensitive to others and environment

— Works to improve in all areas, recognizes strengths and weaknesses
— Healthy relationships with family and friends, capable of giving and receiving love and affection, accepts diversity
— Has strong social support, may need to work on improving social skills/interactions but usually no major problems
— Has occasional emotional "dips" but overall good mental/emotional adaptors

— Shows poorer coping than most, often overwhelmed by circumstances
— Has regular relationship problems, finds that others often disappoint
— Tends to be cynical/critical of others; has friends, but friends tend to be similarly negative/critical
— Lacks focus much of time, hard to keep intellectual acuity sharp
— Quick to anger, a bit volatile in interactions, sense of humor and fun evident less often
— Overly stressed, anxious and pessimistic attitude

— No zest for life; pessimistic/hopeless/cynical most of time; spiritually down
— Laughs, but usually at others, has little fun, no time for self
— Has serious bouts of depression, "down" and "tired" much of time; has suicidal, "life not worth living" thoughts
— A "challenge" to be around, socially isolated
— Developing neurosis/psychosis
— Experiences many illnesses, headaches, aches/pains, gets colds/infections easily

Psychosocially Unhealthy Person (Illness Likely)

Figure 2.2 ■ Characteristics of Psychosocially Healthy and Unhealthy People

ahead. They set realistic goals, think for themselves, and make independent decisions. Acknowledging that change is inevitable, they welcome new experiences.

■ *They curb hate and guilt.* They acknowledge and combat tendencies to respond with anger, thoughtlessness, selfishness, vengeful acts, or feelings of inadequacy. They do not try to knock others aside to get ahead but rather reach out to help others—even those they don't particularly like.

■ *They maintain a positive outlook.* They approach each day with a presumption that things will go well. They look to the future with enthusiasm rather than dread. Reminders of good experiences brighten their day. Fun and making time for themselves are integral parts of their lives.

■ *They value diversity.* They do not feel threatened by those of a different race, gender, religion, sexual orientation, ethnicity, or political party. They are nonjudgmental and do not force their beliefs and values on others.

■ *They appreciate and respect nature.* They take the time to enjoy their surroundings, are conscious of their place in the universe, and act responsibly to preserve their environment.

Of course, none of us ever achieve perfection in these areas. Attaining psychosocial health and wellness involves many complex processes. This chapter will help you understand not only what it means to be psychosocially well, but also why we may run into problems in our psychosocial health. Learning how to assess your own health and taking action to improve your health are important parts of psychosocial health (see the Assess Yourself box).

What Do You Think? Which psychosocial qualities do you value most in your friends? ■ Which of these qualities do you possess yourself? ■ Which area would you most like to improve in yourself?

Assessing Your Psychosocial Health

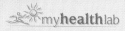

Fill out this assessment online at
www.aw-bc.com/MyHealthLab or www.aw-bc.com/donatelle.

Being psychosocially healthy requires both introspection and the willingness to work on areas that need improvement. Begin by completing the following assessment scale. Use the scale to determine how much each statement describes you. When you've finished, ask someone who is very close to you to take the same test and respond with their perceptions of you. Carefully assess areas where your responses differ from those of your friend or family member. Which areas need some work? Which are in good shape?

	Never	Rarely	Fairly frequently	Most of the time	All of the time
1. My actions and interactions indicate that I am confident in my abilities.	1	2	3	4	5
2. I am quick to blame others for things that go wrong in my life.	1	2	3	4	5
3. I am spontaneous and like to have fun with others.	1	2	3	4	5
4. I am able to give love and affection to others and show my feelings.	1	2	3	4	5
5. I am able to receive love and signs of affection from others without feeling uneasy.	1	2	3	4	5
6. I am generally positive and upbeat about things in my life.	1	2	3	4	5
7. I am cynical and tend to be critical of others.	1	2	3	4	5
8. I have a large group of people whom I consider to be good friends.	1	2	3	4	5
9. I make time for others in my life.	1	2	3	4	5
10. I take time each day for myself for quiet introspection, having fun, or just doing nothing.	1	2	3	4	5
11. I am compulsive and competitive in my actions.	1	2	3	4	5
12. I handle stress well and am seldom upset or stressed out by others.	1	2	3	4	5
13. I try to look for the good in everyone and every situation before finding fault.	1	2	3	4	5
14. I am comfortable meeting new people and interact well in social settings.	1	2	3	4	5
15. I would rather stay in and watch TV or read than go out with friends or interact with others.	1	2	3	4	5
16. I am flexible and can adapt to most situations, even if I don't like them.	1	2	3	4	5
17. Nature, the environment, and other living things are important aspects of my life.	1	2	3	4	5
18. I think before responding to my emotions.	1	2	3	4	5
19. I am selfish and tend to think of my own needs before those of others.	1	2	3	4	5
20. I am consciously trying to be a "better person."	1	2	3	4	5
21. I like to plan ahead and set realistic goals for myself and others.	1	2	3	4	5
22. I accept others for who they are.	1	2	3	4	5

	Never	Rarely	Fairly frequently	Most of the time	All of the time
23. I value diversity and respect others' rights, regardless of culture, race, sexual orientation, religion, or other differences.	1	2	3	4	5
24. I try to live each day as if it might be my last.	1	2	3	4	5
25. I have a great deal of energy and appreciate the little things in life.	1	2	3	4	5
26. I cope with stress in appropriate ways.	1	2	3	4	5
27. I get enough sleep each day and seldom feel tired.	1	2	3	4	5
28. I have healthy relationships with my family.	1	2	3	4	5
29. I am confident that I can do most things if I put my mind to them.	1	2	3	4	5
30. I respect others' opinions and believe that others should be free to express their opinions, even when they differ from my own.	1	2	3	4	5

INTERPRETING YOUR SCORES

Look at items 2, 7, 11, 15, and 19. Add up your score for these five items and divide by 5. Is your average for these items above or below 3? Did you score a 5 on any of these items? Do you need to work on any of these areas? Now look at your scores for the remaining items. (There should be 25 items.) Total these scores and divide by 25. Is your average above or below 3? On which items did you score a 5? Obviously you're doing well in these areas. Now remove these items from this grouping of 25 (scores of 5),

and add up your scores for the remaining items. Then divide your total by the number of items included. Now what is your average?

Do the same for the scores completed by your friend or family member. How do your scores compare? Which ones, if any, are different, and how do they differ? Which areas do you need to work on? What actions can you take now to improve your ratings in these areas?

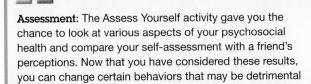

Make It Happen!

Assessment: The Assess Yourself activity gave you the chance to look at various aspects of your psychosocial health and compare your self-assessment with a friend's perceptions. Now that you have considered these results, you can change certain behaviors that may be detrimental to your psychosocial health.

Making a Change: To change your behavior, you need to develop a plan. Follow these steps below and complete your Behavior Change Contract to take action.

1. Evaluate your behavior, and identify patterns and specific things you are doing. What can you change now? What can you change in the near future?
2. Select one pattern of behavior that you'd like to change.
3. Fill out the Behavior Change Contract found at the front of your book. It should include your long-term goal for change, your short-term goals, the rewards you'll give yourself for reaching these goals, potential obstacles along the way, and strategies for overcoming these obstacles. For each goal, list the small steps and specific actions that you can take.

4. Chart your progress in the journal. At the end of one week, consider how successful you were in following your plan.
5. Revise your plan as needed. Are the short-term goals attainable? Are the rewards satisfying?

Example: John assessed himself as a positive and upbeat person, but the assessment his friend gave him rated him as impatient and cynical. John resolved to slow down and become more appreciative of the good things around him. Among his short-term goals: listening to his sister without interrupting her, and expressing a sincere compliment to a family member or friend every other day. John found that paying compliments made him stop to think about the qualities he appreciated in friends and family. While he struggled to listen without interrupting, John found that he was learning a lot about his sister that he had never known before. After several weeks, John's friends commented on his calmer and happier demeanor.

Mental Health: The Thinking You

The term *mental health* is often used to describe the "thinking or rational" part of psychosocial health. It describes your ability to perceive things happening around you in realistic ways, to use reasoning when approaching problems, to interpret what is happening, and to evaluate your situation effectively and react appropriately. In short, you are able to sort through the clutter of events, contradictory messages, and uncertainties of a situation and make sense of it based on experiences, environmental cues, and behaviors. Your values, attitudes, beliefs about your health, relationships with family and others, and your responses to events in your life are usually a reflection of your mental health.

A mentally healthy person is likely to respond to disappointment or frustration without throwing things, outbursts of rage, or blaming others. For example, suppose you decided to spend your spring break with friends on the beaches of Mexico, knowing that you have a major term paper due and an exam on the first day back from vacation. When you return from vacation and quickly throw together your paper and do a quick study session for your exam, you should not fall off the deep end when you get a "D" in the class, blame the instructor or your study-partners for your low grades, and start drinking to drown your sorrows. A mentally healthy student would accept responsibility for the choices he made, learn from mistakes, and try to plan differently next time.

Similarly, people going through difficult break-ups in relationships often are unable to pick themselves up and move on in healthy ways. Learning to acknowledge that it is okay to be sad, unhappy, or frustrated and getting help through counseling or talking with trusted friends is all a part of healthy adapting and coping. Unfortunately, far too many of us get caught up in our emotional upheavals and are unable to pull ourselves out of the deep "funks" we can find ourselves in.

Emotional Health: The Feeling You

The term *emotional health* is often used interchangeably with mental health. Although the two are closely intertwined, emotional health more accurately refers to the feeling, or subjective, side of psychosocial health

---

Mental health The thinking part of psychosocial health, includes your values, attitudes, and beliefs.

Emotional health The feeling part of psychosocial health, includes your emotional reactions to life.

Emotions Intensified feelings or complex patterns of feelings we constantly experience.

---

that includes emotional reactions to life. **Emotions** are intensified feelings or complex patterns of feelings that we experience on a regular basis. Love, hate, frustration, anxiety, and joy are only a few of the many emotions we feel. Typically, emotions are described as the interplay of four components: *physiological arousal, feelings, cognitive (thought) processes,* and *behavioral reactions.* Each time you are put in a stressful situation, you react physiologically as you consciously or unconsciously interpret the situation.

Try it ➤NOW_____

Get used to change! Change is an inevitable part of life, but it can also be a challenge to your psychosocial health. Develop skills to cope with change by creating it. Take a different route to class, study at the coffee shop instead of the library, or commit to trying a new food once a week.

Psychologist Richard Lazarus has indicated that there are four basic types of emotions: emotions resulting from harm, loss, or threats; emotions resulting from benefits; borderline emotions, such as hope and compassion; and more complex emotions, such as grief, disappointment, bewilderment, and curiosity.[5] Each of us may experience any of these feelings in any combination at any time. As rational beings, it is our responsibility to evaluate our individual emotional responses, the environment that is causing them, and the appropriateness of our actions.

Emotionally healthy people usually respond appropriately to upsetting events. Rather than respond in an extreme fashion or behave inconsistently or offensively, they are able to express their feelings, communicate with others, and show emotions in appropriate ways. How many times have you seen someone react with extreme anger by shouting or punching a wall? Ex-lovers who become jealous of new relationships and damage cars or property are classic examples of unhealthy and dangerous emotional reactions. Such violent responses and emotional volatility have become a problem of epidemic proportions in the United States (see Chapter 4).

Emotional health may also affect social health. How many times does someone have to act out in inappropriate ways before nobody wants to be around them anymore? Ironically, when someone is moody, hostile, or withdrawn, it usually is a good indicator that they need emotional support from family and loved ones. However, their actions make support very difficult, often meaning that professional counseling is their only option. Social isolation is just one of the many possible negative consequences of unstable emotional responses.

For students, a more immediate concern is the impact of emotional trauma on academic performance. Have you ever tried to study for an exam after a fight with a close friend or family member? Emotional turmoil can affect your ability to think, focus, reason, and act in rational ways. Many otherwise rational, mentally healthy people do bizarre things when they are going through an emotional crisis. Mental functioning and emotional responses are intricately connected.

Social Health: Interactions with Others

Social health, an important part of the broader concept of psychosocial health, includes your interactions with others on an individual and group basis, your ability to use social resources and support in times of need, and your ability to adapt to a variety of social situations. Socially healthy individuals have a wide range of interactions with family, friends, and acquaintances, and are able to have a healthy interaction with an intimate partner. Typically, socially healthy individuals are able to listen, express themselves, form healthy attachments, act in socially acceptable and responsible ways, and find the best fit for themselves in society. Numerous studies have documented the importance of social health in promoting physical health, mental health, and enhanced longevity.[6]

As social animals, we grow stronger and learn valuable lessons in groups. We depend on others to learn new skills and develop much of our sense of self-worth as a result of our interactions with others. Our adult lives are spent working with others, developing relationships with family and friends, and participating in our community. **Social bonds** reflect the level of closeness and attachment that we develop with individuals. They provide intimacy, acceptance, nurturance, reassurance of one's worth, assistance and guidance. Social bonds take multiple forms, the most common of which are social support and community engagements.

Social support consists of networks of people and services with whom you share ties. These ties can provide tangible support, such as babysitting services or money to help pay the bills, or intangible support, such as encouraging you to share intimate thoughts. Generally, the closer and the higher the quality of the social bond, the more likely a person is to ask for and receive social support. People who are socially isolated, estranged from their families, and have few social connections may not have anyone to turn to when they are in trouble. Psychosocially healthy people create and maintain a network of friends and family with whom they can give and receive support, and they work hard to maintain those relationships even in difficult times.

Social health also reflects the way we react to others. In its most extreme forms, a lack of social health may be represented by aggressive acts of prejudice toward other individuals or groups. In its most obvious manifestations, **prejudice** is reflected in acts of discrimination, hate, and bias, and in purposeful intent to harm individuals or groups.

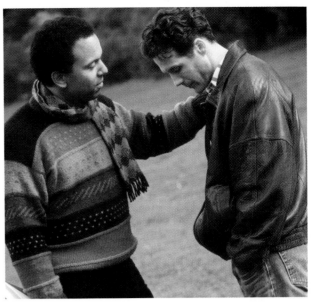
Support from family and friends is a vital component to your social health.

Spiritual Health: An Inner Quest for Well-Being

Although mental and emotional health are key factors in overall psychosocial functioning, it is possible that you could be mentally and emotionally healthy and still find that something is missing in your life. For many people, the difficult-to-describe element that gives zest to life and hope for the future is the spiritual dimension.

Do I have to be religious to be spiritual?

Our spiritual dimension reflects our values, beliefs, and our perceptions of the world and all living things. **Spirituality** may be defined as the way we make sense of and establish meaning in our lives.[7] It is a belief in a unifying force that makes life worthwhile. This unifying force may be nature for some individuals, a god or spiritual symbol, or a feeling of connection to other people.

Social health Aspect of psychosocial health that includes interactions with others, ability to use social supports, and ability to adapt to various situations.

Social bonds Degree and nature of interpersonal contacts.

Social support Network of people and services with whom you share ties and get support.

Prejudice A negative evaluation of an entire group of people that is typically based on unfavorable and often wrong ideas about the group.

Spirituality A belief in a unifying force that gives meaning to life and transcends the purely physical or personal dimensions of existence.

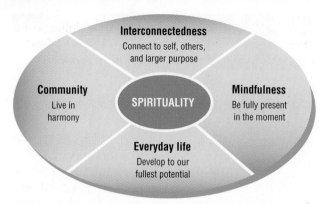

Figure 2.3 ■ Four Major Themes of Spirituality

On a day-to-day basis, many of us focus on acquiring material possessions and satisfying basic needs, but there comes a point when we discover that material possessions do not automatically bring happiness or a sense of self-worth. This realization may be triggered by a crisis. A failed relationship, a terrible accident, the death of a close friend or family member, or other loss often prompts a search for meaning, for the answer to the proverbial question, Is that all there is? Whatever the reason, this search brings new opportunities for understanding ourselves. As we develop into spiritually healthy beings, we recognize our identity as unique individuals. We gain a better appreciation of our strengths and shortcomings and our place in the universe. Perhaps most important, we gain an appreciation for the here-and-now rather than living for aspirations that we may never achieve.

In its purest sense, spirituality addresses four main themes: interconnectedness, the practice of mindfulness, spirituality as a part of everyday life, and living in harmony with the community (Figure 2.3).

- *Interconnectedness.* **Interconnectedness** refers to a sense of belonging and connecting with oneself, with others, and with a larger meaning or purpose of life. Connecting with oneself involves exploring feelings, taking time to consider how you feel in a given situation, assessing your reactions to people and experiences, and taking mental notes when things or people cause you to lose equilibrium. It also

involves considering your values and achieving congruence between your goals and what you can do to achieve them without compromising your values.

- *Practice of mindfulness.* **Mindfulness** refers to the ability to be fully present in the moment. It has been described as a way of nurturing greater awareness and clarity. It is a form of inner flow—a holistic sensation you feel when you are totally involved in the present.[8] According to mindfulness experts, you can achieve this inner flow through an almost infinite range of opportunities for enjoyment and pleasure, either through the use of physical and sensory skills such as athletics, music, or yoga, or through the development of symbolic skills in areas such as poetry, philosophy, or mathematics. The psychologist Abraham Maslow referred to these moments as peak experiences, during which a person feels integrated, synergistic, and at one with the world.

- *Spirituality as a part of daily life.* Spirituality is embodied in the ability to discover and articulate our own basic purpose in life; to learn how to experience love, joy, peace, and fulfillment; and to help ourselves and others achieve their full potential.[9] This ongoing process of growth fosters three convictions: faith, hope, and love. **Faith** is the belief that helps us realize our unique purpose in life; **hope** is the belief that allows us to look confidently and courageously to the future; and **love** involves accepting, affirming, and respecting self and others regardless of who they are.[10]

- *Living in harmony with our community.* Our values are an extension of our beliefs about the world and attitude toward life. They are formed over time through a series of life experiences, and they are reflected in our hopes, dreams, desires, goals, and ambitions.[11] Though most people have some idea of what is important to them, many spend life largely unaware of how their values impact them or those around them until a life-altering event shakes up their perspective on life.

What Do You Think?   What do social, mental, emotional, and spiritual health mean to you? ■ What are your strengths and weaknesses in each area of psychosocial health? ■ What can you do to enhance your strengths? ■ How can you improve areas that are not *strong*?

Spirituality: A Key to Better Health

Although the specific impact of spirituality on health remains elusive, many experts affirm the importance of this dimension in achieving health and wellness. A recent study of spirituality among college students from 46 diverse universities and colleges indicates that spirituality may play a role in student health, their grades, and other aspects of student life.[12] The study found a correlation

---

Interconnectedness   A web of connections, including our relationship to ourselves, to others, and to a larger meaning or purpose in life.

Mindfulness   Awareness and acceptance of the reality of the present moment.

Faith   Belief that helps each person realize a unique purpose in life.

Hope   Belief that allows us to look confidently and courageously to the future.

Love   Acceptance, affirmation, and respect for the self and others.

between spirituality and health achievement, with more spiritually oriented students having better health, better grades, more involvement in charitable organizations or volunteerism, and more interest in helping others. Other recent studies also indicate a correlation between certain elements of spirituality and positive health outcomes. For example, mindfulness therapies have been used effectively to treat depression, to reduce stress in outpatient therapy and in the nursing profession, with anxiety and heart disease treatments, and other problems.[13] Although still in its infancy, this type of research is being rigorously addressed by such groups as the National Center for Complementary and Alternative Medicine (NCCAM) in order to provide a clearer picture of myths and realities.

A Spiritual Resurgence Over recent decades, studies have shown that most adult Americans, like their student counterparts, believe in God and consider spirituality to be important in their lives, although not necessarily in the form of religion.[14] Many find spiritual fulfillment in music, poetry, literature, art, nature, and intimate relationships.[15] Many religious groups have spawned new philosophies that are more inclusive and often influenced by "New Age" ideas, such as using positive thought to achieve your goals and striving to find your rightful place in the world. An estimated 32 million baby boomers have turned to Eastern practices, New Age philosophies, 12-step programs, Greek mythology, shamanistic practices, massage, yoga, and a host of other traditions and practices.[16]

For some, spirituality means a quest for self and selflessness—a form of therapy and respite from a sometimes challenging personal environment. This quest for a life force, which helps people deeply experience the moments of their lives rather than just living through them, has received much scholarly and popular attention. Self-help books that focus on spirituality consistently top the bestseller lists; writers and psychologists such as William James, Carl Jung, Gordon Allport, Erich Fromm, Viktor Frankl, Abraham Maslow, and Rollo May have made spirituality a major focus of their work.

FACTORS INFLUENCING PSYCHOSOCIAL HEALTH

Most of our mental, emotional, and social reactions to life are a direct outcome of our experiences and social and cultural expectations. Our psychosocial health is based, in part, on how we perceive life experiences.

External Factors

While some life experiences are under our control, others are not. External factors in life are those that we do not control, such as who raised us and where we live.

The Family Families have a significant influence on psychosocial development. Children raised in healthy, nurturing, happy families are more likely to become well-adjusted, productive adults. Children raised in **dysfunctional families** in which there is violence, negative behavior, distrust, anger, dietary deprivation, drug abuse, parental discord, or sexual, physical, or emotional abuse may have a harder time adapting to life and run an increased risk of psychosocial problems. In dysfunctional families, love, security, and unconditional trust are so lacking that children often become confused and psychologically bruised. Yet, not all people raised in dysfunctional families become psychosocially unhealthy, and not all children from healthy environments become well adjusted. Obviously, more factors are involved in our "process of becoming" than just our family.

The Wider Environment Although isolated negative events may do little damage to psychosocial health, persistent stressors, uncertainties, and threats can cause significant problems. Drugs, neighborhood crime and threats to safety, injury, school failure, unemployment, financial problems, and a host of other bad things can happen to good people. But it is believed that certain protective factors, such as having a positive role model in the midst of chaos, or certain positive personality traits can help children from even the worst environments remain healthy and well adjusted (see the next section Internal Factors).

Another important influence is access to health services and programs designed to enhance psychosocial health. Going to a support group or seeing a trained therapist is often a crucial first step in prevention and intervention efforts. Individuals from poor socioeconomic environments who cannot afford such services often find it difficult to secure help in improving their psychosocial health.

What Do You Think? ■ Over which external factors does an individual have the most control?
■ Which factors had the greatest impact on making you who you are today?

Internal Factors

Many internal factors also shape a person's development. These factors include hereditary traits, hormonal function, physical health (including neurological function), physical fitness level, and certain elements of mental and emotional health.

> **Dysfunctional families** Families in which there is violence; physical, emotional, or sexual abuse; parental discord; or other negative family interactions.

Self-Efficacy and Self-Esteem During our formative years, successes and failures in school, athletics, friendships, intimate relationships, jobs, and every other aspect of life subtly shape our beliefs about our own personal worth and abilities. These beliefs become internal influences on our psychosocial health.

Psychologist Albert Bandura used the term **self-efficacy** to describe a person's belief about whether he or she can successfully engage in and execute a specific behavior. Prior positive past experiences such as success in academics, athletics, or social interactions will lead to expectations of and efforts to achieve success in the future. Self-efficacious people are more likely to feel a sense of **personal control** over situations, or that their own internal resources allow them to control events. On the other hand, someone with low self-efficacy may give up easily, accept failure, or never even try to change a behavior. Learning new skills and having successful experiences can help improve confidence and add to a "can-do" attitude.

Self-esteem refers to one's sense of self-respect or self-worth. It can be defined as one's evaluation of oneself and one's own personal worth as an individual. People with high self-esteem tend to feel good about themselves and express a positive outlook on life. People with low self-esteem often do not like themselves, constantly demean themselves, and doubt their ability to succeed.

Our self-esteem is a result of the relationships we have with our parents and family during our formative years, with our friends as we grow older, with our significant others as we form intimate relationships, and with our teachers, co-workers, and others throughout our lives. If we felt loved and valued as children, our self-esteem allows us to believe that we are inherently lovable individuals. See the Skills for Behavior Change box for some strategies for increasing your self-esteem.

Learned Helplessness versus Learned Optimism

Psychologist Martin Seligman has proposed that people who continually experience failure may develop a pattern of responding known as **learned helplessness,** in which they give up and fail to take any action to help themselves. Seligman ascribes this in part to society's tendency toward victimology, blaming one's problems on other people and circumstances. Although viewing ourselves as victims may make us feel better temporarily, it does not address the underlying causes of a problem. Ultimately, it can erode self-efficacy and foster learned helplessness by making us feel that we cannot do anything to improve the situation.[17]

Countering this is Seligman's principle of **learned optimism.** Just as we learn to be helpless, so can we teach ourselves to be optimistic. His research provides growing evidence for the central place of mental health in overall positive development.[18]

In one study, university freshmen who had been identified as pessimistic on the basis of a questionnaire were randomly assigned to an experimental group or to a control group. The experimental group attended a 16-hour workshop in which they practiced social and study skills and learned to dispute chronic negative thoughts. The control group did not participate. Eighteen months later, 15 percent of the control group members were experiencing severe anxiety, and 32 percent were suffering from moderate to severe depression. In contrast, only 7 percent of workshop participants suffered from anxiety and 22 percent from depression. Seligman concluded that even relatively brief interventions, such as this workshop, can produce measurable improvements in coping skills.[19]

Personality

Your personality is the unique mix of characteristics that distinguish you from others. Heredity, environment, culture, and experience influence how each person develops. Personality determines how we react to the challenges of life, interpret our feelings, and resolve conflicts.

Most of the recent schools of psychosocial theory promote the idea that we have the power not only to understand our behavior, but also to change it and thus mold our own personalities. Although much has been written about the importance of a healthy personality, there is little consensus on what that concept really means. In general, people who possess the following traits often appear to be psychosocially healthy:[20]

- *Extroversion,* the ability to adapt to a social situation and demonstrate assertiveness as well as power or interpersonal involvement.
- *Agreeableness,* the ability to conform, be likable, and demonstrate friendly compliance as well as love.
- *Openness to experience,* the willingness to demonstrate curiosity and independence (also referred to as inquiring intellect).
- *Emotional stability,* the ability to maintain social control.
- *Conscientiousness,* the qualities of being dependable and demonstrating self-control, discipline, and a need to achieve.[21]

Life Span and Maturity

Our temperaments change as we move through life, as illustrated by the

---

Self-efficacy Belief in one's own ability to perform a task successfully.

Personal control Belief that one's own internal resources can control a situation.

Self-esteem Sense of self-respect or self-confidence.

Learned helplessness Pattern of responding to situations by giving up because of repeated failure in the past.

Learned optimism Teaching oneself to think optimistically.

How can you build self-esteem? Many things you can do daily can have a significant impact on the way you feel about yourself. Practice these tips regularly to bolster your self-esteem.

- *Pay attention to your own needs and wants.* Listen to what your body, your mind, and your heart are telling you.

- *Take good care of yourself.* Eat healthy foods, avoid junk foods, exercise, and plan fun activities for yourself.

- *Take time to do things you enjoy.* Make a list of things you enjoy doing. Then do something from that list every day.

- *Do something that you have been putting off.* Cleaning out your closet, going on a diet, or paying a bill that you've been putting off will make you feel like you've accomplished something.

- *Give yourself rewards.* Acknowledge that you are a great person by rewarding yourself occasionally.

- *Spend time with people.* People who make you feel better about yourself are great self-esteem boosters. Avoid people who treat you badly or make you feel bad about yourself.

- *Display items that you like.* You may have items that remind you of your achievements, your friends, or of special times. Keep those special items close by.

- *Make your meals a special time.* Get rid of distractions like the television and really concentrate on enjoying your meal, whether by yourself or with others.

- *Learn something new every day.* Take advantage of any opportunity to learn something new every day—you'll feel better about yourself and be more productive.

- *Do something nice for another person.* There is no greater way to feel better about yourself than to help someone in greater need. Check out local volunteer opportunities or make a special effort to be nice to those around you such as your parents or siblings.

Sources: A. L. Story, "Self-Esteem and Self-Certainty: A Mediational Analysis," *European Journal of Personality* 18, no. 2 (2004): 115; M. E. Copeland "Building Self-Esteem: A Self-Help Guide," Center for Mental Health Services [online booklet], accessed May 2004, www.mentalhealth.org/publications/allpubs/SMA-3715/default.asp.

extreme emotions experienced by many people in early adolescence. Most of us learn to control our emotions as we advance toward adulthood.

The college years mark a critical transition period for young adults as they move away from families and establish themselves as independent adults. The transition to independence will be easier for those who have successfully accomplished earlier developmental tasks such as learning how to solve problems, make and evaluate decisions, define and adhere to personal values, and establish both casual and intimate relationships. People who have not fulfilled these earlier tasks may find their lives interrupted by recurrent "crises" left over from earlier stages. For example, if they did not learn to trust others in childhood, they may have difficulty establishing intimate relationships as adults.

Resiliency and Developmental Assets

Over the last decade, it has become well established that some people are much better prepared to meet the challenges of life than others. The combination of certain personality traits, coupled with a supportive environment can equip one to deal effectively with life's many challenges. These individuals are able to cope and even thrive in times of great stress or pressure. **Resiliency,** or

protective factors, are terms used to describe those traits or characteristics which protect an individual or community from threat or harm. In a sense, these traits may serve to inoculate one against potential ill health. People with **assets,** whether they be financial, emotional, spiritual, physical, intellectual, or mental, and other positive forces in their lives, are more likely to be resilient and bounce back when facing life's challenges.

STRATEGIES TO ENHANCE PSYCHOSOCIAL HEALTH

As we have seen, psychosocial health involves four dimensions. Attaining self-fulfillment is a lifelong, conscious process that involves enhancing each of these components. Strategies include building self-efficacy

Resiliency An individual's capacity for adapting to change and stressful events in healthy and flexible ways.

Assets Internal and external resources and community supports that help a person be more resilient in difficult times and more likely to make positive choices and respond in positive, healthful ways.

and self-esteem, understanding and controlling emotions, maintaining support networks, and learning to solve problems and make decisions.

Developing and Maintaining Self-Esteem and Self-Efficacy

There are several ways to build self-esteem and self-efficacy. These include finding a support group, completing required tasks, forming realistic expectations, making time for yourself, maintaining your physical health, and examining your problems and seeking help.

Find a Support Group The best way to promote self-esteem is through a support group—peers who share your values. A support group can make you feel good about yourself and force you to take an honest look at your actions and choices. Although you might seek support in a wholly new group, remember that old ties are often the strongest.

Keeping in contact with old friends and important family members can provide a foundation of unconditional love that will help you through the many life transitions ahead. Try to be a support for others, too. Join a discussion, political action, or recreational group. Write more postcards and "thinking of you" notes to people who matter. This will build your own self-esteem and that of your friends.

Complete Required Tasks A good way to boost your self-efficacy is to learn new skills and develop a history of success. Most college campuses provide study groups and learning centers that can help you manage time, develop study skills, and prepare for tests. Poor grades, or grades that do not meet expectations, are major contributors to emotional distress among college students.

Form Realistic Expectations Set realistic expectations for yourself. If you expect perfect grades, a steady stream of Saturday-night dates, and the perfect job, you may be setting yourself up for failure. Assess your current resources and the direction in which you are heading. Set small, incremental goals or steps that are possible for you to meet.

Make Time for You Taking time to enjoy yourself is another way to boost your self-esteem and psychosocial health. View a new activity as something to look forward to and an opportunity to have fun. Anticipate and focus on the fun things you have to look forward to each day.

Insomnia Difficulty in falling asleep or staying asleep.

Maintain Physical Health Regular exercise fosters a sense of well-being. Nourishing meals can help you avoid the weight gain that many college students experience. Several studies support the role of exercise in improved mental health.[22] (See Chapter 9 for information on nutrition and Chapter 10 for information on the role of exercise on health.)

Examine Problems and Seek Help if Necessary Knowing when to seek help from friends, support groups, family, or professionals is another important factor in boosting self-esteem. Sometimes you can handle life's problems alone; at other times, you need assistance.

Sleep: The Great Restorer

Sleep serves at least two biological purposes: conservation of energy so we are rested and ready to perform during daylight hours, and restoration so that neurotransmitters that have been depleted during waking hours can be replenished. Getting enough sleep to prepare for a new day and meet daily challenges is a key factor in physical and psychosocial health.

Insomnia—difficulty in falling asleep quickly, frequent arousals during sleep, or early morning awakening—is a common complaint among 20 to 40 percent of Americans. Insomnia is more common among women than men, and its prevalence is correlated with age and low socioeconomic status.

How much sleep do we need? There is a genetically based need for sleep, and sleep duration is controlled by *circadian rhythms,* which are linked to the hormone *melatonin.* People may also alter sleep patterns by staying up late, drinking coffee, getting lots of physical exercise, eating a heavy meal, or using alarm clocks.

Most of us follow characteristic stages of sleep. The most important period of sleep, known as the time of *rapid eye movement,* or *REM,* is essential to feeling rested and refreshed. In REM sleep, heart rate increases, respiration speeds up, and dreaming tends to occur. If we miss REM sleep, we are left feeling groggy and tired.

Sleepless nights cause many people to turn to over-the-counter sleeping pills, barbiturates, or tranquilizers. The following methods are more effective and less risky.[23]

- *Establish a consistent sleep schedule.* Go to bed and get up at about the same time every day.
- *Evaluate your sleep environment, and change anything that could be keeping you awake.* If it's noise, wear earplugs. If it's light, try room-darkening shades.
- *Exercise regularly.* However, avoid exercise right before bed; activity speeds up your metabolism and makes it harder to fall asleep.
- *Limit caffeine and alcohol.* Caffeine can linger in your body for up to 12 hours and cause insomnia.

While alcohol may make you drowsy at first, it interferes with the normal sleep–wake cycle.

- *Avoid eating a heavy meal or drinking large amounts of liquid before bed.*
- *If you're unable to get to sleep in 30 minutes, get up and do something else for awhile;* return to bed when you feel drowsy.
- *If you nap, do so only during the afternoon* when circadian rhythms make you especially sleepy. Don't let naps interfere with your normal sleep schedule.
- *Establish a relaxing nighttime ritual that puts you in the mood to sleep.* Take a warm shower or listen to relaxing music. This will cue your mind and body that it's time to wind down.[24]

Some people have difficulty getting a good night's sleep due to sleep apnea, an increasingly common and serious disorder. For more on this condition, see Chapter 14.

THE MIND–BODY CONNECTION

Can negative emotions and stress make you sick? Can positive emotions and happiness inoculate you against illness? Although considerable research has attempted to conclusively answer these questions, much remains unknown. For decades we have focused primarily on negative emotions and disease; however, little is known about the role of positive emotions in preserving health and protecting against disease. Many scientists believe that this end of the emotions continuum may hold the key to future advances in health and that mind–body health science may be elevated to new heights as a result of new findings. One area that appears to be particularly promising is the emotion of *happiness.*

> Can negative emotions make me sick?

Happiness and Physical Health

Happiness is defined as a kind of place-holder for a number of positive states in which individuals actively embrace the world around them.[25] As scientists have examined characteristics of happy people, they have found that this emotion can have a profound impact on the body. Researchers have found that happiness or related mental states like hopefulness, optimism, and contentment appear to reduce the risk or limit the severity of cardiovascular disease, pulmonary disease, diabetes, hypertension, colds, and other infections. Laughter can promote increases in heart rate, respiration rate, and reduce levels of stress hormones in much the same way as light exercise. For this reason, it has been promoted as a possible risk reducer for those with hypertension and other forms of cardiovascular disease.[26]

Try it → NOW

Find your flow! **Flow is considered the contentment and happiness you experience when completely absorbed in an activity you enjoy. To find your flow, paint a picture, write a story, or dance to your favorite music. Once you've found your flow, you'll be hooked!**

If happiness is good for your health, how does one "get happy"? **Subjective well-being (SWB)** refers to that uplifting feeling of inner peace or overall "feel-good state," which includes happiness. SWB is defined by three central components:[27]

1. *Satisfaction with present life.* People who are high in SWB tend to like their work and are satisfied with their current personal relationships. They are sociable, outgoing, and willing to open up to others. They also like themselves and enjoy good health and self-esteem.

2. *Relative presence of positive emotions.* People with high SWB more frequently feel pleasant emotions, mainly because they evaluate the world around them in a generally positive way. They have an optimistic outlook, and they expect success in what they undertake.

3. *Relative absence of negative emotions.* Individuals with a strong sense of SWB experience fewer and less severe episodes of negative emotions, such as anxiety, depression, and anger.

Scientists also suggest that people may be biologically predisposed to happiness. Psychologist Richard Davidson suggests that happiness may, in part, be related to actual differences in brain physiology—that *neurotransmitters,* the chemicals that transfer messages between neurons, may function more efficiently in happy people.[28] Other psychologists suggest that we can develop happiness by practicing positive psychological actions.[29]

You do not have to be happy all the time to achieve overall subjective well-being. Everyone experiences disappointments, unhappiness, and times when life seems unfair. But people with SWB are typically resilient, able to look on the positive side, get themselves

---

Happiness Feeling of contentment created when one's expectations and physical, psychological, and spiritual needs have been met and one enjoys life.

Subjective well-being (SWB) That uplifting feeling of inner peace and wonder that we call happiness.

How happy are you?

Read the following statements, and then rate your level of agreement with each one using the 1–7 scale.

1	2	3	4	5	6	7
Strongly disagree	Disagree	Slightly disagree	Neither agree nor disagree	Slightly agree	Agree	Strongly agree

1. In most ways, my life is close to my ideal.
2. The conditions of my life are excellent.
3. I am satisfied with my life.
4. So far I have gotten the important things I want in life.
5. If I could live my life over, I would change almost nothing.

Total score: _____

Scoring:
31–35: You are very satisfied with your life 26–30: Satisfied 21–25: Slightly satisfied
20: You are neither satisfied nor dissatisfied 15–19: Slightly dissatisfied 10–14: Dissatisfied 5–9: Very dissatisfied

Figure 2.4 ■ Satisfaction With Life Scale

Source: W. Pavot and E. Diener, "Review of the Satisfaction with Life Scale," *Psychological Assessment* 5 (1993):164–172.

back on track fairly quickly, and less likely to fall into despair over setbacks. There are several myths about happiness: that it depends on age, gender, race, and socioeconomic status. Take the quiz on happiness and see how satisfied you are with life (Figure 2.4).

Humans are remarkably resourceful creatures. We respond to great loss, such as the death of a loved one or a traumatic event, with an initial period of grief, mourning, and sometimes rage. Yet, with time and the support of loving family and friends, we can brush off the bad times and find satisfaction and peace. Typically, humans learn from suffering and emerge even stronger and more ready to deal with the next crisis. Most find some measure of happiness after the initial shock and pain of loss. Those who are otherwise healthy, in good physical condition, and part of a strong social support network can adapt and cope effectively.

Does Laughter Enhance Psychosocial Health?

Remember the last time you laughed so hard that you cried? Remember how relaxed you felt afterward? Scientists are just beginning to understand the role of humor in our lives and health. For example, laughter has been shown to have the following effects:

■ Stressed-out people with a strong sense of humor become less depressed and anxious than those whose sense of humor is less well developed.

■ Students who use humor as a coping mechanism report that it predisposes them to a positive mood.

■ Telling a joke, particularly one that involves a shared experience, increases our sense of belonging and social cohesion.

Clearly, laughter enhances mental and emotional health. It also promotes social health: people like to be around others who are fun-loving and laugh easily. Learning to laugh puts more joy into everyday experiences and increases the likelihood that fun-loving people will keep company with us.

Psychologist Barbara Fredrickson argues that positive emotions such as joy, interest, and contentment serve valuable life functions. Joy is associated with playfulness and creativity. Interest encourages us to explore our world, which enhances knowledge and cognitive ability. Contentment allows us to savor and integrate experiences, an important step in achieving mindfulness and insight. By building our physical, social, and mental resources, these positive feelings empower us to cope effectively with life's challenges. While the actual emotions may be transient, their effects can be permanent and provide lifelong enrichment.[30]

While positive emotions appear to benefit physical health, evidence is accumulating that negative emotions can impair it. Studies of widowed and divorced people reveal below-normal immune system functioning and higher rates of illness and death than among married people. Other studies have shown unusually high rates of cancer among depressed people.[31]

Psychosocial Health and Overall Well-Being

Do these studies provide conclusive evidence of a mind–body connection? Not necessarily because they do not account for other factors known to be relevant to health. For example, some researchers suggest that people who are divorced, widowed, or depressed are more likely to drink and smoke, use drugs, eat and sleep

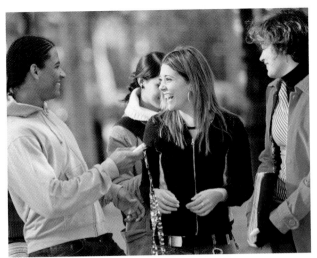

Sharing laughter and having fun with friends improves our social dimension of health and can put more joy into everyday life.

poorly, and be sedentary—all of which may affect the immune system. In fact, the immune system changes measured in studies of the mind–body connection are relatively small. The health consequences of such minute changes are difficult to gauge, and researchers continue to seek the answer to this question.[32]

A large body of evidence points to an association between the emotions and physical health, yet we still have much to learn about this relationship. In the meantime, it appears that happiness and an optimistic mindset don't just feel good—they are also good for you.

WHEN PSYCHOSOCIAL HEALTH DETERIORATES

Sometimes circumstances overwhelm us to such a degree that we need outside assistance to help us get back on track toward healthful living. Abusive relationships, stress, anxiety, loneliness, financial upheavals, and other traumatic events can sap our spirits, causing us to turn inward or to act in ways that are outside of what might be considered normal. Chemical imbalances, drug interactions, trauma, neurological disruptions, and other physical problems also may contribute to these behaviors. **Mental illnesses** are disorders that disrupt thinking, feeling, moods, and behaviors, and cause a varying degree of impaired functioning in daily life. They are believed to be caused by life events in some cases and by actual biochemical and/or brain dysfunction in others.[33] A recent study by the National Institute of Mental Health (NIMH) found that half of all mental illnesses begin by age 14 and that there are often decades of delay between symptoms and treatment. Three-fourths of all mental disorders begin by age 24.[34]

As with physical disease, mental illnesses can range from mild to severe and exact a heavy toll on the

quality of life, both for those with the illnesses and those who come in contact with them. Although mental illness often is not discussed as openly as physical ailments, it is universal. Recent reports by the World Health Organization, the World Bank, and Harvard University indicate that mental illness is the second leading cause of disability and premature death in developed countries—right behind cardiovascular disease and just ahead of cancer.[35] Or consider this from the Mayo Clinic:

> *Studies tell us that, on average, out of every 100 people, 28 have coped with a mental or substance abuse disorder in the past year. Of these, a dozen or so have had symptoms of an anxiety disorder, such as panic disorder or social phobia. Ten have struggled with an addiction, most likely to be alcohol, and about 10 have lived with a mood disorder, perhaps depression or bipolar disorder. These numbers add up to more than 28 because some people experience more than one illness at the same time, just as high blood pressure, diabetes and asthma may occur together. Although these conditions are common, fear of seeming weak or defective makes many people reluctant to acknowledge mental or emotional distress.*[36]

Although there are many types of mental illnesses, we will focus here on those most likely to be experienced by large numbers of college students. For information about other disorders, consult the websites at the end of this chapter or ask your instructor for local resources.

Depression: The Full-Scale Tumble

In a recent meeting of the American Psychological Association, the organization's president remarked, "Depression has been called the common cold of psychological disturbances, which underscores its prevalence, but trivializes its impact."[37] In any one-year period, nearly 10 percent or 20 million American adults suffer from a depressive illness.[38] Many of them are misdiagnosed, underdiagnosed, and not receiving treatment, despite its availability.[39]

Major Depressive Disorder
It is normal to feel blue or depressed in response to certain experiences, such as the death of a loved one, divorce, loss of a job, or an unhappy ending to a long-term relationship.

Mental illnesses Disorders that disrupt thinking, feeling, moods, and behaviors, and impair daily functioning.

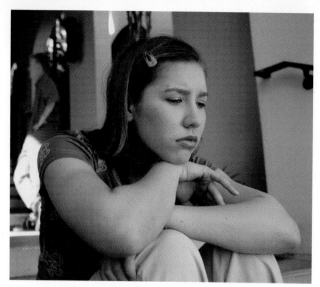

When experiencing depression, it is unwise to try to "go it alone." Supportive family and friends and a qualified therapist can help.

However, people with **major depressive disorder** experience a form of **chronic mood disorder** that involves, on a day-to-day basis, extreme and persistent sadness, despair, and hopelessness. People with this disorder typically feel discouraged by life and circumstances and experience feelings of intense guilt and worthlessness. They may be hypercritical of others and feel disappointed by others most of the time. Usually they show some impairment of social and occupational functioning, although their behavior is not necessarily bizarre. Approximately 15 percent of them eventually attempt suicide or succeed in committing suicide.[40] Untold numbers of others victimize their families, cause disruptions, or display outwardly violent acts.

Depression can strike at any age, but the first episode usually occurs before age 40. (See Table 2.1, which lists common symptoms.) Some people experience one bout of depression and never have problems again, but others suffer recurrences throughout their lives. Stressful life events are often catalysts for these recurrences.

Risks for Depression Major depressive disorder is caused by interaction between biology, learned behavioral responses, and cognitive factors. Chemical and genetic processes may predispose people to depression, and irrational ideas and beliefs can guide them to negative coping behaviors.[41] Because of genetic history, environment, situational triggers and stressors, poor be-

Major depressive disorder Severe depression that entails chronic mood disorder, physical effects such as sleep disturbance and exhaustion, and mental effects such as the inability to concentrate.

Chronic mood disorder Experience of persistent sadness, despair, and hopelessness.

havioral skills, and brain–body chemistry, some people may be particularly vulnerable.

Facts and Fallacies about Depression

Although it is one of the fastest-growing problems in U.S. culture, depression remains one of the most misunderstood. Myths and misperceptions about the disease abound.[42]

- *True depression is not a natural reaction to crisis and loss.* Crisis and loss can lead an already depressed person over the edge to suicide or other problems, but crisis and loss do not inevitably result in depression.

- *People will not snap out of depression by using a little willpower.* Medical intervention in the form of antidepressant drugs and therapy is often necessary for recovery. Understanding the seriousness of the disease and supporting people in their attempts to recover are key elements.

- *Frequent crying is not a hallmark of depression.* Some depressed people bear their burdens in silence, or may even be the life of the party. Some don't cry at all. In fact, biochemists theorize that crying may actually ward off depression by releasing chemicals that the body produces as a positive response to stress.

- *Depression is not "all in the mind." Depression isn't a disease of weak-willed, powerless people.* In fact, research suggests that depressive illnesses originate with an inherited chemical imbalance in the brain. Some physiological conditions, such as thyroid disorders, or certain medications also are known to prompt depressive-like symptoms.

- *In-depth psychotherapy is not the only cure for long-term clinical depression.* No single psychotherapy method works for all cases of depression.

Depression and Gender According to the National Institute of Mental Health (NIMH), women experience depression at nearly two times the rate of men: 8 to 11 percent of men compared to 19 to 23 percent of women. About 6 percent of women and 3 percent of men have experienced episodes severe enough to require hospitalization.[43]

Many hormonal factors may contribute to the increased rates in women, particularly such events as menstrual cycle changes, pregnancy, miscarriage, postpartum period, premenopause, and menopause. In fact, an NIMH study indicated that, in the case of severe premenstrual syndrome (PMS), women with a preexisting vulnerability to PMS experienced relief from mood swings and physical symptoms when their sex hormones were suppressed. Shortly after the hormones were reintroduced, they again developed symptoms of PMS. Women with no history of PMS reported no effects of hormonal manipulation.[44]

Although adolescent and adult females have been found to experience depression at twice the rate of males, the college population seems to represent a notable exception, with equal rates experienced by males and females. Why? Several hypotheses have been suggested:[45]

- The social institutions of the college campus provide more egalitarian roles for men and women.
- College women experience fewer negative events than do high school females. Men in college report more negative events than they experienced in high school.
- College women report smaller and more supportive social networks.

Depression is often preceded by a stressful event. Some psychologists therefore theorize that women are under more stress than men and thus more prone to become depressed. However, women do not report more stressful events than men do.

Finally, researchers have observed gender differences in coping strategies, or the response to certain events or stimuli, and have proposed that some women's strategies make them more vulnerable to depression. Presented with "a list of things people do when depressed," college students were asked to indicate how likely they were to engage in each behavior. Men were more likely to assert that "I avoid thinking of reasons why I am depressed" or "I play sports." Women were more likely to answer "I try to determine why I am depressed" and "I talk to other people about my feelings." In other words, the men tried to distract themselves from a depressed mood whereas the women focused on it. If focusing on negative feelings intensifies them, women who do this may predispose themselves to depression. This hypothesis has not been directly tested, but some supporting evidence suggests its validity.[46]

Overall, the rate of depression among men may be increasing. Certain factors, such as family history, undue stress, loss of a loved one, or serious illness, seem to increase the risk.[47] Men are less likely than women to admit to depression, and doctors are less likely to suspect it. Men's depression is more likely to be hidden by alcohol or drug abuse or by the socially acceptable habit of working long hours. Depression typically shows up in men not as feeling hopeless and helpless, but as being irritable, angry, and discouraged. One marker of the problem is that, although more women attempt suicide, the rate of suicide in men is actually four times that of women. In fact, after age 70, the rate of men's suicide rises, reaching a peak after age 85.[48]

Interestingly, depression seems to be more lethal for men than women in terms of physical health. Although depression is associated with an increased risk of coronary heart disease in both genders, only men suffer a high death rate.[49] Because even men who realize they may be depressed are less likely to seek help than women, encouragement and support from concerned friends and family members are crucial.

Table 2.1

Are You Depressed?

Sadness and despair are the main symptoms of depression. Other common signs include:

- Loss of motivation or interest in pleasurable activities
- Preoccupation with failures and inadequacies; concern over what others are thinking
- Difficulty concentrating; indecisiveness; memory lapses
- Loss of sex drive or interest in close interactions with others
- Fatigue and loss of energy; slow reactions
- Sleeping too much or too little; insomnia
- Feeling agitated, worthless, or hopeless
- Withdrawal from friends and family
- Diminished or increased appetite
- Recurring thoughts that life isn't worth living; thoughts of death or suicide
- Significant weight loss or weight gain

Some depressed people mask their symptoms with a forced, upbeat sense of humor or high energy levels. Communication may cease or seem frantic.

Depression in Selected Populations There are a few exceptions to the findings on depression and gender. Among Jews, males are equally as likely as females to experience major depressive episodes.[50] In recent years, there has also been a noteworthy increase in depression among children, the elderly, and adolescents, particularly adolescent girls, and perhaps in Native American and homosexual young people as well.[51] Writers, composers, and entertainers also seem to have higher than expected rates of major depression, and people experiencing chronic, unrelenting pain have the highest rates of any group.[52]

Depression on Campus Over 15 percent of students seek counseling in college, but there are many more who probably need it and never seek help due to lack of knowledge, worry over stigma associated with mental health therapy, and a host of other reasons.[53] The stressors of college life such as anxiety over relationships, pressure to get good grades and for social acceptance, abuse of alcohol and other drugs, poor diet, and lack of sleep can create a toxic cocktail.[54] It is no surprise depression on college campuses is such a huge problem. According to a longitudinal study of students who sought help at Kansas State University over a 13-year period, sources of depression changed from relationship problems and money problems in the 1980s, to more serious forms of stress-related anxiety in later years, paralleling trends in society as a whole.[55] International students are particularly vulnerable to mental health concerns. Being far from home without the security of family and friends can exacerbate problems and make coping difficult. Most campuses have cultural centers and other services available; however, many students do not use them. Other universities offer relaxation workshops and massage during high stress finals weeks and offer 24-hour counseling for their students. These resources aren't limited to international students though, so if you are feeling unusually blue or overwhelmed, seek out any aid your university may offer. See the Reality Check box for more on how universities are handling student mental health problems.

Treating Depression

The best treatment involves determining the person's type and degree of depression and its possible causes. For clinical (severe and prolonged) depression, drugs and psychotherapy are often recommended. Table 2.2 on page 50 provides an overview of drugs used to treat depression.

In some cases, psychotherapy alone may be the most successful treatment. The two most common psychotherapeutic therapies for depression are cognitive and interpersonal therapy.

Cognitive therapy helps a patient look at life rationally and correct habitually pessimistic thought patterns. It focuses on the here-and-now rather than on analyzing a patient's past. To pull a person out of depression, cognitive therapists usually need 6 to 18 months of weekly sessions that include reasoning and behavioral exercises. *Interpersonal therapy,* which is sometimes combined with cognitive therapy, also addresses the present but focuses on correcting chronic relationship problems. Interpersonal therapists focus on patients' relationships with their families and other people.

Antidepressant drugs relieve symptoms in nearly 80 percent of people with chronic depression. In recent years, Zoloft and Prozac have become such a common part of our vocabulary that it doesn't seem at all unusual to know someone who is taking an antidepressant. Despite how commonplace these medications have become, caution should be taken as with any other prescription medication. Countless emergency room visits occur when people misuse antidepressants, try to quit by going "cold turkey," or suffer reactions to the drugs.

Antidepressants should be prescribed only after a thorough psychological and physiological examination. Recently, the U.S. Federal Drug Administration asked the makers of antidepressant drugs to add a warning to the labels advising that patients taking these drugs should be monitored for "worsening depression or the emergence of suicidality." This warning applies to commonly prescribed drugs such as Prozac, Zoloft, Paxil, Luvox, Celexa, Lexapro, Wellbutrin, Effexor, Serzone, and Remeron.[56]

Other types of the medications known as tricyclics work by preventing excessive absorption of mood-lifting neurotransmitters. Tricyclics can take six weeks to three months to become effective.

Bipolar disorder   Form of depression characterized by alternating mania and depression.

If your doctor suggests an antidepressant, ask these questions first:

- What biological indicators are you using to determine whether I really need this drug? (Beware of the health professional who gives you a five-minute exam, asks you if you are feeling down, and prescribes an antidepressant to fix your problems.)
- What is the action of this drug? What will it do? When will I start to feel the benefits or know it is working?
- What is your rationale for selecting this antidepressant over others?
- What are the side effects of using this drug? What happens if I stop taking it?
- How long can I be on this medication without significant risk to my health?
- How will you follow up or monitor the levels of this drug in my body? How often will I need to be checked?

Clinics have been established in many metropolitan areas to offer group support for depressed people. Some clinics treat all types of depressed people; others restrict themselves to specific groups, such as widows, adolescents, or families and friends of people with depression.

Bipolar Disorder

Also known as manic-depressive illness, **bipolar disorder** is considered another form of depression. It is characterized by alternating emotional highs (mania) and lows (depression). Symptoms can vary from mild to disabling and severe. Bipolar disorder affects more than 2 million adult Americans, about 1 percent of the population. It often begins in adolescence and may persist for life, lasting for weeks or months at a time. In the depression phase, symptoms follow the same pattern as they do in a major depressive syndrome. In the manic phase, symptoms may include feelings of euphoria, extreme optimism, and inflated self-esteem; rapid speech, racing thoughts, agitation, and increased physical activity; poor judgment and recklessness; difficulty sleeping; tendency to be easily distracted; inability to concentrate; and extreme irritability.[57]

Although the exact cause of bipolar disorder is unknown, biological, genetic, and environmental factors seem to be involved in causing episodes of the illness. Evidence indicates that neurotransmitters in people with the disorder differ from those without it. Bipolar disorder tends to run in families, with about 60 percent of cases showing a family history. Thus, a genetic predisposition to have abnormal genes regulating neurotransmitter action may be a risk factor.[58] Factors that are believed to trigger episodes include drug abuse and stressful or psychologically traumatic events. Once diagnosed, persons with bipolar disorder have a number of counseling and pharmaceutical options, and most will be able to live a healthy, functional life while being treated.

Mental Health Problems on Campus: Universities Respond

As students struggle to cope with the escalating pressures of college life, higher education administrators are searching for a way to balance the needs of distressed students with the responsibility of providing a safe learning environment for all. In a recent survey, more than 90 percent of college counseling centers reported seeing increased numbers of students with more serious mental health problems. The increasing incidence of suicide is one major indicator, and schools are jumping to take action to combat the trend. For example, at the Massachusetts Institute of Technology, a series of suicides in the late 1990s and 2000 drove the university to completely overhaul its mental health program. Today, the school offers students therapist support 24-hours-a day, 7-days a week, in addition to seminars and informal gatherings in graduate and professional dorms, awareness training for faculty members, and a web-based suicide prevention program that offers anonymous email counseling.

Other universities have also responded to the dramatic increase in numbers of mental health problems among students. In particular, the option of "student leave" is a growing trend. New York University (NYU), Texas A&M, and Cornell are among the first that have enacted various forms of mandatory 6-month or 1-year "student leave" for those who seem to be at highest risk. In enacting these policies,

colleges and universities are effectively saying that the mental health problems of students are "family" matters—better dealt with in the homes and communities of the student, rather than on campus. Because this is a relatively new policy, statistics on its success and the likelihood of a return to campus by students once their problems are resolved is unknown. Critics argue that such practices are not fair and violate the rights of students to have an education. For students who do not have health insurance, the 6-month to 1-year mandated leave may not be well spent, as access to therapy is a serious challenge.

Student leave and parent intervention are not the only options. Universities are enacting a range of policies, and overburdened counseling centers and student health centers struggle to figure out the best way to help their students cope with psychological problems.

✓ Some institutions, such as the University of Illinois at Urbana-Champaign, mandate counseling for students who are suicidal, requiring a minimum of four therapy sessions following a suicide attempt.

✓ Increasing numbers of institutions offer time management workshops; massage and de-stressing sessions during examinations; and workshops on relationships, coping with loss and grief, and stress management routinely through the academic year.

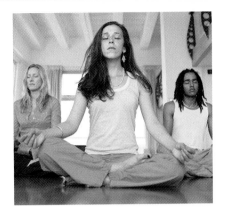

✓ Many institutions have agreements with off-campus counseling centers, fitness centers, and other community-based resources to provide options for students who need help with stress and other problems.

✓ Classes on stress management, coping, relaxation, meditation, yoga, and other mental health strategies are increasingly common on campuses, either as electives or as part of professional curriculum.

✓ Counseling centers with easy access 24-7 are a part of most student health services on campus. Students are encouraged to use them, especially new students who are trying to cope with the challenges of adjusting to life away from home. New-student orientations let students know what kind of help is available on campus.

Source: J. Feirman, "The New College Drop-out," Psychology Today 38, no. 3 (2005): 38–39.

Anxiety Disorders: Facing Your Fears

Anxiety disorders, which are characterized by persistent feelings of threat and anxiousness, are a little-understood yet common psychological problem. Consider John Madden, former head coach of the Oakland Raiders and a true "man's man," who has outfitted his own bus and is driven every weekend across the country to serve as a commentator on NFL football games. What's the reason behind this exhausting schedule? Madden is terrified of getting on a plane.

Anxiety disorders are the number-one mental health problem in the United States. They affect more than 19 million people aged 18 to 54 each year, or about 13 percent of all adults.[59] Some sources place the number as high as 25 percent. Anxiety is also a leading mental health problem among adolescents; it affects

> **Anxiety disorders** Disorders characterized by persistent feelings of threat and anxiousness in coping with everyday problems.

Table 2.2
Drug Treatments for Depression

	SSRI (Selective Serotonin Reuptake Inhibitor)	TCA (Tricyclic Antidepressant)	MAOI (Monoamine Oxidase Inhibitor)
How They Work	An SSRI works by stabilizing levels of serotonin, an important neurotransmitter. Low levels of serotonin have been linked to depression and other mood disorders.	An earlier family of antidepressant drugs, TCAs increase the brain's levels of norepinephrine, a neurotransmitter.	MAOIs increase the levels of epinephrine, norepinephrine, and serotonin in the brain.
Commonly Prescribed Antidepressant Drugs	Zoloft, Prozac, Luvox, Paxil, Paxil CR, Celexa, Lexapro	Adapin, Endep, Norpramin, Pamelor, Sinequan, Effexor	Nardil, Parnate, Remeron
Advantages	Relatively few side effects and no withdrawal symptoms. An SSRI is generally the first choice of most physicians.	Some patients respond better to TCA medication than they do to SSRIs.	May be used if other depression medications fail to treat the condition.
Disadvantages	Can be transferred in breast milk; may cause weight gain, reduced sexual desire. Possible increase in suidical tendencies is under investigation	More side effects than SSRIs. May cause sensitivity to heat, which makes it harder for the body to adapt to temperature changes. Must be discontinued slowly, or withdrawal symptoms may occur.	A strict dietary regime must be followed. Failure to do so can result in hypertensive crisis, which can be fatal. Many other medications react badly with MAOIs.

Source: "Selective Serotonin Reuptake Inhibitors," from Treatment-for-Depression.com. Copyright © NCER, LLC, Oceanside, CA. Reprinted by permission.

13 million youngsters aged 9 to 17. Costs associated with an overly anxious populace are growing rapidly; conservative estimates cite nearly $50 billion a year spent in doctor bills and workplace losses in the United States. According to a study by the World Health Organization, the odds of developing an anxiety disorder have doubled in the past four decades.[60] These numbers don't begin to address the human costs incurred when a person is too fearful to leave the house or talk to anyone outside the immediate family. Anxiety-related ailments include generalized anxiety disorders, panic disorder, specific phobias, and social phobias.

Generalized Anxiety Disorders
Generalized anxiety disorder (GAD) affects over 4 million adults in the United States and is severe enough to significantly interfere with daily life. Generally, the person with this disorder is a consummate worrier who develops a debilitating level of anxiety. Women are more afflicted than men, with nearly twice as many women than men suffering from GAD. Often

multiple sources of worry exist, and it is hard to pinpoint the root cause of the anxiety. A diagnosis of GAD depends on showing at least three of the following symptoms for more days than not during a period of six months:[61]

- Irritability, restlessness, or feeling keyed up or on edge
- Being easily fatigued
- Difficulty concentrating or mind going blank
- Nausea, vomiting
- Muscle tension
- Sleep disturbances (difficulty falling or staying asleep or restless sleep)

Often GAD runs in families and is readily treatable with benzodiazepines such as Librium, Valium, and Xanax, which calm the person for short periods, or antidepressants Zoloft or Paxil. More effective long-term treatments are achieved through individual therapy.

Generalized anxiety disorder (GAD) A constant sense of worry that may cause restlessness, difficulty in concentrating, and tension.

Panic Disorders It can happen at any time: while sleeping, while sitting in traffic, just before you deliver your class presentation. Suddenly and unexpectedly your heart starts to race, your face turns red,

> How do I know if I've had a panic attack?

you can't catch your breath, you feel nauseated, you start to perspire, and you may feel like you are going to pass out.

What you are experiencing could be a **panic attack,** a form of acute anxiety reaction that brings on an intense physical reaction. This reaction may be so severe that you think you are going to have a heart attack and die. Or you may dismiss it as the "jitters" from too much stress. Between 10 and 20 percent of Americans experience panic attacks at some time in their lives. Although it is a highly treatable mental disorder, it is also growing in incidence, particularly among young women. Panic attacks may become debilitating and destructive, particularly if they happen often and lead the person to avoid going out in public or interacting with others.

A panic attack typically starts abruptly, peaks within 10 minutes, lasts about 30 minutes, and leaves the victim tired and drained.[62] In addition to those just described, symptoms can include trembling, dizziness, increased respiration rate, chills, hot flashes, shortness of breath, stomach cramping, chest pain, difficulty swallowing, and a sense of doom or impending death.

Although researchers aren't sure of causation, heredity, stress, and certain biochemical factors may play a role. Your chance of having a panic attack increases if you have a close family member who has them. Some researchers believe that people who have panic attacks are experiencing an over-reactive "fight-or-flight" physical response (see Chapter 3).

As with other forms of anxiety-based disorders, medication and cognitive behavioral therapy are often the keys to treatment. Some individuals are given antidepressants, which often prevent future attacks. In some cases, a medication to relieve anxiety is effective given alone or with other drugs.[63] Cognitive therapy can help sufferers recognize and avoid triggers or deal with triggers through meditation, deep breathing, and other relaxation techniques. Patients usually show improvement within eight to ten sessions.

Specific Phobias
In contrast to panic disorders, **phobias,** or phobic disorders, involve a persistent and irrational fear of a specific object, activity, or situation, which is often out of proportion to the circumstances. Phobias result in a compelling desire to avoid the source of the fear. About 13 percent of Americans suffer from phobias, such as fear of spiders, snakes, and public speaking. Social phobias are perhaps the most common phobic response.[64]

Social Phobias
A **social phobia** is an anxiety disorder characterized by the persistent fear and avoidance of social situations. Essentially, the person dreads these situations for fear of being humiliated, embarrassed, or even looked at.[65] These disorders vary in scope. Some cause difficulty only in specific situations, such as speaking in front of a class. In more extreme cases, a person avoids all contact with others.

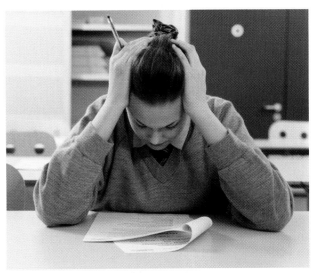

Panic attacks can occur without warning and be precipitated by stressful or uncomfortable situations.

Sources of Anxiety Disorders
Because anxiety disorders vary in complexity and degree, scientists have yet to find clear reasons why one person develops them and another doesn't. The following factors are often cited as possible causes.[66]

- *Biology.* Some scientists trace the origin of anxiety to the brain and brain functioning. Using sophisticated positron emission tomography scans (PET scans), scientists can analyze areas of the brain that react during anxiety-producing events. Families appear to display similar brain and physiological reactivity, so we may inherit our tendencies toward anxiety disorders.

- *Environment.* Anxiety can be a learned response. Though genetic tendencies may exist, experiencing a repeated pattern of reaction to certain situations programs the brain to respond in a certain way. For example, if your mother (or father) screamed whenever a large spider crept into view or if other anxiety-raising events occurred frequently, you might be predisposed to react with anxiety to similar events later in your life. Interestingly, animals also experience such anxieties—perhaps from being around their edgy owners.

- *Social and Cultural Roles.* Cultural and social roles also may be a factor in risks for anxiety. Because men

---

Panic attack Severe anxiety attack in which a particular situation, often for unknown reasons, causes terror.

Phobia A deep and persistent fear of a specific object, activity, or situation that results in a compelling desire to avoid the source of the fear.

Social phobia A phobia characterized by fear and avoidance of social situations.

and women are taught to assume different roles in society (for example, man as protector, woman as victim), women may find it more acceptable to scream, shake, pass out, and otherwise express extreme anxiety. Men, on the other hand, have learned to hide such anxieties rather than act upon them.

Seasonal Affective Disorder

An estimated 6 percent of Americans suffer from **seasonal affective disorder (SAD),** a type of depression, and an additional 14 percent experience a milder form of the disorder known as the *winter blues.* SAD strikes during the winter months and is associated with reduced exposure to sunlight. People with SAD suffer from irritability, apathy, carbohydrate craving and weight gain, increased sleep time, and general sadness. Researchers believe that SAD is caused by a malfunction in the hypothalamus, the gland that regulates responses to external stimuli. Stress also may play a role.

Certain factors seem to put people at risk for SAD. Women are four times more likely to suffer from it than men. Although SAD can occur at any age, people aged 20 to 40 appear to be most vulnerable. Certain families appear to be at risk. Residents of northern states, where there are fewer hours of sunlight during the winter, are more at risk than those living in the South. An estimated 10 percent of the population in Maine, Minnesota, and Wisconsin experience SAD, compared to fewer than 2 percent of those in Florida and New Mexico.

Therapies for SAD are simple but effective. The most beneficial is light therapy, in which patients are exposed to lamps that simulate sunlight. Eighty percent of patients experience relief from their symptoms within four days of treatment. Other treatments for SAD include diet change (eating more complex carbohydrates), increased exercise, stress management techniques, sleep restriction (limiting the number of hours slept in a 24-hour period), psychotherapy, and antidepressants.

Schizophrenia

Perhaps the most frightening of all mental disorders is **schizophrenia,** which affects about 1 percent of the U.S. population. Schizophrenia is characterized by alterations of the senses (including auditory and visual hallucinations); the inability to sort out incoming stimuli and make appropriate responses; an altered sense of self; and radical changes in emotions, movements, and behaviors. Victims of this disease often cannot function in society. Contrary to common misconception, schizophrenia is not the same as split personality, or multiple personality disorder.

For decades, scientists believed that schizophrenia was an environmentally provoked form of madness. They blamed abnormal family interactions or early childhood traumas. Since the mid-1980s, however, when magnetic resonance imaging (MRI) and positron emission tomography (PET) allowed us to study brain function more closely, scientists have recognized that schizophrenia is a biological disease of the brain. The brain damage occurs early in life, possibly as early as the second trimester of fetal development. However, symptoms most commonly appear in late adolescence.

At present, schizophrenia is treatable but not curable. Treatments usually include some combination of hospitalization, medication, and supportive psychotherapy. Supportive psychotherapy, as opposed to more intensive psychoanalysis, can help the patient acquire skills for living in society.

Even though environmental theories on the causes of schizophrenia have been discarded in favor of biological theories, a stigma remains attached to the disease. Families of people with schizophrenia frequently experience anger and guilt. They often need information, family counseling, and advice on how to meet the schizophrenic person's needs for shelter, medical care, vocational training, and social interaction.

Gender Issues in Psychosocial Health

Unfortunately, gender bias can hinder the correct diagnosis of psychosocial disorders. In one study, 175 mental health professionals of both genders were asked to diagnose a patient based upon a summarized case history. Some of the professionals were told that the patient was male, others that the patient was female. The gender of the patient made a substantial difference in the diagnosis (though the gender of the clinician did not). When subjects thought the patient was female, they were more likely to diagnose hysterical personality, which is often thought of as a women's disorder. When they believed the patient to be male, the more likely diagnosis was antisocial personality, often thought of as a male disorder.

PMS: Physical or Mental Disorder? A major controversy is the inclusion of a provisional diagnosis for premenstrual syndrome (PMS) in the American Psychiatric Association's *Diagnostic and Statistical Manual of Mental Disorders* (now in its fourth edition, known as *DSM-IV*). The provisional diagnosis, in an

---

Seasonal affective disorder (SAD)   A type of depression that occurs in the winter months, when sunlight levels are low.

Schizophrenia   A mental illness with biological origins that is characterized by irrational behavior, severe alterations of the senses (hallucinations), and often an inability to function in society.

appendix to *DSM-IV*, indicates that PMS merits further study and may be included as an approved diagnosis in future editions of the *DSM*. In other words, PMS could be considered a mental disorder in the future.

PMS is characterized by depression, irritability, and other symptoms of increased stress typically occurring just prior to menstruation and lasting for a day or two. A more severe case of PMS is known as premenstrual dysphoric disorder (PMDD). Whereas PMS is somewhat disruptive and uncomfortable, it does not interfere with daily function; PMDD does. To be diagnosed with PMDD, a woman must have at least five symptoms of PMS for a week to ten days, with at least one symptom being serious enough to interfere with her ability to function at work or at home. In these more severe cases, antidepressants may be prescribed. The point of contention lies in whether administering this treatment indicates that PMDD is a mental disorder rather than a physical problem.[67] Is it legitimate to attach a label indicating dysfunction and disorder to symptoms experienced only once or twice a month? Further controversy stems from the possible use (or misuse) of the diagnostic label to justify exclusion of women from certain desirable jobs.

SUICIDE: GIVING UP ON LIFE

Each year there are over 35,000 reported suicides in the United States. Experts estimate that there may actually be closer to 100,000 cases, due to the difficulty in determining the causes of many suspicious deaths. More lives are lost to suicide than to any other single cause except cancer and cardiovascular disease. Suicide often results from poor coping skills, lack of social support, lack of self-esteem, and the inability to see one's way out of a bad situation.

College students are more likely than the general population to attempt suicide; suicide is the third leading cause of death in people between the ages of 15 and 24. In fact, this age group now accounts for nearly 20 percent of all suicides.[68] The pressures, joys, disappointments, challenges, and changes of the college environment are believed to be partially responsible. However, young adults who choose not to go to college but who are searching for direction in careers, relationships, and other life goals are also at risk.

Risk factors for suicide include a family history of suicide, previous suicide attempts, excessive drug and alcohol use, prolonged depression, financial difficulties, serious illness in the suicide contemplator or in his or her loved ones, and loss of a loved one through death or rejection. Societal pressures often serve as a catalyst.

In most cases, suicide does not occur unpredictably. In fact, 75 to 80 percent of people who commit suicide give a warning of their intentions.

Warning Signs of Suicide

Common signs of possible suicide include:[69]

- Recent loss and a seeming inability to let go of grief
- Change in personality, such as sadness, withdrawal, irritability, anxiety, tiredness, indecisiveness, apathy
- Change in behavior, such as inability to concentrate, loss of interest in classes, or a sudden, unexplained demonstration of happiness following a period of depression
- Diminished sexual interest, such as impotence, menstrual abnormalities
- Expressions of self-hatred and excessive risk taking or an "I don't care what happens to me" attitude
- Change in sleep patterns
- Change in eating habits
- A direct statement about committing suicide, such as, "I might as well end it all."
- An indirect statement, such as, "You won't have to worry about me anymore."
- Final preparations, such as writing a will, repairing poor relationships with family or friends, giving away prized possessions, or writing revealing letters
- A preoccupation with themes of death
- Marked changes in personal appearance

What Do You Think?
■ If your roommate showed warning signs of suicide, what action would you take? ■ Who would you contact first? ■ Where on campus might your friend get help? ■ What if someone in class whom you hardly know gave warning signs of suicide? ■ What would you do then?

Taking Action to Prevent Suicide

Most people who attempt suicide really want to live but see suicide as the only way out of an intolerable situation. Crisis counselors and suicide hotlines may help temporarily, but the best way to prevent suicide is to get rid of conditions and substances that may precipitate attempts, including alcoholism, drugs, loneliness, isolation, and access to guns.

If someone you know threatens or displays warning signs of suicide, take the following actions.

- *Monitor the warning signals.* Keep an eye on the person, or ensure there is someone around the person as much as possible.
- *Take threats seriously.* Don't brush them off.

- *Let the person know how much you care about him or her.* State that you are there if he or she needs help.
- *Listen.* Try not to discredit or be shocked by what the person says. Empathize, sympathize, and keep the person talking. Talk about stressors, and listen to the responses.
- *Ask directly, "Are you thinking of hurting or killing yourself?"*
- *Do not belittle the person's feelings or say that he or she doesn't really mean it or couldn't succeed at suicide.* To some people, these comments offer the challenge of proving you wrong.
- *Help the person think about alternatives.* Offer to go for help together. Call your local suicide hotline and use all available community and campus resources. Recommend a counselor or other person to talk to.
- *Remember that your relationships with others involve responsibilities.* Give of yourself by staying with the person, taking the person to a health care facility, or providing support.
- *Tell your friend's spouse, partner, relatives, or counselor.* Do not keep your suspicions to yourself.

Don't let a suicidal friend talk you into keeping your discussions confidential. If your friend succeeds in a suicide attempt because you kept a promise not to tell others of the danger, you may find that others will question your decision, just as you may blame yourself.

SEEKING PROFESSIONAL HELP

A physical ailment will readily send most of us to the nearest health professional, but many people view seeking professional help for psychosocial problems as an admission of personal failure. However, increasing numbers of Americans are turning to mental health professionals, and nearly one in five seeks such help. Researchers cite breakdown in support systems, high societal expectations of the individual, and dysfunctional families as three major reasons why more people are asking for assistance than ever before.

Consider seeking help if:

- You feel like you need help.
- You experience wild mood swings or inappropriate emotional responses.
- A problem is interfering with your daily life.
- Your fears or feelings of guilt frequently distract your attention.

> **Psychiatrist** A licensed physician who specializes in treating mental and emotional disorders.

- You begin to withdraw from others.
- You feel inadequate, worthless, or that life is not worth living.
- Your daily life seems to be nothing but repeated crises.
- You feel you can't "get your act together."
- You are considering suicide.
- You turn to drugs or alcohol to escape from your problems.
- You feel out of control.

Getting Evaluated for Treatment

If you are considering treatment for a psychosocial problem, schedule a complete evaluation first. Consult a credentialed health professional for a thorough examination, which should include three parts.

- A physical checkup, which will rule out thyroid disorders, viral infections, and anemia—all of which can result in depressive-like symptoms—and a neurological check of coordination, reflexes, and balance to rule out brain disorders
- A psychiatric history, which will attempt to trace the course of the apparent disorder, genetic or family factors, and any past treatments
- A mental status examination, which will assess thoughts, speaking processes, and memory, and will include an in-depth interview with tests for other psychiatric symptoms[70]

Once physical factors have been ruled out, you may decide to consult a professional who specializes in psychosocial health.

Mental Health Professionals

How can I choose the right therapist for me?

Several types of mental health professionals are available to help you. The most important criterion is not how many degrees this person has, but whether you feel you can work together. Table 2.3 presents fundamental criteria to help you choose the best therapist for your needs.

Psychiatrist A **psychiatrist** is a medical doctor. After obtaining a medical doctor (MD) degree, a psychiatrist spends up to 12 years studying psychosocial health and disease. As a licensed MD, a psychiatrist can prescribe medications for various mental or emotional problems and may have admitting privileges at a local hospital. Some psychiatrists are affiliated with hospitals, while others are in private practice.

Psychologist A **psychologist** usually has a doctor of philosophy (PhD) degree in counseling or clinical psychology. Many states also require licensure. Psychologists are trained in various types of therapy, including behavior and insight therapy. Most can conduct both individual and group counseling sessions. Psychologists may be trained in certain specialties, such as family counseling or sexual counseling.

Psychoanalyst A **psychoanalyst** is a psychiatrist or psychologist with special training in psychoanalysis. This is a type of therapy that helps patients remember early traumas that have blocked personal growth. Facing these traumas helps them resolve conflicts and lead more productive lives.

Clinical/Psychiatric Social Worker A **social worker** has at least a master's degree in social work (MSW) and two years of experience in a clinical setting. Many states require an examination for accreditation. Some social workers work in clinical settings, whereas others have private practices.

Counselor A **counselor** often has a master's degree in counseling, psychology, educational psychology, or related human service. Professional societies recommend at least two years of graduate course work or supervised practice as a minimal requirement. Many counselors are trained to do individual and group therapy. They often specialize in one type of counseling, such as family, marital, relationship, children, drug, divorce, behavioral, or personal counseling.

Psychiatric Nurse Specialist Although all registered nurses can work in psychiatric settings, some continue their education and specialize in psychiatric practice. A **psychiatric nurse specialist** can be certified by the American Nursing Association in adult, child, or adolescent psychiatric nursing.

What to Expect in Therapy

Many different types of counseling exist, ranging from individual therapy, which involves one-on-one work between therapist and client, to group therapy, in which two or more clients meet with a therapist to discuss problems. The first trip to a therapist can be difficult. Most of us have misconceptions about what therapy is and what it can do. That first visit is a verbal and mental sizing up between you and the therapist. You may not accomplish much in that first hour. If you decide that this professional is not for you, you will at least have learned how to present your problem and what qualities you need in a therapist.

Before meeting, briefly explain your needs. Ask what the fee is. Arrive on time, wear comfortable clothing, and expect to spend about an hour during your first

---

Table 2.3

Questions to Ask When Choosing a Therapist

A qualified mental health professional should be willing to answer all your questions during an initial consultation. Questions to ask include the following.

- Can you interview the therapist before starting treatment? An initial meeting will help you determine whether this person will be a good fit for you.
- Do you like the therapist as a person? Can you talk to him or her comfortably?
- Is the therapist watching the clock or easily distracted? *You* should be the main focus of the session.
- Does the therapist demonstrate professionalism? Be concerned if your therapist is frequently late or breaks appointments, suggests social interactions outside your therapy sessions, talks inappropriately about himself or herself, has questionable billing practices, or resists releasing you from therapy.
- Will the therapist help you set your own goals? A good professional should evaluate your general situation and help you set small goals to work on between sessions. The therapist should not tell you how to help yourself but help you discover the steps.

Remember, in most states, the use of the title *therapist* or *counselor* is unregulated. Make your choice carefully.

---

visit. The therapist will want to take down your history and details about the problems that have brought you to therapy. Answer as honestly as possible. Many will ask how you feel about aspects of your life. Do not be embarrassed to acknowledge your feelings. It is critical to the success of your treatment that you trust this person enough to be open and honest.

Do not expect the therapist to tell you what to do or how to behave. The responsibility for improved behavior lies with you. Ask if you can set your own therapeutic goals and timetables.

If after your first visit (or even after several visits) you feel you cannot work with this person, say so. You have the right to find a therapist with whom you feel comfortable.

Psychologist A person with a PhD degree and training in psychology.

Psychoanalyst A psychiatrist or psychologist with special training in psychoanalysis.

Social worker A person with an MSW degree and clinical training.

Counselor A person with a variety of academic and experiential training who deals with the treatment of emotional problems.

Psychiatric nurse specialist A registered nurse specializing in psychiatric practice.

Taking Charge

Summary

- Psychosocial health is a complex phenomenon involving mental, emotional, social, and spiritual health.

- Many factors influence psychosocial health, including life experiences, family, the environment, other people, self-esteem, self-efficacy, and personality. Some of these are modifiable; others are not.

- Developing self-esteem and self-efficacy and getting enough sleep are key to enhancing psychosocial health.

- Many people believe spirituality is important to wellness. Though the exact reasons have not been established, many studies show a connection between the two.

- Happiness is a key factor in determining overall reaction to life's challenges. The mind–body connection is an important link in overall health and well-being.

- Indicators of deteriorating psychosocial health include depression. Identifying depression is the first step in treating this disorder.

- Other common psychosocial problems include bipolar disorder, anxiety disorders, panic disorders, phobias, seasonal affective disorder, and schizophrenia.

- Suicide is a result of negative psychosocial reactions to life. People intending to commit suicide often give warning signs of their intentions. Such people often can be helped.

- Mental health professionals include psychiatrists, psychoanalysts, psychologists, clinical/psychiatric social workers, counselors, and psychiatric nurse specialists. Many therapy methods exist, including group and individual therapy. It is wise to interview a therapist carefully before beginning treatment.

Chapter Review

1. The practice of mindfulness is a theme of
   a. social health.
   b. mental health.
   c. emotional health.
   d. spiritual health.

2. Marty flunked a math class twice and does not believe that he is good at math. He has resigned himself to not being able to graduate because he will never pass a required math class. This is known as
   a. external locus of control.
   b. learned helplessness.
   c. post-traumatic stress disorder.
   d. exogenous depression.

3. All of the following traits have been identified as characterizing psychosocially healthy people *except*
   a. conscientiousness.
   b. introversion.
   c. openness to experience.
   d. agreeableness.

4. What hormone is linked to circadian rhythms?
   a. dopamine
   b. serotonin
   c. GABA
   d. melatonin

5. Subjective well-being has all of the following components *except*
   a. psychological hardiness.
   b. satisfaction with present life.
   c. relative presence of positive emotions.
   d. relative absence of negative emotions.

6. Zoloft and Prozac, commonly prescribed drug treatments for depression, are classified as
   a. tricyclic antidepressants (TCAs).
   b. monoamine oxidase inhibitors (MAOIs).
   c. selective serotonin reuptake inhibitors (SSRIs).
   d. electroconvulsive therapy (ECT).

7. What are the two most common psychotherapeutic therapies for depression?
   a. humanistic therapy and gestalt therapy
   b. cognitive therapy and interpersonal therapy
   c. psychodynamic therapy and family therapy
   d. cognitive therapy and psychodynamic therapy

8. What is the number-one mental health problem in the United States?
   a. depression
   b. anxiety disorders
   c. alcohol dependence
   d. schizophrenia

9. Every winter, Stan suffers from irritability, apathy, carbohydrate craving, weight gain, increased sleep time, and sadness. He most likely has
   a. panic disorder.
   b. generalized anxiety disorder.
   c. seasonal affective disorder.
   d. chronic mood disorder.

10. A person with a PhD in counseling psychology and training in various types of therapy is a
   a. psychiatrist.
   b. psychologist.
   c. social worker.
   d. psychoanalyst.

Answers to these questions can be found on page A-1.

Questions for Discussion and Reflection

1. What is psychosocial health? What indicates that you are or aren't psychosocially healthy? Why might the college environment provide a challenge to your psychosocial health?

2. Discuss the factors that influence your overall level of psychosocial health. Which factors can you change? Which ones may be more difficult to change?

3. What steps could you take today to improve your psychosocial health? Which steps require long-term effort?

4. What are four main themes of spirituality, and how are they expressed in daily life?

5. Why is laughter therapeutic? How can humor help you better achieve wellness?

6. What factors appear to contribute to psychosocial difficulties and illnesses? Which of the common psychosocial illnesses is likely to affect people in your age group?

7. What are the warning signs of suicide? Of depression? Why is depression so pervasive among young Americans today? Why are some groups more vulnerable to suicide and depression than are others? What would you do if you heard a friend in the cafeteria say to no one in particular that he was going to "do the world a favor and end it all"?

8. Discuss the different types of health professionals and therapies. If you felt depressed about breaking off a long-term relationship, which professional and therapy do you think would be most beneficial? Explain your answer. What services does your student health center provide? What fees are charged to students?

9. What psychosocial areas do you need to work on? Which are most important to you, and why? What actions can you take today?

Accessing Your Health on the Internet

The following websites explore further topics and issues related to personal health. For links to the websites below, visit the Companion Website for *Health: The Basics,* Seventh Edition at www.aw-bc.com/donatelle.

1. *American Psychological Association Help Center.* Includes information on psychology at work, the mind–body connection, psychological responses to war, and other topics.

2. *Anxiety Disorders Association of America.* Offers links to treatment resources, self-help tools, information on clinical trials, and other information.

3. *National Alliance for the Mentally Ill.* A support and advocacy organization of families and friends of people with severe mental illnesses. More than 1,200 state and local affiliates; local branches often can help with finding treatment.

4. *National Institute of Mental Health (NIMH).* Overview of mental health information and new research relating to mental health.

5. *National Mental Health Association.* Works to promote mental health through advocacy, education, research, and services.

Further Reading

Dalai Lama and H. C. Cutler. *The Art of Happiness: A Handbook for Living.* New York: Riverhead, 1998.

Through a series of interviews, the authors explore questions of meaning, motives, and the interconnectedness of life, including why so many people are unhappy, and offer strategies for becoming happy.

Norem, J. *The Positive Power of Negative Thinking.* New York: Basics Books, 2002.

Explores reasons for negative thinking and mechanisms for changing the way you think. Includes self-tests and analysis for helping you retrain your thinking processes.

References

1. H. Marano, "A Nation of Wimps," *Psychology Today* 37, no. 6 (2004): 58–68.
2. S. Benton et al., "Changes in Counseling Center Problems across 13 Years," *Professional Psychology: Research and Practice* 34, no. 1 (2003): 65–69.
3. Marano, "A Nation of Wimps."
4. National Institute of Mental Health, 2005, www.nimh.gov.
5. R. Lazarus, *Stress and Emotion: A New Synthesis* (New York: Springer Publishing Company, 1999).
6. A. F. Jorm, "Social Networks and Health: It's Time for an Intervention Trial," *Journal of Epidemiology and Community Health* 59 (2005): 537–539; C. Huang, "Elderly Social Support System and Health Status in the Urban and Rural Areas" (Paper presented at the American Public Health Association Annual Meeting, New Orleans, LA, 2005); C. Alarie, *The Impact of Social Support on Women's Health: A Literature Review,* Women's Center of Excellence, www.pwhce.ca/limpactDuSupport.htm.
7. C. Westlake and K. Dracup, "Role of Spirituality in Adjustment of Patients with Advanced Heart Failure," *Progressive Cardiovascular Nursing* 16, no. 3 (2001): 119–125.
8. J. A. Astin et al., "Mind-Body Medicine: State of the Science, Implications for Practice," *Journal of the American Board of Family Practice* 16 (2003): 131–147; J. Bishop et al., "Mindfulness: A Proposed Operational Definition," *Clinical Psychology* 11 (2004): 230–241.
9. Ibid., Bishop.
10. Ibid.
11. Ibid.
12. A. Astin et al., "Spirituality in Higher Education: A National Study of College Students' Search for Meaning and Purpose," 2004, www.spirituality.ucla.edu.
13. Z. Segal et al., *Mindfulness-Based Cognitive Therapy for Depression: A New Approach to Preventing Relapse* (New York: Guilford Publications, 2001); M. Weiss, J. W. Nordlie, and E. P. Siegel, "Mindfulness-based Stress Reduction as an Adjunct to Outpatient Psychotherapy," *Psychotherapy and Psychosomatics* 74, no. 2 (2005): 108–112; J. Cohen-Katz et al., "The Effects of Mindfulness-Based Stress Reduction on Nurse Stress and Burnout, Part II:

A Quantitative and Qualitative Study," *Holistic Nurse Practice* 1, (2005): 26–35; A. Tacon et al., "Mindfulness Meditation, Anxiety Reduction, and Heart Disease: A Pilot Study," *Family and Community Health* 26, 1 (2003): 25–33.

14. D. Elkins, *Beyond Religion—A Personal Program for Building a Spiritual Life Outside the Walls of Traditional Religion* (Wheaton, IL: Quest Books, 1998).

15. Ibid.

16. D. Elkins, "Spirituality: It's What's Missing in Mental Health," *Psychology Today* 32, no. 5 (1999): 48.

17. P. McGuire, "Seligman Touts the Art of Arguing with Yourself," *The APA Monitor Online* 29, no. 10 (October 1998).

18. M. Seligman, *Learned Optimism* (New York: Knopf, 1990).

19. S. Proffit, "Pursuing Happiness with a Positive Outlook, Not a Pill," *Los Angeles Times,* January 24, 1999, www.apa.org/releases/pursuing.html; APA HelpCenter: Mind/Body Connection, "Learned Optimism Yields Health Benefits," 1996, http://helping.apa.org.

20. P. Zimbardo, A. Weber, and R. Johnson, *Psychology* (Boston: Allyn and Bacon, 2000), 403.

21. G. Wilson et al., *Abnormal Psychology* (Boston: Allyn and Bacon, 1996), 137.

22. D. Brown and C. Blanton, "Physical Activity, Sports Participation, and Suicidal Behavior Among College Students," *Medicine & Science in Sports & Exercise* 34, no. 7 (2002): 1087–1096.

23. National Institutes of Health, "National Center on Sleep Disorders Research," 2004, www.nhlbi.nih.gov/about/ncsdr/index.htm.

24. Ibid.

25. M. Lemonick, "The Biology of Joy," *Time Magazine* 165, no. 3 (2005): A12–A14.

26. J. Kluger, "The Funny Thing about Laughter," *Time Magazine* 165, no. 3 (2005): A25–A29.

27. Ibid.

28. R. Davidson et al., "The Privileged Status of Emotion in the Brain," Proceedings of the National Academy of Sciences of the United States of America 101, no. 33, 2004.

29. E. Diener and M. E. P. Seligman, "Beyond Money: Toward an Economy of Well-Being," *Psychological Science in the Public Interest* 5 (2004): 1–31; C. Peterson and M. Seligman, *Character Strengths and Virtues* (London: Oxford University Press, 2004).

30. B. Fredrickson, "Cultivating Positive Emotions to Optimize Health and Well-Being," *Prevention and Treatment* 3 (March 7, 2000), Article 0001a.

31. Grady, "Think Right, Stay Well," *American Health* 11 (1992): 50–54.

32. L. Cool, "Is Mental Illness Catching?" *American Health for Women* 16 (1997).

33. MayoClinic.com, "Mental Health Definitions," 2003, www.mayoclinic.com.

34. R. Kessler et al., "Mental Illness Exacts Heavy Toll," *Archives of General Psychiatry* 62, no. 6: 593–602.

35. World Health Organization, "GBD 2001 Estimates by Region," www.who.int/en; Burden of Disease Unit, *The Global Burden of Disease: A Comprehensive Assessment of Mortality and Disability from Diseases, Injuries, and Risk Factors in 1990 and Projected to 2020* (Cambridge, MA: Harvard University Press, 1996).

36. MayoClinic.com, "Lifting the Curtain on Mental Illness: Growing Awareness of a Common Problem," April 19, 2001, www.mayoclinic.com.

37. L. A. Lefton, *Psychology,* 8th ed. (Boston: Allyn and Bacon, 2002), 542.

38. M. Sullivan, "Widespread Effects of Depression," *NIH Word on Health* newsletter, April 2003, www.nih.gov/news/WordonHealth/apr2003/depression.htm.

39. R. Hirshchfeld et al., "The National Depressive and Manic Depression Association Consensus Statement on the Undertreatment of Depression," *Journal of the American Medical Association* 277, no. 4 (1997): 333–340.

40. Ibid.

41. Ibid.

42. Adapted by permission of the author from K. R. Gertz, "Mood Probe: Pinpointing the Crucial Differences between Emotional Lows and the Gridlock of Depression," *Self* (November 1990): 165–168.

43. S. Scott, "Biology and Mental Health: Why Do Women Suffer More Depression and Anxiety?" *Maclean's,* January 12, 1998, 62–64.

44. National Institute of Mental Health, "Real Men. Real Depression," 2003, 6. www.menanddepression.nimh.nih.gov/.

45. Ibid.

46. A. K. Ferketick et al., "Depression as an Antecedent to Heart Disease among Women and Men in the NHANES I Study. National Health and Nutrition Examination Survey," *Archives of Internal Medicine* 160, no. 9 (2002): 1261–1268.

47. I. Levav et al., "Vulnerability of Jews to Affective Disorders," *American Journal of Psychiatry* 154 (1997): 941–947.

48. S. Wood and E. Wood, *The World of Psychology* (Boston: Allyn & Bacon, 1999), 513.

49. S. Banks and R. Kerns, "Explaining High Rates of Depression in Chronic Pain: A Diathesis–Stress Framework," *Psychological Bulletin* 119 (1996): 995–110.

50. Ibid.

51. Adapted by permission of the author from K. R. Gertz, "Mood Probe," 165–168, 204.

52. S. Banks and R. Kerns, "Explaining High Rates of Depression; National Institute of Mental Health (NIH Publication No. 00-4779), "Depression: What Every Woman Should Know" 2000, www.nimh.nih.gov/publicat/depwomenknows.cfm#ptdep4.

53. B. Jonas and A. Looker, "More College Students Seeking Mental Health Services," *Mental Health Weekly* 14, no. 13 (2004): 7.

54. R. Voelker, "Stress, Sleep Loss and Substance Abuse Create Potent Recipe for College Depression," *Journal of the American Medical Association* 291, no. 18 (2004): 2172–2174.

55. S. Benton et al., "Changes in Counseling Center Client Problems."

56. U.S. Food and Drug Administration (FDA), "FDA Issues Public Health Advisory on Cautions for Use of Antidepressants in Adults and Children" (FDA Talk Paper, T04–08), March 22, 2004, www.fda.gov/bbs/topics/ANSWERS/2004/ANS01283.html; Center for Drug Evaluation and Research, "Antidepressant Use in Children, Adolescents, and Young Adults," March 22, 2004, www.fda.gov/cder/drug/antidepressants/default.htm.

57. MayoClinic.com, "Bipolar Disorder," 2005, www.mayoclinic.com.

58. Ibid.

59. National Institute of Mental Health, "The Numbers Count: Mental Disorders, 2005, www.nimh.nih.gov.

60. M. Z. Lerner, "Anxiety Disorders," *USA Weekend,* October 12, 2000, 12.

61. National Institute of Mental Health, "Generalized Anxiety Disorder, GAD," February, 2005, www.nimh.nih.gov/healthinformation/gadmenu.cfm.

62. Ibid.

63. Ibid.

64. Ibid.

65. Ibid.

66. Ibid.

67. R. Saltus, "The PMS Debate," *Boston Globe Magazine,* July 25, 1999, 8–9.

68. National Institute of Mental Health, "Depression" (NIMH Publication No. 00-3561), 2000, www.nimh.nih.gov/publicat/depression.cfm.

69. K. Kendler and C. Gardner, "Boundaries of Major Depression: An Evaluation of DSM-IV Criteria," *The American Journal of Psychiatry* 155 (1998): 172–176.

70. Lefton, *Psychology,* 542.

Why do I feel so "pumped up" when I am in a stressful situation?

How can I cope more effectively with daily pressures?

Why do I always catch a cold during finals week?

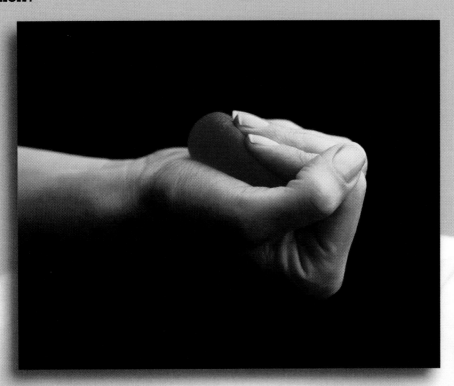

How can I prioritize everything I try to do in a day?

3

Managing Stress
Coping with Life's Challenges

Objectives

- **Define** stress, and examine the potential impact of stress on the dimensions of health.
- **Describe** the phases of the general adaptation syndrome and the physiological changes that occur.
- **Examine** the health risks that may occur with chronic stress.
- **Discuss** sources of stress, and examine ways in which you might reduce risks from these stressors or inoculate yourself against stressful situations.
- **Examine** the special stressors that affect college students and strategies for reducing risk.
- **Discuss** techniques for coping with or reducing exposure to stress and using positive stressors to enrich life experiences.

Rising tuition, too much noise, no privacy, long lines at the bookstore, pressure to get good grades, never enough money, worries over war and terrorism. STRESS! You can't run from it, you can't hide from it, and it invades your waking and sleeping hours. Exposure to stressful situations is among the most common of life experiences, ranging from unexpected calamities to routine daily exposures.

Often, stress is insidious, and we don't even notice the things that affect us. As we sleep, it encroaches on our psyche through noise or incessant worries over things that need to be done. While we work at the computer, stress may interfere in the form of a headache, strain on our eyes, and tension in our backs. The precise toll stress exacts from us during a lifetime is unknown, but it is much more than an annoyance. Rather, it is a significant health hazard that can rob the body of needed nutrients, damage the cardiovascular system, raise blood pressure, and weaken the immune system, leaving us vulnerable to infections and disease. It can drain our emotional reserves, contribute to depression, anxiety, and irritability, and punctuate social interactions with hostility and anger.

Stress is a major concern in the United States, and it appears to be getting worse: according to a national survey conducted annually by the Higher Education Research Institute, almost a third of college freshman report feeling "frequently overwhelmed by all they have to do," up from a low of 16 percent when the question was first asked in 1985.[1] Although much has been written about stress, we are only beginning to understand the multifaceted nature of the stress response and its tremendous potential for harm or benefit.

WHAT IS STRESS?

Often, we think of stress as an externally imposed factor. For most of us, stress results from an *internal* state of emotional tension that occurs in response to the vari-

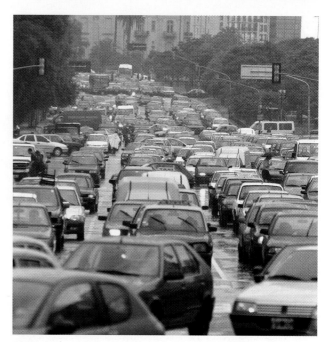

Traffic jams are a modern stressor and an example of the daily strains that can add up and jeopardize our health.

ous demands of living. Most current definitions state that **stress** is the mental and physical response of our bodies to the changes and challenges in our lives. Inherent in these definitions is the idea that we sometimes take ourselves too seriously: that we should loosen up, worry less, and gain greater control over our minds as well as our bodies.

A **stressor** is any physical, social, or psychological event or condition that causes the body to adjust to a specific situation. Several factors influence your response to stressors, including characteristics of the stressor (can you control it? is it predictable? does it occur often?), biological factors (i.e., your age or gender), and past experiences.[2] Stressors may be tangible, such as getting in a car accident, or intangible, such as the mixed emotions associated with meeting your significant other's parents for the first time. **Adjustment** is the attempt to cope with a given situation. **Strain** is the wear and tear the body and mind sustain in adjusting to or resisting a stressor.

Stress and strain are associated with most daily activities. Generally, positive stress, or stress that presents the opportunity for personal growth and satisfaction, is called **eustress.** Getting married, starting school, beginning a career, developing new friendships, and learning a new physical skill all give rise to eustress. **Distress,** or negative stress, is caused by events that result in debilitative stress and strain including financial problems, the death of a loved one, academic difficulties, and the breakup of a relationship. Distress can have a negative effect on health.

We cannot get rid of distress entirely: like eustress, it is a part of life. However, we can train ourselves to

---

Stress   Mental and physical response of our bodies to the changes and challenges of our lives.

Stressor   A physical, social, or psychological event or condition that causes the body to adjust to a specific situation.

Adjustment   The attempt to cope with a given situation.

Strain   The wear and tear the body and mind sustain in adjusting to or resisting a stressor.

Eustress   Positive stress that presents opportunities for personal growth.

Distress   Negative stress that can have a detrimental effect on health.

recognize the events that cause distress and to anticipate our reactions to them. We can learn coping skills and strategies that will help us manage stress more effectively.

THE BODY'S RESPONSE TO STRESS

The Fight-or-Flight Response

Whenever we're surprised by a sudden stressor, such as someone swerving into our lane of traffic, our emotional reactions trigger the adrenal glands (two almond-sized glands sitting atop the kidneys) to secrete adrenaline and other hormones into the bloodstream. As a result, the heart speeds up, breathing rate increases, blood pressure elevates, and the flow of blood to the muscles increases with a rapid release of blood sugars into the bloodstream. This sudden burst of energy and strength is believed to provide the extra edge that has helped generations of humans survive during adversity. Known as the **fight-or-flight response,** this physiological reaction is one of our most basic, innate survival instincts.[3] When activated, our bodies go on the alert to either fight danger or escape from it. The series of behavioral, neurological, and immunological changes that occur are designed to help us; however, if overtaxed, the response can be damaging to our bodies.

The General Adaptation Syndrome

What has just been described in very general terms is a complex physiological response to stress in which our bodies move from **homeostasis,** a level of functioning in which the body's systems operate smoothly and maintain equilibrium, to one of crisis as the body attempts to return to homeostasis, after responding to a stressor. This adjustment is referred to as an **adaptive response.** First characterized by Hans Selye in 1936, this internal fight to restore homeostasis is known as the **general adaptation syndrome (GAS)** (Figure 3.1). The GAS has three distinct phases: alarm, resistance, and exhaustion.[4]

Alarm Phase When the body is exposed to a real or perceived stressor, the fight-or-flight response kicks into gear. Stress hormones flow into the body, and it prepares to do battle. The subconscious perceptions and appraisal of the stressor stimulate the areas in the brain responsible for emotions. This emotional stimulation triggers the physical reactions we associate with stress (Figure 3.2 on page 62). The entire process takes only a few seconds.

Suppose that you are walking to your dormitory after a night class on a dimly lit campus. As you pass a

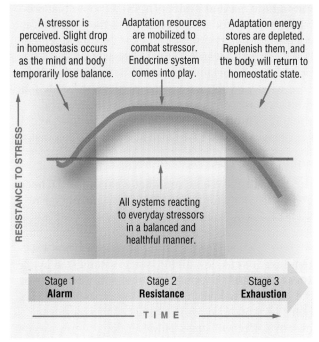

Figure 3.1 ■ The General Adaptation Syndrome

particularly dark area, you hear someone cough behind you and sense that this person is fairly close. You walk faster, only to hear the quickened footsteps of the other person. Your senses become increasingly alert, your breathing quickens, your heart races, and you begin to perspire. The stranger is getting closer and closer. In desperation you stop, clutching your book bag in your hands, determined to use force if necessary to protect yourself. You turn around quickly and let out a blood-curdling yell. To your surprise, the only person you see is your classmate Cindy, who has been trying to stay close to you out of her own anxiety about walking alone in the dark. She screams and jumps back, only to trip and fall. You look at her in startled embarrassment. You both have just experienced the alarm phase of GAS.

When the mind perceives a real or imaginary stressor, the cerebral cortex, the region of the brain that interprets the nature of an event, is called to attention. If the cerebral cortex perceives a threat, it triggers an

---

Fight-or-flight response Physiological reaction in which the body prepares to combat or escape a real or perceived threat.

Homeostasis A balanced physical state in which all the body's systems function smoothly.

Adaptive response Form of adjustment in which the body attempts to restore homeostasis.

General adaptation syndrome (GAS) The pattern followed in the physiological response to stress, consisting of the alarm, resistance, and exhaustion phases.

autonomic nervous system (ANS) response that prepares the body for action. The ANS is the portion of the central nervous system that regulates bodily functions that we do not normally consciously control, such as heart function, breathing, and glandular function. When we are stressed, the activity rate of all these bodily functions increases dramatically to give us the physical strength to protect ourselves or to make the physiological changes needed to respond and mobilize internal forces.

The ANS has two branches: sympathetic and parasympathetic. The **sympathetic nervous system** energizes the body for fight or flight by signaling the release of several stress hormones that speed the heart rate, increase the breathing rate, and trigger many other stress responses. The **parasympathetic nervous system** functions to slow all the systems stimulated by the stress response—in effect, it counteracts the actions of the sympathetic branch. In a healthy person, these two branches work together in a balance that controls the negative effects of stress. However, long-term stress can strain this balance, and chronic physical problems can occur as stress reactions become the dominant forces in a person's body.

The responses of the sympathetic nervous system to stress involve a series of biochemical exchanges between different parts of the body. The **hypothalamus,** a structure in the brain, functions as the control center of the sympathetic nervous system and determines the overall reaction to stressors. When the hypothalamus perceives that extra energy is needed to fight a stressor, it stimulates the adrenal glands, located near the top of the kidneys, to release the hormone **epinephrine,** also called adrenaline. Epinephrine causes more blood to be pumped with each beat of the heart, dilates the bronchioles (air sacs in the lungs) to increase oxygen intake, increases the breathing rate, stimulates the liver to release more glucose (which fuels muscular exertion), and dilates the pupils

> Why do I feel so "pumped up" when I am in a stressful situation?

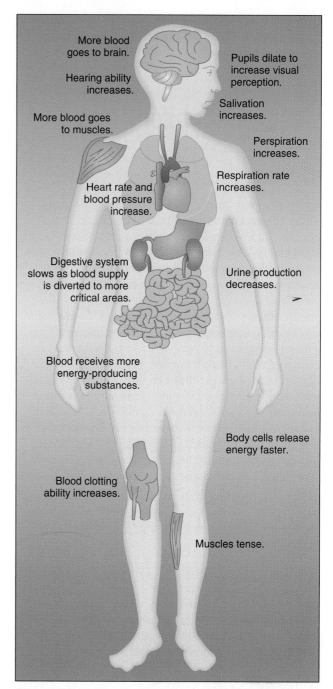

Figure 3.2 ■ The General Adaptation Syndrome: Alarm Phase

to improve visual sensitivity. The body is then poised to act immediately.

As epinephrine secretion increases, blood is diverted away from the digestive system, which might cause nausea and cramping if the distress occurs shortly after a meal, and drying of nasal and salivary tissues, which produces dry mouth. The alarm phase also provides for longer-term reaction to stress. At the same time, the hypothalamus uses chemical messages to trigger the *pituitary gland* within the brain to release the powerful hormone, *adrenocorticotrophic hormone*

Autonomic nervous system (ANS) The portion of the central nervous system that regulates bodily functions that a person does not normally consciously control.

Sympathetic nervous system Branch of the autonomic nervous system responsible for stress arousal.

Parasympathetic nervous system Part of the autonomic nervous system responsible for slowing systems stimulated by the stress response.

Hypothalamus A section of the brain that controls the sympathetic nervous system and directs the stress response.

Epinephrine Also called adrenaline, a hormone that stimulates body systems in response to stress.

(ACTH). ACTH signals the adrenal glands to release **cortisol,** a hormone that makes stored nutrients more readily available to meet energy demands. Finally, other parts of the brain and body release endorphins, the body's naturally occurring opiates, which relieve pain that a stressor may cause.

Resistance Phase The resistance phase of the GAS is similar to the alarm phase in that the same organs and systems are mobilized but at a less intense level. The body tries to return to homeostasis but, because some perceived stressor still exists, complete rest is never achieved. Instead, the body stays activated or aroused at a level that causes a higher metabolic rate in some organ tissues. These that and systems of resistance are working "overtime" and after prolonged stress will become depleted to the point where they cannot function effectively.

Exhaustion Phase In the exhaustion phase of the GAS, the physical and emotional energy used to fight a stressor has been depleted. The toll it takes on the body depends on the type of stress or the period of time spent under stress. Short-term stress probably would not deplete all of a person's energy reserves in an otherwise healthy person, but chronic stress experienced over a period of time can create continuous states of alarm and resistance, resulting in total depletion of energy and susceptibility to illness. The key to warding off the effects of stress lies in what many researchers refer to as **adaptation energy stores,** the physical and mental foundations of our ability to cope with stress.

As the body adjusts to chronic unresolved stress, the adrenal glands continue to release cortisol, which remains in the bloodstream for longer periods of time due to slower metabolic responsiveness. Over time, without relief, cortisol can reduce **immunocompetence,** or the ability of the immune system to respond to various assaults.[5] Blood pressure can remain dangerously elevated, we may catch colds more easily, or our body's ability to control blood glucose levels is affected.

STRESS AND YOUR HEALTH

Although much has been written about the negative effects of stress, researchers have only recently begun to untangle the complex web of physical and emotional interactions that can break down the body over time. Stress is often described as a disease of prolonged arousal that leads to other negative health effects. Nearly all body systems become potential targets, and the long-term effects may be devastating.

Studies indicate that 40 percent of deaths and 70 percent of disease in the United States is related, in whole or in part, to stress.[6] The list of ailments related to chronic stress is endless and includes heart disease, diabetes, can-

cer, headaches, ulcers, low back pain, depression, and the common cold. Alarming increases in rates of suicide, homicide, and domestic violence across the United States are additional symptoms of a nation under stress.

In a landmark study, M. D. Jeremko observed that chronic, unresolved stress can result in headaches, asthma, hypertension, ulcers, lower back pain, impairments of the immune system and other medical conditions, a finding substantiated by a meta-analysis of over 100 similar studies.[7] Numerous studies have concluded that mental health is a key predictor of physical health.[8] While the battle over the legitimacy of these observations continues to be waged in research labs across the country, the theory that chronic stress increases susceptibility to certain illnesses and infectious diseases has gained credibility.

Stress and Cardiovascular Disease Risks

Perhaps the most studied and documented health consequence of unresolved stress is cardiovascular disease. Since Friedman and Rosenman's classic study of Type A and Type B personalities and heart disease (discussed later in this chapter), researchers have tried to definitively link personality, emotions, and a host of other variables to heart disease.[9] Results of numerous meta-analyses that summarize many studies have consistently pointed to a correlation between chronic, unresolved stress and prolonged elevations in heart rate and blood pressure. This increased pressure can cause turbulence in the blood flow and is believed to damage the inner lining of blood vessels. Once this damage occurs, fatty substances seem to stick to this site more readily, which leads to atherosclerotic plaque buildup. A large number of epidemiological studies have related the incidence of heart disease deaths and sudden myocardial infarction (heart attack) to prolonged stress in the environment.[10] Individuals with certain types of employment, particularly those in which a person is subject to many demands and has very little control in decision making, are suspected to be at increased risk of death from cardiovascular disease (CVD).[11]

Historically, the increased risk of CVD due to chronic stress has been linked to increased plaque buildup due to elevated cholesterol, hardening of the

---

Cortisol Hormone released by the adrenal glands that makes stored nutrients more readily available to meet energy demands.

Adaptation energy stores The physical and mental foundations of our ability to cope with stress.

Immunocompetence The ability of the immune system to respond to assaults.

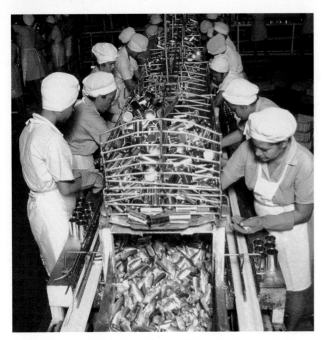

Studies indicate that those who have little control or decision-making powers in their employment are at an increased risk for stress-related CVD.

arteries, alterations in heart rhythms, increased and fluctuating blood pressure, and difficulties in cardiovascular responsiveness due to all of the above. While these continue to be considered major risks, recent research points to some type of inflammation in the vessels, perhaps due to lingering viral effects, as a major contributor to heart disease.[12] (For more information about CVD, see Chapter 12.)

Stress and Impaired Immunity

A growing area of scientific investigation known as **psychoneuroimmunology (PNI)** analyzes the intricate relationship between the mind's response to stress and the ability of the immune system to function effectively. A review of research linking stress to adverse health consequences suggests that too much stress over a long period can negatively regulate various aspects of the cellular immune response.[13] In particular, stress disrupts bidirectional communication networks between the nervous, endocrine, and immune systems. When these networks fail, messenger systems that regulate hormones, blood cell formation, and a host

> Why do I always catch a cold during finals week?

Psychoneuroimmunology (PNI) Science of the interaction between the mind's response to stress and the immune system.

of other health-regulating systems begin to falter or send faulty information.[14] During prolonged stress, elevated levels of adrenal hormones destroy or reduce the ability of the white blood cells, known as killer T cells, to aid the immune response. When killer T cells are suppressed and other regulating systems aren't working correctly, illness may occur.

For example, research indicates that students' disease-fighting mechanisms are weaker during high-stress times, such as exam weeks and on days when they are upset. In one experiment, a stressful event increased the severity of symptoms in a group of volunteers who were knowingly infected with a cold virus. In another, 47 percent of subjects living high-stress lives developed colds after a virus was dropped into their noses, but only 27 percent of those living relatively stress-free lives caught these colds.[15]

Other studies that link stress with infectious diseases include the following:

- People with self-reported high stress levels were much more likely to develop upper respiratory infections than those who reported lower levels of stress.[16]
- People with high stress levels who skip breakfast and consume a high level of fat catch many more colds than those who eat healthily and have low stress levels.[17]
- Certain changes in lifestyle may increase resistance to infectious diseases. These changes include broadening one's social involvement (e.g., joining social or spiritual groups, having a confidant, spending time with supportive friends) and maintaining healthful practices, such as proper diet, exercise, and sleep.[18]

We are only beginning to understand the relationship between high stress and increased risk for disease. Some research indicates that other factors, such as genetics and environmental stimuli, may be involved. However, in spite of questions, studies supporting the relationship between high stress and increased risk for disease outnumber those that don't.[19]

Stress and Diabetes

The effect of stress on blood sugar levels makes its impact on diabetes management crucial. People under lots of stress often don't get enough sleep, don't eat well, and may drink alcohol or take other drugs to help them get through a stressful time. All of these behaviors can alter blood sugar levels. Blood sugar levels also rise to ensure that extra fuel is available to fight or flee. In a person with diabetes, the pancreas is not functioning properly so that insulin, a hormone that controls our blood sugar levels, isn't produced sufficiently or is less effective. High blood sugar may damage body organs such as the kidneys and blood vessels in the extremities and eyes. Both mental and physical stress can cause blood sugar levels to rise precipitously.[20] While an occasional stress reaction might not be harmful, high-pressure jobs, unresolved problems, and chronic stress can make it extremely difficult for diabetics to control blood sugar.

Controlling stress levels is critical for both short- and long-term diabetes management. Exercise, maintaining a healthy weight, and relaxation techniques are particularly important strategies for controlling diabetes. Being at a healthy weight and at least light exercise contributes to overall glucose control and prevents the stress that people feel when they are overweight. Getting enough sleep and practicing the stress management techniques provided throughout this chapter are also important glucose control strategies. For more information on diabetes, see Chapter 14.

Stress and the Mind

Stress may be one of the single greatest contributors to mental disability and emotional dysfunction in the United States. Whether stress results in lost work productivity, difficulties in relationships, substance abuse, displaced anger and aggressive behavior, or a host of other problems, the net toll is staggering. Clearly, stress does much more than cause the heart rate to soar and blood pressure to go up. Substantial research supports a strong relationship between stress and the potential for negative mental health reactions. Consider the following:[21]

- Among college students, low self-esteem or depression and concerns about stress and health were identified as unresolved problems for 35 percent and 20 percent of the respondents, respectively.

- People with high nervous tension have increased risk for mental illness, suicide, and coronary heart disease.

- The high incidence of suicide among college students is assumed to be indicative of societal stress in the lives of young people.[22]

- A recent national study of Americans aged 15 to 54 found that almost half will suffer a mental and addictive disorder during their lifetime.

- College counseling centers report an 85 percent increase in the number of students they see with severe psychological problems—problems largely related to stress and adjustment difficulties.[23]

- People who regularly suffer from overload, frustration, and disappointment may eventually experience **burnout,** a state of physical and mental exhaustion caused by excessive stress. People involved in the helping professions, such as teaching or social work, or emergency services, such as police, firefighters, and medical professions, experience higher levels of burnout than others.

Try it →NOW_____

Write it down! **Journal writing is a great method to cleanse the mind, release emotions, and draft strategies for resolution. The next time an event or situation activates your stress response, identify the emotions that accompany it, and then list several options to bring closure to the event. This can be an effective means to cope with stressors.**

SOURCES OF STRESS

Both eustress and distress have many sources that include psychosocial factors, environmental stressors, and self-imposed stress.

Psychosocial Sources of Stress

Psychosocial stress refers to the factors in our daily lives that cause stress (see the Assess Yourself box on page 70). Interactions with others, the subtle and unsubtle expectations we and others have of ourselves, and the social conditions we live in force us to readjust constantly. Key psychosocial stressors include change, hassles, pressure, inconsistent goals and behaviors, conflict, overload, and discrimination.

Change Any time good or bad change occurs in your normal routine, you will experience stress. The more changes you experience and the more adjustments you must make, the greater the stress effects may be. Although many other factors must be considered, in general, the more of these stressors you experience, the more you need to change your behaviors or situation before problems occur. In 1967, Drs. Thomas Holmes and Richard Rahe analyzed the social readjustments experienced by more than 5,000 patients and noted which events seemed to occur just prior to disease onset.[24] They determined that certain positive and negative events were predictive of increased risk for illness. They called their scale for predicting stress overload and the likelihood of illness the Social Readjustment Rating Scale (SRRS).[25] The SRRS since has served as the model for scales that measure the stress levels of certain groups, including student populations. Table 3.1 shows the Student Stress Scale, one example of a scale based on the SRRS.

Burnout A state of physical and mental exhaustion caused by excessive stress.

Table 3.1
The Student Stress Scale

The Student Stress Scale represents an adaptation of Holmes and Rahe's Social Readjustment Rating Scale (SRRS). The SRRS has been modified to college-age adults and provides a rough indication of stress levels and health consequences for instructional purposes.

In the Student Stress Scale, each event is given a score that represents the amount of readjustment a person has to make as a result of the life change. To determine your stress score, check each event that you have experienced in the last 12 months, and then sum the number of points corresponding to each event.

1. Death of a close family member	_____	100
2. Death of a close friend	_____	73
3. Divorce between parents	_____	65
4. Jail term	_____	63
5. Major personal injury or illness	_____	63
6. Marriage	_____	58
7. Firing from a job	_____	50
8. Failure of an important course	_____	47
9. Change in health of a family member	_____	45
10. Pregnancy	_____	45
11. Sex problems	_____	44
12. Serious argument with close friend	_____	40
13. Change in financial status	_____	39
14. Change of major	_____	39
15. Trouble with parents	_____	39
16. New girlfriend or boyfriend	_____	37
17. Increase in workload at school	_____	37
18. Outstanding personal achievement	_____	36
19. First quarter/semester in school	_____	36
20. Change in living conditions	_____	31
21. Serious argument with an instructor	_____	30
22. Lower grades than expected	_____	29
23. Change in sleeping habits	_____	29
24. Change in social activities	_____	29
25. Change in eating habits	_____	28
26. Chronic car trouble	_____	26
27. Change in number of family gatherings	_____	26
28. Too many missed classes	_____	25
29. Change of college	_____	24
30. Dropping of more than one class	_____	23
31. Minor traffic violations	_____	20
Total:	_____	

Scoring: If your score is 300 or higher, you may be at high risk for developing a stress-related illness. If your score is between 150 and 300, you have approximately a 50:50 chance of experiencing a serious health problem within the next two years. If your score is below 150, you have a 1 in 3 chance of experiencing a serious health change in the next few years.

The following can help you to reduce your risk:

- Watch for early warning signs such as irritable bowels.
- Avoid negative thinking.
- Exercise regularly and eat nutritiously.
- Practice some form of relaxation regularly.
- Ask for help when necessary.

Source: Reproduced from: R. Blonna, "The Social and Spiritual Basis of Stress," *Coping with Stress in a Changing World,* 3rd ed., ed. R. Blonna (Boston: McGraw Hill, 1995), 99–100. *Original source:* T. Holmes and R. H. Rahe, "The Social Readjustment Rating Scale," *Journal of Psychosomatic Research* 11 (1967): 213.

What Do You Think?

Think about the changes that you have made during the past couple of years. Which of them would you regard as positive? ■ As negative? ■ How did you react to them initially? ■ Did your reactions change later? ■ What are the most important changes that students must make as they enter college? ■ What can they do to cope with unexpected changes?

Hassles While Holmes and Rahe examined major stressors, early psychologists such as Richard Lazarus and Susan Folkman focused on petty annoyances and frustrations, collectively referred to as hassles.[26] Minor hassles—losing your keys, slipping and falling in front of everyone as you walk to your seat in a new class, finding that you went through a whole afternoon with spinach stuck in your front teeth—seem unimportant. However, their cumulative effects have been shown to be harmful in the long run.[27] In fact, hassles are related to subsequent illness and disease to a greater degree than are major life events.[28]

Pressure Pressure occurs when we feel forced to speed up, intensify, or shift the direction of our behavior to meet a higher standard of performance.[29] Pressures can be based on our personal goals and expectations, concern about what others think, or on outside influences. Among the most significant outside influences are society's demands that we compete and be all that we can be. The forces that push us to compete for the best grades, nicest cars, most attractive significant others, and highest-paying jobs create significant pressure to personify American success.

Inconsistent Goals and Behaviors For many of us, the negative effects of stress are magnified when there is a disparity between our goals (what we value or hope to obtain in life) and our behaviors (actions that may or may not lead to these goals). For instance, you may want good grades—and your family may expect them—but if you party and procrastinate throughout the term, your behaviors are inconsistent with your goals. Significant stress in the form of guilt, last-minute frenzy before exams, and disappointing grades may result. On the other hand, if you dig in, work, and remain committed to getting good grades, much of your negative stress may be eliminated. Thwarted goals can lead to frustration, and frustration has been shown to be a significant disrupter of homeostasis.

Determining whether behaviors are consistent with goals is an essential component of maintaining balance in life. If we consciously strive to attain our goals, we greatly improve our chances of success.

Conflict Conflict occurs when we are forced to make difficult decisions between competing motives, behaviors, or impulses or when we are forced to face incompatible demands, opportunities, needs, or goals.[30] What if your best friends all choose to smoke marijuana, and you don't want to smoke but fear rejection? Conflict often occurs as our values are tested. College students who are away from home for the first time often face conflict between parental values and their own set of developing beliefs.[31]

Overload Excessive time pressure, too much responsibility, high expectations of yourself and those around you, and lack of support can lead to **overload,** a state of being overburdened. Have you ever felt you had so many responsibilities that you couldn't possibly fulfill them all? Have you longed for a weekend when you could just take time out with friends and not feel guilty? These feelings are symptoms of overload. Students suffering from overload may experience depression, anxiety about tests, poor self-concept, a desire to drop classes or drop out of school, and other problems. Significant numbers of students resort to excessive use of alcohol and other drugs in response to overload. Binge drinking (see Chapter 8) is one of the leading problems on college campuses today.[32]

"Isms" Today's racially and ethnically diverse group of students, faculty members, and staff enriches everyone's educational experience yet also challenges us to deal with differences. Often, students who act, speak, dress, or appear different face additional pressures that do not affect students considered more typical. Students perceived as different may become victims of subtle and not-so-subtle bigotry; insensitivity; and harassment, or hostility because of their race, ethnicity, religious affiliation, age, sexual orientation, or other "isms."

Evidence of the health effects of excessive stress in minority groups abounds. For example, African Americans suffer higher rates of hypertension, CVD, and most cancers than their white counterparts do. Although poverty and socioeconomic status have been blamed for much of the spike in hypertension rates for African Americans and other marginalized groups, this chronic, physically debilitating stress may reflect real and perceived status in society more than it reflects actual poverty. Feeling that you occupy a position of low status due to living conditions, financial security, or job status can be a source of stress. The problem is exacerbated

for those who are socially disadvantaged early in life and grow up without a nurturing environment.[33]

Imagine what it would be like to find yourself isolated, lacking friends, and ridiculed on the basis of who you are or how you look. In addition to making the grade in classes, these individuals must deal with hidden fears, suffering, and difficulties caused by intolerant factions on campus. (Chapter 4 focuses on violence and its incidence and prevalence on campus.)

What Do You Think?
What are your greatest sources of stress right now? ■ On a scale of 1 to 10, with 10 being the highest level, how stressed are you? ■ Have you noticed any symptoms of stress? ■ How can you reduce it?

Environmental Stress

Environmental stress results from events occurring in the physical environment as opposed to social surroundings. Environmental stressors include natural disasters, such as floods and hurricanes, and human-made disasters, such as chemical spills and explosions. Often as damaging as one-time disasters are **background distressors,** such as noise, air, and water pollution, although we may be unaware of them and their effects may not become apparent for decades. As with other challenges, our bodies respond to environmental stressors with the GAS. People who cannot escape background distressors may exist in a constant resistance phase, which can contribute to stress-related disorders.

Self-Imposed Stress

Appraisal and Stress We encounter many different types of life demands and potential stressors—some biological, some psychological, and others sociological. In any case, it is our appraisal of these demands, not the demands themselves, that results in the experience of stress. **Appraisal** is defined as the interpretation and evaluation of information provided to the brain by the senses. As new information becomes available, appraisal helps us recognize stressors, evaluate them on the basis of past experiences and emotions, and make decisions regarding how to cope with them.

Overload   A state in which a person feels overburdened by demands.

Background distressors   Environmental stressors of which people are often unaware.

Appraisal   The interpretation and evaluation of information provided to the brain by the senses.

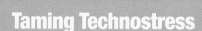
Cell phones that ring constantly; e-mail lists that grow on your computer desktop like an out-of-control fungus; laptop computers that somehow end up in your luggage when you go on vacation; voice message systems that don't allow you to talk to a live person; and slow, slow, slow downloading of information. Can you feel your heart rate speeding up just thinking about these situations?

On college campuses across the country, students, faculty, and administrators are using electronic organizers, the Internet, and other forms of technology. E-mail, the World Wide Web, and personal digital assistants (PDAs) are no longer flashy new tools but are as commonplace as the backpack. Unfortunately, many people feel frustrated and distressed in their struggle to adapt to increasingly complex technology. As many as 85 percent of us have at least some level of discomfort around technology.

If you are like millions of people today, you find that technology is often a daily terrorizer that raises your blood pressure, frustrates you, and prevents you from ever really getting away from it all. In short, you may be a victim of stressors that previous generations only dreamed (or had

nightmares) about. Known as *techno-stress,* this problem is defined as "personal stress generated by reliance on technological devices . . . a panicky feeling when they fail, and a state of near-constant stimulation, or being perpetually 'plugged in.'" When technostress grabs you, it may interact with other forms of stress to create a synergistic, never-ending form of stimulation that keeps your stress response reverberating all day.

Part of the problem, ironically, is that technology enables us to be so productive. Because it encourages polyphasic activity, or "multitasking," people are forced to juggle multiple thoughts and actions at the same time, such as driving and talking on cell phones or checking handheld devices for appointments. People who multitask, however, are actually less efficient than those who focus on one project at a time. Moreover, there is clear evidence that multitasking contributes to auto accidents and other harmful consequences, including short-term memory loss. What is less clear is what happens to someone who is always plugged in.

What are the symptoms of technology overload? It evokes typical stress

responses by increasing heart rate and blood pressure and causing irritability and memory disturbances. Over time, many stressed-out people lose the ability to relax and find that they feel nervous and anxious when they are supposed to be having fun. Headaches, stomach and digestive problems, skin irritations, frequent colds, difficulty in wound healing, lack of sleep, ulcers, and other problems may result. Other red flags include gaps in your attentiveness and changes in your ability to concentrate. A study conducted by Yale University indicates that chronic stress may even thicken the waistline; increased secretions of cortisol caused even slender women to store added fat in the abdomen.

Authors Michelle Weil and Larry Rosen describe *technosis,* a syndrome in which people get so immersed in technology that they risk losing their own identity. If you answer "yes" to questions such as "Do you rely on preprogrammed systems to contact others?" and "Do you feel stressed if you haven't checked your e-mail within the last 12 hours?" you may be too dependent on technology.

When an individual appraises his or her coping resources as sufficient to meet life demands, little or no stress is experienced. On the other hand, if an individual appraises life demands as exceeding his or her coping resources, strain and distress are likely to occur. Several coping resources that contribute to stressful appraisals, including self-esteem and self-efficacy, are discussed below.

Self-Esteem As you learned in Chapter 2, self-esteem refers to a sense of positive self-regard or how you feel about yourself; it is a variable entity that can continually change.[34] When we feel good about our self we are less likely to respond to or interpret an event as stressful. Conversely, if we place little or no value on our self and believe we have inadequate coping skills, we become susceptible to stress and strain.[35]

Self-esteem is closely related to the emotions engendered by past experiences. Low self-esteem can lead to helpless anger. People suffering helpless anger usually have learned that they are wrong to feel anger, so instead of expressing it in healthy ways they turn it inward. They may swallow their rage in food, alcohol, or other drugs, or they may act in other self-destructive ways. Of particular concern, research with high school and college students has found that low self-esteem and stressful life events significantly predict suicidal ideation, a desire to die and thoughts about suicide.[36] Several methods to develop and maintain self-esteem were discussed in Chapter 2.

Self-Efficacy Self-efficacy, also introduced in Chapter 2, is another important factor in one's ability to cope with life's challenges. Self-efficacy refers to one's

Tips for Fighting Technostress

- *Enjoy the natural environment.* Get away from any form of technology. Try to find a place that has few people and little noise—that usually means outdoors.

- *Become aware of what you are doing.* Log the time you spend on e-mail, voice mail, etc. Set up a schedule to limit your use of technology. For example, spend no more than a half-hour per day answering e-mails.

- *Give yourself more time for everything you do.* If you are surfing the Web for resources for a term paper, start early rather than the night before the paper is due.

- *Manage the telephone—don't let it manage you.* Rather than interrupting what you're doing to answer, screen calls with an answering machine or caller ID. Get rid of call waiting, which forces you to juggle multiple calls, and subscribe to a voice mail service that takes messages when you're on the phone.

- *Set "time out" periods when you don't answer the phone, listen to the stereo, use the computer, or watch TV.* Switch off e-mail notification systems so you aren't beeped during these periods.

- *Take regular breaks.* Even when working, get up, walk around, stretch, do deep breathing, or get a glass of water, every hour.

- *If you are working on the computer, look away from the screen and focus on something far away every 30 minutes.* Stretch your shoulders and neck periodically as you work. Playing soft background music can help you relax.

- *Resist the urge to buy the newest and fastest technology.* Such purchases not only cause financial stress, but also add to stress levels with the typical glitches that occur when installing and adjusting to new technology.

- *Do not take laptops, hand-held devices, or other technological gadgets on vacation.* If you must take a cell phone for emergencies, turn it and your voice messaging system off, and use the phone only in true emergencies.

- *Back up materials on your computer at regular intervals.* Writing a term paper only to lose it during a power outage will send you into hyperstress very quickly.

- *Expect technological change.* The only constant with technology is

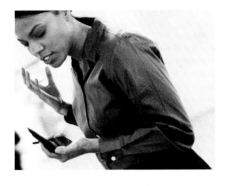

improvement and change. No matter how at ease you are with your current computer, cell phone, PDA, etc., at some point you will need to move on to a new one.

Sources: D. Zielinski, "Techno-stressed?," *Presentations* 18, no. 2 (2004): 28–34; Dr. L. D. Rosen and Dr. M. M. Weil, *TechnoStress: Coping with Technology @Work@Home@Play* (New York: John Wiley & Sons, 1997). Copyright © 1997. Material used by permission of John Wiley & Sons; M. Weil and L. Rosen, "Technostress: Are You a Victim of Technosis?," 2004, www.technostress .com/tstechnosis.htm; Yale University, "Stress May Cause Excess Abdominal Fat in Otherwise Slender Women, Study Conducted at Yale Shows," *ScienceDaily,* November 23, 2000; MayoClinic.com, "Are You a Slave to the Telephone?," November 1, 2000, www.mayoclinic .com/; S. Shellenbarger, "Multitasking Makes You Stupid: Studies Show Pitfalls of Doing Too Much at Once," *The Wall Street Journal* (February 27, 2003): D1.

belief or confidence in personal skills and performance abilities.[37] If they have succeeded in mastering similar problems in the past, they will be more likely to believe in their own effectiveness. Similarly, people who have repeatedly tried and failed may lack confidence in their abilities to deal with life's problems. In some cases, this insecurity may prevent them from trying to cope.

External versus Internal Locus of Control
People who believe they lack control in a situation may become easily frustrated and give up. Those who feel they have no personal control tend to have an external locus of control and a low level of self-efficacy. People who are confident their behavior will influence the outcome tend to have an internal locus of control. Individuals who feel that they have limited control over their lives often show higher levels of stress.[38]

Type A Personality and Hostility
Personality may contribute to the kind and degree of self-imposed stress we experience. In 1974, physicians Meyer Friedman and Ray Rosenman identified two stress-related personality types: Type A and Type B.[39] Type A personalities are hard-driving, competitive, anxious, time-driven, impatient, quick-tempered, and perfectionistic. Type B personalities are relaxed and noncompetitive. According to Rosenman and Friedman, people with Type A characteristics are more prone to heart attacks than are their Type B counterparts. Because some Type A behavior is learned, it can be modified. Some Type As are able to slow down and become more tolerant and patient. Unfortunately, many people

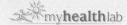

Fill out this assessment online at
www.aw-bc.com/myhealthlab or www.aw-bc.com/donatelle.

How Stressed Are You?

Each of us reacts differently to life's little challenges. Faced with a long line at the bookstore, most of us will get anxious for a few seconds before we start grumbling or shrug and move on. For others—the one in five of us whom researchers call hot reactors—such incidents are part of a daily health assault. These individuals may get outwardly angry or appear calm and collected. It is what is going on under the surface that affects health. Surges in blood pres-sure, increases in heart rate, nausea, sweating, and other hot reactor indicators may occur. Completing the following assessment will help you think about the nature and extent of stress in your life and how you respond to daily stressors. Although this survey is just an indicator of what stress levels might be, it will help you focus on areas that you may need to work on to reduce stress.

Part One: What Is Stressing You Out?

For each statement, indicate how often the following stressful situations or feelings are a part of your daily life.

	Never	Rarely	Sometimes	Often	All the Time
1. I find that there are not enough hours in the day to finish everything I have to do.	1	2	3	4	5
2. I am anxious about how I am performing in my classes.	1	2	3	4	5
3. People don't seem to notice whether or not I do a good job.	1	2	3	4	5
4. I am tired and feel like I don't have the energy to do everything that I need to get done.	1	2	3	4	5
5. I seem to be easily irritated by things that people do.	1	2	3	4	5
6. I worry about what is happening in my family (health of a loved one, financial problems, relationship problems, etc.).	1	2	3	4	5
7. I'm worried about my finances and having enough money to pay my bills.	1	2	3	4	5
8. I don't have enough time for fun.	1	2	3	4	5
9. I am unhappy with my body (weight, fitness level, etc.).	1	2	3	4	5
10. My family and friends count on me to help them with their problems.	1	2	3	4	5
11. I am concerned about my current relationship (or lack of a relationship).	1	2	3	4	5
12. I am impatient/intolerant of the weaknesses of others.	1	2	3	4	5
13. My house/apartment is a mess, and I'm embarrassed to have others see it.	1	2	3	4	5
14. I worry about whether I'll get a job and be able to support myself after graduation.	1	2	3	4	5
15. I worry that people don't like me.	1	2	3	4	5

Your Total Score: _____

ANALYZING THIS SECTION

Scores of 60–75: Your stress level is probably quite high. Prioritize the areas where you scored 5s, and list two to three things for each area that you could do to reduce your stress level. Note any increase in headaches, backaches, or insomnia; your body is telling you to lighten your load. Plan at least one fun thing to do for yourself each day. Make yourself more of a daily priority.

Scores of 45–60: Your stress level is moderate. Look at those areas that are 5s and list two to three things that you would like to change now to help yourself reduce stress. Practice at least one stress management technique each day. Make more time for yourself.

Scores of 30–45: You seem to have a lower level of stress. This is good. However, there are still areas that you could work on. Think about what these are, and list things you could do now to reduce stress.

Scores below 30: You seem to be doing a great job. Whatever your problems, stress isn't one of them. Even when stressful events do occur—and they will—your health probably won't suffer.

Remember, each of us has "stress slips" along the way. Think about your reactions to situations like those above. Whenever possible, make conscious choices to reduce stress.

Part Two: How Do You Respond to Stress?

Respond to each of the following statements with a rating of how likely you are to react to a given stressful event.

	Never	Rarely	Some of the Time	Usually or Always

SCENARIO 1

You've been waiting 20 minutes for a table in a crowded restaurant, and the hostess seats a group that arrived after you.

	Never	Rarely	Some of the Time	Usually or Always
1. You feel your anger rise as your face gets hot and your heart beats faster.	1	2	3	4
2. You yell "Hey! I was here first" in an irritated voice to the hostess.	1	2	3	4
3. You angrily confront the people who are being seated in front of you and tell them you were there first.	1	2	3	4
4. You say, "Excuse me" in a polite voice and inform the other group and/or the hostess that you were there first.	1	2	3	4
5. You note it, but don't react. It's no big deal, and the hostess obviously didn't notice the order of arrival.	1	2	3	4

SCENARIO 2

You get to a movie theater early so that you and a friend can get great seats. You strategically pick a seat that will give you a good view. Although the theater is nearly empty, a large, tall man plops himself in the seat directly in front of you. Try as you might, you cannot see the screen.

	Never	Rarely	Some of the Time	Usually or Always
1. You say in a very loud voice: "There's a whole theater, and he has to sit right in front of us!"	1	2	3	4
2. You yell directly at the man, saying, "Can't you sit somewhere else? I can't see!"	1	2	3	4
3. You tap the man on the shoulder and say, "Excuse me, I wonder if you could slide down a seat. I can't see."	1	2	3	4
4. You calmly nudge your friend and decide to move.	1	2	3	4
5. You aren't bothered by the person in front of you. This is just part of going to the movies, and it is no big deal.	1	2	3	4

OTHER SCENARIOS

How would you respond to the following?

	Never	Rarely	Some of the Time	Usually or Always
1. Your sister calls out of the blue and starts to tell you how much you mean to her. Uncomfortable, you change the subject without expressing what you feel.	1	2	3	4
2. You come home to find the kitchen looking like a disaster area and your spouse/roommate lounging in front of the TV. You tense up and can't seem to shake your anger, but you decide not to bring it up.	1	2	3	4
3. Faced with a public speaking event, you get keyed up and lose sleep for a day or more, worrying about how you'll do.	1	2	3	4

(continues)

(continued)

	Never	Rarely	Some of the Time	Usually or Always
4. Your boyfriend/girlfriend/partner is seen out with another person and appears to be acting quite close to the person. You are a trusting person and decide not to worry about it. If your significant other has anything to tell you, you know he/she will talk to you.	1	2	3	4
5. You aren't able to study as much as you'd like for an exam, yet you think that you really "nailed" the exam once you take it. When you get it back, you find that you did horribly. You make an appointment to talk with the professor and determine what you can do to improve on the next exam. You acknowledge that you are responsible for the low grade this time but vow to do better next time. You are disappointed, but you don't let it bother you.	1	2	3	4

ANALYZING THIS SECTION

Look carefully at each of these scenarios. Obviously, none of us is perfect, and we sometimes react in ways that we later regret. The key here is to assess how you react the majority of the time.

If stressful events occur and you remain calm, do not experience increases in heart rate or blood pressure, or avoid excess anxiety, anger, or frustration, you are probably a cool reactor who tends to roll with the punches when a situation is out of your control. This usually indicates a good level of coping; overall, you will suffer fewer health consequences when stressed. The key here is that you really are not stressed, and you really are calm and unworried about the situation.

If you fret and stew about a stressor, can't sleep, or tend to react with hostility, anger, or other negative physiological overreactions, you probably are a hot reactor who responds to mildly stressful situations with a fight-or-flight adrenaline rush that drives up blood pressure and can lead to heart rhythm disturbances, accelerated clotting, and damaged blood vessel linings. Some hot reactors can seem cool on the outside, but inside their bodies are silently killing them. They may be on edge or jumpy or unable to sleep, even though most people would never suspect that they are in trouble. Before you honk or make obscene gestures at the guy who cuts you off in rush hour traffic, remember that getting angry can destroy thousands of heart muscle cells within minutes. Robert S. Eliot, author of *From Stress to Strength,* says hot reactors have no choice but to calm themselves down with rational thought. Look at ways to change your perceptions and cope more effectively. Ponder the fact that the only thing you'll hasten by reacting is a decline in health. "You have to stop trying to change the world," Eliot advises, "and learn to change your response to it."

Make It Happen!

Assessment: The Assess Yourself activity gave you the chance to look at your stress levels and identify situations in your life that particularly cause stress. Now that you are aware of these patterns, you can change a behavior that leads to increased stress.

Making a Change: In order to change your behavior, you need to develop a plan. Follow these steps:

1. Evaluate your behavior, and identify patterns.
2. Select one pattern of behavior that you want to change.
3. Fill out the Behavior Change Contract found at the beginning of your book. It should include your long-term goal for change, your short-term goals, the rewards for reaching these goals, potential obstacles along the way, and strategies for overcoming these obstacles.
4. Chart your progress in a journal.
5. Revise your plan as needed: Are the short-term goals attainable? Are the rewards satisfying?

Example: Kim discovered that much of her stress was caused by school deadlines. She wanted to learn how to manage her time more efficiently. Kim filled out a Behavior Change Contract, with a goal of finishing her history term paper five days before its due date to give herself enough time to study for her biology final. She broke the paper-writing process into manageable steps of research, writing, revising, and proofreading. Each time she finished a stage she rewarded herself with a movie or a trip to the local coffeehouse. She fell behind when her sister unexpectedly visited her for two days, but she got back on schedule when she worked on her paper instead of watching her afternoon soap opera. Kim completed her paper in plenty of time, was able to study efficiently for her biology exam, and didn't come down with her usual finals-period cold.

do not decide to modify their Type A habits until after they become ill or suffer a heart attack. Prevention of stress-related health problems requires recognizing and changing dangerous behaviors before damage is done.

Researchers today believe that more needs to be discovered about personality types. Most people are not one personality type all the time, and other unexplained variables must also be explored. For example, researchers at Duke University contend that the Type A personality may be more complex than previously described. They have identified a "toxic core" in some Type A personalities, which makes them angry, distrustful of others, and cynical—a collection of characteristics commonly referred to as **hostility.**[40] It may be this toxic core rather than the hard-driving nature of the Type A personality that makes people more vulnerable to self-imposed stress.[41] People who are hostile often have below-average levels of self-esteem and social support and other increased risks for ill health. A wide range of studies have identified hostility as an independent risk factor for coronary heart disease (CHD), hypertension, and premature mortality.

Psychological Hardiness According to psychologist Susanne Kobasa, **psychological hardiness** may negate self-imposed stress associated with Type A behavior. Psychologically hardy people are characterized by control, commitment, and challenge.[42] People with a sense of control are able to accept responsibility for their behaviors and change those that they discover to be debilitating. People with a sense of commitment have good self-esteem and understand their purpose in life. People with a sense of challenge see change as a stimulating opportunity for personal growth. The concept of hardiness has been studied extensively and many researchers believe it is the foundation of an individual's ability to cope with stress and remain healthy.[43]

STRESS AND THE COLLEGE STUDENT

College students thrive under a certain amount of stress, but excessive stress can leave them overwhelmed and underenthused about their classes and social interactions. Some 32 percent of students surveyed for the National College Health Assessments reported that stress was the number-one factor affecting their individual academic performance, followed closely by stress-related problems such as cold/flu/sore throats (25 percent) and sleep difficulties (24 percent).[44]

A recent study by UCLA's (University of California–Los Angeles) Higher Education Research Institute reported that current college freshmen are more stressed than any class of freshmen before them. These researchers define **psychological stress** as the relationship between a person and the environment that the

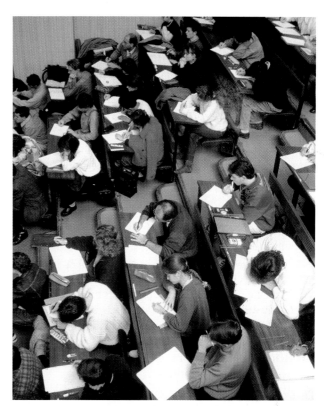

College can be a stressful time for students, whether they are young people choosing a career path or older adults returning to school to change directions later in life.

person judges to be beyond his or her resources and jeopardizes his or her well-being.[45] Freshmen seem to be the most vulnerable to the negative effects of psychological stress, with relationships, school events, safety, and feeling deviance from school norms noted as being particularly distressful. Not only did freshmen report more problems with these issues, they also reported more emotional reactivity in the form of anger, hostility, and frustration and a greater sense of being out of control. Sophomores and juniors reported fewer problems with these issues, and seniors reported the fewest problems, which perhaps indicates progressive emotional growth through experience, maturity, increased awareness of support services, and more social connections.[46]

In a study of chronic stressors, male and female college students differed significantly in the things they perceived to be significant stressors.[47] Women

Hostility The cognitive, effective, and behavioral tendencies toward anger, distrust, and cynicism.

Psychological hardiness A personality trait characterized by control, commitment, and challenge.

Psychological stress Stress caused by being in an environment perceived to be beyond one's control and endangering one's well-being.

indicated that among their most frequent stressors were trying to diet, having an overload of school work, and gaining weight. Men, in contrast, tended to list the following items as major stressors: being underweight, problems relating to commuting to school, not having enough sex, being behind in schoolwork, not having enough friends, and concerns about drug or alcohol use.[48]

College students may be especially vulnerable because they are in a period of transition, often being away from home for the first time, striking out on their own, and forging new relationships. From the moment they start packing, these transitions cause them to face key developmental tasks as their lives begin to make dramatic changes, such as achieving emotional independence from family; choosing and preparing for a career; preparing for a major relationship, or commitment; facing economic independence; and developing their own values and ethical system. These tasks require that the college student develop new social roles and modify old ones. Such changes can result in persistent stress and strain as students attempt to adapt to new roles and form new identities.

If you experience any of the stressors listed in the Student Stress Scale in Table 3.1, act promptly to reduce their impact. Most colleges offer stress management workshops through health centers or student counseling departments. Do not ignore the symptoms of stress overload, which include a vague sense of anxiety or nervousness; changes in sleep, diet, or exercise patterns; headaches; dizziness; short temper; increased negativism, cynicism, anger, or frustration; recurring colds and minor illnesses; persistent time pressures; increased difficulty in completing tasks; inability to concentrate; wanting to get away from others; and less tolerance of petty annoyances.

According to researchers, many mental health problems may be traced to stress-related trauma that occurs at key periods of life, particularly during the college years. Consider these facts:[49]

- The Centers for Disease Control relates that 7.8 percent of men and 12.3 percent of women aged 18 to 24 report frequent mental distress; and in a recent national survey, 10 to 13 percent of college students said they have been diagnosed with depression.

- In 2000, almost 7 percent of college students reported experiencing anxiety disorders within the previous year. Women are five times as likely to experience anxiety disorders as men.

- More than 30 percent of college freshmen report feeling overwhelmed a great deal of the time, and about 38 percent of college women report feeling frequently overwhelmed.

MANAGING YOUR STRESS

Acknowledging that stress is causing some difficulties in your life—be it physical or psychosocial—is often the first step toward making positive change. Being on your own in college poses many challenges. However, it also lets you evaluate your unique situation and take steps that fit your own schedule and lifestyle to reduce negative stressors in your life.

One of the most effective ways to combat stressors is to build skills and coping strategies that will help inoculate you against them. Such efforts are known collectively as *stress management techniques;* they may range from doing something as simple as taking 20 minutes each day to be alone, to developing an elaborate time management plan. Any strategy that you select should be developed in a series of steps; do not change too many things at once or your new stress management program will stress you out!

Building Skills to Reduce Stress

Dealing with stress involves assessing all aspects of a stressor, examining your response and how you can change it, and learning to cope. Often we cannot change the requirements at our college, assignments in class, or unexpected stressors. Inevitably, we will be stuck in classes that bore us and for which we find no application in real life. We feel powerless when a loved one dies. Although the facts cannot be changed, we can change our reactions to them.

> How can I cope more effectively with daily pressures?

Assess Your Stressors After recognizing a stressor, evaluate it. Can you alter the circumstances to reduce the amount of distress you are experiencing or must you change your behavior and reactions to reduce stress levels? For example, you may have five term papers due for five different courses during the semester, but your professors are unlikely to drop such requirements. However, you can change your behavior by beginning the papers early and spacing them over time to avoid last-minute panic.

Change Your Responses Changing your responses requires practice and emotional control. If your roommate is habitually messy and this causes you stress, you can choose from among several responses. You can express your anger by yelling; you can pick up the mess and leave a nasty note; or you can defuse the situation with humor. The first reaction that comes to mind is not always the best. Stop before reacting to gain the time you need to find an appropriate response. Ask yourself, "What is to be gained from my response?"

Many people change their responses to potentially stressful events through cognitive coping strategies. These strategies help them prepare through gradual exposure to increasingly higher stress levels.

Learn to Cope Everyone copes with stress in different ways. Some people drink or take drugs; others seek help from counselors; and still others try to forget about it or engage in positive activities, such as exercise. **Stress inoculation** helps people prepare for stressful events ahead of time. For example, suppose you are petrified about speaking in front of a class. Practicing in front of friends or in front of a video camera may inoculate you and prevent your freezing up on the day of the presentation. The assumption is that, by dealing with smaller fears, a person gathers resistance so that larger fears do not seem so overwhelming. Some health experts compare stress inoculation to a vaccine given to protect against a disease. Regardless of how you cope with a situation, your conscious effort to deal with it is an important step in stress management.

Try it ➤NOW_____

Think triple A! **Feeling overwhelmed? Experiencing overload? If the answer is yes, try the three As of coping—Avoid, Alter, and Abolish.[50] If your school workload is causing distress, you may chose to avoid taking more than 15 credits, alter your schedule so that you attend classes in the morning when you are most alert, or abolish a few of your social events to devote more time to studying.**

Consider Downshifting Today's lifestyles are hectic and pressure-packed, and stress often comes from trying to keep up. Many people are questioning whether "having it all" is worth it, and they are taking a step back and simplifying their lives. This trend is known as **downshifting.** Moving from a large urban area to a smaller town, leaving a high-paying, high-stress job for one that makes you happy, and a host of other changes in lifestyle typify downshifting.

Downshifting involves a fundamental alteration in values and honest introspection about what is important in life. When you consider any form of downshift or perhaps even start your career this way, it's important to move slowly and consider the following.

- *Determine your ultimate goal.* What is most important to you, and what will you need to reach that goal? What can you do without?
- *Make a short-term and a long-term plan for simplifying your life.* Set up your plan in doable steps, and work slowly toward each step. Begin saying no to requests for your time, and determine those people with whom it is important for you to spend time. Clear out clutter or material items you don't need or use.

- *Complete a financial inventory.* How much money will you need to do the things you want to do? Will you live alone or share costs with roommates? Do you need a car, or can you rely on public transportation? Pay off your debt and get used to paying with cash. If you don't have the cash, don't buy. Remember, your lifestyle as a student will be different than living at home.
- *Plan for health care costs.* Make sure that you budget for health insurance and basic preventive health services if you're not covered under your parents' plan. Understand your coverage. This should be a top priority.
- *Select the right career.* Look for work that you enjoy. Can you be happy taking a lower-paying job that is less stressful and allows you the opportunity to have a life?
- *Consider options for saving money.* Downshifting doesn't mean you renounce money; it means you choose not to let money dictate your life. It's still important to save. If you're just getting started, you need to prepare for emergencies and for future plans.

Managing Social Interactions

As you plan a stress management program, don't underestimate the importance of social networks and social bonds. Consider the nature and extent of your friendships. Do you have someone with whom you can share intimate thoughts and feelings? Do you trust your friends to be supportive? Will your friends be honest with you if you are doing something risky or inappropriate? Friendships are an important aspect of inoculating yourself against harmful stressors. Studies have demonstrated the importance of social support in buffering individuals from the effects of stress.[51] It isn't necessary to have a large number of friends. However, different friends often serve different needs, so having more than one is usually beneficial. As you work to develop and cultivate friendships, look for individuals who possess the following traits listed on page 76.

Stress inoculation Stress management technique in which a person consciously tries to prepare ahead of time for potential stressors.

Downshifting Conscious attempt to simplify life in an effort to reduce the stresses and strains of modern living.

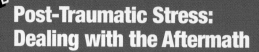

Post-Traumatic Stress: Dealing with the Aftermath

For many college students, war, national threats, and devastating natural disasters were something studied in history classes—until the events of September 11, 2001, the recent bombings on the London underground system, Hurricane Katrina, and the war in Iraq. For most, these were our first brushes with threats to a secure world, and reactions such as fear, anxiety, anger, and depression were not uncommon. These reactions are exacerbated in situations where individuals have suffered personal losses or are separated from their families and loved ones due to impending threats.

It is important to know that each person, whether directly or indirectly affected by traumatic events, will react differently and that a range of responses is normal. Emotional responses can appear immediately or sometimes develop months later. According to the National Mental Health Association, common responses to disaster and its consequences include:

- Disbelief and shock
- Fear and anxiety about the future
- Disorientation, difficulty making decisions or concentrating
- Inability to focus on schoolwork and extracurricular activities
- Irritability and anger
- Extreme mood swings
- Feelings of powerlessness
- Changes in eating patterns; loss of appetite
- Crying for no apparent reason
- Headaches and stomach problems
- Difficulty sleeping
- Excessive use of drugs or alcohol

Post-Traumatic Stress Disorder

In severe cases, an individual's response may be considered **post-traumatic stress disorder (PTSD).** PTSD generally develops within the first hours or days after a traumatic event, but occasionally symptoms do not begin until months or years later. Typically, persons suffering from PTSD were soldiers returning from war, particularly those who saw friends killed or mangled or who experienced terrible suffering and pain themselves. Other extreme traumatic events include rape or other severe physical attacks, near-death experiences in accidents, witnessing a murder or death, being caught in a natural disaster, or falling victim to terrorist attacks.

Symptoms of PTSD include:

- Dissociation, or perceived detachment of the mind from the emotional state or even the body. The person may have a sense of the world as a dreamlike or unreal place and have poor memory of the events—a form of dissociative amnesia.

- Acute anxiety or nervousness, in which the person is hyperaroused; may cry easily or experience mood swings; and experience flashbacks, nightmares, and recurrent thoughts or visual images. They may sense vague uneasiness or feel like the event is happening again and again. Some may experience intense physiological reactions, such as shaking or nausea when something reminds them of the event. In some cases, they may have difficulty returning to areas that remind them of the trauma. For example, an individual who has been assaulted in a parking garage may have difficulty entering a parking garage again, be extremely fearful when walking in dark places when there is no one around, or suffer from recurring nightmares.

Persistent Stress Symptoms

Sufferers may have two or more of these symptoms:

- Difficulty falling or staying asleep
- Irritability or outbursts of anger or other emotions

- have values and interests that are similar to your own (as well as those with different interests that force you to grow and explore new ideas).

- are good listeners, give and share freely, are tolerant, and do not rush to judgment.

- are trustworthy and have your best interests at heart.

- are not unusually critical, negative, selfish, or only bring you down. Avoid people who enjoy "stirring things up" and always seem to be in some crisis themselves; they often precipitate rather than reduce stress responses.

- are responsible, value doing well in school, but also know when and how to have fun.

- are willing to be exercise and diet buddies or study partners with a mutual interest in a healthy lifestyle.

- know how to laugh, cry, engage in meaningful conversation, and feel comfortable with silence.

Just as it is important to find these characteristics in your friends, it is also important for you to bring these qualities to your friendships. Sometimes, focusing on others can help you get your own problems into better focus and control.

If you do not have a close friend or support group, find out where to turn when the pressures of life seem

Post-traumatic stress disorder (PTSD) An anxiety disorder that can occur after exposure to a terrifying event or major trauma and is accompanied by symptoms severe enough to impair the person's daily life.

- Difficulty concentrating
- Hypervigilance
- Exaggerated startle response

If these symptoms last more than one month, PTSD may be diagnosed, either as acute (less than three months' duration) or chronic (longer than three months). A delayed onset form of PTSD may appear months after the event. If feelings of sadness or depression persist, seek help. In most people, symptoms disappear within six months.

Tips for Coping

The National Institutes of Health indicates that as many as 5 to 8 percent of the American public may have chronic PTSD, with women having almost twice the prevalence of men. It is important to acknowledge the trauma and to address its effects. Ways to recover include:

- Talking about it and encouraging others to share their perspectives.

- Taking care of yourself. Get plenty of rest and exercise. Do things you find relaxing and soothing. Limit your exposure to media reports and images of the tragedy. As soon as possible, get back to normal routines.

- Staying connected to friends and family. Make plans to visit family or others who can offer reassurance and stability. If you can't travel or are nervous about it, use phone or e-mail contact.

- Doing something positive that will help you gain a greater sense of control, such as giving blood, taking a first aid class, or donating food or clothing. Get involved with campus activities planned in response to a disaster, such as candlelight vigils, benefits, or discussion groups and speakers.

- Asking for help if you are feeling overwhelmed or out of control. It's not a sign of weakness. Talk with a trusted friend or faith leader. Use on-campus resources such as the counseling center or student health center. If you don't know where to go, talk with your health professor about options.

Therapies designed to help trauma victims recover are increasingly effective as our knowledge about this disorder grows. Schools, communities, and workplaces now routinely bring in crisis experts immediately after an event to help survivors talk through their feelings and gain support from others. A supportive family, employer, and friends and access to professional counseling are important in the

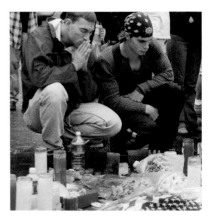

recovery process. New generations of anti-anxiety drugs can help individuals who have difficulties. Sleep aids and other options are available to ease short-term symptoms.

Sources: Posttraumatic Stress Disorder Society, "Posttraumatic Stress Disorder," 2003, www .mentalhealth.com/dis/p20-an06.html; National Center for Post Traumatic Stress, 2004, www.ncptsd.org; National Mental Health Association, "Coping with Disaster," 2001. www.nmha .org/ reassurance/collegetips.cfm; "Mental Health: A Report of the Surgeon General," www.surgeongeneral.gov/library/mentalhealth/; E. L. MacGeorge et al., "Stress, Social Support, and Health Among College Students after September 11, 2001," *Journal of College Student Development* 45 (2004): 655–670.

overwhelming. Family members are often a steady base of support on which you can rely. But if friends or family are unavailable, most colleges and universities offer counseling services at no cost for short-term crises. Clergy, instructors, and dorm supervisors also may be excellent resources. If university services are unavailable, or if you are concerned about confidentiality, most communities offer low-cost counseling through mental health clinics.

Taking Mental Action

Stress management calls for mental action in two areas. First, positive self-esteem, which can help you cope with stressful situations, comes from learned habits and responses to people and events. Successful stress management involves mentally developing and practicing self-esteem skills, focusing on positive thinking about yourself, and examining self-talk to reduce irrational responses. Focus on the here and now rather than on past problems.

Second, because you can't always anticipate what the next stressor will be, you need to develop the mental skills necessary to manage your reactions after it has occurred. The ability to react productively and appropriately comes with time, practice, patience, and experience with a variety of stressful situations.

Change the Way You Think As noted earlier our appraisals, thoughts, and ideas of people and situations are what make these things stressful, not the people or situations themselves. To combat negative

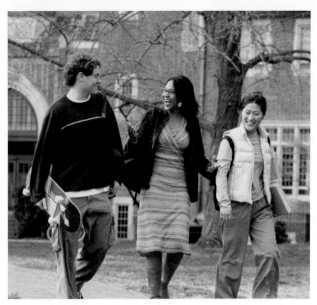

Spending time with friends is an important part of stress reduction.

self-talk, we must first become aware of it, then stop it, and finally replace the negative thoughts with positive ones—a process referred to as **cognitive restructuring.** Several types of negative self-talk exist, but among the most common are pessimism, or focusing on the negative; perfectionism, or expecting super-human standards; "should-ing," or reprimanding yourself for items that you should have done; blaming yourself or others for circumstances and events; and dichotomous thinking, where everything is either black or white (good or bad) instead of gradations.[52] Once you realize that some of your thoughts may be irrational or overreactive, interrupt this self-talk by saying aloud or subvocally "stop," and make a conscious effort to adjust your thinking. Focus on more positive patterns. If we can learn to view potential stressors more positively we can reduce our stress levels without having to remove the potential stressors. Here are specific actions you can take to develop these mental skills.

- *Worry constructively.* Don't waste time and energy worrying about things you can't change or events that may never happen.

- *Look at life as being fluid.* If you accept that change is a natural part of living and growing, the jolt of changes will become less stressful.

- *Consider alternatives.* Remember, there is seldom only one appropriate action. Anticipating options will help you plan for change and adjust more rapidly.

Cognitive restructuring   The modification of thoughts, ideas, and beliefs that contribute to stress.

- *Moderate your expectations.* Aim high, but be realistic about your circumstances and motivation.

- *Weed out trivia.* Cardiologist Robert Eliot offers two rules for coping with life's challenges: "Don't sweat the small stuff," and remember that "It's all small stuff."

- *Don't rush into action.* Think before you act.

- *Tolerate mistakes by yourself and others.* Rather than getting angry or frustrated by mishaps, evaluate what happened and learn from them.

- *Live simply.* Eliminate unnecessary things and obligations. Prioritize. Commitments should be to things you have to and want to do.

Once you have improved your mental outlook and gained a more positive perspective on life, you will find it easier to cope with stressors.

Try it ▸NOW

A penny for your thoughts! Negative self-talk can contribute to feelings of stress. Try this exercise now to see how often you have negative emotional responses. Place a handful of pennies in your right-hand pocket and each time you catch yourself having a negative thought, remove a penny from your right pocket and place it in your left pocket. After this exercise, resolve to replace negative thoughts with a positive or optimistic statement that boosts your self-esteem.

Managing Emotional Responses

Have you ever gotten all worked up about something only to find that your perceptions were totally wrong? We often get upset, not by realities but by our faulty perceptions. For example, suppose you found out that everyone except you is invited to a party. You might easily begin to wonder why you were excluded. Does someone dislike you? Have you offended someone? Such thoughts are typical. However, the reality of the situation may have absolutely nothing to do with your being liked or disliked. Perhaps you were sent an invitation, and it didn't get to you.

Stress management requires that you examine your self-talk and your emotional responses to interactions with others. With any emotional response to a stressor, you are responsible for the emotion and the resultant behaviors. Learning to tell the difference between normal emotions and those based on irrational beliefs can help you stop the emotion or express it in a healthy and appropriate way.

Table 3.2
Strategies for Anger Control

1. **Calm yourself.** There are many relaxation techniques. Find one that works for you and bring yourself back to a level feeling.
2. **Change your thoughts about the situation.** When angry, many people act out in verbally abusive or other dramatic ways. Instead of screeching and yelling, tell yourself that you are justified in being angry and that you have a right to be upset, but don't act overtly. Remember that "get it all out of your system" impulse is really not productive. It only makes you feel good for a bit, and then you realize that you have hurt others and said much more than you should have—and in the end, nothing is changed. Avoid thoughts or statements such as "never" or "always." Stay in the present.
3. **Improve your communication with the person who has made you angry or frustrated.** Talk with them when you are calm. Be direct and assertive. Let them know how you feel without being aggressive or attacking them. Social psychologist Carol Tavris, in her book *Anger: The Misunderstood Emotion,* says that anger should be expressed directly at the person or object that is perceived to have violated personal space, values, or identity, not randomly. If you can't express it immediately, try writing down your feelings and thoughts in a journal and describe what you'd like to see changed. Be clear when you talk with the person and try to keep your comments to "I" rather than

"you" statements (e.g., "I feel like I have been insulted in some way," rather than "You insulted me").
4. **Don't fight back. It is natural to get upset if you feel attacked or criticized.** Instead of reacting with anger, listen to what the person is saying, ask clarifying questions, and keep your cool. When the person has finished talking, acknowledge that you have heard and then express your own feelings.
5. **Use humor if possible.** Sometimes, the sheer volatility of a situation requires a bit of defusing, similar to the comic relief that accompanies a long dramatic passage in a movie or play. Try to defuse the situation if possible, and don't allow it to escalate. However, this doesn't mean sitting there with a smirk on your face or laughing at the other person or being sarcastic. Try to get the other person to laugh with you.
6. **Recognize that certain situations may cause little things to blow out of proportion.** Drinking, not enough sleep, responses to loss, and other situations may make people short fused. Avoid conflict when you are tired or too drained to respond appropriately, and respect these needs in others.
7. **Seek help.** If you feel about yourself or have others telling you that you are a chronically hostile or angry person, seek help. Your school has counselors who are able to help you. Talk with them or someone else you trust.

Source: C. Tavris, *Anger: The Misunderstood Emotion* (Carmichael, CA: Touchstone Books, 1989).

Fighting the Anger Urge Anger usually results when we feel we have lost control of a situation and/or are frustrated by a situation that we can do little about. The five main sources of anger are related to threats to (1) safety and well-being; (2) power; (3) perfectionism and pride; (4) self-sufficiency and autonomy; and (5) self-esteem and status.[53]

Anger may vary in intensity from mild irritation to rage and may be acted out as cynicism, sarcasm, intimidation, frustration, impatience, quick flaring of temper, distrust, or anxiety. Not all anger is inherently bad. Sometimes, it can give us the energy we need to fight back if attacked or the resolve to work even harder to accomplish a goal. It is unresolved anger, the kind that festers and clouds our reasoning and our reactions, that we need to control.

Each of us has learned by this point in our lives that we have three main approaches to dealing with anger: expressing it, suppressing it, or calming it. You may be surprised to find out that *expressing* your anger is probably the healthiest thing to do in the long run, particularly if you express anger in an assertive rather than aggressive way. However, it's a natural reaction to want to respond aggressively, and that is what we must learn to keep at bay. To be able to do this, there are several things that you can do (see also Table 3.2):[54]

- Understand what anger is and how you tend to express it.
- Develop an awareness and acceptance of your own tendency to anger.
- Recognize your anger patterns: When do you get angry and how often? Who makes you angry?
- Learn and practice good communication.
- Respect others and yourself.

Taking Physical Action

Physical activities can complement the emotional and mental strategies of stress management.

Exercise Exercise reduces stress by raising levels of endorphins—mood-elevating, pain-killing hormones—in the bloodstream. Exercise increases energy, reduces hostility, and improves mental alertness. It also can be a source of social interaction, which further reduces stressor effects.

Most of us have relieved stress by engaging in vigorous physical activity: joining a kick-boxing class is one example. Exercise performed as an immediate response can help alleviate stress symptoms. However, a regular exercise program yields even more substantial benefits. Try to engage in at least 25 minutes of aerobic exercise three or four times a week. Although it may not improve your aerobic capacity, a quiet walk can refresh your mind, calm your stress response, and replenish your adaptation energy stores. Plan walking breaks alone or with friends, or stretch after prolonged periods of study at your desk. A short period of physical exercise may provide the break you really need. For more information on the beneficial effects of exercise, see Chapter 11.

Relax Like exercise, relaxation can help you cope with stressful feelings, preserve adaptation energy stores, dissipate excess hormones associated with the fight-or-flight response, and refocus your energies. Relaxation techniques that involve both the mind and body are great stress reducers for college students.[55] Yoga and other exercises that increase flexibility also aid in relaxation (see Chapter 11). Practice relaxation daily until it becomes a habit. You probably will find that you enjoy it.

Once you have learned simple relaxation techniques, you can use them at any time—before or during a tough exam or when faced with a stressful confrontation or assignment, for example. As your body relaxes, your heart rate slows, your blood pressure and metabolic rate decrease, and many other body-calming effects occur, all of which allow you to channel energy appropriately. (See the Skills for Behavior Change box on page 82 on relaxation techniques.)

Eat Right Is food really a de-stressor? Whether foods can calm us and nourish our psyches is a controversial question. High-potency supplements that are supposed to boost resistance against stress-related ailments are nothing more than gimmicks. But it is clear that eating a balanced, healthful diet will help provide the stamina you need to get through problems and will stress-proof you in ways that are not fully understood. It also is known that undereating, overeating, and eating the wrong kinds of foods can create distress in the body. In particular, food substances that produce (or mimic) stress-like responses, called **sympathomimetics,** should be avoided. The most common sympathomimetic is caffeine, commonly found in colas, coffee, tea, and chocolate. Sugar is often considered a sympathomimetic, but much of what has been published about hyperactivity and its relation to the consumption of sweets has been shown to be scientifically invalid. For more information about the benefits of sound nutrition, see Chapter 9.

Sympathomimetics Food substances that can produce stress-like responses.

Managing Your Time

How can I prioritize everything I try to do in a day?

Time. Everybody needs more of it, especially students trying to balance the demands of classes, social life, earning money for school, and family obligations. Keep a journal for one week to become aware of your time patterns (Figure 3.3) and use the following time management tips in your stress management program.

- *Take on only one thing at a time.* Don't try to pay bills, wash clothes, and write your term paper all at once. Stay focused.

- *Clean off your desk.* Go through the things on your desk, toss the unnecessary papers, and put into folders the papers for tasks that you must do. When bills come in, take care of them immediately. Write a check and hold it for mailing. Read your mail, and file it or toss it.

- *Find a clean, comfortable place to work.* Go someplace where you won't be distracted.

- *Prioritize your tasks.* Make a daily "to do" list, and try to stick to it. Categorize the things you must do today, the things that you have to do but not immediately, and the things that it would be nice to do. Only consider the Nice to Do items if you finish the others or if the Nice to Do list includes something fun. Give yourself a reward as you finish each task.

- *Don't be afraid to say no.* All too often, we do things out of fear of what someone may think. Set your school and personal priorities and live according to your own agenda, values, and goals.

- *Avoid interruptions.* When you've got a project that requires total concentration, schedule uninterrupted time. Don't answer the phone; close your door and post a Do Not Disturb sign; go to a quiet room in the library or student union where no one will find you.

- *Reward yourself for being efficient.* Did you finish a task early? Take some time for yourself. See a movie or go for a walk. Differentiate between rest breaks and work breaks. Work breaks simply mean switching tasks for awhile. Rest breaks give you time to yourself to help you recharge and refresh your energy levels.

- *Use time to your advantage.* If you're a morning person, schedule activities to coincide with the time when you're at your best. Take a short nap or break when you need it.

- *Break overwhelming tasks into small pieces, and allocate a certain amount of time to each.* If you are floundering in a task, move on and come back to it when you're refreshed.

- *Remember that time is precious.* Many people learn to value their time only when they face a terminal

Activity	Monday	Tuesday	Wednesday	Thursday	Friday	Saturday	Sunday	Total Hours
Getting ready								
On the road								
In class								
Working for pay								
Exercising								
Eating (meals & snacks)								
Studying								
Watching TV, videos								
Using computer (school-related)								
Using computer (recreational)								
Spending time with friends								
Leisure activities								
Other (specify)								
Total Hours								

Figure 3.3 ■ How Do You Spend Your Time?

Fill in your daily activities for a week, and assess where you spend time. Are there any activities you could cut back or that you would like to increase?

illness. Try to value each day. Time spent not enjoying life is a tremendous waste of potential.

Alternative Stress Management Techniques

Popular stress fighters include visualization, hypnosis, massage therapy, meditation, and biofeedback.

Visualization Often it is our own thoughts and imagination that provoke distress by conjuring up worst-case scenarios and exaggerating the significance of situations. Our imagination, however, can be an asset as well as a liability. **Visualization,** or the creation of mental scenes, works by engaging one's imagination of the physical senses of sight, sound, smell, taste, and feel to replace stressful stimuli with peaceful or pleasurable thoughts. The choice of mental images is unlimited, but natural settings such as ocean beaches and mountain lakes are often used because they simulate vacation locations where people typically go to escape the stress of home, school, or work environments.[56] So the next time you are feeling stressed, close your eyes, imagine yourself at some tranquil location full of color, fresh air,

soothing sounds, and other elements of nature, and take a mini mental vacation to allow your mind and body a chance to unwind.

Hypnosis **Hypnosis** is a process that requires a person to focus on one thought, object, or voice, thereby freeing the right hemisphere of the brain to become more active. The person then becomes unusually responsive to suggestion. Whether self-induced or induced by someone else, hypnosis can reduce certain types of stress.

Massage Therapy If you have ever had someone massage your stiff neck or aching feet, you know that massage is an excellent way to relax. Massage techniques vary from vigorous Swedish massage to the gentler acupressure and Esalen massage. Before selecting a

Visualization The creation of mental images to promote relaxation.

Hypnosis A process that allows people to become unusually responsive to suggestion.

Relaxation techniques for stress reduction have been practiced for centuries, and there is a wide selection from which to choose.

Yoga

An estimated 20 million adults in America actively engage in yoga, an ancient tradition that combines meditation, stretching, and breathing exercises designed to relax, refresh, and rejuvenate. There are several popular versions.

Classical yoga is the ancestor of nearly all forms of yoga practiced today. Breathing, poses, and verbal mantras are often part of classical yoga.

Kripalu is a gentle, introspective practice in which much emphasis is placed on breathing techniques and releasing emotional blockages. Initially practitioners concentrate mainly on poses and deep breathing followed by emotional exercises. In later stages, practitioners focus primarily on poses. Kripalu is particularly suited for those who want to go slowly and gently or who have underlying injuries or problems.

Ashtanga yoga is designed to improve sport performance with deep breathing and a progressive series of postures. Less well-known than other forms, this type of yoga is growing in popularity.

Hot yoga, also known as *bikram yoga*, differs from traditional yoga in that classes are held in rooms where the temperatures are up to 105 degrees Fahrenheit. After going through up to 26 poses, students emerge from these classes drained of energy, drenched in sweat, and feeling cleansed. Although bikram centers have sprung up across the country, there have been reports of heat exhaustion, dehydration, and other problems. This style of yoga is risky for those with hypertension, certain respiratory conditions, and other cardiovascular risks. If you feel weak, dizzy, nauseated, or have other ill effects, use caution. Before attending a class, speak with your doctor if you have questions or concerns, and make sure you go to a reputable facility with qualified staff.

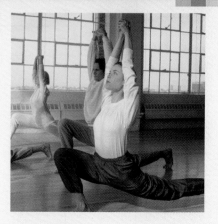

Qigong

Qigong (pronounced *chee-kong*) is one of the fastest-growing and most widely accepted forms of mind–body health exercises. Qigong taps into a complex system of internal pathways called meridians, which are thought to run along the length of the body. According to Chinese medicine, meridians carry *chi,* or vital energy, throughout your body. If your chi becomes stagnant or blocked, you'll feel sluggish or powerless. Thus, a series of flowing movements, mental visualization exercises, and

massage therapist, check his or her credentials carefully. The therapist should have training from a reputable program that teaches scientific principles for anatomic manipulation and should be certified through the American Massage Therapy Association. Chapter 18 provides more information about the benefits of massage as well as other body-based methods such as acupressure and shiatsu.

Meditation There are many different forms of **meditation.** Most involve sitting quietly for 15 to 20 minutes, focusing on a particular word or symbol, controlling breathing, and getting in touch with the inner self. Practiced by Eastern religions for centuries, meditation is believed to be an important form of introspection and personal renewal. As a stress management tool, it can calm the body and quiet the mind, creating a sense of peace.

> **Meditation** A relaxation technique that involves focusing on a word or symbol, controlling breathing, and getting in touch with the inner self.
>
> **Biofeedback** A technique that involves self-monitoring by machine of physical responses to stress and attempts to control the responses.

Biofeedback **Biofeedback** involves self-monitoring by machine of physical responses to stress and attempts to control these responses. The machine records perspiration, heart rate, respiration, blood pressure, surface body temperature, muscle tension, and other stress responses. Various relaxation techniques are employed while the person is hooked up to a biofeedback machine and, through trial-and-error and signals from the machine, the person learns to lower his or her stress response. Eventually, the person develops the ability to recognize and lower stress responses without using the machine.

vocalizations of healing sounds such as "shhhuuu" are designed to integrate and refresh through easy-to-perform techniques.

Diaphragmatic or Deep Breathing

Typically, we breathe only using the upper chest and thoracic region rather than involving the abdominal region. Simply stated, diaphragmatic breathing is deep breathing that maximally expands the chest by involving the movement of the lower abdomen. This technique is commonly used in yoga exercises. The diaphragmatic breathing process occurs in three stages.

Stage 1: Assume a comfortable position. Whether sitting or lying down on your back, find the most natural position to be in. Close your eyes, unbutton your shirt or binding clothes, remove your belt, or unbutton your pants. Often it works best to fold your hands over your abdomen and get used to feeling the rise and fall of your stomach.

Stage 2: Concentrate on the act of breathing. Shut out external noise. Focus on inhaling, exhaling, and the route the air is following. Try saying to yourself, "Feel the warm air coming into your nose, warming your windpipe, and flowing into your lungs. Feel your stomach rise and fall as you inhale slowly and exhale slowly, noting the air flowing out of your nose or mouth." Repeat this action several times.

Stage 3: Visualize. The above stages seem to work best when combined with visualization. A common example is to visualize clean, fresh, invigorating air slowly entering the nose and being exhaled as gray, stale air that has accumulated in the body. Such processes, particularly when they involve the whole body, seem to help deep breathers become more refreshed from their experience.

Progressive Muscle Relaxation

Progressive muscle relaxation involves systematically contracting and relaxing each of several muscle groups; proper breathing and concentration are part of this process. Again, find a comfortable position similar to that discussed in the deep breathing section above, and begin a deep breathing cycle. The difference from diaphragmatic breathing is that, as you concentrate on inhaling, you also contract a particular muscle group (for example, the hand and fingers). Hold that position for a short period and then, as you exhale, slowly release the muscles that you have been contracting. Repeat and add more muscle groups. You might start with a hand, then move to the forearm, the entire arm, the neck, to the shoulders, back, buttocks, foot, and thigh. You can add components of other relaxation techniques to this experience by saying, "My hands are getting warmer, my arm is getting warmer," and so on as you work to gain maximum control of blood flow and muscle tension in a region.

Source: Paragraph on qigong from C. Dold, "The New Yoga," *Health* (May 2004): 73–77.

DEVELOPING YOUR SPIRITUAL SIDE: MINDFULNESS

In discussions of spirituality, the concept of mindfulness often emerges. As a meditative technique, **mindfulness**—the ability to be fully present in the moment—can aid relaxation; reduce emotional and physical pain; and help us connect more effectively with ourselves, with others, and with nature. The practice of mindfulness includes strategies and activities that contribute to overall health and wellness. In fact, mindfulness and wellness are interconnected and can be developed concurrently, each reinforcing the other. In addition to the themes of spirituality discussed in Chapter 2, we can think of spirituality as encompassing four dimensions: physical, emotional, social, and intellectual.

The Physical Dimension: Moving in Nature

A delightful way to strengthen the body, build endurance, and bring peace of mind is to interact with the natural environment. Activities such as walking, jogging, biking, and swimming foster this interaction, providing sensory experience (feeling, smelling, touching, listening, and hearing) while strengthening muscles and the cardiovascular system. By focusing on the birdsong or the crunch of your shoes on freshly fallen snow, you can free yourself of worry or anxious thoughts. Appreciating and absorbing the beauty of nature allow us to unwind emotionally even as our bodies are at work.

Mindfulness The ability to be fully present in the moment.

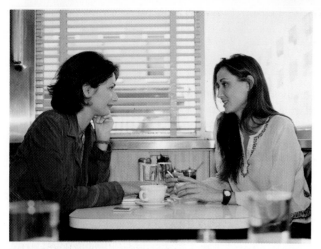

Healthy and effective communication is an important element to our social dimension of spiritual health.

The Emotional Dimension: Dealing with Negative Feelings

Each of us has positive and negative emotions that govern moods and behaviors throughout the day. We often take joy, happiness, and contentment for granted since we tend not to notice the *absence* of stress and distress. However, we typically are aware of negative emotions, such as jealousy, hatred, and anger, because they deplete our energy reserves and cause us problems in interacting with others.

To improve our emotional health and access our spiritual side, we must take notice of the situations that trigger negative emotions (see the Type A Personality and Hostility and the Fighting the Anger Urge sections earlier in this chapter). By stopping in the midst of anger and concentrating on physical reactions, we realize the full extent of the damage we inflict upon ourselves when we allow negativity to get the best of us. We might ask ourselves, Is it worth it? And probably we will conclude: "I don't like allowing this kind of hit on my body. I've got to get a handle on this before I hurt myself or someone else." By practicing thought-stopping, blocking negative thoughts, and focusing on positive emotions via self-talk and other methods of diversion, we can help ourselves through a negative experience.

Equally important as the control of negative emotions is the development of spiritual wholeness characterized by faith, hope, and love, the beliefs mentioned in Chapter 2. These beliefs contribute to spiritual growth and also lessen the negative effects of stress.

The Social Dimension: Interacting, Listening, and Communicating

Developing the spiritual side is not just an internal process. It is also a social process that enhances relationships with others. The ability to give and take, speak and listen, forgive and move on are all integral to spiritual development.

Today, life is busier than ever. While constantly juggling responsibilities, it is easy to get so caught up in the stresses of our own lives that we find it difficult to give to others. Being too self-enmeshed can affect relationships and the ability to communicate with others. Communication is a two-way process in which listening is every bit as important as speaking. Learning to listen actively is a potent asset. Active listeners take note of content, intent, and feelings being expressed. They listen to all levels of the communication. Sensitivity and honesty are also essential to the give and take of communication. Ask questions, rephrase the speaker's ideas, and focus genuine attention on the speaker. Through such active participation, we gain a greater insight into the other person, who in turn will be encouraged to share more. Sharing becomes more intimate and relationships more connected when people feel that others care and are genuinely interested in their well-being. Both parties benefit from such an interchange. For more on communication, see Chapter 5.

The Intellectual Dimension: Sharpening Intuition

Take the time to assess events in life, their causes, and your own involvement in them. This often involves putting aside our emotional dimension for a moment to reflect, read, and ponder. Sometimes this process leads to startling new insights. Such moments mean so much, but few people include this mental activity in daily rituals. Examining the past, how we've gotten to where we are in the present, and what actions might have changed the course of events is a critical element of spiritual growth. By using our minds for objective reasoning, we develop the intellectual dimension of spiritual health.

Taking Charge

Summary

- Stress is an inevitable part of our lives. Eustress refers to stress associated with positive events, distress to negative events.

- The alarm, resistance, and exhaustion phases of the general adaptation syndrome involve physiological responses to both real and imagined stressors and cause a complex cascade of hormones to rush through the body. Prolonged arousal due to stress may be detrimental to health.

- Undue stress for extended periods of time can compromise the immune system and result in serious health consequences. Psychoneuroimmunology is the science that analyzes the relationship between the mind's reaction to stress and the function of the immune system. While increasing evidence links disease susceptibility to stress, much of this research remains controversial. However, stress has been linked to numerous health problems, including CVD, diabetes, cancer, and increased susceptibility to infectious diseases.

- Multiple factors contribute to stress and the stress response. Psychosocial factors include change, hassles, pressure, inconsistent goals and behaviors, conflict, overload, and burnout. Other factors are environmental stressors and self-imposed stress. Persons subjected to discrimination or bias due to "isms" may face unusually high levels of stress.

- College can be especially stressful. Recognizing the signs of stress is the first step toward better health. Learning to reduce test anxiety and cope with multiple stressors is also important.

- Managing stress begins with learning simple coping mechanisms: assessing stressors, changing responses, and learning to cope. Finding out what works best for you—probably some combination of managing emotional responses, taking mental or physical action, downshifting, learning time management, or using alternative stress management techniques—will help you better cope with stress in the long run.

- Developing the spiritual side involves practicing mindfulness and its many dimensions. These include the physical dimension (moving in nature); the emotional dimension (identifying and controlling negative feelings); the social dimension (interacting, listening, and communicating); and the intellectual dimension (sharpening intuition).

Chapter Review

1. Even though André experienced stress when he graduated from college and moved to a new city, he viewed it as an opportunity for growth. What is André's stress called?
   a. strain
   b. distress
   c. eustress
   d. adaptive response

2. The branch of the autonomic nervous system that is responsible for energizing the body for either fight or flight and for triggering many other stress responses is the
   a. central nervous system.
   b. parasympathetic nervous system.
   c. sympathetic nervous system.
   d. endocrine system.

3. During what phase of the general adaptation syndrome has the physical and psychological energy used to fight the stressors been depleted?
   a. alarm phase
   b. resistance phase
   c. endurance phase
   d. exhaustion phase

4. A state of physical and mental exhaustion caused by excessive stress is called
   a. conflict.
   b. overload.
   c. hassles.
   d. burnout.

5. At Bev's new job, there is excessive time pressure and responsibility coupled with a lack of support by co-workers. Bev risks suffering from
   a. hassles.
   b. overload.
   c. conflict.
   d. burnout.

6. Suzanne Kobasa characterized psychologically healthy people as having all of the following, *except*
   a. control.
   b. charm.
   c. commitment.
   d. challenge.

7. Losing your keys is an example of what psychosocial source of stress?
   a. pressure
   b. inconsistent behaviors
   c. hassles
   d. conflict

8. After five years of 70-hour work weeks, Tom decided to leave his high-paying, high-stress law firm and lead a simpler lifestyle. What is this trend called?
   a. adaptation
   b. conflict resolution
   c. burnout reduction
   d. downshifting

9. Deep breathing is also known as
   a. qigong.
   b. yoga.
   c. diaphragmatic breathing.
   d. progressive muscle relaxation.

10. What stress-fighting technique is a process that allows people to become unusually responsive to suggestion?
   a. meditation
   b. hypnosis
   c. massage
   d. biofeedback

Answers to these questions can be found on page A-1.

Questions for Discussion and Reflection

1. Compare and contrast distress and eustress. Are both types of stress potentially harmful?

2. Describe the alarm, resistance, and exhaustion phases of the general adaptation syndrome and the body's physiological response to stress. Does stress lead to more irritability or emotionality, or does emotionality lead to stress? Provide examples.

3. What are some of the health risks that result from chronic stress? How does the study of PNI link stress and illness?

4. What major factors seem to influence the nature and extent of a person's susceptibility to stress? Explain how social support, self-esteem, and personality may make a person more or less susceptible.

5. Why are some students more vulnerable to stress than others? What services are available on your campus to help you deal with excessive stress?

6. What can college students do to inoculate themselves against negative stress effects? What actions can you take to manage your stressors? How can you help others manage their stressors more effectively?

7. How does anger affect the body? Discuss the steps you can take to fight your own anger and help your friends control theirs.

8. What can you do to develop the dimensions of spirituality in your life? How can you apply the social dimension of spirituality to your current relationships?

Accessing Your Health on the Internet

The following websites explore further topics and issues related to personal health. For links to the websites below, visit the Companion Website for *Health: The Basics,* Seventh Edition at www.aw-bc.com/donatelle.

1. *American College Counseling Association.* This website of the professional organization for college counselors offers useful links and articles.

2. *American College Health Association.* Provides information and data from the National College Health Assessment survey.

3. *Center for Anxiety and Stress Treatment.* Provides resources and services regarding a broad range of stress-related topics.

4. *Hampden-Sydney College.* Provides links to helpful tips for dealing with stressful issues college students commonly experience.

5. *Mind Tools.* Focuses on all aspects of stress and stress management.

6. *National Institute of Mental Health.* A resource for information on all aspects of mental health, including the effects of stress.

Further Reading

"Health and Stress: The Newsletter of the American Institute of Stress," www.stress.org/news.htm

Excellent monthly resource on stress. Reports on latest developments in all areas of stress research. Each issue contains a listing of meetings of interest and a book review.

Greenberg, J. S. *Comprehensive Stress Management,* 9th ed. New York: McGraw-Hill, 2004.

An overview of current perspectives on stress and the influence of personal control and behavior on health. Discusses stress management as a factor in controlling pain, anxiety, and depression. An excellent resource for health professionals.

Romas, J. A. and M. Sharma. *Practical Stress Management,* 4th ed. San Francisco: Benjamin Cummings, 2007.

An accessible text that combines theory and principles with hands-on exercises to manage stress. Includes an audio CD with guided relaxation techniques such as progressive muscle relaxation, deep breathing, and visual imaging.

Seaward, B. *Managing Stress: Principles and Strategies for Health and Well-Being,* 4th ed. Sudbury, MA: Jones and Bartlett, 2004.

Spirituality and stress expert provides complete overview of stress and health effects, as well as strategies for reducing risk.

Weil, A. *Ask Dr. Weil.* New York: Random House, 2003.

Weil, a holistic doctor, has written this and other books giving overviews of mind–body health and alternative strategies for coping with life's challenges.

References

1. L. J. Sax et al., *The American Freshman: National Norms for Fall 2004* (Los Angeles: Higher Education Research Institute, 2005).

2. H. Anisman and Z. Merali, "Understanding Stress: Characteristics and Caveats," *Alcohol Research & Health* 23, no. 4 (1999): 241–249.

3. W. B. Cannon, *The Wisdom of the Body* (New York: W. W. Norton, 1932).

4. H. Selye, "A Syndrome Produced by Diverse Nocuous Agents," *Nature* 138, no. 32 (1936).

5. S. Dickerson and M. Kemeny, "Acute Stressors and Cortisol Responses: A Theoretical Integration and Synthesis of Laboratory Research," *Psychological Bulletin* 130, no. 3 (2005): 355–360.

6. A. Mokdad et al., "Actual causes of death in the United States 2000," *Journal of the American Medical Association* 291 (2004): 1238–1245.

7. M. D. Jeremko, "Stress Inoculation Training: A Generic Approach for the Prevention of Stress-Related Disorders," *The Personal and Guidance Journal* 62 (1984): 544–550; H. S. Freidman and S. Booth-Kewley, "The Disease-Prone Personality: A Meta-Analytic View of the Construct," *American Psychologist* 42 (1987): 539–555; S. Segerstrom and G. Miller, "Psychological Stress and the Human Immune System: A Meta-Analysis Study of 30 Years of Inquiry," *Psychological Bulletin* 130, no. 4 (2004): 601.

8. G. E. Vaillant, *Adaptation to Life* (Boston: Little, Brown, 1977); National Center for Chronic Disease Prevention and Health Promotion, "Bridging the Gap Between Physical and Mental Illness," *Chronic Disease Notes and Reports* 16, no. 1 (2003).

9. S. A. Lyness, "Predictions of Differences between Type A and B Individuals in Heart Rate and Blood Pressure Reactivity," *Psychological Bulletin* 114 (1993): 266–295; J. C. Barefoot and M. Schroll, "Symptoms of Depression, Acute Myocardial Infarction, and Total Mortality in a Community Sample, 1976–1980," *Circulation* 93 (1996); G. Schiraldi, T. Spalding, and C. Holford, "Expanding Health Educators' Roles to Meet Critical Needs in Stress Management and Mental Health," *Journal of Health Education* 70 (1998).

10. M. Greer, "Mental Stress Wreaks Havoc on Workers." (Paper presented at the International Commission on Occupational Health's Fourth International Conference on Work Environment and Occupational Diseases, Newport Beach, CA, March 9–11, 2005).

11. Ibid.

12. J. R. Hapuarachchi et al., "Changes in Clinically Relevant Metabolites with Psychological Stress Parameters," *Behavioral Medicine* 29 (2003): 52–60; C. N. Merz et al., Psychosocial Stress and Cardiovascular Disease: Pathophysiological Links," *Behavioral Medicine* 27 (2002): 141–148.

13. Segerstrom, "Psychological Stress and Human Immune System."

14. M. E. Kemeny, "The Psychobiology of Stress," *Current Directions in Psychological Science* 12 (2003): 124–130.

15. S. Cohen et al., "Social Ties and Susceptibility to the Common Cold," *The Journal of the American Medical Association* 277 (1997): 1940–1944.

16. R. Glaser et al., "The Influence of Psychological Stress on the Immune Response to Vaccines," *Annals of the New York Academy of Sciences* 840 (1998): 649–655.

17. A. Smith, "Breakfast, Stress, and Catching Colds," *Journal of Family Health Care* 13, no. 1 (2003).

18. S. Cohen et al., "Types of Stressors That Increase Susceptibility to the Common Cold in Adults," *Health Psychology* 17 (1998): 214–223.

19. R. Kessler, "The Effects of Stressful Life Events on Depression," *Annual Reviews of Psychology* 48 (1997): 191–214.

20. American Diabetes Association, "Stress," 2004, www.diabetes.org/type-1-diabetes/stress.jsp.

21. G. R. Schiraldi, T. W. Spalding, and C. W. Hofford, "Expanding Health Educators' Role to Meet Critical Needs in Stress Management and Mental Health," *Journal of Health Education* 29 (1998): 68–77.

22. V. R. Wilburn and D. E. Smith, "Stress, Self-Esteem, and Suicidal Ideation in Late Adolescents," *Adolescence* 40 (2005): 33–46.

23. "The Doctors Are 'In'," *Newsweek* 140 (October 2002), 58.

24. T. Holmes and R. Rahe, "The Social Readjustment Rating Scale," *Journal of Psychosocial Research* _____ (1967): 213–217.

25. Ibid., 214.

26. R. Lazarus, "The Trivialization of Distress," in *Preventing Health Risk Behaviors and Promoting Coping with Illness*, eds. J. Rosen and L. Solomon (Hanover, NH: University Press of New England, 1985), 279–298.

27. D. J. Maybery and D. Graham, "Hassles and Uplifts: Including Interpersonal Events," *Stress and Health* 17 (2001): 91–104.

28. R. Blonna, *Coping with Stress in a Changing World*, 3rd ed. (Boston: McGraw Hill, 2005).

29. L. Lefton, *Psychology* (Boston: Allyn and Bacon, 1994), 471.

30. M. Kenny and K. Rice, "Attachment to Parents and Adjustment in College Students: Current Status, Applications, and Future Considerations," *The Counseling Psychologist* 23 (1995): 433–456.

31. T. Bartlett, "Freshman Pay Mentally and Physically as They Adjust to Life in College," *Chronicle of Higher Education (*February 1, 2002): 4.

32. C. Park et al., "The Daily Stress and Coping Process and Alcohol Use Among College Students," *Journal of Studies on Alcohol* 65, no. 1 (2004): 126–130.

33. T. LaVeist, *Minority Populations and Health: An Introduction to Health Disparities* (San Francisco, CA: Jossey Bass, 2006); T. Lewis, "Discrimination, Black Americans, and Health: Results of the SWAN Study" (Paper presented at the American Heart Association, 45th Annual Conference on Cardiovascular Disease Epidemiology and Prevention. Washington, DC, 2005).

34. K. J. Karren et al., *Mind/Body Health: The Effects of Attitudes, Emotions, and Relationships*, 3rd ed. (San Francisco: Benjamin Cummings, 2006).

35. B. L. Seaward, *Managing Stress: Principles and Strategies for Health and Well-Being*, 4th ed. (Boston: Jones & Bartlett, 2004); Wilburn and Smith, "Stress, Self-Esteem, and Suicidal Ideation."

36. Ibid., Wilburn and Smith.

37. K. Glanz, B. Rimer, and F. Levis, F. (eds.), *Health Behavior and Health Education: Theory, Research, and Practice*, 3rd ed. (San Francisco, CA: Jossey Bass, 2002).

38. J. M. Twenge, Z. Liqing, and C. Im, "It's Beyond My Control: A Cross-Temporal Meta-Analysis of Increasing Externality in Locus of Control, 1960–2002," *Personality and Social Psychology Review* 8 (2004): 308–320.

39. M. Friedman and R. H. Rosenman, *Type A Behavior and Your Heart* (New York: Knopf, 1974).

40. Karren et al., "Mind/Body Health."

41. R. Ragland and R. Brand, "Distrust, Rage May Be Toxic Cores That Put Type A Person at Risk," *Journal of American Medical Association* 261 (1989): 813, 814; J. C. Barefoot, W. G. Dahlstrom, and R. B. Williams, "Hostility, CHD Incidence, and Total Mortality: A 25 Year Follow-up Study of 255 Physicians," *Psychosomatic Medicine* 51 (1983): 46–57; J. C. Barefoot et al., "Hostility Patterns and Health Implications: Correlates of Cook-Medley Hostility Scale Scores in a National Survey," *Health Psychology* 10 (1991): 18–24.

42. S. Kobasa, "Stressful Life Events, Personality, and Health: An Inquiry into Hardiness," *Journal of Personality and Social Psychology* 37 (1979): 1–11.

43. B. J. Crowley, B. Hayslip, and J. Hobdy, "Psychological Hardiness and Adjustment to Life Events in Adulthood," *Journal of Adult Development* 10 (2003): 237–248; S. R. Maddi, "The Story of Hardiness: Twenty Years of Theorizing, Research, and Practice," *Consulting Psychology Journal: Practice and Research* 54 (2002): 173–186.

44. American College Health Association, "National College Health Assessment Web Summary," updated June 2004, www.acha.org/projects_programs/ncha_sampledata_public.cfm.

45. L. Reisberg, "Student Stress Is Rising, Especially Among Women," *Chronicle of Higher Education* 46 (2000): A49–A50; L. J. Sax et al., *The American Freshman: National Norms for Fall 2004* (Los Angeles: Higher Education Research Institute, 2005).

46. P. Jackson and M. Finney, "Negative Life Events and Psychological Distress among Young Adults," *Social Psychology Quarterly,* (2003), www.homepages.Indiana.edu/101201/text/stress.html.

47. L. Towbes and L. Cohen, "Chronic Stress in the Lives of College Students: Scale Development and Prospective Prediction of Distress," *Journal of Youth and Adolescence* 25 (1996): 206–217.

48. C. Crandell, J. Preisler, and J. Ausspring, "Measuring Life Event Stress in the Lives of College Students: The Undergraduate Stress Questionnaire (USQ)," *Journal of Behavioral Medicine* 15 (1992): 627–642.

49. National Mental Health Association, "Finding Hope and Help: College Student and Depression Pilot Initiatives," 2004, www.nmha.org/camh/college/index.cfm.

50. Blonna, *Coping with Stress.*

51. S. Levine, D. M. Lyons, and A. F. Schatzberg, "Psychobiological Consequences of Social Relationships," *Annals of the New York Academy of Science* 89, no. 7 (1999): 210–218; M. G. Marmot et al., "Contributions of Psychosocial Factors to Socioeconomic Difference in Health," *Milbank Quarterly* 76 (1998): 403–448; D. P. Phillips, T. E. Ruth, and L. M. Wagner, "Psychology and Survival," *The Lancet* 342 (1993): 1142–1145; D. Ornish et al., "Intensive Lifestyle Changes for Reversal of Coronary Heart Disease," *Journal of the American Medical Association* 280 (1998): 2001–2007; D. Spiegel, "Healing Words: Emotional Expression and Disease Outcome," *Journal of the American Medical Association* 281 (1999): 1328–1329.

52. Seaward, *Managing Stress.*

53. P. Holmes, "Managing Anger: Understanding the Dynamics of Violence, Abuse and Control," SIUC Mental Health Web Site, 2004, www.siu.edu/offices/counsel/anger.htm.

54. Ibid.

55. G. R. Deckro et al., "The Evaluation of Mind/Body Intervention to Reduce Psychological Distress and Perceived Stress in College Students," *Journal of American College Health* 50, no. 6 (May 2002): 281–287.

56. Ibid.

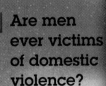

Is there anything I can do to protect myself from terrorism?

What can I do if I think I am being stalked?

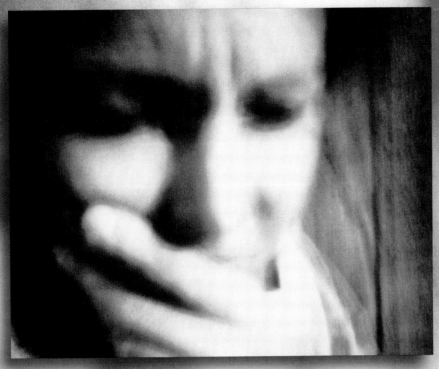

Are men ever victims of domestic violence?

Can my university do anything to make me feel safer?

Violence and Abuse
Creating Healthy Environments

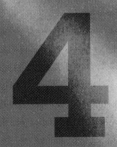

Objectives

- *Differentiate* between intentional and unintentional injuries.
- *Discuss* factors that contribute to homicide, domestic violence, sexual victimization, and other intentional acts of violence in American society.
- *Explain* how terrorism can affect individuals and populations, and summarize practical steps to lower your risk from terrorist attacks.

- *Discuss* strategies to prevent intentional injuries and reduce their risk of occurrence.
- *Explain* how the campus community, law enforcement officials, and individuals can prevent common campus crimes.
- *Discuss* the impact of unintentional injuries on American society, and identify actions that contribute to personal risk of injuries.

"Across the land, waves of violence seem to crest and break, terrorizing Americans in cities and suburbs, in prairie towns, and mountain hollows."

"To millions of Americans few things are more pervasive, more frightening, more real today than violent crime. . . . The fear of being victimized by criminal attack has touched us all in some way."

"Among urban children ages 10–14, homicides are up 150 percent, robberies are up 192 percent, assaults are up 290 percent."

You might think these are statements from today's newspapers or television news. They're not. The first quotation comes from President Herbert Hoover's 1929 inauguration speech, the second from the 1860 Senate report on crime, and the third from a 1967 report on children's violence.[1] Clearly, violence has been a part of U.S. history since our country's early days.

The term **violence** indicates a set of behaviors that produce injuries, regardless of whether they are **intentional injuries** (committed with intent to harm) or **unintentional injuries** (committed without intent to harm, often accidentally). Any definition of violence implicitly includes the use of force, regardless of the intent; however, it is important to realize that some forms of violence are also extremely subtle.

In this chapter, we focus on the various types of intentional and unintentional injuries, the underlying causes of or contributors to these problems, strategies to reduce risk of encountering violence, and possible methods for preventing violence. Although certain indicators of violence, such as murders and deadly assaults, seem to be on the decline, other forms of violence, such as rape and hate crimes, are on the increase. Even more important is that, for all we know about the incidence and prevalence of violence, a great deal remains unknown. Just how many people suffer in silence, failing to report violent acts because of fear of repercussions or because they accept violence as the way life is, remains unknown.

Violence A set of behaviors that produce injuries, as well as the outcomes of these behaviors (the injuries themselves).

Intentional injuries Injuries committed with intent to harm.

Unintentional injuries Injuries committed without intent to harm, often accidentally.

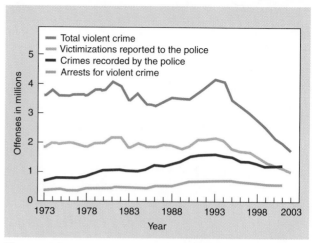

Figure 4.1 ■ Changes in Crime Rates, 1973–2003
Total serious violent crime is the number of homicides recorded by police plus the number of rapes, robberies, and aggravated assaults reported in the National Crime Victimization Survey. Victimization is the number of homicides recorded by police plus other serious crimes that respondents to the survey said were reported to police. Crimes recorded by police and arrests are based on law enforcement reports to the FBI.

Source: Bureau of Justice Statistics, "Key Crime and Justice Facts at a Glance," August 2003, www.ojp.usdoj.gov/bjs/glance.htm.

VIOLENCE IN THE UNITED STATES

Although violence has long been a concern in American society, the U.S. Public Health Service did not formally identify violence as a leading public health problem that contributed significantly to death and disability rates until 1985. The Centers for Disease Control and Prevention (CDC) created the Division of Violence Prevention and considers violence a chronic disease that is pervasive at all levels of American society. Vulnerable populations, such as children, women, black males, and the elderly, were listed as being at high risk for certain types of crime, while older teens and young adults have the highest rates of both violent crime victimization and offending rates.[2]

Recent numbers indicate that rates of most major crime are on the decline (Figure 4.1). In 2003, overall rates of crime continued to decline. It is important to note that over 70 percent of all deaths among persons aged 10 to 24 have violent elements and stem from just four causes: motor vehicle crashes (particularly where alcohol is involved), other unintentional injuries, homicide, and suicide.[3]

Why should we be concerned about a violence-prone society? Violence affects all of us, directly or indirectly. Although the direct victims of violence and those close to them obviously suffer the most, others suffer in various ways because of the climate of fear that violence generates. Women are afraid to walk alone at night. The elderly are often afraid to go out even in the daytime. After terrorist episodes such as the 2001

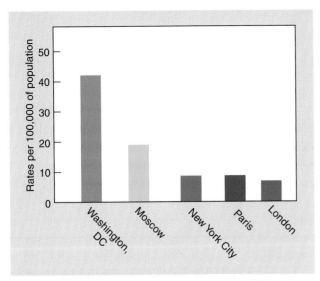

Figure 4.2 ■ International Capital Murder Rates

Is it any wonder the international community views the United States as a violent place?

Source: Home Office of the United Kingdom International Comparisons of Criminal Justice Statistics 2001 (London: Home Office, 2003).

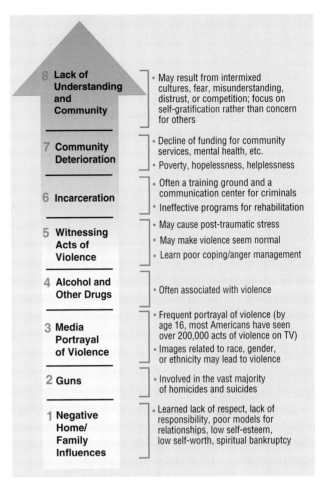

Figure 4.3 ■ Correlates to Violence

World Trade Center attack and the Madrid and London subway attacks, some people are afraid to use mass transportation, work in tall buildings, or travel to popular international destinations. The cost of homeland security is staggering. You might be surprised to learn that international travelers often fear coming to the United States in much the same way that some Americans fear traveling to other regions of the world; tourists fear being robbed at gunpoint, and stories of children dodging bullets while playing in city neighborhoods or of drivers being carjacked contribute to their fear. Many of these reports are carried in the international news media and depict the United States as a violent nation compared to many other international cities. Even people who live in supposedly safe areas can become victims of violence within their own homes or at the hands of family members. Figure 4.2 demonstrates how American cities compare internationally in terms of homicide.

SOCIETAL CAUSES OF VIOLENCE

Several social, cultural, and individual factors increase the likelihood of violent acts (Figure 4.3), including:[4]

■ *Poverty.* Low socioeconomic status and poor living conditions can create an environment of hopelessness; people view violence as the only way to obtain what they want.

■ *Unemployment.* It is a well-documented fact that when the economy goes sour, violent and nonviolent crimes increase.

■ *Parental influence.* Children raised in environments in which shouting, hitting, and other forms of violence are commonplace are more apt to act out these behaviors as adults. Recent research has substantiated this cycle of violence.

■ *Cultural beliefs.* Cultures that objectify women and empower men to be tough and aggressive show higher rates of violence in the home.

■ *The media.* A daily dose of murder and mayhem can take a toll on even resistant minds.

■ *Discrimination/oppression.* Whenever one group is oppressed by another, seeds of discontent are sown, and hate crimes arise.

■ *Religious beliefs and differences.* Religious persecution has been a part of the human experience since earliest times. Strong beliefs can foster martyrdom, often expressed in such actions as suicide bombings.

■ *Political differences.* Civil unrest and differences in political party affiliations and beliefs have historically been triggers for violent acts.

■ *Breakdowns in the criminal justice system.* Overcrowded prisons, lenient sentences, early releases from prison, and trial errors subtly encourage violence in a number of ways.

- *Heavy use of alcohol and other substances.* Alcohol and drug abuse are often catalysts for violence, and other crimes.[5]

In addition to these broad, societally based factors, many personal factors also can lead to violence.[6]

Personal Precipitators of Violence

If you are like most people, you probably acted out your anger more readily as a child than you do today. With increasing maturity, most people learn to control outbursts of anger in a socially acceptable and rational manner. Yet others go through life acting out their aggressive tendencies in much the same ways they did as children or as their families did. Why do two children from the same neighborhood, or even from the same family, go in different directions when it comes to violence? There are several predictors of future aggressive behavior.

Anger Anger is a spontaneous, usually temporary, biological feeling or emotional state of displeasure that occurs most frequently during times of personal frustration. As we learned in Chapter 2, life is stressful, and anger becomes a part of daily experience. Anger can range from slight irritation to rage, a violent and extreme form of anger.[7] When it is acted out at home or on the road, the consequences can be deadly.

What makes some people flare at the slightest provocation? Causes may vary. Often, people who anger quickly have a low tolerance for frustration and believe that they should not have to put up with inconvenience or petty annoyances—the cause may be genetic or physiological; there is evidence that some people are born unstable, touchy, or easily angered.[8] Sociocultural factors may play a role because many people are taught not to express anger in public so do not know how to handle it when it reaches a level that cannot be hidden. Family background may be the most important factor. Typically, anger-prone people come from families that are disruptive, chaotic, and unskilled in emotional expression.[9] In fact, the single largest predictor of future violence is past violence.[10]

Aggressive behavior is often a key aspect of violent interactions. **Primary aggression** is goal-directed, hostile self-assertion that is destructive in nature. **Reactive aggression** is more often part of an emotional reaction

---

brought about by frustrating life experiences. Whether aggression is primary or reactive, it is most likely to flare in times of acute stress, during relationship difficulties or loss, or when a person is so frustrated that the only recourse is to strike out at others.

What Do You Think? What are some examples of primary aggression? ■ Reactive aggression? ■ Can both of them result in the same degree of harm? ■ Do you think our laws are more lenient when violent acts result from reactive aggression? Why?

Substance Abuse Although much has been written about a strong link between substance abuse and violence, many violent episodes are in fact carefully planned actions that involve no alcohol or drug abuse. In other situations, however, psychoactive substances appear to be a form of ignition for violence.

- Consumption of alcohol—by perpetrators of the crime, the victim, or both—immediately preceded over half of all violent crimes, including murder.[11]
- Criminals using illegal drugs commit robberies and assaults more frequently than nonusing criminals and do so especially during periods of heavy drug use.[12]
- In domestic assault cases, over 90 percent of the assailants and over half of victims reported using alcohol at the time of the attack. Nearly 20 percent of victims and assailants reported using cocaine or methamphetamine at the time of the attack.[13]
- Ninety-two percent of assailants and 42 percent of victims reported having used alcohol or other drugs on the day of the assault.[14]

INTENTIONAL INJURIES

Any time someone sets out to harm other people or their property, the incident may be referred to as intentional violence. Though nonviolent crime is more common, violent crime occurs all too often (Figure 4.4). The resulting intentional injuries cause pain and suffering at the very least, and death and disability at the worst.

Gratuitous Violence

Violence can manifest itself in many ways. Often the most shocking or gratuitous crimes gain the greatest attention, such as stories of innocent victims of drive-by shootings or young students who turn their rage on family, classmates, and teachers.

Primary aggression   Goal-directed, hostile self-assertion that is destructive in character.

Reactive aggression   Emotional reaction brought about by frustrating life experiences.

Homicide Death that results from intent to injure or kill—**homicide**—accounts for over 19,000 premature deaths in the United States.[15] These numbers are down significantly from recent years but still represent a significant contributor to life lost in certain segments of the population. Although homicide was the nineteenth leading cause of death in the United States among all age groups in 2002, it was the second leading cause of death for persons age 15 to 24.[16] Homicide is an area in which disparities among races are particularly clear. Asian/Pacific Islander, Hispanic or Latino, and African American groups all list homicide among the top ten causes of death, while homicide is not among the top ten killers of whites or American Indians.

As measured by years of potential life lost, homicide exacts a heavy toll (Table 4.1 on page 94). For every violent death, at least 100 nonfatal injuries are caused by violence. In 2003, an estimated 29,730 firearm-related deaths occurred, including large numbers of homicides and suicides.[17] For every person shot and killed by a firearm, almost three others were treated annually for nonfatal shootings, many of them children under age 10.[18]

For an American, the average lifetime probability of being murdered is 1 in 153—but the average masks large differences for specific segments of the population. For white women, the risk of murder is 1 in 450; for a black man in the 20- to 22-year-old age group, the risk is 1 in 3. Combined across races, males represent 77 percent of all murder and nonnegligent manslaughter victims. Black males are 1.14 times more likely than white males to be murder victims; white females are 1.5 times more likely than black females to be victims.[19] Over half of all homicides occur among people who know one another. In two-thirds of these cases, the perpetrator and the victim are friends or acquaintances; in one-third, they belong to the same family.[20]

Bias and Hate Crimes

In spite of national efforts in workplaces, schools, and communities to promote understanding and diversity-related appreciation, intolerance of differences continues to smolder in many parts of U.S. society. The well-publicized murders of homosexual men such as Matthew Shepard, and the arson attacks on several U.S. synagogues remind Americans that violence based on race and other "-isms" still occurs. International terrorist acts often reflect the hatred of one religious or political group for another that is considered to be of less value due to differences in religion, language, or other characteristics. Acts of violence against different racial groups by police, beatings in public schools and on the streets that are racially motivated gang events, and other hate crimes are common events on the nightly news.

According to the most recent Hate Crime Statistics Report of the Federal Bureau of Investigation (FBI), 8,715 bias-motivated crimes were reported in 2003. Of the total reported incidents, 52 percent were motivated by racial bias, 16 percent by religious bias, 16 percent by sexual orientation bias, and 14 percent by ethnicity/national origin bias.[21]

Since the 2001 terrorist attacks in the United States and the conflicts in Iraq and Afghanistan, reports of hate-related incidents, beatings, and other physical and verbal assaults have escalated, even as other rates of violent crime decreased. In particular, persons of Muslim or Middle-Eastern descent reported civil rights violations at work, in mass transit, and in communities throughout the United States. Many believe that the actual numbers of bias/hate-related crimes are much higher, but people do not report them out of fear of possible retaliation.

Hate crimes vary along two dimensions: (1) the way they are carried out and (2) their effects on victims. Vicious gossip, nasty comments, and devilish pranks may not make headlines, but they can hurt nonetheless. Generally, about 30 percent of all hate crimes are against property; the other 70 percent are against the person in the form of intimidation or assault. Recent studies have identified three additional characteristics of hate crimes:[22]

■ Excessive brutality often at random on total strangers

■ Perpetrated by multiple offenders

■ Offenders are young: 46 percent are under the age of 18

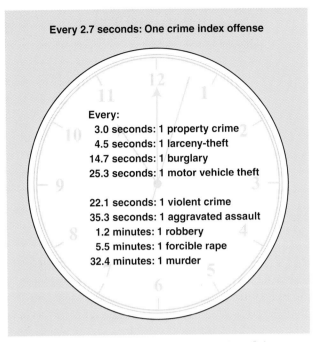

Every 2.7 seconds: One crime index offense

Every:
3.0 seconds: 1 property crime
4.5 seconds: 1 larceny-theft
14.7 seconds: 1 burglary
25.3 seconds: 1 motor vehicle theft

22.1 seconds: 1 violent crime
35.3 seconds: 1 aggravated assault
1.2 minutes: 1 robbery
5.5 minutes: 1 forcible rape
32.4 minutes: 1 murder

Figure 4.4 ■ Crime Clock: How Often Is a Crime Committed?

Source: Federal Bureau of Investigation, "Crime in the U.S.," 2002, www.fbi.gov.

Homicide Death that results from intent to injure or kill.

Table 4.1
Years of Potential Life Lost (per 100,000)

Years of Potential Life Lost (YPLL) is a rough measure of the impact of a specific disease or societal event/ condition on a given population. It is calculated by subtracting the age at death of a person from the expected life expectancy for this person. In this table, the total years are those lost before age 75 per 100,000 population under the age of 75. It provides a glimpse of the overall impact of a problem on the lives of particular populations.

Some questions to consider: Where are the greatest disparities in YPLL among males? Among females? What factors do you think contribute to the low rates of suicide in some groups? High rates of assault?

	Unintentional Injury	Suicide	Assault (Homicide)
Male			
White	1,475.9	624.7	253.9
African American	1,888.7	388.1	1,753.5
American Indian/Alaska Native	2,771.7	850.8	568.3
Asian/Pacific Islander	637.1	308.8	210.2
Hispanic	1,536.8	346.6	676.8
White, non-Hispanic	1,440.8	657.6	167.1
Female			
White	586.8	154.4	95.0
African American	676.9	67.0	370.2
American Indian/Alaska Native	1,276.8	219.7	205.8
Asian/Pacific Islander	309.6	102.5	80.2
Hispanic	461.8	306.3	121.9
White, non-Hispanic	599.1	164.4	88.2

Note: The groups of white, African American, Asian/Pacific Islander, and American Indian/Alaska Native include persons of Hispanic and non-Hispanic origin. Conversely, persons of Hispanic origin may be of any race.
Source: Department of Health and Human Services, National Institutes of Health, Centers for Disease Control and Prevention, 2001, www.cdc.gov.

The perpetrators tend to be motivated by thrill, defensive feelings, or a hate-mongering mission.

Academic settings are not immune to hatred and bias. Students bring with them attitudes and beliefs from past family and life experiences. According to a report in the *Chronicle of Higher Education,* nearly one-third of our nation's campuses have reported hate crimes. Among these crimes, 57 percent were motivated by race, 18 percent by anti-Semitism, and 16 percent by sexual orientation.[23] Sadly, many minor assaults go unreported, so this may be only part of the picture.

The tendency toward violent acts on campus that are based on prejudice and discrimination might best be defined as campus **ethnoviolence,** a term that reflects relationships among groups in the larger society. Although ethnoviolence often is randomly directed at persons affiliated with a particular group, the group itself is specifically targeted apart from other people, and that differentiation is usually based on ethnicity. Typically, the perpetrators agree that the group is an "acceptable target." For example, in a largely Christian community, Jews and Muslims may be considered acceptable targets.

Prejudice and discrimination are always at the base of ethnoviolence. **Prejudice** is a set of negative attitudes toward a group of people. To say that a person is prejudiced against some group is to say that the person holds a set of beliefs about the group, has an emotional reaction to or way of thinking about the group, and is motivated to behave in a certain way toward the group. **Discrimination** constitutes actions often based on bias and prejudice that deny equal treatment or opportunities to a group of people.

Ethnoviolence Violence directed randomly at persons affiliated with a particular group.

Prejudice A set of negative attitudes and beliefs or an emotional reaction or way of thinking about a group of people.

Discrimination Actions often based on bias and prejudice that deny equal treatment or opportunities to a group.

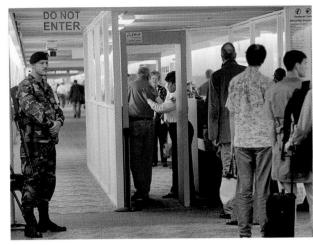

The threat of terrorism has affected many aspects of our
daily lives.

Gang Violence The growing influence of street
gangs has had a harmful impact on our country. Drug
abuse, gang shootings, beatings, thefts, carjackings, and
the possibility of being caught in the crossfire have
caused entire neighborhoods to be held hostage by gang
members. Once thought to occur only in inner-city
areas, gang violence now also appears in rural and sub-
urban communities, particularly in the Southeast, the
Southwest, and the West.

Why do young people join gangs? Although the
reasons are complex, gangs seem to meet many of their
needs. Gangs provide a sense of belonging to a family
that gives them self-worth, companionship, security,
and excitement. In other cases, gangs provide economic
security through criminal activity, drug sales, or prosti-
tution. Once young people become involved in the gang
subculture, it is difficult for them to leave. Threats of
violence or fear of not making it on their own dissuade
even those who are most seriously trying to get out.

Who is at risk for gang membership? The age range
of gang members is typically 12 to 22 years. Risk factors include low self-esteem, academic problems, low
socioeconomic status, alienation from family and society, a history of family violence, and living in gang-
controlled neighborhoods.

Terrorism: Increased Risks from Multiple Sources

Not so long ago, Americans thought acts of terrorism
occurred only in distant cities, seldom amounting to
more than a blip on the evening news. On September
11, 2001, terrorist attacks on the World Trade Center
and Pentagon revealed the vulnerability of our nation to
domestic and international threats. The terms *terrorist
attack, bioterrorism,* and *biological weapons* catapulted
us into the new millennium with an emotional reaction
unlike any ever seen. An undercurrent of fear and anxiety about potential threats from faceless strangers shook
many of us in ways that we had never even considered.
Today, the specter of a terrorist attack looms ever present. Any time there is a national holiday or occasion
where many Americans gather, we worry about a terrorist event.

What Is Terrorism? According to the FBI,
terrorism is the use of unlawful force or violence against
persons or property to intimidate or coerce a government,
the civilian population, or any segment thereof, in further-
ance of political or social objectives. Typically, there are
two major types of terrorism. *Domestic terrorism* involves
groups or individuals whose terrorist activities are directed at elements of our government or population without foreign direction. *International terrorism* involves
groups or individuals whose terrorist activities are for-
eign-based, transcend national boundaries, and are directed by countries or groups outside the United States.

Clearly, terrorist activities may have immediate impact in terms of loss of lives and resources. Worldwide
attacks can also have more long-term impact, affecting
world economies, the airline industry, and transportation systems. Perhaps most damaging in the aftermath
of the 2001 and more recent European subway system
attacks is the fear, anxiety, and altered behavior of
countless individuals. How many people will fear traveling on a plane or train or working in a skyscraper for
years to come? Will concern about future terrorist attacks disrupt our lives and our interactions with others?

As the media spurs our anxieties about germ,
chemical, and nuclear warfare and the multitude of
ways that terrorists can breach our defenses, is it any
wonder that an already stressed American public is
demonstrating increasing concern? What can we do to
reduce our risk of terrorist attack?

> **Terrorism** The use of unlawful force or violence
> against persons or property to intimidate or coerce a gov-
> ernment, the civilian population, or any segment thereof,
> in furtherance of political or social objectives.

Be assured that the U.S. Department of Health and Human Services has a wide range of ongoing programs and services designed to help Americans respond to terrorist threats and prepare for possible attacks. Information is available on their CDC website and is updated regularly. The Department of Homeland Security, FBI, and other government agencies also have prepared a sweeping set of procedures and guidelines for ensuring citizen safety. Below are some things you can do to help reduce anxiety and harm related to terrorist attacks. These tips can also apply to damage brought on by a natural disaster, like Hurricane Katrina.

> **Is there anything I can do to protect myself from terrorism?**

- *Be aware of your own reactions to stress, anxiety, and fear.* Is your fear justifiable or a product of media sensationalism? Determine the source of your stressors or anxiety, and react as prudently as possible.

- *Be conscious of your surroundings.* If you note suspicious activities or irregularities, report them to a person in authority.

- *Stay informed and seek information.* Try to stay on top of the news and understand the underlying roots of violent activity. Understand your government's stance on current key issues.

- *Seek understanding.* Whenever communication between two opposing groups breaks down, hate, bigotry, and anger may occur. Tolerance of other cultures and keeping a line of communication open are good steps to avoiding separation.

- *Know what to do in an emergency.* How would you access local and regional assistance? Do you have the necessary provisions for basic survival—food, water, first aid—in case of an attack?

Try it ▶ NOW _____

Have an emergency plan. An emergency plan can make you feel more at ease and eliminate anxiety. Get together with your family, friends, or roommates and make a plan for a natural disaster or terrorist attack. Keep an emergency kit on hand containing several days worth of food and water, flashlights, batteries, and even a small radio. Determine a meeting spot in case there are no phones or other ways to get in touch with each other.

Domestic violence The use of force to control and maintain power over another person in the home environment, including both actual harm and the threat of harm.

Domestic Violence

Domestic violence refers to the use of force to control and maintain power over another person in the home environment. It can involve emotional abuse, verbal abuse, threats of physical harm, and actual physical violence ranging from slapping and shoving to beating, rape, and homicide. How bad is the problem? There are over half a million victims of domestic violence each year. Over 1 million women are stalked, and one-third of female homicide victims are murdered by an intimate partner.[24]

Women as Victims While young men are more apt to become victims of violence from strangers, women are much more likely to become victims of violent acts perpetrated by spouses, lovers, ex-spouses, and ex-lovers. Domestic violence is the single greatest cause of injury to women, surpassing rape, mugging, and automobile accidents combined. Women often know their attacker: 40 percent of offenders were described as friends, 20 percent as intimates, and 7 percent as relatives—this leaves only 31 percent in the "stranger" category.[25] Six of every 10 women in the United States will be assaulted at some time in their lives by someone they know.[26] Every year, approximately 12 percent of married women are the victims of physical aggression perpetrated by their husbands.[27] This aggression often includes pushing, slapping, and shoving, but it can take more severe forms.

Acts of aggression by a husband or boyfriend are one of the most common causes of death for young women globally, with at least one in three women being beaten, coerced into sex, or otherwise abused in her lifetime.[28] These acts of violence are spread across races, with women of any race being equally vulnerable to attack.[29]

The following U.S. statistics indicate the seriousness of this long-hidden problem:[30]

- Every 15 seconds, someone batters a woman; 1 in every 250 such assaults is reported.

- Over a third of female victims of domestic violence are severely abused on a regular basis.

- Three of every four women murdered are killed by their husbands.

- Pregnant women are more likely to be victims of homicide than to die from any other cause.

Murder is not the only devastating result of these acts of violence. Depression, panic attacks, disordered eating, migraine and other headaches, sexually transmitted infections, ulcers, and social isolation can all be results of domestic violence.

How many times have you heard of a woman who is beaten repeatedly by her partner and wondered, "Why doesn't she just leave him?" There are many reasons why some women find it difficult to break their ties with their abusers. Many women, particularly those with small children, are financially dependent on their partners. Others fear retaliation against themselves or their children. Some women hope that the situation will change with time (it rarely does); others stay because their cultural or religious beliefs forbid divorce. Finally, though it is hard to understand, some women still love the abusive partner.

Psychologist Lenore Walker developed a theory known as the "cycle of violence" to explain how women can get caught in a downward spiral without knowing what is happening to them.[31] The cycle has three phases.

1. *Tension building.* In this phase, minor battering occurs, and the woman may become more nurturant and more intent on pleasing the spouse in order to forestall more violence. She assumes guilt for doing something to provoke him and tries hard to avoid doing it again.

2. *Acute battering.* At this stage, pleasing her man doesn't help, and she can no longer control or predict the abuse. Usually, the spouse is trying to "teach her a lesson," and when he feels he has inflicted enough pain, he'll stop. Violence may include forced sexual relations and psychological and economic abuse, as well as beatings. When the acute attack is over, he may respond with shock and denial about his own behavior. Both batterer and victim may soft-pedal the seriousness of the attacks.

3. *Remorse/reconciliation.* During this "honeymoon" period, the batterer may be kind, loving, and apologetic, swearing he will never act violently again. He may stop his violent behavior for several weeks or months, and the woman may come to question whether she overreacted.

When the tension that precipitated past abuse resurfaces, the man beats the woman again. Unless some form of intervention breaks this downward cycle of abuse, it will repeat itself again and again and perhaps end only with the woman's or, rarely, the man's death.

It is very hard for most women who get caught in this cycle of violence to summon the resolution to extricate themselves. Most need effective outside intervention.

Men as Victims Are men also victims of domestic violence? Some women do abuse and even kill their partners. Approximately 12 percent of men reported that their wives had engaged in physically aggressive behavior against them in the past year—nearly the same percentage of claims reported from women. The difference between male and female batterers is twofold. First, although the frequency may be similar, the impact is drastically different: women are much more likely to sustain serious injury or die at the hands of a partner. Women do engage in moderate

> Are men ever victims of domestic violence?

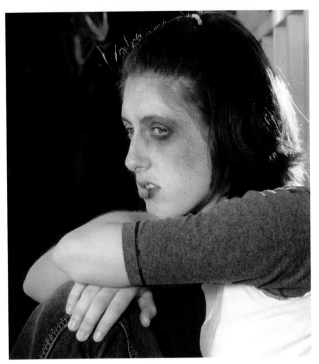

Despite obvious physical and psychological injury, it can be difficult for a person to leave an abusive partner.

aggression, such as pushing and shoving, at rates almost equal to those of men, but severe aggression that is likely to land a victim in the hospital is almost always male against female. Second, a woman who is physically abused by a man is generally intimidated by him: she fears that he will use his power and control over her in some fashion. Men, however, generally report that they do not live in fear of their wives.

Causes of Domestic Violence There is no single explanation for why people tend to be abusive in relationships. Although alcohol abuse often is associated with such violence, marital dissatisfaction, differences in communication patterns, rigid gender roles, poor skills for coping with anger, and other factors contribute to violent actions. Often, patterns of aggression are influenced by family and begin in youth. The tendency for violent behavior is further aggravated by stress and uncertainty in our lives.

Regardless of the cause, the dynamics that both people bring to a relationship result in violence and allow it to continue. Community support and counseling services can help determine underlying problems and allow the victim and the batterer to break the cycle. The Assess Yourself box on page 98 may help you determine if you are a victim of abuse.

Child Abuse and Neglect These are defined as any recent act or failure to act on the part of parent or caretaker that results in imminent risk of death, serious physical or emotional harm, sexual abuse, or exploitation.[32]

Relationship Violence: Are You at Risk?

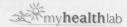
Fill out this assessment online at
www.aw-bc.com/myhealthlab or www.aw-bc.com/donatelle.

Although we all want to have healthy relationships, many of us get caught in patterns of behavior that are a direct result of things we've learned or haven't learned in our past. Sometimes we don't even recognize that we are acting inappropriately; other times we know we should act in a particular way, but we get caught up in our own emotions and act out in ways that are physically or emotionally abusive to others. If you have been a victim of emotional or physical violence, you may have become so used to certain behaviors that you might not recognize them as inappropriate. To prevent violence, we have to be able to recognize it, deal with it in appropriate ways, and/or take action to avoid it. One place to start is to examine our intimate interpersonal relationships. Answer the following questions about your current or past relationships.

How often does your partner:

		Never	Sometimes	Often
1.	Criticize you for your appearance (weight, dress, hair, etc.)?	❏	❏	❏
2.	Embarrass you in front of others by putting you down?	❏	❏	❏
3.	Blame you or others for his or her mistakes?	❏	❏	❏
4.	Curse at you, say mean things, or mock you?	❏	❏	❏
5.	Demonstrate uncontrollable anger?	❏	❏	❏
6.	Criticize your friends, family, or others who are close to you?	❏	❏	❏
7.	Threaten to leave you if you don't behave in a certain way?	❏	❏	❏
8.	Manipulate you to prevent you from spending time with friends or family?	❏	❏	❏
9.	Express jealousy, distrust, and anger when you spend time with other people?	❏	❏	❏
10.	Tell you that you are crazy, irrational, or paranoid?	❏	❏	❏
11.	Call you names to make you lose confidence in yourself?	❏	❏	❏
12.	Make all the significant decisions in your relationship?	❏	❏	❏
13.	Intimidate or threaten you, making you fearful or anxious?	❏	❏	❏
14.	Make threats to harm others you care about?	❏	❏	❏
15.	Prevent you from going out by taking your car keys?	❏	❏	❏
16.	Control your telephone calls, listen in on your messages, or read your e-mail?	❏	❏	❏
17.	Punch, hit, slap, or kick you?	❏	❏	❏
18.	Gossip about you to turn others against you or make them think bad things about you?	❏	❏	❏
19.	Make you feel guilty about something?	❏	❏	❏
20.	Use money or possessions to control you?	❏	❏	❏
21.	Force you to have sex or perform sexual acts that make you uncomfortable?	❏	❏	❏
22.	Threaten to kill himself or herself if you leave?	❏	❏	❏
23.	Control your money and make you ask for what you need?	❏	❏	❏
24.	Set many rules that you must abide by?	❏	❏	❏
25.	Follow you, call to check on you, or demonstrate a constant obsession with what you are doing?	❏	❏	❏

Now look at your responses to the above questions. If you answered "sometimes" to one or more of these questions, you may be at risk for emotional or physical abuse. If you answered "often" to any question, you may need to talk with someone about immediate threats to your emotional or physical health. Typically, such potentially abusive patterns only get worse over time as a person gains control and power in a relationship. If you are anxious about talking to your partner, seek counseling through your campus counseling center, student health center, or community services.

Make It Happen!

Assessment: The Assess Yourself activity gave you a chance to consider symptoms of abuse. If any of the symptoms describe a relationship experienced by you or someone you know, you should consider taking action.

Making a Change: In order to change your behavior, you need to develop a plan. Follow these steps below and complete your Behavior Change Contract to take action.

1. Evaluate your behavior and identify patterns and specific things you are doing. What can you change now? What can you change in the near future?
2. Select one pattern of behavior that you want to change.
3. Fill out the Behavior Change Contract found at the front of your book. It should include your long-term goal for change, your short-term goals, the rewards you'll give yourself for reaching these goals, potential obstacles along the way, and strategies for overcoming these obstacles. For each goal, list the small steps and specific actions that you will take.

If you don't know where to go, ask your professor for possible options.

After you have completed the test about your partner's behavior, you should ask the same questions about your own behavior. If any of the questions describe your actions in a relationship, you should seek help to change these behavioral patterns. These actions are not conducive to healthy relationships and may result in harm to you or your loved ones. Seek help now to insure healthier relationships in the future.

4. Chart your progress in a journal. At the end of a week, consider how successful you were in following your plan. What helped you be successful? What made change more difficult? What will you do differently next week?
5. Revise your plan as needed. Are the short-term goals attainable? Are the rewards satisfying?

Example: Sondra thought that her roommate Jessie was experiencing several symptoms of abuse. Jessie's boyfriend Carl sometimes belittled her in front of her friends. He once broke her cell phone by throwing it against a wall toward Jessie and seemed resentful when she spent time with anyone but him. When Sondra talked to Jessie about her perceptions, Jessie was surprised and very defensive at first. The more she thought about it, though, she realized that sometimes she was afraid of Carl's actions. She started to consider what she could do about the situation. As a first step, Sondra helped Jessie make immediate appointments at the school counseling center, one for herself and one for her and Carl together.

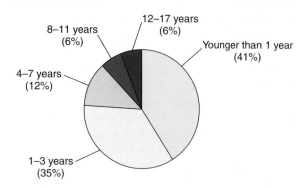

Figure 4.5 ■ Child Abuse and Neglect Fatalities, by Age, 2002

Source: U.S. Department of Health and Human Services, Bureau of Justice Statistics, "National Child Abuse and Neglect Data," 2002, http://nccanch.acf.hhf.gov/pubs/factsheets/fatality.cfm.

It is a myth to think that child abuse is the result of some stranger lurking in the bushes who snatches a child. **Child abuse** refers to the systematic harm of a child by a caregiver, most typically a parent. In fact, 80 percent of the perpetrators are parents, with other relatives and unmarried partners of a parent accounting for 10 percent of the crimes. The remaining 10 percent include persons with other (camp counselor, school employee, etc.) or unknown relationships to the child victims. The abuse may be sexual, psychological, physical, emotional, or any combination of the above.[33]

Neglect includes failure to provide for a child's basic needs for food, shelter, clothing, medical care, education, or proper supervision. How serious is the problem (Figure 4.5)? In 2004, 2.6 million reports concerning the welfare of approximately 4.5 million children were made to child protective service agencies in the United States.[34] In about two-thirds of these cases, sufficient abuse was detected to prompt investigation—resulting in over 896,000 cases (2,450 cases per day)![35] Of these cases, 60 percent of victims experienced neglect.

There is no single profile of a perpetrator of fatal child abuse. Frequently, the perpetrator is a young adult in his or her mid-twenties without a high school diploma, living at or below the poverty level, depressed, and who may have difficulty coping with stressful situations. In many instances, the perpetrator has experienced violence. Most fatalities from *physical abuse* are caused by fathers and other male caretakers. Mothers are most often held responsible for deaths resulting from *neglect.* However, in some cases this may be because women are the ones who spend the most time with the children and whom society deems responsible for their care. While it is difficult to measure long-term consequences of abuse, an average of nearly four children die every day as a result of abuse or neglect.[36]

Child Sexual Abuse
Sexual abuse of children by adults or older children includes sexually suggestive conversations; inappropriate kissing; touching; petting; oral, anal, or vaginal intercourse; and other kinds of sexual interaction. The most frequent abusers are a child's parents or their parents' companions or spouses. The next most frequent abusers are grandfathers and siblings. Girls are more commonly abused than boys, although young boys are also frequent victims, usually of male family members. Between 20 and 30 percent of all adult women report an unwanted childhood sexual encounter with an adult male, usually a father, uncle, brother, or grandfather. It is a myth that male deviance or mental illness accounts for most of these incidents: "Stories of retrospective incest patients typically involved perpetrators who are 'Everyman'—attorneys, mental health practitioners, businessmen, farmers, teachers, doctors, and clergy."[37]

Most sexual abuse occurs in the child's home. The risk is higher in the following situations:[38]

1. The child lives without one of his or her biological parents.
2. The mother is unavailable because she is disabled, ill, or working outside the home.
3. The parents' marriage is unhappy.
4. The child has a poor relationship with his or her parents or is subjected to extremely punitive discipline.
5. The child lives with a stepfather or mother's boyfriend.

Many abused children bear spiritual, psychological, and/or physical scars. Clinical psychologist Marjorie Whittaker has found that "of all forms of violence, incest and childhood sexual abuse are considered among the most 'toxic' because of their violations of trust, the confusion of affection and coercion, the splitting of family alignments, and serious psychological and physical consequences."[39] Parents and caretakers of children should be aware of behavioral changes that may signal sexual abuse.[40] Such changes may include noticeable fear of a certain person or place, drawings that show sexual acts or attempts to get other children to perform sexual acts, abrupt changes in behavior

---

Child abuse The systematic harming of a child by a caregiver, typically a parent.

Neglect Failure to provide for a child's basic needs such as food, shelter, medical care, and clothing.

Sexual abuse of children Sexual interaction between a child and an adult or older child. Includes, but is not limited to, sexually suggestive conversations; inappropriate kissing; touching; petting; and oral, anal, or vaginal intercourse.

such as bed-wetting, or sudden or unusual awareness of genitals or sexual acts.

Not all child violence is physical. Health can be severely affected by psychological violence—assaults on personality, character, competence, independence, or general dignity as a human being. The negative consequences of this kind of victimization can be harder to discern and therefore harder to combat. They include depression, low self-esteem, and a pervasive fear of doing something that will offend the abuser.

What Do You Think? ■ What factors in society lead to child abuse and neglect? ■ Why are family members often the perpetrators of child abuse and child sexual abuse? ■ What actions can be taken to prevent such behaviors?

Sexual Victimization

As with all forms of violence, men and women alike are susceptible to sexual victimization. However, sexual violence against women is of epidemic proportions, so we will focus on women; in the United States, it occurs more frequently than car accidents, muggings, and rapes combined.[41] Physical battering and emotional abuse associated with sexual battery often leave psychological as well as physical scars.

Sexual Assault and Rape

Sexual assault is any act in which one person is sexually intimate with another person without that other person's consent. This may range from simple touching to forceful penetration. It may include such acts as ignoring indications that intimacy is not wanted, threatening force or other negative consequences, and actually using force.

Rape, the most extreme form of sexual assault, is defined as penetration without the victim's consent.[42] Whether committed by an acquaintance, a date or spouse, or a stranger, rape is a criminal activity that usually has serious psychological and physical consequences for the victim. Typically, victims are young females, with 29 percent under 11 years of age, 32 percent between the ages of 11 and 17, and 22 percent between ages 18 and 24.[43]

One of the most startling aspects of sex crimes is how many go unreported, usually out of a belief that this is a private matter, fear of reprisal by the assailant, or unwarranted feelings of guilt and responsibility. It is thought that one out of every three women is the victim of an attempted or completed rape in her lifetime. Although as many as two-thirds of all rapes are never

reported, there were over 683,000 reported cases of rape, attempted rape, or sexual assault in 2003.[44]

Incidents of rape generally fall into one of two types—aggravated or simple. An **aggravated rape** involves multiple attackers, strangers, weapons, or physical beatings. A **simple rape** is perpetrated by one person, whom the victim knows, and does not involve a physical beating or use of a weapon. Most incidents are classified as simple rapes, with one report suggesting that 82 percent of female rape victims have been victimized by acquaintances (53 percent), current or former boyfriends (16 percent), current or former spouses (10 percent), or other relatives (3 percent). With a criminal justice system that lets sex offenders off with minimal punishment, exemplified by almost half of all rape charges dismissed before the cases reach trial, and a perceived lack of male understanding of how rape affects women, it's easy to understand why experts feel that simple rape is seriously underreported and ignored.

Acquaintance or Date Rape Although the terms *date rape, friendship rape,* and *acquaintance rape* have become standard terminology, they typically are misused. Not all rapes occur on dates, not all the relationships are friendships, and sometimes the term *acquaintance* is used all too loosely. Many acquaintance rapes occur as the result of incidental contact at a party or when people congregate at one person's house. These are crimes of opportunity, not necessarily the result of a prearranged date. This is an important distinction because the term *date* suggests some type of reciprocal interaction arranged in advance. While most date or acquaintance rapes happen to women aged 15 to 21 years, the 18-year-old new college student is the most likely victim. For more information, see the following section Crime on Campus.

Marital Rape Marital rape is any unwanted intercourse or penetration (vaginal, anal, or oral) obtained by force, threat of force, or when the wife is unable to consent.[45] Some researchers estimate that marital rape may account for 25 percent of all rapes; rape in marriage may be an extremely prevalent form of sexual violence. Although this problem has undoubtedly been

Sexual assault Any act in which one person is sexually intimate with another person without that other person's consent.

Rape Sexual penetration without the victim's consent.

Aggravated rape Rape that involves multiple attackers, strangers, weapons, or a physical beating.

Simple rape Rape by one person, usually known to the victim, that does not involve a physical beating or use of a weapon.

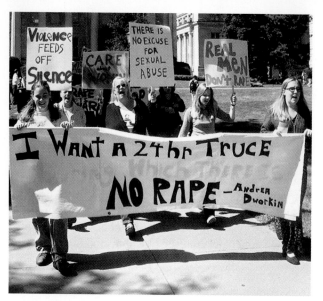
College students can organize vigils, marches, and educational programs to raise awareness about violence against women.

common since the earliest origins of marriage as a social institution, it is noteworthy that marital rape did not become a crime in all 50 states until 1993. Even more noteworthy is the fact that in 33 states there are still exemptions from rape prosecution, which means that the judicial system may treat it as a lesser crime.

Who is most vulnerable to marital rape? In general, women under the age of 25 and those who are from lower socioeconomic groups are at highest risk. Women from homes where other forms of domestic violence are common and where there is a high rate of alcoholism and/or substance abuse also tend to be victimized at greater rates than others. Women who are subjected to marital rape often report multiple offenses over a period of time; these events are likely to be forced anal and oral experiences.[46]

Abuse of power and a need to control and dominate seem to be key factors in the husband-rapist profile. Marital rape can have devastating short- and long-term consequences for women, including injuries to the vaginal and anal areas, lacerations, soreness, bruising, torn muscles, fatigue, panic attacks, sexually transmitted infections, broken bones, wounds, and other emotional and physical scars.

What Do You Think? Why do you think women are often reluctant to report sexual harassment? ■ Why do you think so many men report that they were unaware of their own sexually harassing behaviors? ■ What can be done to increase awareness in this area?

Social Contributors to Sexual Assault

According to many experts, certain common assumptions in our society prevent both the perpetrator and the public from recognizing the true nature of sexual assault. These assumptions include the following.

■ *Minimization and trivialization.* It is often assumed that sexual assault of women is rare because official crime statistics, including the Uniform Crime Reports of the FBI, show very few rapes per thousand population. However, rape is the most underreported of all serious crimes.

■ *Blaming the victim.* Many discussions of sexual violence against women display a sometimes unconscious assumption that the woman did something to provoke the attack—that she dressed revealingly, for example, and that men just can't control themselves when faced with temptation.

Over the years, psychologists and others have proposed several theories to explain why many males sexually victimize women. In one of the first major studies to explore this issue, almost two-thirds of the male respondents had engaged in intercourse unwanted by the woman, primarily because of male peer pressure.[47] By all indicators, these trends continue today. Peer pressure is certainly a strong factor, but a growing body of research suggests that sexual assault is encouraged by the socialization processes that males experience daily, including the belief that rape is something women secretly desire, and by norms that often portray women as the targets of male aggression.[48]

What Do You Think? What factors make men likely to commit sexual assault or rape? ■ What measures might be effective in preventing such behaviors?

Crime on Campus: Victims and Perpetrators

It is not unusual for parents to send their sons and daughters away to colleges and universities with some trepidation. Parents worry that their children will have trouble adjusting to college life, drink too much and party too hard, and not eat right or sleep enough. Few realize that the 16 million students enrolled in some 4,200 colleges and universities in the United States face risks from campus violence that can cause significant physical and mental problems for their children The term *campus violence* include acts of physical violence such as homicide, suicide, rape, assault, dating violence, harassment and stalking, hazing, and hate crimes.[49]

The results of the *Violent Victimization of College Students* report details that between 1995 and 2002 students aged 18 to 24 were victims of approximately 479,000 violent crimes annually.[50] Of the victims who participated in the study:

- Approximately 93 percent of crimes against students occurred off-campus.
- White college students had somewhat higher rates of violent victimization overall than students of other races. Blacks are more likely to experience simple assault.
- Alcohol was a factor in nearly half of all violent crimes on campus.
- Simple assault accounted for about two-thirds of college student violent crimes (63 percent).
- Data from the spring 2004 American College Health Association-National College Health Assessment (ACHA-NCHA) indicates that out of a sample of 47,202 students, 17 percent of women and 10 percent of men report being in an emotionally abusive relationship within the last school year.[51]

However, these statistics represent only the tip of the iceberg. The sad fact is that fewer than 25 percent of campus crimes are reported to *any* authority.[52] Why would students fail to report such crimes? The typical reasons are that the crimes were too minor and not worth the hassle; privacy concerns; not clear it was a crime; ashamed, embarrassed; feeling overwhelmed, lack of support.[53]

In 1992, Congress passed the Campus Sexual Assault Victim's Bill of Rights, known as the Ramstad Act. The act gives victims the right to call in off-campus authorities to investigate serious campus crimes. In addition, universities must set up educational programs and notify students of available counseling. More recent provisions of the act specify received notification procedures and options for victims, rights of victims and the accused perpetrators, and consequences if schools do not comply. It also requires the Department of Education to publish campus crime statistics annually.

Sexual Violence on Campus

Sexual harassment is unwelcome sexual conduct that is related to any condition of employment or evaluation of student performance. It includes unwarranted sex-related comments, sexually explicit comments or graphics, unwelcome touching, etc.[54] Although often not thought of as harassment by many, making derogatory jokes based on sex or appearance, speaking in crude or offensive language, spreading rumors about a person's sexuality, placing compromising photos on the Web, or ogling are common forms of sexual harassment. Commonly, people only think of harassment as involving faculty members or persons in power, where sex is used to exhibit control of a situation. However, peers can harass one another too. Harassment can occur at many

Table 4.2 **Strategies for Preventing or Stopping Harassment**	
Tell the harasser to stop.	Be clear and direct about what is bothering you and why you are upset.
Document the harassment.	Make a record of the incident. If the harassment becomes intolerable, a record of exactly what occurred (and when and where) will help make your case.
Complain to a higher authority.	Talk to your instructor, adviser, or counseling center about what happened. If they don't take you seriously, investigate your school's internal grievance procedures.
Remember that you have not done anything wrong.	You will likely feel awful after being harassed (especially if you have to complain to superiors). However, feel proud that you are not keeping silent. The person who is harassing you is wrong, not you.

levels and can be extremely detrimental to those who are involved. Although exact numbers of cases of sexual harassment are difficult to determine, it is widely perceived to be a major problem on college campuses, forcing administrators to enact strict guidelines about interpersonal relationships between students and instructors or co-workers. A study by the Institute of Social and Economic Research at Cornell University found that 61 percent of upperclass and graduate students have experienced "unwanted sexual attention from someone of authority within the university."[55] Table 4.2 details strategies for handling harassment.

What Do You Think?
What policies does your school have regarding consensual relationships between faculty members and students? ■ Should consenting adults have the right to interact, regardless of their positions within a system or workplace? ■ What are the potential dangers of such interactions?

Sexual harassment   Any form of unwanted sexual attention.

Sexual Assault Earlier in this chapter, you learned about rape and sexual assault. Rape, acquaintance rape, sodomy, unwanted touching, and other forms of sexual assault occur daily on campuses throughout the United States, and, like other forms of violence, these crimes have particularly high rates of nonreporting.[56] Sexual assault often involves force sufficient to cause serious injury, and psychological trauma may be substantial. A recent study found that the incidence of rape and attempted rape in female college students within the last academic year was 5.8 percent, with nearly 12 percent reporting unwanted sexual touching. The majority of rapes occurred in living quarters.[57] Studies of sexual assaults vary considerably; however, over the years, college men have consistently acknowledged forced intercourse at a rate of 5 to 15 percent and college sexual aggression at a rate of 15 to 25 percent.[58]

Stalking The "willful, repeated, and malicious following, harassing, or threatening of another person is **stalking**."[59] The most common form of stalking and that which poses the greatest risk of violence occurs following the termination of romantic relationships.[60] However, stalking may be more subtle, particularly with the use of modern technology. For example, cell phone–stalkers can keep track of a victim's actions by calling repeatedly, asking questions about what you are doing, who you are with, and other seemingly harmless checks on activity. If this persists, let the person know it's not appropriate behavior and ask that they stop calling. Although stalking occurs in virtually all populations, research suggests that stalking rates may be higher among female college students than in the general population.[61]

What can I do if I think I am being stalked?

Researchers suggest several reasons for stalking: (1) stalkers may have deficits in social skills, (2) they are young and have not yet learned how to deal with complex social relationships and situations, (3) they may not realize their behavior is stalking, (4) they have a flexible schedule and free time, and (5) they are not accountable to authority figures for their daily activities.[62] How prevalent is stalking on campus? As with other violent acts, stalking behaviors are believed to be widely underreported; however, estimates are that

between 25 and 30 percent of college women and between 11 and 17 percent of college men have been stalked.[63]

Campus Dating Violence Actual or threatened physical or sexual violence or psychological and emotional abuse directed toward a current or former dating partner is known as campus dating violence. Intimate partners may be heterosexual, bisexual, or homosexual.[64] Studies of campus dating violence indicate that 15 percent of women and 9.2 percent of men reported being in emotionally abusive relationships during the last year, and 2.4 percent of women and 1.3 percent of men reported physically abusive relationships. Sexually abusive relationships were reported by 1.7 percent of women and 1.0 percent of men.[65] Like many forms of campus violence, alcohol use is frequently involved. See the Reality Check box for more on drug use and rape.

Other Forms of Campus Violence Violent assaults and sexual violence are not the only types of campus violence that can inflict pain and suffering on students. **Hazing** refers to "activities expected of someone joining a group (or to maintain status in the group) that humiliate, degrade, or risk emotional and/or physical harm, regardless of the person's willingness to participate."[66] Hazing can range from verbal abuse that embarrasses a student, to forced consumption of alcohol or other vile substances, or to branding or burning. Although most fraternities and sororities have rules against it, hazing continues to be a problem on many campuses.

REDUCING YOUR RISK

After a violent act is committed against someone we know, we acknowledge the horror of the event, express sympathy, and go on with our lives. But the person who has been brutalized may take months or years to recover. Campus communities have taken action to help, but there is much more you can do to keep yourself safe.

Self-Defense against Rape

Rape can occur no matter what preventive actions you take, but commonsense self-defense tactics can lower the risk. Self-defense is a process that includes learning increased awareness, self-defense skills, taking reasonable precautions, and having the judgment necessary to respond to different situations. The Skills for Behavior Change box on page 106 identifies practical tips for preventing personal assaults.

Taking Control Most rapes by unknown assailants are planned in advance. They are frequently preceded by a casual, friendly conversation. Although

Stalking The willful, repeated, and malicious following, harassing, or threatening of another person.

Hazing Activities expected of someone joining a group (or to maintain status in the group) that humiliate, degrade, or risk emotional and/or physical harm, regardless of the person's willingness to participate.

Of the over 600,000 sexual assaults and rapes that occur each year in the United States, many involve drugs or alcohol. In the late 1990s, rape crisis centers became alarmed about reports of drugs being used to immobilize victims and make them unable to defend themselves from sexual attacks. These drugs are typically slipped into the drinks of unsuspecting women, who wake up after being raped and can remember few details of the assault. Two of the most common drugs used are Rohypnol and GHB. Although these drugs are often called "date rape" drugs, their use is often unrelated to a date. Many times, they are slipped into the drinks of women whose only meeting with the male perpetrator is to be bought a drink at a bar or handed a drink at a party. There is no date involved—just an opportunity to gain control and remove any chance of resistance.

Although not approved for sale in the United States, Rohypnol (flunitrazepam) is widely available in other countries as a sleep aid. Street names for it include Roaches, LaRocha, rope, Rib Roche, Roches, roofies, Ruffies, Mexican Valium, and roach-2. When dissolved in a drink, Rohypnol produces a sedative-hypnotic effect that includes muscle relaxation and amnesia. Generally, sedative effects occur within 20 to 30 minutes and incapacitation within 1 to 2 hours, often lasting

for hours. People who take it may appear drunk or sleepy, dizzy, or confused. Tablets are white and contain the name "Roche" and an encircled "1" or "2" on one side indicating dosage. The manufacturer has now released a new, lower dose blue tablet designed to be impossible to slip into a drink without detection. Tests are available at rape crisis centers and emergency rooms and through law enforcement agencies to see if Rohypnol has been administered.

GHB (gamma-hydroxybutyrate) is known as Liquid E, Liquid Ecstasy, Liquid X, Grievous Bodily Harm, and Easy First. Illicitly used for its euphoric, sedative, and anabolic (body-building) effects, today GHB is more commonly used than Rohypnol in sexual assaults. GHB is usually a colorless, odorless liquid that may taste salty. Used as a surgical anesthetic in Europe, it is not legal in the United States and can induce short-term coma, slowed heart rate, decreased breathing, seizures, and death.

A drug that has recently appeared and that causes similar reactions is Burundanga, a light yellow powder that has no taste and an immediate effect. Burundanga affects the central nervous system and can be highly dangerous.

Each year, there are several deaths from these rape-facilitating drugs. Survivors must cope with the fact that

they have been violated without a chance to defend themselves. To reduce your risk, follow these guidelines:

✓ Do not accept drinks from strangers. In fact, do not take any beverages or open-container drinks from anyone you do not know well and trust.

✓ Never leave a drink unattended. If you get up to dance, have someone watch your drink or take it with you.

✓ At a bar or club, accept drinks only from the bartender or wait staff. Watch the bartender pour the drink and keep the drink in sight until it's in your hand.

✓ Be alert to the behavior of friends. If they seem disproportionately "out of it" in relation to what they've had to drink, stay with them and watch them carefully.

✓ Go out with friends and leave with friends. Make a rule never to leave a bar or party with someone you don't know well.

✓ If you think you may have been slipped something in a drink, tell a friend and have him or her get you to an emergency room. Call 911 if anyone appears to be unusually "out of it" or experiences seizures, difficulty breathing, or other complications.

Source: National Institute of Drug Abuse, "NIDA Info Facts: Rohypnol and GHB," July 15, 2005, www.nida.nih.gov/infofax/RohypnolGHB.html.

---

many women have said that they started to feel uneasy during such a conversation, they denied the possibility of an attack until it was too late.

Listen to your feelings, and trust your intuition. Be assertive and direct to someone who is getting out of line or threatening—this may convince the would-be rapist to back off. Stifle your tendency to be nice, and don't fear making a scene. Let him know that you mean what you say and are prepared to defend yourself. Consider the following.

■ *Speak in a strong voice.* Use statements such as "Leave me alone" rather than questions such as "Will

you please leave me alone?" Avoid apologies and excuses. Sound like you mean it.

■ *Maintain eye contact with the would-be attacker.* This keeps you aware of the person's movements and conveys an aura of strength and confidence.

■ *Stand up straight, act confident, and remain alert.* Walk as if you own the sidewalk.

Many rapists use certain ploys to initiate their attacks. Examples include asking for help, offering help, a deliberate "accident" such as bumping into you, or posing as policeman or other authority figure.

There are many steps you can take to protect yourself from personal assaults, whether you are home alone or on a date. Implement these steps to increase your awareness and reduce your risk of a violent attack.

When dating

- Set limits. If the situation feels like it is getting out of control, stop and talk, say no directly and don't be coy or worry about hurting feelings. Be firm.

- Most rapes are committed by someone you know. If you feel uncomfortable, protect yourself or get away.

- Date in couples or groups when dating someone new.

- Pay attention to your date's actions. If there is too much teasing and all of the decisions are made for you, it may mean trouble.

- Trust your intuitions. Talk and try to get a sense of the person's history with others, what they say were issues with their past relationships, etc.

- Stick with your friends. Agree to keep an eye out for one another at parties and have a plan for leaving together and checking in with each other. Never leave a bar or party alone with a stranger.

- Avoid drinking too much. Never accept drinks from strangers and don't leave drinks unattended.

When You're Outside Alone

- Carry a cell phone, but stay off of it. Many people are attacked as they get in their cars or are out walking and on their cells and not paying attention.

- Be aware of what is happening around you. Look, listen, and notice what is happening and how close people are to you. Avoid areas where people can lurk in bushes, etc.

- If you are being followed, don't go home. Head for a location where there are other people. If you decide to run, run fast and scream loudly to alert attention.

- Vary your routes; walk or jog with others at a steady pace. Walk with or stay close to others.

- Park near lights; avoid dark areas where people could hide.

- Carry pepper spray or other deterrents. Consider using your campus escort service.

- Tell others where you are going, and when you expect to be back.

While in Your Car

- Lock your doors.

- Purchase cars with alarm systems and remote entry with a light that goes on.

- If someone hits you while you are driving, stay in your car until help comes. Do not open your doors or windows to strangers.

- Call for help from police or road service.

- Never leave your keys in your vehicle, and have your keys ready as you approach your car.

- Never leave a purse or package out in plain view in your car, even if it is locked.

- Be alert to cars that appear to be following you. Do not drive home. Drive to the nearest police station.

While at Home

- Check doors and windows. Make sure locks work.

- Lock doors when at home during the day. Home invasions while residents are at home are becoming more common.

- Keep your garage door locked and closed.

- Don't leave a spare key outside or in the garage.

- When you move into a new residence, pay a locksmith to change the keys and locks.

- If your residence is broken into, don't enter—and call the police.

If you are attacked, act immediately. Draw attention to yourself and your assailant. Scream "fire!" loudly. Research has shown that passersby are much more likely to help if they hear the word *fire* rather than just a scream. Your attacker also may be caught off-balance by the action.

What to Do if a Rape Occurs

If you are a rape victim, report the attack. This gives you a sense of control. Follow these steps.

- Call 911 (if a phone is available).

- Do not bathe, shower, douche, clean up, or touch anything the attacker may have touched.

- Save the clothes you were wearing, and do not launder them. They will be needed as evidence. Bring a clean change of clothes to the clinic or hospital.
- Contact the rape assistance hotline in your area, and ask for advice on therapists or counseling if you need additional help.

If a friend is raped, here's how you can help.

- Believe her, and don't ask questions that may appear to implicate her in the assault.
- Recognize that rape is a violent act and the victim was not looking for this to happen.
- Encourage her to see a doctor immediately because she may have medical needs but feel too embarrassed to seek help on her own. Offer to go with her.
- Encourage her to report the crime.
- Be understanding, and let her know you will be there for her.
- Recognize that this is an emotional recovery, and it may take six months to a year for her to bounce back.
- Encourage her to seek counseling.

A Campus-Wide Response to Violence

Can my university do anything to make me feel safer?

Increasingly, campuses have become microcosms of the greater society, complete with the risks, hazards, and dangers people face in the world. Many college administrators have been proactive in establishing violence prevention policies, programs, and services.[67]

Changing Roles To increase student protection, campus law enforcement has changed over the years in both numbers and authority to prosecute student offenders. Campus police are responsible for emergency responses to situations that threaten safety, human resources, the general campus environment, traffic and bicycle safety, and other dangers. They have the power to enforce laws with students in the same way they are handled in the general community. In fact, many campuses now hire state troopers or local law enforcement officers to deal with campus issues rather than maintain a separate police staff.

Many of these law enforcement groups follow a community policing model in which officers have specific responsibilities for certain areas of campus, departments, or events. By narrowing the scope of each officer's territory, officers get to know people in the area and are better able to anticipate and prevent risks. This differs from earlier safety policies in which campus security typically swooped down only in times of trouble.

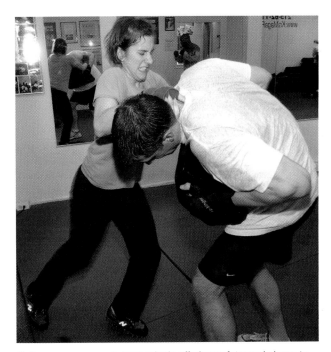

College campuses are increasingly offering safety workshops to equip students with skills to protect themselves from violent acts.

Prevention Efforts Many universities now hire crime prevention and safety specialists. They commonly offer activities such as rape awareness programs, safety workshops, anti-theft programs, and grounds safety measures such as good lighting, escort services, and emergency call boxes. What types of resources are available to you on your campus?

The Role of Student Affairs Although there may be some overlap with law enforcement activities, student affairs offices need to play a vital role in all on-campus programs, both to prevent trouble and to resolve problems that do occur. Student groups should monitor progress, identify potential threats, and advocate for improvements in any areas found to be deficient. A student affairs office can play a key role in making sure that mental health services, student assistance programs, and other services are high quality, easily accessible, and meet student needs. A human services or student affairs office should seek to involve the wider student body and ensure that all are acutely aware of its services. If these programs are not visible or proactive in ensuring campus safety, their roles and responsibilities should be carefully assessed. Student leaders can play a major role in shaping such services and advocating for the campus population.

UNINTENTIONAL INJURIES

As stated previously, unintentional injuries occur without planning or intending to harm. Examples of unintentional injuries include car accidents, falls, water

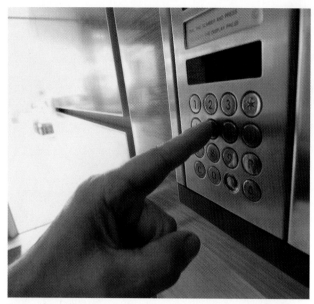

Security systems that control access can make dormitories and apartment buildings safer but are not a substitute for other safety precautions.

accidents, accidental gunshots, recreational accidents, and workplace accidents. None of them happen on purpose, yet they may result in pain, suffering, and possibly even death. Most efforts to prevent unintentional injuries focus on changing something about the person, the environment, or the circumstances (policies, procedures) that put people in harm's way.

Residential Safety

Injuries within the home typically occur in the form of falls, burns, or intrusions by others. Some populations, such as the elderly, are particularly vulnerable. However, older adults are not the only victims; each year, hundreds of children suffer severe burns or die from accidental fires, falls, and other home-based injuries. To reduce the risk of accidents, consider the following.

Fall-Proof Your Home Falls are a common source of home injury. Eliminate objects you may stumble over, especially in the dark. Take the following measures to prevent falls:

- Leave nothing lying around on the floor and use rubberized mats or strips to fasten rugs to the floor.
- Train your pets to stay away from your feet.
- Install slip-proof mats, treads, or decals in showers and tubs and on the stairs.

Avoid Burns and Fires Prevent injury from fires and take precautions to prevent fires from starting in the first place. Tips to prevent the risk of fires and related injury include the following.

- Extinguish all cigarettes in ashtrays before bed, and never smoke in bed at any time!
- Set all lamps away from drapes, linens, and paper.
- Be cautious in the kitchen. Keep hotpads and kitchen cloths away from stove burners, avoid reaching over hot pans, and use caution when lighting barbecue grills.
- Keep candles under control and away from combustibles. Never leave candles unattended or burning while you sleep.
- Avoid overloading electrical circuits with appliances and cords. Older buildings are at particular risk for fire from such overloads.
- Be prepared. Have the proper fire extinguishers ready in case of fire and replace batteries in and test smoke detectors periodically.

Prevent Intruders Take precautions such as the following to ensure your safety when you are home:

- Close blinds and drapes whenever you are away and in the evening when you are home. Remove obstructions from around your windows and doors so that anyone lurking outside will be visible. Consider a low-cost home alarm system.
- Install dead-bolt locks on all doors, including a screen door, and locks on windows. Put a peephole in the main entryway to your home, and do not let anyone in without checking to see who it is. Be cautious of pet doors and skylights.
- Rent apartments that require a security code or clearance to gain entry, and avoid easily accessible apartments such as first-floor units.
- Don't let repair people in without asking for their identification. Preferably, landlords should inform you about such visits well in advance. Have someone else with you when repairs are being made in your home or apartment. Just because a person is licensed to fix refrigerators does not mean he or she can be trusted.
- Avoid dark parking structures, laundry rooms, etc. Try to use these areas only when others are around.
- Use initials for first names on mailboxes and in phone listings. Keep your address out of phone books.
- Keep a cell phone near your bed, and program it to dial 911. Intruders commonly pick up the receiver in another room, thereby disabling a bedroom phone.
- Get to know your neighbors. Organize a neighborhood watch.
- When you are away, put the lights in different rooms on timers set to come on and go off at different times. Stop your mail and newspaper delivery.

Although no amount of security will prevent all threats of intrusion, following these precautions and actively searching for well-maintained housing in low-crime areas are good steps toward preventing break-ins. Usually intruders enter searching for items to sell. If you encounter an intruder, it is far better to give up your money than to fight.

Try it → NOW

Make a safety plan. **Take safety precautions in your home or dorm to prevent intruders. Using the information above, check your living space tomorrow. Identify places where a thief could break in, and write down a list of emergency phone numbers to keep by the phone. Get your roommates in on the plan, and spend a day "safety proofing."**

Workplace Safety

American adults spend most of their waking hours on the job. While most job situations are pleasant and productive, others pose physical and emotional hazards. Stress, burnout, hostile or abusive interactions, discrimination, power struggles, sexual harassment, and a host of other threats are possible whenever people are cloistered together for prolonged periods of time. The nature of the job itself, the corporate culture, and the policies and procedures that characterize certain professions can add to workplace stress.

Fatal Work Injuries Certain industries are inherently more hazardous than others; outdoor occupations show the highest fatality and injury rates. Although workplaces have instituted programs and services to reduce risks, the following statistics indicate a continuing problem:[68]

- In 2003, 5,534 people lost their lives at work. Rates had been decreasing slightly until 2002 but continued to rise in 2003, surpassing most previous fatality reports. There were 1.4 million injuries that required time off work.

- Highway crashes were the leading cause of on-the-job fatalities and accounted for over 25 percent of fatal work injury totals in 2003. Most involved truck drivers.

- Sixteen percent of worker fatalities resulted from other types of transportation-related incidents, such as tractors and forklifts overturning in fields or warehouses, workers being struck by vehicles, aircraft and railway crashes, and water vehicles crashing or capsizing.

- Workplace homicides were higher in 2003 and continue to be a major cause of workplace danger, accounting for 631 murders at work in 2003. Workplace suicides are also on the rise.

Nonfatal Work Injuries Although deaths capture media attention, other workers may be seriously injured or disabled at their jobs. Chronic, debilitating pain and other injuries can cause great economic strain on organizations due to workers' compensation claims and days lost from work. Injuries that cause the greatest number of lost-work days include carpal tunnel syndrome, hernia, amputation of a limb, fractures, sprains and strains (often of the back), cuts or lacerations, and chemical burns. For example, nearly half of all workers with carpal tunnel syndrome miss 30 days or more of work each year. Because so many work injuries are due to repetitive motion, overexertion, or inappropriate motion, they are largely preventable through training and techniques designed to reduce employees' risks.

■ Taking Charge

Summary

- Intentional injuries result from actions committed with intent to harm. Unintentional injuries are the result of actions involving no intent to harm. Many factors lead people to be violent. Among them are anger; substance abuse; and root causes of oppression, mental health, and economic difficulties.

- Acts of terrorism are becoming more common in the United States. In addition to their immediate impact, terrorist activities can exert damaging long-term effects by fostering an atmosphere of fear and anxiety.

- Violence affects everyone in society—from the direct victims to those who live in fear, to those who pay higher taxes and insurance premiums. Over half of all homicides are committed by people who know their victims. Bias and hate crimes divide people, but teaching tolerance can reduce risks. Gang violence continues to grow but can be combated by programs that reduce the problems that lead to gang membership. Violence on campus may be increasing, but victims' rights also have increased as a result of major legislation.

- Prevention begins with avoiding situations in which harm may occur. There are several avenues available for reducing risks, including community, school, workplace, and individual strategies. Many crimes committed in general society are now commonplace at universities and colleges, including personal assaults, sexual assaults, harassment, hate crimes, and even murder.

■ Unintentional injuries frequently occur in homes and at worksites and can produce serious consequences, including death. By following commonsense guidelines, you can significantly reduce your risk of falls, burns, and other injuries.

Chapter Review

1. Which of the following does *not* characterize hate crimes?
   a. They are perpetrated by multiple offenders.
   b. Offenders tend to be older adult males.
   c. Thirty percent of all hate crimes are against property, with the other 70 percent being against the person.
   d. They are excessively brutal and perpetrated at random on total strangers.

2. For an African American man in the 20- to 22-year age group, the probability of being murdered is
   a. 1 in 3.
   b. 1 in 28.
   c. 1 in 153.
   d. 1 in 450.

3. Emotional reaction brought about by frustrating life experiences is called
   a. reactive aggression.
   b. primary aggression.
   c. secondary aggression.
   d. tertiary aggression.

4. When Jane began her new job with all male co-workers, her supervisor told her that he enjoyed having an attractive woman in the workplace and winked at her. His comment constitutes
   a. acquaintance rape.
   b. sexual assault.
   c. sexual harassment.
   d. sexual battering.

5. Psychologist Lenore Walker developed a theory known as the
   a. aggression cycle.
   b. sexual harassment cycle.
   c. cycle of child abuse.
   d. cycle of violence.

6. What is the single greatest cause of injury to women?
   a. rape
   b. mugging
   c. auto accidents
   d. domestic violence

7. In a sociology class, a group of students were discussing sexual assault. One student commented that some women dress too provocatively. The social assumption this student made is
   a. minimization.
   b. trivialization.
   c. blaming the victim.
   d. "boys will be boys."

8. Jack beats his wife Melissa "to teach her a lesson." Afterwards, he denies attacking her. The phase of the cycle of violence that this illustrates is
   a. acute battering.
   b. chronic battering.
   c. remorse/reconciliation.
   d. tension building.

9. Eighty percent of perpetrators of child abuse are
   a. parents.
   b. unmarried partners of a parent.
   c. camp counselors.
   d. school employees.

10. Rape of a person known to the victim and that does not involve a physical beating or use of a weapon is called
    a. simple rape.
    b. sexual assault.
    c. simple assault.
    d. aggravated rape.

Answers to these questions can be found on page A-1.

Questions for Discussion and Reflection

1. What major types of crimes are committed in the United States? What is the difference between primary and reactive aggression?

2. What major factors lead to violent acts?

3. Who tends to be susceptible to the appeal of gang membership?

4. What is terrorism, and why does it occur? What can you do to protect yourself against terrorist attacks?

5. Compare domestic violence against men and against women. What are the differences? What are the similarities? What causes domestic violence?

6. What conditions put a child at risk for abuse? What can be done to prevent or decrease child abuse?

7. What is sexual harassment, and what factors contribute to it in the workplace?

8. What factors increase risk for sexual assault?

9. What are the most effective violence prevention strategies on your campus?

10. What steps can you take to lower your risk of injury from unintentional violence?

Accessing Your Health on the Internet

The following websites explore further topics and issues related to personal health. For links to the websites below, visit the Companion Website for *Health: The Basics,* Seventh Edition at www.aw-bc.com/donatelle.

1. *Communities against Violence Network.* An extensive, searchable database for information about violence against women, with articles, legal information, and statistics.

2. *Crimes on College Campuses.* Comprehensive source of information and statistics of colleges and universities across America.

3. *Men Can Stop Rape.* Practical suggestions for men interested in helping to protect women from sexual predators and assault.

4. *National Center for Injury Prevention and Control.* The WISQARS database of this Centers for Disease Control and Prevention (CDC) section provides statistics and information on fatal and nonfatal injuries, both intentional and unintentional.

5. *National Center for Victims of Crime.* Provides information and resources for victims of crimes ranging from hate crimes to sexual assault.

6. *National Institute for Occupational Safety and Health.* Excellent reference for national statistics on injury and violence, both in the community and in the workplace.

7. *National Sexual Violence Resources Center.* An excellent resource for victims of sexual violence.

8. *Workplace Solutions.* Provides information that helps promote well-being by helping people understand the nature of interpersonal conflict, stress, and violence at work.

Further Reading

Hines, D. and K. Malley-Morrison. *Family Violence in the United States: Defining, Understanding, and Combating Abuse.* Thousand Oaks, CA: Sage Publications, 2005.

Overview of violence statistics, risk factors for various types of violence, and strategies for control and prevention.

Kruttschnitt, C., B. McLauglin, and C. Petrie. *Advancing the Federal Research Agenda on Violence Against Women.* Washington, DC: National Research Council, 2004.

Provides key statistics on the epidemic of violence against women, suspected contributors, and areas where more research is needed.

Ottens, A. and K. Hotelling, eds. *Sexual Violence on Campus: Policies, Programs, and Perspectives.* New York: Springer Publishing, 2001.

Overview of trends, causes, and contributors to violence on campus, as well as policies and programs designed to prevent violence.

Wellford, C., J. Pepper, and C. Petrie. *Firearms and Violence: A Critical Review.* National Academic Press, 2004.

Overview of firearm violence and exploration of key issues to violence.

References

1. D. Zucchio, "Today's Violent Crime Is an Old Story with a New Twist," *San Jose Mercury News,* November 21, 1994.
2. Bureau of Justice Statistics, "Homicide Trends in the U.S.," September 2004, www.ojp.usdoj.gov/bjs/homicide/teens.htm.
3. Bureau of Justice Statistics, "Crime and Victims Statistics: Summary Findings," 2004, www.ojp.usdoj.gov/bjs.
4. D. P. Barash, *Understanding Violence* (Boston: Allyn & Bacon, 2001), 118–122.
5. K. Maguire and A. L. Pastore, eds. *Sourcebook of Criminal Justice Statistics,* 2002, www.albany.edu/sourcebook/.
6. National and Regional Crime Statistics from 1970–2003: Summary Findings.
7. M. Leeds, "Violence Prevention," (Summer Institute, Oregon State University, Corvallis, OR, 2005).
8. Ibid.
9. Ibid.
10. Ibid.
11. Ibid.
12. Ibid.
13. G. Stuart et al., "Relationship Aggression and Substance Use Among Women with Court Deferred Domestic Violence Programs," *Addictive Behaviors* 28, no. 9, (2003): 1603–1610; E. Bacskai et al., "Drinking and Intimate Partner Violence in a Changing Society," *American Journal of Public Health* 95 (2005): 1092–1093.
14. Ibid.
15. Federal Bureau of Investigation, "Uniform Crime Reports, January–December 2003," 2004, www.fbi.gov/ucr/ucr.htm.
16. U.S. Center for Health Statistics, "Table 32: Leading Causes of Death and Numbers of Deaths by Age," *Health United States, 2003* (Atlanta: Centers for Disease Control and Prevention (CDC), 2004).
17. National Center for Health Statistics, Table 7 in "Deaths and Death Rates for the 10 Leading Causes of Death by Age: U.S. Preliminary Data, 2003," *National Vital Statistics Report* 53, no. 15 (2005).
18. Ibid., Table 2.
19. C. Branas, "Firearm Deaths: Not Just a Big City Problem," *American Journal of Public Health* 94 (2004): 1750–1755.
20. R. Lacyo, "Still Under the Gun?" *Time,* July 6, 1998, 32–56.
21. Federal Bureau of Investigation, "Hate Crimes Statistics Report, 2003," 2004, www.fbi.gov/ucr/hatecrime2003.pdf.
22. Ibid.
23. S. Wessler and M. Moss, *Hate Crimes on Campus: The Problem and Efforts to Confront It* (NCJ Publication No. 187249) (Washington, DC: U.S. Department of Justice , 2001).
24. D. Stewart (Director of the Office on Violence Against Women) in statement made before the U.S. Senate Judiciary Committee concerning the reauthorization of the Violence Against Women Act, July 19, 2005.
25. C. Renninson and M. Rand, "National Crime Victimization Survey, 2002," U.S. Department of Justice, Bureau of Crime Statistics, 2003, www.ojp.usdoj.gov/bis.
26. National Center for Injury Prevention and Control, *Intimate Partner Violence,* Fact Sheet Updated (Atlanta: Centers for Disease Control and Prevention, November 30, 2004).
27. Ibid.
28. L. Heise et al., "Ending Violence Against Women," *Population Reports,* series L, no. 11, 1999.
29. C. Rennison, *Bureau of Justice Statistics Crime Data Brief: Intimate Partner Violence, 1993–2001* (NCJ Publication No. 197838) (Washington DC: U.S. Department of Justice, February 2003).
30. Ibid.

31. N. West, "Crimes against Women," *Community Safety Quarterly* 5 (1992): 3.

32. National Clearinghouse on Child Abuse and Neglect Information, "*What Is Child Abuse and Neglect,*" 2004, http://nccanch.acf.hhs .gov/pubs/factsheets/whatiscan.cfm.

33. American Academy of Pediatrics, "Child Abuse and Neglect," 2004, www.aap.org/healthtopics/childabuse.cfm.

34. Administration for Children and Families, "An Issue Facing All Communities: The National Scope of the Problem," February 4, 2005, http://nccanch.acf.hhs.gov/topics/prevention/childabuse_ neglect/scope.cfm.

35. Ibid.

36. Ibid.

37. M. Whittaker, "The Continuum of Violence against Women: Psychological and Physical Consequences," *Journal of American College Health 40* (1992): 155. Reprinted with permission of the Helen Dwight Reid Education Foundation. Published by Heldref Publications, 1319 Eighteenth Street NW, Washington, DC 20036-1802. Copyright © 1992.

38. U.S. Department of Health and Human Services. Administration on Children, Youth, and Families, National Clearinghouse on Child Abuse and Neglect Information, "Summary of Child Maltreatment," 2003, http://nccanch.acf.hhs.gov (Washington DC: Government Printing Office, 2005).

39. Whittaker, "The Continuum of Violence," 152.

40. American Academy of Pediatrics, "Child Abuse and Neglect."

41. Ibid.

42. A. Berkowitz, "College Men as Perpetrators of Acquaintance Rape and Sexual Assault: A Review of Recent Literature," *Journal of American College Health 40* (1992): 175.

43. National Women's Health Information Center, "Sexual Assault," January 2005, www.4woman.gov/faq/sexualassault.htm

44. Rennison, "National Crime Victimization Survey, 2002."

45. R. K. Bergen, "Violence against Women Online Resources," 2004, www.vaw.umn.edu/Vawnet/mrape.htm.

46. Ibid.

47. Berkowitz, "College Men as Perpetrators of Acquaintance Rape," 177.

48. J. Katz, "Tough Guize" (presentation at the Violence Prevention Summer Institute, Oregon State University, Corvallis, OR, 2003).

49. U.S. Department of Education, *Summary of Campus Crime and Security Statistics: Criminal Offenses,* 2004, 2005, www.ed.gov/ admins/lead/safety/crime/criminaloffenses/index.html.

50. K. Baum and P. Klaus, *Violent Victimization of College Students, 1995–2002* (NCJ Publication No. 206836) (Washington, DC: U.S. Department of Justice, 2005).

51. American College Health Association, *Security on Campus Update: American College Health Association Calls for Better Response to Campus Violence* 4, no. 10, February 13, 2004, www.securityoncampus.org/update/v04n10.html. updated 7-14-2005; J. L. Carr, *American College Health Association Campus Violence White Paper* (Baltimore, MD: American College Health Association February, 2005).

52. A. Hoffman et al., eds. *Violence on Campus: Defining the Problems, Strategies for Action* (Gaithersburg, MD: Aspen Publishers, 1998), 1–40.

53. Ibid.

54. Ibid.

55. Bureau of Justice Statistics, "College Students Victimized Less by Violent Crime than Non-Students According to New Justice Department Study," (press release) December 7, 2003, www.ojp .usdoj.gov/bjs/pub/press/vvcs00pr.htm; Hoffman et al., *Violence on Campus.*

56. J. Carr and K. Van Deusen, "Risk Factors for Male Sexual Aggression on College Campuses," *Journal of Family Violence* 19, no. 5, (2004): 279–289.

57. B. Fisher, F. Cullen, and M. Turner, *The Sexual Victimization of College Women* (NCJRS Publication No. 182369) (Washington, DC: U.S. Department of Justice, 2000).

58. E. Dersinger, C. Cychosz, and C. Jaeger, "Strategies for Dealing with Campus Violence" in Hoffman et al., eds. *Violence on Campus,* 248; L. Hong, "Understanding and Preventing Violence on Our Campuses: A Comprehensive Student Affairs Initiative (paper presented at the annual meeting of the American College Health Association, Washington DC, 2002).

59. H. Melton, "Stalking: A Review of the Literature and Direction for the Future," *Criminal Justice Review* 25, no. 2 (2000): 246–252.

60. K. A. Roberts, "Associated Characteristics of Stalking Following the Termination of Romantic Relationships," *Applied Psychology in Criminal Justice* 1, no. 1 (2005):15-35.

61. Fisher et al., *Sexual Victimization of College Women;* Roberts, "Associated Characteristics of Stalking."

62. V. Ravensberg and C. Miller, "Stalking Among Young Adults: A Review of the Preliminary Research," *Aggression and Violent Behavior* 8 (2003): 455–469.

63. Baum et al., *Violent Victimization of College Students.*

64. Ibid.

65. Ibid.

66. StopHazing.org, "Hazing Defined," 2005, www.stophazing.org/ definition.html.

67. Desinger et al., "Strategies for Dealing with Campus Violence"; Fisher et al., *Sexual Victimization of College Women;* Hong, "Understanding and Preventing Violence."

68. U.S. Center for Health Statistics, *Health: United States 2004*; U.S. Department of Labor, Bureau of Labor Statistics, *Injuries, Illnesses and Fatalities* (Atlanta: Centers for Disease Control and Prevention, 2005).

How can I become a more effective communicator?

What can I do to cope with a bad breakup?

Does an intimate relationship have to be sexual?

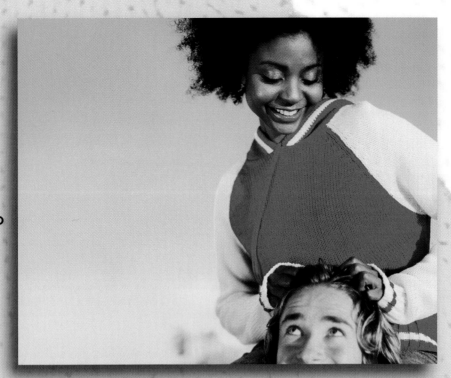

Do men and women have the same sexual response?

5 Healthy Relationships and Sexuality
Making Commitments

Objectives

- *Discuss* ways to improve communication skills and interpersonal interactions.
- *Describe* the characteristics of each type of intimate relationship, common challenges, and how to deal with relationship problems.
- *Examine* factors that affect life decisions, such as whether to have children.

- *Define* sexual identity, and discuss the role of gender identity.
- *Identify* major features and functions of sexual anatomy and physiology.
- *Classify* sexual dysfunctions and describe major disorders.

Humans are social beings—we have a basic need to belong and to feel loved, appreciated, and wanted. We can't live without relating to others in some way. In fact, a study done by researchers at the Harvard School of Public Health shows that the ability to relate well with people, as well as give and receive love and support throughout your life, can have almost as much impact on your health as exercise and good nutrition.[1]

All relationships involve a degree of risk. However, only by taking these risks can we grow and truly experience all that life has to offer. By looking at our intimate and nonintimate relationships, components of sexual identity, gender roles, and sexual orientation, we will come to better understand who we are.

COMMUNICATING: A KEY TO GOOD RELATIONSHIPS

From the moment of birth, we struggle to be understood. We flail our arms, cry, scream, smile, frown, and make sounds and gestures to attract attention, get a reaction from someone we care about, or have someone understand what we want or need from them. By the time we enter adulthood, each of us has developed a unique way of communicating to others with gestures, words, expressions, and body positions. No two of us communicate in the exact same way or have the same need for connecting with others. Some are outgoing and quick to express our emotions and thoughts. Others are quiet, reluctant to talk about feelings, and may prefer to spend time alone rather than with others.

Different cultures not only have different languages and dialects, but also different ways of expressing themselves and using body language to communicate information.[2] Some cultures gesture wildly; others maintain a closed and rigid means of speaking. Some cultures are offended by apparent "fixed and dilated" staring, while others welcome a steady look in the eyes.

Although people differ in the way they communicate, this doesn't mean that one sex, culture, or group is better or should be a model for the others. We have to be willing to accept differences and work to keep communication lines open and fluid. Appearing interested, actively engaged in the interaction, and open and willing to exchange ideas and thoughts is something that we typically learn with practice and hard work.

Communicating How You Feel

Do you find it easy to convey how much you care about friends and family members with hugs and verbal expressions of appreciation and love? If you are comfortable telling them you love them and that they mean a lot

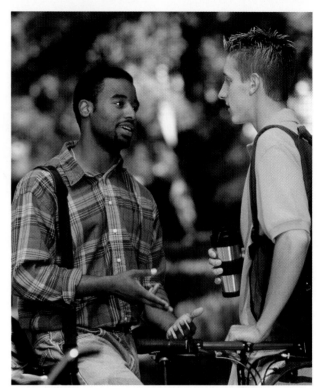

"The better part of one's life consists of his friendships."
—Abraham Lincoln

to you, chances are that you also will be able to tell them when you are feeling bad, disappointed, angry, or frustrated. However, it's important to realize that some people were not raised in affectionate families, do not readily discuss feelings or emotions, and sometimes may struggle to find the right words for expressing what they feel.

When two people begin a relationship, they bring their past communication styles with them.[3] How often have you heard someone say, "We just can't communicate," or "You're sending mixed messages"? These exchanges occur regularly as people start relationships or work through ongoing communication problems in an existing relationship. Because communication is a process, our every action, word, facial expression, gesture, or body posture becomes part of our shared history and part of the evolving impression we make on others. If we are angry in our responses, others will be reluctant to interact with us. If we bring "baggage" from past bad interactions to new relationships, we may be cynical, distrustful, and guarded in our exchanges with others. If we are positive, happy, and share openly with others, they will be more likely to communicate openly with us. This ability to communicate assertively is an important skill in relationships (see the Assess Yourself box on page 138). Assertive communicators are in touch with their feelings and values and are able to directly and honestly communicate their needs or defend choices in a positive manner.

Improving Communication Skills Because people have such different ways of communicating, there is no recipe for how to communicate best in a

How can I become a more effective communicator?

given situation. At times, silence may be the best approach. However, there are things that each of us can do to become better communicators and to encourage and assist others in their attempts to interact with us.

Learning Appropriate Self-Disclosure

Sharing personal information with others is called **self-disclosure.** If you are willing to share personal information with others, they will likely share personal information with you. In other words, if you want to learn more about someone, you have to be willing to share parts of your personal self with that person. Self-disclosure is not storytelling or sharing secrets; rather, it is revealing how you are reacting to the present situation and giving any information about the past that is relevant to the other person's understanding of your current reactions.[4]

Self-disclosure can be a double-edged sword, for there is risk in divulging personal insights and feelings. If you sense that sharing feelings and personal thoughts will result in a closer relationship, you will likely take such a risk. But if you believe that the disclosure may result in rejection or alienation, you may not open up so easily. If the confidentiality of previously shared information has been violated, you may hesitate to disclose yourself in the future.

Being a Better Listener

Listening is a vital part of interpersonal communication; it allows us to share feelings, express concerns, communicate wants and needs, and let our thoughts and opinions be known. We must do the necessary work to improve both our speaking and listening skills, which will enhance our relationships, improve our grasp of information, and allow us to interpret more effectively what others say. We listen best when (1) we believe that the message is somehow important and relevant to us, (2) the speaker holds our attention through humor, dramatic effect, use of media, or other techniques, and (3) we are in the mood to listen (free of distractions and worries). When we really listen effectively, we try to understand what people are thinking and feeling from their perspective. We not only hear the words, but we try to understand what is really being said. How many times have you been caught pretending to be listening when you were not? After several moments of nodding and saying "uh-huh," your friend finally asks you a question, and you haven't a clue about what she has been saying. Sometimes this tuned-out behavior is due to a lack of sleep, stress overload, being preoccupied, having too much to drink, or being under the influence of drugs. Other times it's because speakers are motor-mouths who talk for the sake

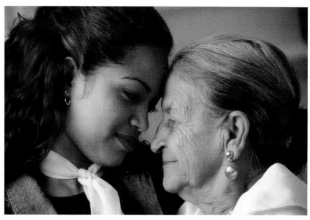

The emotional bonds that characterize intimate relationships often span the generations and help individuals gain insight and understanding into each other's worlds.

of talking or you find them or what they are talking about is boring. Some of the most common listening difficulties are things that we can work to improve. See the Skills for Behavior Change box on the next page for suggestions for improving your listening.

Try it ➤NOW

Change the "You" to "I." **Think about the last time you had a disagreement with a friend, sibling, or roommate. On a piece of paper, rewrite the statement using an "I" message (such as "I feel . . .") instead. The next time you have a similar disagreement with the same person, use the "I" message. Notice how the other person's response changed, and how the conversation became less hostile and more solution oriented.**

CHARACTERISTICS OF INTIMATE RELATIONSHIPS

We can define **intimate relationships** in terms of four characteristics: behavioral interdependence, need fulfillment, emotional attachment, and emotional availability. Each of these characteristics may be related to interactions with family, close friends, and romantic partners.

Self-disclosure Sharing personal feelings or information with others.

Intimate relationships Relationships with family members, friends, and romantic partners, characterized by behavioral interdependence, need fulfillment, emotional attachment, and emotional availability.

Most of us have lamented the fact that someone "never listens" and seems to monopolize the entire conversation. Although we are quick to recognize such flaws in others, we are often less likely to spot listening problems of our own. On a daily basis, we all have times when we just "tune out." When a professor drones on about a subject we don't relate to, we begin doodling or put on a fake interested facial expression, even though we are thinking about dinner or what to wear to the movies that night. When that boring friend tells the same story over and over again, we say "uh-huh"—and worry that we'll be caught when he asks a question and we don't have a clue what he is talking about. We grimace at the thought of certain people calling but dash for the phone when the caller ID indicates that it is someone we love to talk with. What is the difference? Why do we tune out when some people speak and tune in for others?

We gravitate toward those who seem to understand us and with whom we have fun and interesting interactions. If the truth be told, most of us are only mediocre listeners. What does it take to be an excellent listener? Practicing the following skills and consciously using them on a daily basis is an important part of improved communication.

■ *Be present in the moment.* Contrary to what is often believed, good listeners don't just sit back with their mouths shut. They participate and acknowledge what the other person is saying. (Nodding, smiling, saying "yes" or "uh-huh," and asking questions at appropriate times are all part of this. Take care, however, not to numbly say "uh-huh" to every word, which is distracting and conveys insincerity.)

■ *Use positive body language and voice tone.* Show that you are "with" the speaker by turning toward him or her and staying focused (wandering eyeballs are a sure sign that your mind is elsewhere). Avoid barrier gestures such as shaking your head "no," making negative faces, or folding your arms; smile at appropriate times and maintain appropriate eye contact (deadpan stares can also be distracting). Voice tone, posture, and an attitude that conveys interest are all key.

■ *Show empathy and sympathy.* Watching for verbal and nonverbal clues to the other person's feelings and trying to relate can be very useful. For example, saying, "That must have been really hard for you" can encourage the speaker to talk and feel more comfortable with you as an understanding listener.

■ *Ask for clarification.* If you aren't sure what the speaker means, indicate that you're not sure you understand, or paraphrase what you think you heard. This kind of feedback is invaluable in avoiding misinterpretation and lapses in overall communication. As a speaker, you may ask, "What did you think I was just saying?" but be sure to say this in a nonthreatening manner.

■ *Control that deadly desire to interrupt.* Some people start nodding and gesturing before you ever get a word out of your mouth. If you are like that, squelch it, even if you have to put an inconspicuous hand over your mouth. Try taking a deep breath for two seconds, then hold your breath for another second and really listen to what is being said as you slowly exhale. Don't be so enthusiastically empathetic that you finish speakers' sentences or put words in people's mouths.

■ *Avoid snap judgments based on what other people look like or are saying.* If you notice some strange mannerism, try to focus on what is being said, not how it is being said. Avoid stereotyping or labeling.

■ *Resist the temptation to "set the other person straight."* Control your urge to correct errors or react defensively. Listen and hear without reacting or trying to rationalize what the speaker is trying to say.

■ *Try to focus on the speaker.* Sometimes it is very tough to listen to someone who is trying to talk about a painful situation, especially if we are experiencing or have recently experienced the same thing. Hold back the temptation to "tell all" and fly off into your own rendition of a similar situation. Give the speaker the moment and later, after he or she is done talking, you may want to discuss your own experience as a way of validating the feelings expressed. Don't tell him how he is feeling or how he should feel.

■ *Be tenacious.* Stick with the speaker and try to stay on the topic. If they seem to wander, gently nudge them back by saying, "You were just saying . . ." Offer your thoughts and suggestions, but remember that you should only advise up to a certain point. Clarify statements with "this is my opinion" as a reminder that it is only opinion, rather than fact.

Behavioral interdependence refers to the mutual impact that people have on each other as their lives and daily activities intertwine. What one person does influences what the other person wants to do and can do. Behavioral interdependence may become stronger over time to the point that each person would feel a great void if the other were gone.

Intimate relationships also fulfill psychological needs and so are a means of *need fulfillment*. Through relationships with others, we fulfill our needs for:

■ *Intimacy* —someone with whom we can share our feelings freely.

- *Social integration*—someone with whom we can share worries and concerns.
- *Nurturance*—someone whom we can take care of and who will take care of us.
- *Assistance*—someone to help us in times of need.
- *Affirmation*—someone who will reassure us of our own worth and tell us that we matter.

In rewarding intimate relationships, partners and friends meet each other's needs. They disclose feelings, share confidences, and provide support and reassurance. Each person comes away from interactions feeling better for the experience and validated by the other person.

In addition to behavioral interdependence and need fulfillment, intimate relationships involve strong bonds of *emotional attachment,* or feelings of love. When we hear the word intimacy, we often think of a sexual relationship. Although sex can play an important role in emotional attachment, a relationship can be very intimate and yet not sexual. Two people can be emotionally intimate (they share feelings) or spiritually intimate (they share spiritual beliefs and meanings), or they can be intimate friends. The intimacy level two people experience cannot be judged easily by those outside the relationship.

> **Does an intimate relationship have to be sexual?**

Emotional availability, the ability to give to and receive from others emotionally without fear of being hurt or rejected, is the fourth characteristic of intimate relationships. At times, all of us may limit our emotional availability. For example, after a painful breakup we may decide not to jump into another relationship immediately, or we may decide not to talk about it with every friend. Holding back can offer time for introspection and healing, as well as for considering the lessons learned. However, because of intense trauma, some people find it difficult ever to be fully available emotionally. This limits their ability to experience intimate relationships.

FORMING INTIMATE RELATIONSHIPS

In the early years of life, families provide the most significant relationships. Gradually, the circle widens to include friends, coworkers, and acquaintances. Ultimately, most of us develop romantic or sexual relationships with significant others. Each of these relationships plays a significant role in psychological, social, spiritual, and physical health.

Families: The Ties That Bind

A **family** is typically thought of as people (two or more) related to one another by blood, marriage/long-term committed relationships, or adoption. Yet, the family is

Table 5.1

Today's Changing Families

The United States is a melting pot of family types. The estimated percentages of school-age children living in various family structures is listed below and are based on data from the U.S. Census Bureau, 2002.

Family Structure	School-age children living in identified family structure (%)
Nuclear family: husband and wife plus biological offspring	58
Stepparent family: one biological parent plus one stepparent	10
Blended family: parents plus children born to several families	5
Adoptive family: two parent	2
Single mother, never married	10
Single mother, divorced	10
Single father, divorced and never remarried	5

a dynamic institution that is constantly changing as society changes. The specific functions and expectations of a family may differ from one culture to another.

The United States is a melting pot of family types. The U.S. Census Bureau has identified seven family structures (Table 5.1). Today, family units may include unmarried, same-or other-sex couples with or without children; one-parent families including never married, widowed, or single-parent households of divorced or separated spouses; *reconstituted families,* or stepfamilies consisting of children from multiple marriages; and *blended families* in which either or both partners bring children to the family, and they may also have additional children together. *Extended families* including grandparents, aunts, uncles, cousins, and other relatives are also common in today's society. About 2 percent of school aged-children live with their grandparents alone, and 7 percent of school-aged children live in extended families that may include grandparents, one of their parents, and other relatives.[5] Regardless of family structure, the central focus of families should be to care, protect, love, and socialize with one another. Healthy families provide children the opportunity to

> **Family** People (two or more) related to one another by blood, marriage/long-term committed relationships, or adoption and have common values, attitudes, behaviors, and belief systems.

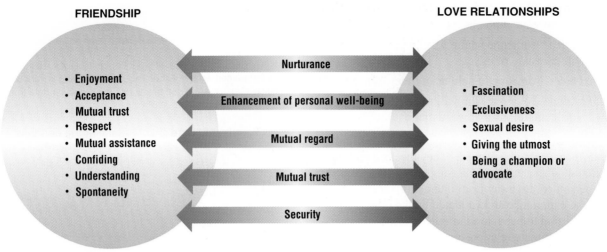

FRIENDSHIP

- Enjoyment
- Acceptance
- Mutual trust
- Respect
- Mutual assistance
- Confiding
- Understanding
- Spontaneity

Nurturance

Enhancement of personal well-being

Mutual regard

Mutual trust

Security

LOVE RELATIONSHIPS

- Fascination
- Exclusiveness
- Sexual desire
- Giving the utmost
- Being a champion or advocate

Figure 5.1 ■ Common Bonds of Friends and Lovers

learn to communicate effectively; influence values, attitudes, and behaviors; and cultivate spiritual belief systems.[6]

Children of healthy families are likely to become emotionally connected adults. If the home environment provides stability and safety, it is likely that the children will learn to express feelings and develop intimacy skills. Sibling interactions provide a way to learn and practice interpersonal skills. When the family itself is healthy, people can practice positive behaviors and learn the consequences of negative behaviors in a safe and nonjudgmental environment. However, in unhealthy family environments there is often little positive communication, and a lack of affection. Children are less likely to share feelings out of fear and frequent arguments may fail to teach children problem-solving skills. Children raised in unhealthy families may have significant problems with later relationships, as we will discuss in this chapter.

Friendship and Love

Friendship and love give life meaning. They connect us in significant ways to others, provide for emotional growth and development, and help us weather life's stress. It is interesting, but not surprising, that best-friend relationships and spouse/lover relationships are more similar than they are different. Both rely on high levels of respect, trust, self-disclosure, understanding, mutual acceptance, and shared interests and values. Communication and trust are key to identifying and maintaining boundaries in both types of relationships. In fact, friendship is often the best foundation for a strong love relationship. What separates friends from lovers is often the nature of the attraction and the degree of exclusiveness one feels with a partner versus a friend; with lovers, passion and emotional intimacy alter the nature of a relationship, creating new expectations and possibilities.[7]

Friendships are more likely to last if two people have real or perceived similarities in attitudes, opinions, and backgrounds.[8] Strong, lasting friendships result when both people nurture the relationship; taking the time to be the best friend you are looking for in another person is key.[9]

Establishing Friendships

True friends have the ability to make us feel like we matter and can give us the strength and support needed to get through just about anything. Not only do friends enrich our lives, but there are real health benefits to having strong social bonds. Social support has been shown to boost the immune system, improve the quality of and even lengthen life, and reduce the risks of heart disease.[10]

What are the characteristics of a good friendship? Though little research has been done on this subject, there are some common characteristics that make a good friendship.[11] These characteristics include enjoyment of each other's company, acceptance, mutual trust and assistance, respect, ability to confide in one another, and mutual understanding.

Significant Others, Partners, and Couples

Most people choose at some point to enter into an intimate sexual relationship with another person. Most partners fit into one of four categories: married heterosexual couples, cohabiting heterosexual couples, lesbian couples, and gay male couples. These groups are discussed in greater detail later in this chapter.

Love relationships in each of these four groups typically include all the characteristics of friendship as well as the following characteristics related to passion and caring (Figure 5.1).[12]

- *Fascination.* Lovers tend to pay attention to the other person even when they should be involved in other activities. They are preoccupied with the other and want to think about, talk to, or be with the other.

- *Exclusiveness.* Lovers have a special relationship that usually precludes having the same relationship with a third party. The love relationship takes priority over all others.

- *Sexual desire.* Lovers desire physical intimacy and want to touch, hold, and engage in sexual activities with the other.

- *Giving the utmost.* Lovers care enough to give the utmost when the other is in need, sometimes to the point of extreme sacrifice.

- *Being a champion or advocate.* Lovers actively champion each other's interests and attempt to ensure that the other succeeds.

THIS THING CALLED LOVE

What is love? This four-letter word has been written about and engraved on walls; it has been the theme of countless novels, movies, and plays. There is no single definition of love, and the word may mean different things to people, depending on cultural values, age, gender, and situation. Yet, we all know what it is when it strikes.

Many social scientists maintain that love may be of two kinds: companionate and passionate. Companionate love is a secure, trusting attachment, similar to what we may feel for family members or close friends. In companionate love, two people are attracted, have much in common, care about each other's well-being, and express reciprocal liking and respect. Passionate love, in contrast, is a state of high arousal filled with the ecstasy of being loved and the agony of being rejected.[13] In this next section, we will explore what passionate love is.

Theories of Love

How and why love develops is not an easy question to answer. Several theories have been proposed to help provide insight into the process. Sternberg's Triangular Theory of Love (Figure 5.2) suggests three key components to loving relationships.[14]

- *Intimacy*—the emotional component, which involves closeness, sharing, and mutual support.

- *Passion*—the motivational component, which includes lust, attraction, sexual arousal, and sharing.

- *Commitment*—the cognitive component, which includes the decision to be open to love in the short term and the commitment to the relationship in the long term.

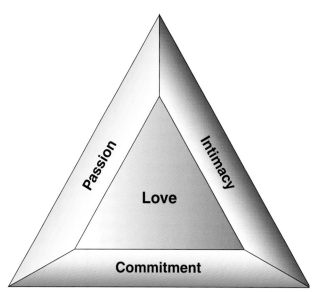

Figure 5.2 ■ Sternberg's Triangular Theory of Love

The quality of love relationships is reflected by the level of intimacy, passion, and commitment each brings to the relationship over time.

A second theory of love and attraction, based upon brain circuitry and chemistry, is quite different from that of Sternberg. Anthropologist Helen Fisher (and others) hypothesizes that attraction and falling in love follow a fairly predictable pattern based on (1) *imprinting,* in which our evolutionary patterns, genetic predispositions, and past experiences trigger a romantic reaction; (2) *attraction,* in which neurochemicals produce feelings of euphoria and elation; (3) *attachment,* in which endorphins—natural opiates—cause lovers to feel peaceful, secure, and calm; and (4) *production of a cuddle chemical,* in which the brain secretes the chemical *oxytocin,* thereby stimulating sensations during love-making and eliciting feelings of satisfaction and attachment.[15]

Lovers who claim that they are swept away by passion may not be far from the truth. Why? Because the love-smitten person's endocrine system secretes chemical substances such as dopamine, norepinephrine, and phenylethylamine (PEA), which are chemical cousins to amphetamines.[16] Although attraction may in fact be a "natural high," this hit of passion loses effectiveness over time as the body builds up a tolerance. Many people may become attraction junkies, seeking the intoxication of love much as the drug user seeks a chemical high.[17] Fisher speculates that PEA levels drop significantly over a three- to four-year period, leading to the "four-year itch" that shows up in the peaking fourth-year divorce rates present in over 60 cultures. Romances that last beyond the four-year mark are influenced by another set of chemicals, known as endorphins, soothing substances that give lovers a sense of security, peace, and calm.[18]

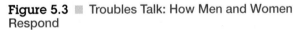

Men

- Talk is primarily a means of preserving independence and negotiating and maintaining status.

- Men are more likely to give advice, tell a joke, change the subject, or remain silent when trouble arises.

- When women offer sympathy to men, men may feel that they are being placed in a lower-status position and find it condescending.

- Men are more likely to be avoidant.

Women

- Talk is primarily a means of rapport, a way of establishing connections and negotiating relationships. Emphasis is on displaying similarities and matching experiences.

- Women are more likely to share a similar problem or openly express sympathy and to expect sympathy in return.

- When men give advice, women feel that their feelings are being invalidated, their problems are being minimized, or that the simple "fix" provided is condescending.

- Women are likely to be supportive.

Figure 5.3 ■ Troubles Talk: How Men and Women Respond

Source: S. L. Michaud and R. Warner, "Gender Differences in Self-Reported Responses in Troubles Talk," *Sex Roles: A Journal of Research* 37, no. 7–8 (1997): 527.

In another theory, researchers describe the first stage as the *lust phase,* in which our biological and genetic histories converge to pique our interest and intensity of response. In the lust phase, if someone comes into our range of awareness, a chemical surge can trigger our enthusiastic response. Known as *pheromones* and said to be as unique as our fingerprints, these triggers are scent-infused chemicals found in perspiration under the armpits. They trigger a unique sensory reaction in the nose and result in attraction if their producer is a match for you.[19] Following these pheromone triggers comes the *attraction phase,* often labeled the

falling in love phase, and then the *attachment phase.* The two hormones that are most important in this last phase are oxytocin and vasopressin. Oxytocin increases the bond between lovers, is released by both sexes during orgasm, and is one of the chemicals responsible for contractions during childbirth, milk expression when breastfeeding. Scientists suspect vasopressin to be the chemical responsible for creating the desire to be monogamous with another person. The science behind this is relatively new, but the implications are interesting. The theory suggests that the more sex a couple have, the greater the bond between them.[20]

GENDER ISSUES IN RELATIONSHIPS

When it comes to relationships, are men really from Mars and women from Venus? If they are not planets apart, how far apart are they, and what are the implications of the disparities? In her landmark book *You Just Don't Understand: Women and Men in Conversation,* psychologist Deborah Tannen coined the term **genderlect** to characterize differences in word choices, interruption patterns, questioning patterns, language interpretations and misinterpretations, and vocal influences based on gender.[21] Tannen is not alone in her research; communication patterns between women and men have been studied for generations with similar results. Recent research validates much of this work and indicates that women tend to be more expressive, relationship oriented, and concerned with creating and maintaining intimacy; men tend to be more instrumental, task oriented, and concerned with gathering information or establishing and maintaining social status or power.[22] Unlike women, men tend to believe that they are not supposed to show emotions and are brought up to believe that "being strong" is often more important than having close friendships. As a result, men are generally less likely to share their innermost thoughts. Figure 5.3 summarizes some of these characteristics.

What Do You Think? Who are the people with whom you feel most comfortable talking about personal issues? ■ Do you talk with both males and females about these issues, or do you tend to gravitate toward just one sex? ■ Why do you think you do this?

Styles in Decision Making

According to classic research conducted by Harvard professor Carol Gilligan, men and women may make very different decisions when facing ethical dilemmas.[23] Gilligan believes that women tend to think and

---

Genderlect The "dialect," or individual speech pattern and communication style, of each gender.

speak differently from men because of the two genders' contrasting images of self: there is a feminine ethic of *care* and a masculine ethic of *justice*.[24] Following this line of thinking, she suggests that women view sensitivity to others, loyalty, responsibility, self-sacrifice, and peacemaking as key factors to consider in making ethical decisions. In contrast, men are more interested in individual rights, equality before law, and fair play—factors that are much more impersonal. Because such gender differences would affect both the encoding and decoding of messages, difficulties in communication might result.[25] Today, as gender differences have become less pronounced, decisions are influenced more by past experiences and behaviors. Men are more likely than ever to express caring ethics and women to express justice ethics.

Picking Partners

For both males and females, the choice of partners is influenced by more than just chemical and psychological processes. One important factor is *proximity,* or being in the same place at the same time. The more you see a person in your hometown, at social gatherings, or at work, the more likely that interaction will occur. Thus, if you live in New York, you'll probably end up with another New Yorker. (With the advent of the Internet, however, geographic proximity is not always important.)

You also pick a partner based on similarities (attitudes, values, intellect, interests); the old adage that "opposites attract" usually isn't true. If your potential partner expresses interest or liking, you may react with mutual regard known as *reciprocity.* The more you express interest, the safer it is for someone else to return the regard, and the cycle spirals onward.

A final factor that plays a significant role in selecting a partner is physical attraction. Whether such attraction is caused by a chemical reaction or a socially learned behavior, males and females appear to have different attraction criteria. Men tend to select their mates primarily on the basis of youth and physical attractiveness. Although physical attractiveness is an important criterion for women in mate selection, they tend to place higher emphasis on partners who are somewhat older, have good financial prospects, and are dependable and industrious.[26]

What Do You Think?
What factors do you consider the most important in a potential partner? ▪ Which are absolute musts? ▪ Are there any differences between what you believe to be important in a relationship and the things your parents feel are important?

Sharing Feelings

Although men tend to talk about intimate issues with women more frequently than with men, women still complain that men do not communicate enough about what is really on their minds. This may reflect the powerfully different socialization processes experienced by women and men, which influence their communication styles. Throughout their lives, females are offered opportunities to practice sharing their thoughts and feelings with others. In contrast, males receive strong societal messages to withhold their feelings. The classic example of this training in very young males is the familiar saying, "Big boys don't cry." Men learn early that certain emotions are not to be shared, with the result that they are more information-focused and businesslike in their conversations. Understandably, such differences in communication styles contribute to misunderstandings and conflict.

Although men are often perceived as being less emotional than women, do they really feel less or do they just have more difficulty expressing their emotions? In one study, when men and women were shown scenes of people in distress, the men exhibited little outward emotion, whereas the women communicated feelings of concern and distress. However, physiological measures of emotional arousal (such as heart rate and blood pressure) indicated that the male subjects were as affected emotionally as the female subjects but inhibited the expression of their emotions; the women openly expressed them. In other studies, men and women responded very differently to the same test.[27]

When men are angered, they tend to interpret the cause of their anger as something or someone in their environment and are likely to turn their anger outward in an aggressive manner. Women, on the other hand, tend to see themselves as the source of the problem and turn their anger inward, suppressing direct expression of it.[28]

OVERCOMING BARRIERS TO INTIMACY

Obstacles to intimacy include lack of personal identity, emotional immaturity, and a poorly developed sense of responsibility. The fear of being hurt, low self-esteem, mishandled hostility, chronic "busyness" (and its attendant lack of emotional presence), a tendency to "parentify" loved ones, and a conflict of role expectations may be equally detrimental. Individual insecurities and difficulties in recognizing and expressing emotional needs also can create obstacles. These barriers to intimacy may have many causes, including a dysfunctional family background and jealousy.

Dysfunctional Families

As noted earlier, the ability to sustain genuine intimacy is largely developed in the family of origin. If you were to examine even the most pristine family under a microscope, you would likely find some problems. No group of people can interact perfectly all the time, but this does not necessarily make them dysfunctional. In a truly **dysfunctional family,** interaction between family members inhibits psychological growth, self-love, emotional expression, and individual development. Negative interactions are the norm rather than the exception. It is important to note that dysfunctional families are found in every social, ethnic, religious, economic, and racial group.

Children raised in dysfunctional settings tend to face tremendous obstacles to growing up healthy. Coming to terms with past hurts may take years. However, with support from loved ones, and counseling when needed, children from even the most dysfunctional homes have proven to be remarkably resilient. Many are able to forget the past, focus on the future, and develop into healthy, well-adjusted adults.

Jealousy in Relationships

"Jealousy is like a San Andreas fault running beneath the smooth surface of an intimate relationship. Most of the time, its eruptive potential lies hidden. But when it begins to rumble, the destruction can be enormous."[29] **Jealousy** has been described as an aversive reaction evoked by a real or imagined relationship involving one's partner and a third person.

Contrary to what many of us may believe, jealousy is not a sign of intense devotion. Instead, jealousy often indicates underlying problems that may prove to be a significant barrier to a healthy intimate relationship. Often, jealousy in a relationship is rooted in a past relationship in which an individual experiences deception or from observing patterns among our friends. Causes of jealousy typically include the following.

- *Overdependence on the relationship.* People who have few social ties and rely exclusively on their significant others tend to be fearful of losing them.
- *High value on sexual exclusivity.* Those who believe sexual exclusivity is a crucial indicator of love are more likely to become jealous.

> **Dysfunctional family** A family in which the interaction between family members inhibits rather than enhances psychological growth, self-love, emotional expression, and individual development.
>
> **Jealousy** An aversive reaction evoked by a real or imagined relationship involving one's partner and a third person.

- *Severity of the threat.* People may feel uneasy if someone with stunning good looks and a great personality appears interested in their partners.
- *Low self-esteem.* The underlying question that torments people with low self-esteem is "Why would anyone want me?" People who feel good about themselves and that they are a good "catch" are less likely to fear that someone else is going to snatch their partners.
- *Fear of losing control.* Some people need to feel in control of the situation. Feeling that they may be losing the attachment of or control over a partner can cause jealousy.

In both sexes, jealousy is related to the expectation that it would be difficult to find another relationship if the current one ends. For men, jealousy is positively correlated with self-evaluative dependency, the degree to which the man's self-esteem is affected by his partner's judgments. Though a certain amount of jealousy can be expected in any loving relationship, it doesn't have to threaten a relationship as long as partners communicate openly about it.[30]

What Do You Think? "Jealousy is not a barometer by which the depth of love can be read. It merely records the depth of the lover's insecurity" (anthropologist Margaret Mead, 1901–1978). Do you agree or disagree with this statement? ■ What other factors may play a role in jealousy?

COMMITTED RELATIONSHIPS

Commitment in a relationship means that there is intent to act over time in a way that perpetuates the well-being of the other person, oneself, and the relationship. Polls show that the majority of Americans—as many as 96 percent—strive to develop a committed relationship, even though many have difficulty maintaining them. These relationships can take several forms, including marriage, cohabitation, and gay and lesbian partnerships.

Marriage

In many societies around the world, traditional committed relationships take the form of marriage. In the United States, marriage means entering into a legal agreement that includes shared financial plans, property, and responsibility for raising children. Many Americans also view marriage as a religious sacrament that emphasizes certain rights and obligations for each spouse.

Historically, close to 90 percent of Americans marry at least once during their lifetime. In recent years, Americans have become less likely to marry. From 1970 to 2004, annual marriages of adult women declined 50 percent.[31] This decrease may be due to several factors, including delay of first marriages, increase in cohabitation, and a small decrease in the number of divorced persons who remarry. In 1970, the median age for first marriage was 22.5 years for men and 20.6 years for women; in 2004, the median age of first marriage was 26 for females and 27 for males.[32]

Many Americans believe that marriage involves **monogamy,** or exclusive sexual involvement with one partner. In fact, the lifetime pattern for many Americans appears to be **serial monogamy,** which means that a person has a monogamous sexual relationship with one partner before moving on to another monogamous relationship. However, some people prefer to have an **open relationship,** or open marriage, in which the partners agree that there may be sexual involvement for each person outside their relationship.

Marriage is socially sanctioned and highly celebrated in our culture, so there are numerous incentives for couples to formalize their relationship with a wedding ceremony. A healthy marriage provides emotional support by combining the benefits of friendship and a loving committed relationship. A happy marriage also provides stability for both the couple and for those involved in the couple's life. However, traditional marriage does not work for everyone, and is not the only path to a happy and successful committed relationship.

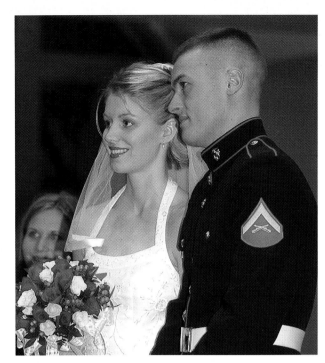

For many people, marriage or commitment ceremonies serve as the ultimate symbol of commitment between two people and validate their love for each other.

Try it → NOW

Create an ideal partner checklist. **After class, make a list of factors you have used or think would be useful in choosing a partner for a committed relationship. Then review the information on common myths associated with marriage and choosing a partner found in the Reality Check box on page 124. Were you surprised when you compared the information on your list with current research findings?**

by living together.[33] Cohabitation can serve as a prelude to marriage, but for some it is an alternative to marriage. Cohabitation is more common among those of lower socioeconomic status, those who are less religious, those who have been divorced, and among those who have experienced high levels of parental conflict or parental divorce during childhood. Many people believe that living together before marriage is a good way to find out how compatible you are with your partner and possibly avoid a bad marriage; however, current data does not support this belief. The long-term outcomes or implications of living together may be related more to who chooses to cohabitate rather than the experience of cohabitating itself.

Cohabitation

Cohabitation is defined as two unmarried people with an intimate connection who live together in the same household. For a variety of reasons, increasing numbers of Americans are choosing cohabitation. In some states, cohabitation that lasts a designated number of years (usually seven) legally constitutes a **common-law marriage** for purposes of purchasing real estate and sharing other financial obligations.

Between 1960 and 2004, the number of cohabiting adults in America increased by over 1,000 percent. In fact, today over half of all first marriages are preceded

Monogamy   Exclusive sexual involvement with one partner.

Serial monogamy   A series of monogamous sexual relationships.

Open relationship   A relationship in which partners agree that sexual involvement can occur outside the relationship.

Cohabitation   Living together without being married.

Common-law marriage   Cohabitation lasting a designated period of time (usually seven years) that is considered legally binding in some states.

For many young adults the idea of marriage conjures images of their parents, and other older adults they may know. What does marriage mean to you? Marriage is the great unknown for many young people, and it is possible that you wonder when Mr. or Mrs. Right will come along, where you'll find your lifetime partner, or if there is such a thing as the "perfect" marriage.

The National Marriage Project, a research initiative at Rutgers University in New Jersey, is taking the topic of marriage to task by researching the attitudes of young adults toward marriage and working to educate young adults on how to prepare for marriage in the future. The following facts and myths are the result of the National Marriage Project's current research findings.

Fact—*The most likely way to find a future marriage partner is through an introduction by family, friends, or acquaintances.* Despite the romantic notion that people meet and fall in love through chance or fate, the evidence suggests that social networks are important in bringing together individuals of similar interests and backgrounds, especially when it comes to selecting a marriage partner. According to a large-scale national survey of sexuality, almost 60 percent of married people were introduced by family, friends, coworkers, or other acquaintances.

Myth—*Marriage benefits men much more than women.* Contrary to earlier and widely publicized reports, recent research finds men and women benefit about equally from marriage, although in different ways. Both men and women live longer, happier, healthier, and wealthier lives when they are married. Husbands typically gain greater health benefits while wives gain greater financial advantages.

Fact—*The more similar people are in their values, backgrounds, and life goals, the more likely they are to have a successful marriage.* Opposites may attract, but they may not live together harmoniously as married couples. People who share common backgrounds and similar social networks are better suited as marriage partners than people who are very different in their backgrounds and networks.

Myth—*Couples who live together before marriage, and are thus able to test how well suited they are for each other, have more satisfying and longer-lasting marriages than couples who do not.* Many studies have found that those who live together before marriage have less satisfying marriages and a considerably higher chance of eventually breaking up. One reason is that people who cohabit may be more skittish of commitment and more likely to call it quits when problems arise. The very act of living together may lead to attitudes that make happy marriages more difficult. The findings of one recent study, for example, suggest "there may be less motivation for cohabiting partners to develop their conflict resolution and support skills." (One important exception: cohabiting couples who are already planning to marry each other in the near future have just as good a chance at staying together as couples who don't live together before marriage.)

Fact—*For large segments of the population, the risk of divorce is far below 50 percent.* Although the overall divorce rate in America remains close to 50 percent of all marriages, it has been dropping gradually over the past 20 years. The risk of divorce is far below 50 percent for educated people going into their first marriage and lower still for people who wait to marry until at least their mid-twenties, haven't lived with many different partners prior to marriage, or are strongly religious and marry someone of the same faith.

Myth—*Married people have less satisfying sex lives and less sex than single people.* According to a large-scale national study, married people have both more and better sex than do their unmarried counterparts. Not only do they have sex more often, but they enjoy it more, both physically and emotionally.

Source: D. Popenoe, "The Top Ten Myths of Marriage," The National Marriage Project Ten Things to Know Series, 2004, http://marriage.rutgers.edu; D. Popenoe, "Ten Important Research Findings on Marriage and Choosing a Marriage Partner: Helpful Facts for Young Adults," The National Marriage Project, 2004, http://marriage.rutgers.edu.

Although cohabitation has its advantages, it also has some drawbacks. In 1996, Congress reaffirmed tax advantages for married couples and effectively blocked cohabiting heterosexual and homosexual couples from these benefits through the "Defense of Marriage Bill." Today, controversy continues over whether traditional marriage should remain the only means of eligibility for tax deductions, health insurance, and other benefits.

Gay and Lesbian Partnerships

Most adults want intimate, committed relationships, whether they are gay or straight, men or women. Lesbians and gay men seek the same things in primary relationships that heterosexual partners do: friendship, communication, validation, companionship, and a sense of stability.

The 2000 U.S. Census revealed a significant increase in the number of same-sex partner households across the country—more than three times the total reported in the 1990 Census. The states with the most reported same-sex households are California, New York, Florida, Illinois, and Georgia. According to Lee Badgett, research director of the Institute for Gay and Lesbian Strategic Studies, the actual number of households is probably much higher. Many gay and lesbian partners hesitate to report their relationship because of concerns about discrimination.[34]

Studies of lesbian couples indicate high levels of attachment and satisfaction and a tendency toward monogamous, long-term relationships. Much like their heterosexual counterparts, gay men tend to form committed, long-term relationships, especially as they age.

Challenges to successful lesbian and gay male relationships often stem from discrimination and difficulties dealing with social, legal, and religious doctrines. For lesbian and gay couples, obtaining the same level of "marriage benefits," such as tax deductions, power-of-attorney, child custody, and other rights, continues to be a challenge. However, commitment ceremonies and marriage ceremonies are becoming more frequent in some U.S. cities and in several countries. In 2004, courts in Massachusetts legalized marriages between same-sex partners. Worldwide, same-sex marriages are legal in the Netherlands, Belgium, Spain, and Canada.

STAYING SINGLE

Increasing numbers of adults of all ages are electing to marry later or to remain single altogether. Data from 2004 indicates that the percentage of women aged 20 to 24 who have never been married is 75 percent. Likewise, men in this age group postponed marriage in increasing numbers, with over 86 percent of this group remaining unmarried in 2004.[35] According to the most recent figures from the U.S. Census Bureau and National Center for Health Statistics, the number of unmarried women aged 15 and older will soon surpass the number of married women.[36] The number of unmarried men is also increasing. Other changes are reflected in the following facts:

- Over 10 percent of all people say they would never marry.
- People marrying today have about a 50 percent chance of divorcing.
- As more women enjoy financial independence, they are less likely to remarry after divorce.
- Increasing numbers of widows and widowers are opting not to remarry.

Today, large numbers of people prefer to remain single or to delay marriage. Singles clubs, social outings arranged by communities and religious groups, extended family environments, and many social services support the single lifestyle. Many singles live rich, rewarding lives and maintain a large network of close friends and families. Although sexual intimacy may or may not be present, the intimacy achieved through other interactions with loved ones is a key aspect of the single lifestyle.

What Do You Think? Although there are advantages and disadvantages to marriage, many people feel that it is a desirable option. Are there advantages to remaining single? ■ Are there potential disadvantages? ■ Are there any societal or organizational supports for the single lifestyle?

SUCCESS IN RELATIONSHIPS

Most people's definition of success in a relationship is based on whether a couple stays together over the years. Learning to communicate, respecting each other, and sharing a genuine fondness are crucial to relationship success. Many social scientists agree that the happiest committed relationships are flexible enough to allow the partners to grow throughout their lives.

Partnering Scripts

Parents often believe that their children will achieve happiness by living much as they have. Accordingly, most children are reared with a very strong script for what is expected of them as adults. Each group in society has its own partnering script that prescribes standards regarding sex, age, social class, race, religion, physical attributes, and personality types. By adolescence, people generally know exactly what type of person they are expected to befriend or date. By which partnering script were you raised? Just picture whom you could or couldn't bring home to meet your family.

Society provides constant reinforcement for traditional couples, but it may withhold this reinforcement from couples of the same sex, mixed race, mixed religion, or mixed age. People who have not chosen a traditional partner are subject to a great deal of external stress. In addition to denying recognition to such couples, friends and family often blame the nontraditional nature of the couple if the relationship fails.

Nonetheless, many nontraditional relationships survive and flourish. For example, the number of interracial marriages has quadrupled since the late 1960s, and the number of same-sex partner households has grown from 145,130 to almost a half-million over the past ten years.[37]

Being Self-Nurturant

It is often stated that you must love yourself before you can love someone else. What does this mean? Learning how you function emotionally and how to nurture yourself through all life's situations is a lifelong task. You should certainly not postpone intimate connections with others until you have achieved this state. However, a certain level of individual maturity helps in maintaining a committed relationship. For example, divorce rates are much higher for couples under age 30 than for older couples.

Two concepts that are especially important to a good relationship are accountability and self-nurturance. **Accountability** means that both partners in a relationship see themselves as responsible for their own decisions, choices, and actions. They don't hold the other person responsible for positive or negative experiences.

Self-nurturance, which goes hand in hand with accountability, means developing individual potential through a balanced and realistic appreciation of self-worth and ability. In order to make good choices in life, a person needs to balance many physical and emotional needs, including sleeping, eating, exercising, working, relaxing, and socializing. When the balance is disrupted, as it will inevitably be, self-nurturing people are patient with themselves and try to put things back on course. It is a lifelong process to learn to live in a balanced and healthy way. Two people who are on a path of accountability and self-nurturance together have a much better chance of maintaining a satisfying relationship.

HAVING CHILDREN . . . OR NOT?

When a couple decides to raise children, their relationship changes. Resources of time, energy, and money are split many ways, and the partners no longer have each other's undivided attention. Babies and young children do not time their requests for food, sleep, and care to the convenience of adults. Therefore, individuals or couples whose own basic needs for security, love, and purpose are already met make better parents. Any stresses existing in a relationship will be further accentuated when parenting is added to the responsibilities. Having a child does not save a bad relationship—in fact, it only seems to compound the problems that already exist. A child cannot and should not be ex-

Accountability Accepting responsibility for personal decisions, choices, and actions.

Self-nurturance Developing individual potential through a balanced and realistic appreciation of self-worth and ability.

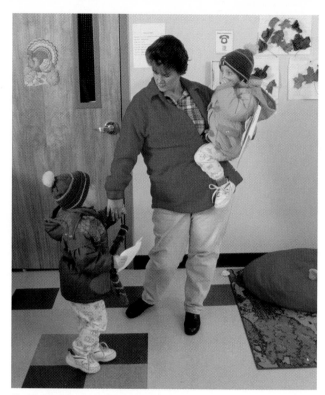

Single parents face additional challenges in juggling their work and family responsibilities. Many use community resources, such as after-school day care centers.

pected to provide the parents with self-esteem and security.

Changing patterns in family life affect the way children are raised. In modern society, it is not always clear which partner will adjust his or her work schedule to provide the primary care of children. Nearly half a million children each year become part of a blended family when their parents remarry; remarriage creates a new family of stepparents and stepsiblings. In addition, an increasing number of individuals are choosing to have children in a family structure other than a heterosexual marriage (see Table 5.1). Single women or lesbian couples can choose adoption or alternative insemination as a way to create a family. Single men can choose to adopt or obtain the services of a surrogate mother. According to the 2002 census, over 25 percent of all school aged children were living in families headed by a man or woman raising a child alone, reflecting a growing trend in America and in the international community. Regardless of the structure of the family, certain factors remain important to the well-being of the unit: consistency, communication, affection, and mutual respect.

Some people become parents without a lot of forethought. Some children are born into a relationship that was supposed to last and didn't. This does not mean it is too late to do a good job of parenting. Children are amazingly resilient and forgiving if parents show respect and communicate about household activities that affect their lives. Even children who grew up in a household of conflict can feel loved and respected if the parents treat them fairly. This means that parents must take responsibility for their own emotions and make it clear to children that they are not the reason for the conflict.

Finally, consider the financial implications of deciding to have a child. Today, many families find that two incomes are needed just to make ends meet. For more on family planning and financial evaluation, see Chapter 6.

WHEN RELATIONSHIPS FALTER

Breakdowns in relationships usually begin with a change in communication, however subtle. Either partner may stop listening and cease to be emotionally present for the other. In turn, the other feels ignored, unappreciated, or unwanted. Unresolved conflicts increase, and unresolved anger can cause problems in sexual relations.

When a couple who previously enjoyed spending time alone together find themselves continually in the company of others, spending time apart, or preferring to stay home alone, it may be a sign that the relationship is in trouble. Of course, the need for individual privacy is not a cause for worry—it's essential to health. If, however, a partner decides to change the amount and quality of time spent together without the input or understanding of the other, it may be a sign of hidden problems.

College students, particularly those who are socially isolated and far from family and hometown friends, may be particularly vulnerable to staying in unhealthy relationships. They may become emotionally dependent on a partner for everything from eating meals to recreational and study time; mutual obligations such as shared rental arrangements, transportation, and child care can make it tough to leave.

It's also easy to mistake unwanted sexual advances for physical attraction or love. Without a network of friends and supporters with whom a student can talk, obtain validation for feelings, or share concerns, he or she may feel stuck in a relationship that is headed nowhere.

Honesty and verbal affection are usually positive aspects of a relationship. In a troubled relationship, however, they can be used to cover up irresponsible or hurtful behavior. "At least I was honest" is not an acceptable substitute for acting in a trustworthy way. "But I really do love you" is not a license for acting inconsiderate or rude.

Most communities have trained therapists who specialize in relationship difficulties, and most student health centers offer these services at reduced fees for students. If you are unaware of such services, ask your instructor for suggestions.

When and Why Relationships End

The lifetime probability for divorce or separation of a recently married couple in the United States is between 40 and 50 percent. While this is still high, it does represent a small decline from previous decades. This small decrease may be related to an increase in the age at which persons first marry and to a higher level of education among those that are marrying—both contribute to marital stability.[38]

While the divorce rate may seem alarming, the actual number of failed relationships is probably much higher. Many people never go through a legal divorce process so are not counted in these statistics. Cohabitors and unmarried partners who raise children, own homes together, and exhibit all the outward appearances of marriage without the license are also not included.

Why do relationships end? There are many reasons, including illness, financial concerns, and career problems. Other breakups arise from unmet expectations. Many people enter a relationship with certain expectations about how they and their partner will behave. Failure to communicate these beliefs can lead to resentment and disappointment. Differences in sexual needs may also contribute to the demise of a relationship.

Under stress, communication and cooperation between partners can break down. Conflict, negative interactions, and a general lack of respect between partners can erode even the most loving relationship. One of the greatest predictors of divorce appears to be husband dissatisfaction in the first five years of marriage.

Coping with Failed Relationships

No love relationship comes with a guarantee, no matter how many promises have been made by partners to be together forever. Losing a love is as much a part of life as falling in love. That being said, the uncoupling process can be very painful. Whenever we risk getting close to another, we also risk being hurt if things don't work out. Remember that knowing, understanding, and feeling good about oneself before entering the relationship waters is very important. Consider these tips for coping with a failed relationship.[39]

What can I do to cope with a bad breakup?

1. *Recognize and acknowledge your feelings,* which may include grief, loneliness, rejection, anger, guilt, relief, or sadness. Seek professional help and support as needed.

2. *Find healthful ways to express your emotions,* rather than turning them inward. Go for a walk, talk to friends, listen to music, work out at the gym,

volunteer with a community organization, or write in a journal.

3. *Spend time with current friends or reconnecting with old friends.* Get reacquainted with yourself and what you enjoy doing.

4. *Don't rush into a "rebound" relationship.* You need time to resolve your past experience rather than escape from it. You can't be trusting and intimate in a new relationship if you are still working on getting over a past relationship.

BUILDING BETTER RELATIONSHIPS

Most relationships start with great optimism and true love. So why do so many run into trouble? "We just don't know how to handle the negative feelings that are the unavoidable by-product of the differences between two people, the very differences that attract them to each other in the first place. Think of it as the friction any two bodies would generate rubbing against each other countless times each day," says Howard Markman, PhD, professor of psychology at the University of Denver.[40] According to Markman, most unhappy couples don't need therapy; they need education in how relationships work and the special skills that make them work well. Markman and others promote **psychoeducation,** the teaching of crucial psychological skills that give people knowledge so they can help themselves. Psychoeducation courses aren't therapy per se, but they typically have a therapeutic effect on couples.

Elements of Healthy Relationships

Satisfying and stable relationships share certain identifiable traits such as good communication, intimacy, friendship, and other factors discussed in this chapter

---

Psychoeducation   The teaching of crucial psychological skills that give people knowledge so they can help themselves.

Trust   The degree of confidence partners feel in a relationship.

Sexual identity   Recognition of oneself as a sexual being; a composite of biological sex, gender roles, gender identity, and sexual orientation.

Intersexuality   Not exhibiting exclusively male or female secondary sex characteristics.

Gonads   The reproductive organs in a male (testes) or female (ovaries).

(Table 5.2). A key ingredient is **trust,** the degree of confidence partners feel in a relationship. Without trust, intimacy will not develop, and the relationship could fail. Trust includes three fundamental elements.

- *Predictability* means that you can predict your partner's behavior, based on the knowledge that your partner acts in consistently positive ways.

- *Dependability* means that you can rely on your partner to give support in all situations, particularly those in which you feel threatened with hurt or rejection.

- *Faith* means that you feel absolutely certain about your partner's intentions and behavior.

Trust can develop even when it is initially lacking. This requires opening yourself to others, which carries the risk of hurt or rejection.

YOUR SEXUAL IDENTITY

Sexual identity, the recognition and acknowledgment of oneself as a sexual being, is determined by a complex interaction of genetic, physiological, environmental, and social factors. The beginning of sexual identity occurs at conception with the combining of chromosomes that determine sex. The biological father determines whether a baby will be a boy or a girl. All eggs (ova) carry an X sex chromosome; sperm may carry either an X or a Y chromosome. If a sperm carrying an X chromosome fertilizes an egg, the resulting combination of sex chromosomes (XX) provides the blueprint to produce a female. If a sperm carrying a Y chromosome fertilizes an egg, the XY combination produces a male.

However, nature does not always get it right though. **Intersexuality** may occur as often as one in 100 live births. This refers to a medical condition in which a person is born with sex chromosomes, external genitalia, and/or an internal reproductive system that has both male and female components. Some of these individuals may not even be aware that their internal reproductive organs are unusual, while others may have external evidence. There is great variation in the manifestations of intersexuality.

The genetic instructions included in the sex chromosomes lead to the differential development of male and female **gonads** (reproductive organs) at about the eighth week of fetal life. Once the male gonads (testes) and the female gonads (ovaries) are developed, they play a key role in all future sexual development because the gonads are responsible for the production of sex hormones. The primary sex hormones produced by females are estrogen and progesterone. In males, the sex hormone of primary importance is testosterone. The release of testosterone in a maturing fetus signals the development of a penis and other male genitals. If no testosterone is produced, female genitals form.

Table 5.2
Healthy versus Unhealthy Relationships

Being in a *healthy relationship* means . . .	If you are in an *unhealthy relationship* . . .
Loving and taking care of yourself before and while in a relationship.	You care for and focus on another person only and neglect yourself or you focus only on yourself and neglect the other person.
Respecting individuality, embracing differences, and allowing each person to "be themselves."	You feel pressure to change to meet the other person's standards, you are afraid to disagree, and your ideas are criticized. Or, you pressure the other person to meet your standards and criticize his/her ideas.
Doing things with friends and family and having activities independent of each other.	One of you has to justify what you do, where you go, and who you see.
Discussing things, allowing for differences of opinion, and compromising equally.	One of you makes all the decisions and controls everything without listening to the other's input.
Expressing and listening to each other's feelings, needs, and desires.	One of you feels unheard and is unable to communicate what you want.
Trusting and being honest with yourself and each other.	You lie to each other and find yourself making excuses for the other person.
Respecting each other's need for privacy.	You don't have any personal space and have to share everything with the other person.
Sharing sexual histories and sexual health status with a partner.	Your partner keeps his/her sexual history a secret or hides a sexually transmitted infection from you, or you do not disclose your history to your partner.
Practicing safer sex methods.	You feel scared of asking your partner to use protection or he or she has refused your requests for safer sex. Or, you refuse to use safer sex methods after your partner has requested, or you make your partner feel scared.
Respecting sexual boundaries and being able to say no to sex.	Your partner has forced you to have sex or you have had sex when you don't really want to. Or, you have forced or coerced your partner to have sex.
Resolving conflicts in a rational, peaceful, and mutually agreed upon way.	One of you yells and hits, shoves, or throws things at the other in an argument.
Having room for positive growth, and learning more about each other as you develop and mature.	You feel stifled, trapped, and stagnant. You are unable to escape the pressures of the relationship.

Source: Advocates for Youth, "Healthy versus Unhealthy Relationships," 2005. www.advocatesforyouth.org/youth/health/relationships/healthy.htm.

At the time of **puberty,** sex hormones again play major roles in development. Hormones released by the **pituitary gland,** called gonadotropins, stimulate the testes and ovaries to make appropriate sex hormones. The increase of estrogen production in females and testosterone production in males leads to the development of **secondary sex characteristics.** Male secondary sex characteristics include deepening of the voice, development of facial and body hair, and growth of the skeleton and musculature. Female secondary sex characteristics include growth of the breasts, widening of the hips, and the development of pubic and underarm hair.

Thus far, we have described sexual identity only in terms of a person's biology. While biology is an important facet of sexual identity, the relationship of biology and culture is much more complicated than the popular notion of sex as referring to biology and gender to social issues. In other words, *sex* simply refers to the biological condition of being male or female based on physiological and hormonal differences.

Gender is the practice of behaving in masculine or feminine ways as defined by the society in which one

---

Puberty   The period of sexual maturation.

Pituitary gland   The endocrine gland controlling the release of hormones from the gonads.

Secondary sex characteristics   Characteristics associated with gender but not directly related to reproduction, such as vocal pitch, degree of body hair, and location of fat deposits.

Gender   The psychological condition of being feminine or masculine as defined by the society in which one lives.

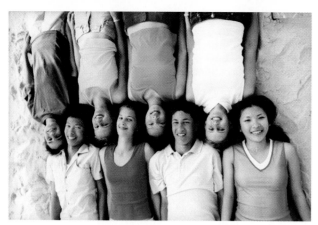

Signs of physical maturity are not always indicators of emotional adulthood.

lives and as a component of our identity, while sex is more related to physical form and function. In this sense, gender is a performance, something we do rather than something we have, and we learn gender through the process of **socialization.** Through interactions with family, peers, teachers, media, and other social

organizations, we learn to act in ways that society deems appropriate. Think about the television shows you watch. Do the characters play out traditional gender roles?

Each of us expresses our maleness or femaleness to others on a daily basis by the **gender roles** we play. **Gender identity** refers to the personal sense or awareness of being masculine or feminine, a male or a female. It may sometimes be difficult to express one's true sexual identity because of the bounds established by **gender-role stereotypes,** or generalizations about how males and females should express themselves and the characteristics each possesses. Our traditional sex roles are an example of gender-role stereotyping. Men are thought to be independent, aggressive, better in math and science, logical, and always in control of their emotions. Women, on the other hand, are traditionally expected to be passive, nurturing, intuitive, sensitive, and emotional.

Androgyny refers to the combination of traditional masculine and feminine traits in a single person. Androgynous people choose behaviors based on the given situation rather than following traditional sex roles. Other people consider themselves to be **transgendered.** These people refuse to follow the sexual and gender scripts prescribed to them based on their biology and resist the division of gender into two distinct categories.[41] **Transsexuality**, also known as gender dysphoria, refers to a condition in which a person is in a state of conflict between gender identity and physical sex. Simply stated, a transsexual is a mind physically trapped in the body of the opposite sex. The condition is not related to sexual orientation, nor should it be confused with transvestism, or cross-dressing.

By now you can see that defining sexual identity is not a simple matter. It is a lifelong process of growing and learning. Your sexual identity is made up of the unique combination of your biology, gender identity, chosen gender roles, sexual orientation, and personal experiences. No other person on this earth is exactly like you, and it is up to you to take every opportunity to get to know and like yourself so that you may enjoy your life to the fullest.

What Do You Think?
How often do you challenge existing gender-role stereotypes? ■ What is the outcome? ■ Do you think men and women have the same degree of freedom in gender-role expression?

Sexual Orientation

Sexual orientation refers to a person's enduring emotional, romantic, sexual, or affectionate attraction to other persons. You may be primarily attracted to members of the other sex (**heterosexual**), your same sex (**homosexual**), or both sexes (**bisexual**).

Socialization   Process by which a society communicates behavioral expectations to its individual members.

Gender roles   Expression of maleness or femaleness in everyday life.

Gender identity   Personal sense or awareness of being masculine or feminine, a male or a female.

Gender-role stereotypes   Generalizations about how males and females should express themselves and the characteristics each possesses.

Androgyny   Combination of traditional masculine and feminine traits in a single person.

Transgendered   Refusing to follow the sexual and gender scripts prescribed based on biology and resisting the division of gender into two distinct categories.

Transsexuality   Condition in which a person is psychologically of one sex but physically of the other; also called gender dysphoria.

Sexual orientation   A person's enduring emotional, romantic, sexual, or affectionate attraction to other persons.

Heterosexual   Experiencing primary attraction to and preference for sexual activity with people of the other sex.

Homosexual   Experiencing primary attraction to and preference for sexual activity with people of the same sex.

Bisexual   Experiencing attraction to and preference for sexual activity with people of both sexes.

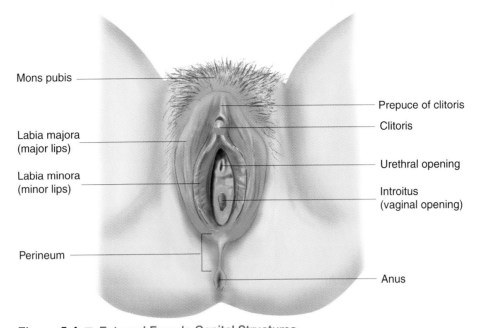

Figure 5.4 ■ External Female Genital Structures

Source: R. D. McAnulty and M. M. Burnette, *Exploring Human Sexuality: Making Healthy Decisions* (Boston: Allyn & Bacon, 2001). Copyright © 2001 by Pearson Education.

Many homosexuals prefer the terms *gay* and *lesbian* to describe their sexual orientations, as these terms go beyond the exclusively sexual connotation of the term *homosexual. Gay* applies to both men and women, but *lesbian* refers specifically to women.

Most researchers today agree that sexual orientation is best understood using a multifactorial model, which incorporates biological, psychological, and socioenvironmental factors. Biological explanations focus on research into genetics, hormones (perinatal and postpubertal), and differences in brain anatomy, while psychological and socioenvironmental explanations examine parent–child interactions, sex roles, and early sexual and interpersonal interactions. Collectively, this growing body of research suggests that the origins of homosexuality, like heterosexuality, are complex. To diminish the complexity of sexual orientation to "a choice" is a clear misrepresentation of current research. Homosexuals do not "choose" their sexual orientation any more than heterosexuals do.

Irrational fear or hatred of homosexuality creates antigay prejudice and is expressed as **homophobia.** Homophobic behaviors range from avoiding hugging same-sex friends to name-calling and physical attacks. Herek and colleagues surveyed 2,259 gay and lesbian people and found that one in five women and one in four men had been victimized in the preceding five years because of their sexual orientation.[42]

What Do You Think? Why is sexual orientation controversial in our society? ■ Do you ever display homophobic behavior? ■ What can you do to help prevent hate crimes?

SEXUAL ANATOMY AND PHYSIOLOGY

An understanding of the functions of the male and female reproductive systems will help you derive pleasure and satisfaction from your sexual relationships, be sensitive to your partner's wants and needs, and make responsible choices regarding your own sexual health.

Female Sexual Anatomy and Physiology

The female reproductive system includes two major groups of structures, the external genitals (Figure 5.4) and the internal genitals. The **external female genitals** include all structures that are outwardly visible; they are

Gay Sexual orientation involving primary attraction to people of the same sex; usually but not always applies to men attracted to men.

Lesbian Sexual orientation involving primary attraction of women to other women.

Homophobia Irrational hatred or fear of homosexuals or homosexuality.

External female genitals The mons pubis, labia majora and minora, clitoris, urethral and vaginal openings, and the vestibule of the vagina and its glands.

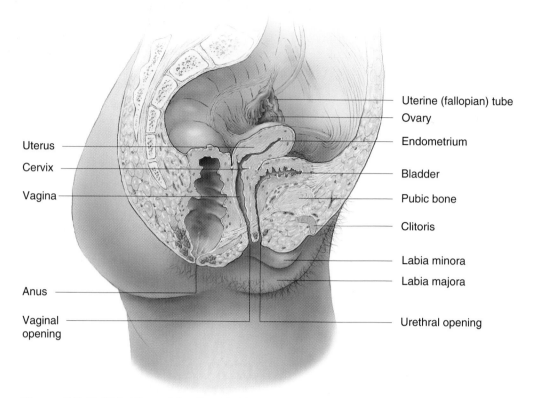

Figure 5.5 ■ Side View of the Female Reproductive Organs

Labels on figure:
Uterus
Cervix
Vagina
Anus
Vaginal opening

Uterine (fallopian) tube
Ovary
Endometrium
Bladder
Pubic bone
Clitoris
Labia minora
Labia majora
Urethral opening

referred to as the vulva. Specifically, the **vulva,** or external genitalia, includes the mons pubis, the labia minora and majora, the clitoris, the urethral and vaginal openings, and the vestibule of the vagina and its glands.

Vulva   The female's external genitalia.

Mons pubis   Fatty tissue covering the pubic bone in females; in physically mature women, the mons is covered with coarse hair.

Labia minora   "Inner lips," or folds of mucous membrane just inside the labia majora.

Labia majora   "Outer lips," or folds of skin and erectile tissue that cover the female sexual organs.

Clitoris   A pea-sized nodule of tissue located at the upper end of the labia minora.

Urethral opening   The opening through which urine is expelled.

Hymen   Thin membrane covering the vaginal opening.

Perineum   Tissue between the vulva and the anus.

Internal female genitals   The vagina, uterus, uterine tubes, and ovaries.

Vagina   The passageway in females that leads from the uterus to the vulva.

The **mons pubis** is a pad of fatty tissue covering the pubic bone. The mons protects the pubic bone, and after onset of puberty it becomes covered with coarse hair. The **labia minora** are inner lips or folds of mucous membrane, and the **labia majora** are folds of skin and erectile tissue that enclose the urethral and vaginal openings. The labia minora are found just inside the labia majora.

The **clitoris** is the female sexual organ whose only known function is sexual pleasure. It is located at the upper end of the labia minora and beneath the mons pubis. Directly below the clitoris is the urethral opening through which urine is expelled from the body. Below the **urethral opening** is the vaginal opening, or opening to the vagina. In some women, the vaginal opening is covered by a thin membrane called the **hymen.** It is a myth that an intact hymen is proof of virginity. The **perineum** is the tissue between the vulva and the anus. Although not technically part of the external genitalia, the tissue in this area has many nerve endings and is sensitive to touch; it can play a part in sexual excitement.

The **internal female genitals** of the reproductive system include the vagina, uterus, uterine (fallopian) tubes, and ovaries (Figure 5.5). The **vagina** is a tubular organ that serves as a passageway from the uterus to the outside of a female's body. This passageway allows menstrual flow to exit from the uterus during a woman's monthly cycle, receives the penis during intercourse, serves as the birth canal. The **uterus** (or **womb**) is a hollow, muscular, pear-shaped organ. Hormones acting on the soft, spongy matter that makes up the inner lining of the uterus, called the **endometrium,** either prepare the uterus for implantation and development of a fertilized egg or signal that no fertilization has taken place, in which case the endometrium deteriorates and becomes menstrual flow.

The lower end of the uterus, the **cervix,** extends down into the vagina. The ovaries are almond-sized structures suspended on either side of the uterus. The **ovaries** produce the hormones estrogen and progesterone and are the reservoir for developing eggs. All the eggs a female will ever have are present in the ovaries at birth. Eggs mature and are released from the ovaries in response to hormone levels. Extending from the upper end of the uterus are two thin, flexible tubes called the **uterine (fallopian) tubes.** The sperm and egg meet in the uterine tubes, and fertilization takes place. The uterine tubes then serve as the passageway to the uterus, where the fertilized egg becomes implanted and development continues.

The Onset of Puberty and the Menstrual Cycle
With the onset of puberty, the female reproductive system matures, and the development of secondary sex characteristics transforms young girls into young women. The first sign of puberty is the development of breast buds, which occurs around age 11. Under the direction of the endocrine system, the pituitary gland, **hypothalamus,** and ovaries all secrete hormones that act as chemical messengers among them. Working in a feedback system, hormonal levels in the bloodstream act as the trigger mechanism for release of more or different hormones.

Around age 9½ to 11½, the hypothalamus receives the message to begin secreting **gonadotropin-releasing hormone (GnRH).** The release of GnRH in turn signals the pituitary gland to release hormones called gonadotropins. Two gonadotropins, **follicle-stimulating hormone (FSH)** and **luteinizing hormone (LH),** signal the ovaries to start producing **estrogens** and **progesterone.** Estrogens regulate the menstrual cycle, and increased estrogen levels assist in the development of female secondary sex characteristics. Progesterone helps keep the endometrium developing in order to nourish a fertilized egg and helps maintain pregnancy.

The normal age range for the onset of the first menstrual period, the **menarche,** is 9 to 17 years, with the average age being 11½ to 13½ years. Body fat heavily influences the onset of puberty, and increasing rates of obesity in children may account for the fact that girls here and in other countries seem to be reaching puberty much earlier than they used to.[43] Very thin girls, such as young athletes, tend to start menstruating later.

The average menstrual cycle is 28 days and consists of two phases: the menstrual/proliferative (also known as the follicular) phase, and the secretory or luteal phase (Figure 5.6). During the proliferative phase, the pituitary gland releases FSH and LH. The FSH acts on the ovaries to stimulate the maturation process of several **ovarian follicles (egg sacs),** areas within the ovaries in which individual eggs develop. These follicles secrete estrogen, which stimulates the *endometrium* to grow and develop. The inner walls of the uterus become coated with a thick, spongy lining composed of blood and mucus. If fertilization occurs, this endometrial tissue will become a nesting place for the developing embryo. The increased estrogen level also signals the pituitary to slow down FSH production but increase LH secretion. Of the several follicles developing in the ovaries, only one each month normally reaches complete maturity. Under the influence of LH, this follicle rapidly matures; on about the fourteenth day of the proliferative phase, it releases an ovum into the uterine tube—a process called **ovulation.** Just prior to

---

Uterus (womb) Hollow, muscular, pear-shaped organ whose function is to contain the developing fetus.

Endometrium Soft, spongy matter that makes up the uterine lining.

Cervix Lower end of the uterus, which extends down into the vagina.

Ovaries Almond-sized organs suspended on either side of the uterus that house developing eggs and produce hormones.

Uterine (fallopian) tubes Two thin, flexible tubes that extend from the ovaries to the uterus; the sperm and the egg meet here, and fertilization takes place.

Hypothalamus An area of the brain located near the pituitary gland; works in conjunction with the pituitary gland to control reproductive functions.

Gonadotropin-releasing hormone (GnRH) Hormone that signals the pituitary gland to release gonadotropins.

Follicle-stimulating hormone (FSH) Hormone that signals the ovaries to prepare to release eggs and to begin producing estrogens.

Luteinizing hormone (LH) Hormone that signals the ovaries to release an egg and to begin producing progesterone.

Estrogens Hormones that control the menstrual cycle.

Progesterone Hormone secreted by the ovaries; helps keep the endometrium developing in order to nourish a fertilized egg; also helps maintain pregnancy.

Menarche The first menstrual period.

Ovarian follicles (egg sacs) Areas within the ovary in which individual eggs develop.

Ovulation The point of the menstrual cycle at which a mature egg ruptures through the ovarian wall.

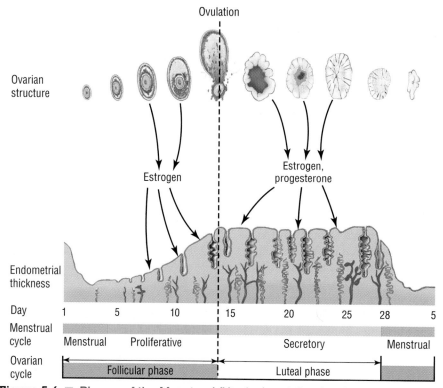

Ovulation

Ovarian structure

Estrogen

Estrogen, progesterone

Endometrial thickness

Day	1	5	10	15	20	25	28	5

Menstrual cycle: Menstrual | Proliferative | Secretory | Menstrual

Ovarian cycle: Follicular phase | Luteal phase

Figure 5.6 ■ Phases of the Menstrual (Uterine) and Ovarian Cycle

Source: R. D. McAnulty and M. M. Burnette, *Exploring Human Sexuality: Making Healthy Decisions* (Boston: Allyn & Bacon, 2001). Copyright © 2001 by Pearson Education.

ovulation, the mature egg's follicle begins to increase secretion of progesterone, the primary function of which is to spur the addition of further nutrients to the developing endometrium.

After ovulation, the secretory phase begins. The ovarian follicle is converted into the *corpus luteum,* or yellow body, which continues to secrete estrogen and progesterone but in decreasing amounts. In addition, FSH also falls back to preproliferative levels. Essentially, the woman's body is waiting to see whether fertilization will occur. During this time, LH declines and progesterone levels begin to rise, which causes additional tissue growth in the endometrium.

If fertilization takes place, cells surrounding the developing embryo release a hormone called **human chorionic gonadotropin (hCG).** The HCG increases estrogen and progesterone secretion, which maintains

the endometrium while signaling the pituitary gland not to start a new menstrual cycle.

When fertilization does not occur, the egg disintegrates within approximately 72 hours. The corpus luteum gradually becomes nonfunctional, which causes levels of progesterone and estrogen to decline. As hormonal levels decrease, the endometrial lining of the uterus loses its nourishment, dies, and is sloughed off as menstrual flow.

For more information on issues associated with menstruation, such as premenstrual syndrome, toxic shock syndrome, and dysmenorrhea (painful menstruation), see Chapter 14.

Menopause Just as menarche signals the beginning of a woman's reproductive years, **menopause**—the permanent cessation of menstruation—signals the end. Generally occurring between the ages of 40 and 60, and at age 51 on average in the United States, menopause results in decreased estrogen levels, which may produce troublesome symptoms in some women. Decreased vaginal lubrication, hot flashes, headaches, dizziness, and joint pains all have been associated with the onset of menopause.

Hormones, such as estrogen and progesterone, have long been prescribed as **hormone replacement therapy (HRT)** to relieve menopausal symptoms and reduce the risk of heart disease and osteoporosis. (The National Institutes of Health prefers the term

Human chorionic gonadotropin (hCG) Hormone that calls for increased levels of estrogen and progesterone secretion if fertilization has taken place.

Menopause The permanent cessation of menstruation.

Hormone replacement therapy (HRT), or menopausal hormone therapy Use of synthetic or animal estrogens and progesterone to compensate for decreases in estrogens in a woman's body.

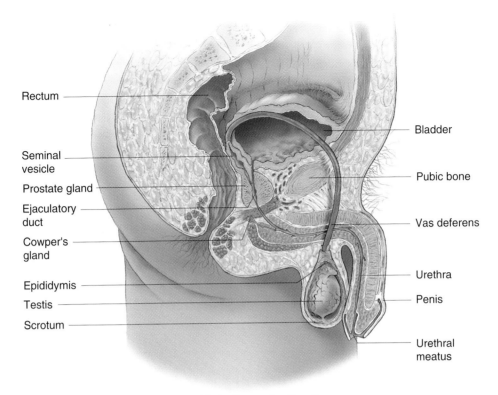

Figure 5.7 ▪ Side View of the Male Reproductive Organs

Labels (from figure): Rectum, Seminal vesicle, Prostate gland, Ejaculatory duct, Cowper's gland, Epididymis, Testis, Scrotum, Bladder, Pubic bone, Vas deferens, Urethra, Penis, Urethral meatus

menopausal hormone therapy, since hormone treatment is not a replacement and does not restore the physiology of youth.) However, some studies, including results from the Women's Health Initiative (WHI), suggest that hormone therapy may actually do more harm than good. In fact, the WHI terminated this research ahead of schedule due to concerns about participants' increased risk of breast cancer, heart attack, stroke, blood clots, and other health problems.[44] All women need to discuss the risks and benefits of menopausal hormone therapy with their health care provider and come to an informed decision. It is crucial to find a doctor who specializes in women's health and keeps up to date with the latest research findings. Certainly a healthy lifestyle, such as regular exercise, a balanced diet, and adequate calcium intake, can also help protect postmenopausal women from heart disease and osteoporosis.

Male Sexual Anatomy and Physiology

The structures of the male sexual system may be divided into external and internal genitals (Figure 5.7). The penis and the scrotum make up the **external male genitals.** The **internal male genitals** include the testes, epididymides, ductus deferentia, urethra, and three

other structures—the seminal vesicles, the prostate gland, and the bulbourethral glands—that secrete components that, with sperm, make up semen. These three structures are sometimes referred to as the **accessory glands.**

The **penis** serves as the organ that deposits sperm in the vagina during intercourse. The urethra, which passes through the center of the penis, acts as the passageway for both semen and urine to exit the body. During sexual arousal, the spongy tissue in the penis becomes filled with blood, making the organ stiff (erect). Further sexual excitement leads to **ejaculation,** a series of rapid, spasmodic contractions that propel semen out of the penis.

External male genitals   The penis and scrotum.

Internal male genitals   The testes, epididymides, vasa deferentia, ejaculatory ducts, urethra, and accessory glands.

Accessory glands   The seminal vesicles, prostate gland, and bulbourethral glands.

Penis   Male sexual organ that releases sperm into the vagina.

Ejaculation   The propulsion of semen from the penis.

Situated behind the penis and also outside the body is a sac called the **scrotum.** The scrotum protects the testes and also helps control the temperature within the testes, which is vital to proper sperm production. The **testes** (singular: *testis*) are egg-shaped structures that manufacture sperm and **testosterone,** the hormone responsible for the development of male secondary sex characteristics.

The development of sperm is referred to as **spermatogenesis.** Like the maturation of eggs in the female, this process is governed by the pituitary gland. Follicle-stimulating hormone (FSH) is secreted into the bloodstream to stimulate the testes to manufacture sperm. Immature sperm are released into a comma-shaped structure on the back of the testis called the **epididymis** (plural: *epididymides*), where they ripen and reach full maturity.

The epididymis contains coiled tubules that gradually "unwind" and straighten out to become the **ductus (vas) deferens.** The two ductus deferentia, as they are called in the plural, make up the tubular transportation system whose sole function is to store and move sperm. Along the way, the **seminal vesicles** provide sperm with nutrients and other fluids that compose **semen.**

The ductus deferentia eventually connect each epididymis to the ejaculatory ducts, which pass through the prostate gland and empty into the urethra. The **prostate gland** contributes more fluids to the semen, including chemicals that aid the sperm in fertilizing an ovum and neutralize the acidic environment of the vagina to make it more conducive to sperm motility (ability to move) and potency (potential for fertilizing an ovum).

Just below the prostate gland are two pea-shaped nodules called the **bulbourethral (Cowper's) glands.** The bulbourethral glands secrete a fluid that lubricates the urethra and neutralizes any acid that may remain in the urethra after urination. Urine and semen do not come into contact with each other. During ejaculation of semen, a small valve closes off the tube to the urinary bladder.

Debate continues over the practice of **circumcision,** the surgical removal of a fold of skin covering the end of the penis known as the foreskin. Most circumcisions are performed for religious or cultural reasons or because of hygiene concerns. (Uncircumcised males must regularly clean the area under the foreskin.) The American Academy of Pediatrics does not consider the procedure medically necessary; if it is performed, the infant should be given pain relief.[45]

Human Sexual Response

> **Do men and women have the same sexual response?**

Psychological traits greatly influence sexual response and sexual desire. Thus, you may find a relationship with one partner vastly different from experience with other partners.

Sexual response is a physiological process that generally follows a pattern. Both males' and females' sexual responses are somewhat arbitrarily divided into four stages: excitement/arousal, plateau, orgasm, and resolution. Researchers agree that each individual has a personal response pattern that may or may not conform to these phases. Regardless of the type of sexual activity (stimulation by a partner or self-stimulation), the response stages are the same.

During *excitement/arousal-stage,* **vasocongestion** (increased blood flow that causes swelling in the genitals) stimulates male and female genital responses. The vagina begins to lubricate in preparation for penile penetration, and the penis becomes partially erect. Both sexes may exhibit a "sex flush," or light blush all over their bodies. Excitement/arousal can be generated through fantasy or by touching other parts of the body, kissing, viewing films or videos, or reading erotic literature.

During the *plateau phase,* the initial responses intensify. Voluntary and involuntary muscle tensions increase. The female's nipples and the male's penis become erect. The penis secretes a few drops of pre-ejaculatory fluid, which may contain sperm.

During the *orgasmic phase,* vasocongestion and muscle tensions reach their peak, and rhythmic

---

Scrotum   Sac of tissue that encloses the testes.

Testes   Two organs, located in the scrotum, that manufacture sperm and produce hormones.

Testosterone   The male sex hormone manufactured in the testes.

Spermatogenesis   The development of sperm.

Epididymis   A comma-shaped structure atop the testis where sperm mature.

Ductus (vas) deferens   A tube that transports sperm toward the penis.

Seminal vesicles   Storage areas for sperm where nutrient fluids are added to them.

Semen   Fluid containing sperm and nutrient fluids that increase sperm viability and neutralize vaginal acid.

Prostate gland   Gland that secretes nutrients and neutralizing fluids into the semen.

Bulbourethral (Cowper's) glands   Glands that secrete a fluid that lubricates the urethra and neutralizes any acid remaining in the urethra after urination.

Circumcision   Surgical removal of a fold of skin covering the end of the penis known as the foreskin.

Vasocongestion   The engorgement of the genital organs with blood.

contractions occur through the genital regions. In females, these contractions are centered in the uterus, outer vagina, and anal sphincter.

In males, the contractions occur in two stages. First, contractions within the prostate gland begin propelling semen through the urethra. In the second stage, the muscles of the pelvic floor, urethra, and anal sphincter contract. Semen usually, but not always, is ejaculated from the penis. In both sexes, spasms in other major muscle groups also occur, particularly in the buttocks and abdomen. Feet and hands may also contract, and facial features often contort.

Muscle tension and congested blood subside in the *resolution phase,* as the genital organs return to their pre-arousal states. Both sexes usually experience deep feelings of well-being and profound relaxation. Following orgasm and resolution, many females can become aroused again and experience additional orgasms. However, some men experience a refractory period, during which their systems are incapable of subsequent arousal. This refractory period may last from a few minutes to several hours and tends to lengthen with age.

Men and women experience the same stages in the sexual response cycle; however, the length of time spent in any one stage varies. Thus, one partner may be in the plateau phase while the other is in the excitement or orgasmic phase. Such variations in response rates are entirely normal. Some couples believe that simultaneous orgasm is desirable for sexual satisfaction. Although simultaneous orgasm is pleasant, so are orgasms achieved at different times.

Sexual pleasure and satisfaction are also possible without orgasm or even intercourse. Expressing sexual feelings for another person involves many pleasurable activities, of which intercourse and orgasm may be only a part.

EXPRESSING YOUR SEXUALITY

Finding healthy ways to express your sexuality is an important part of developing sexual maturity. Many avenues of sexual expression are available.

Sexual Behavior: What Is "Normal"?

Most of us want to fit in and be identified as normal, but how do we know which sexual behaviors are considered normal? What or whose criteria should we use? These are not easy questions.

Every society sets standards and attempts to regulate sexual behavior. Boundaries arise that distinguish good from bad, acceptable from unacceptable, and result in criteria used to establish what is viewed as

normal or abnormal. Some of the common sociocultural standards for sexual behavior in Western culture today include:[46]

- *The heterosexual standard.* Sexual attraction should be limited to members of the other sex.
- *The coital standard.* Penile/vaginal intercourse (coitus) is viewed as the ultimate sex act.
- *The orgasmic standard.* All sexual interaction should lead to orgasm.
- *The two-person standard.* Sex is an activity to be experienced by two.
- *The romantic standard.* Sex should be related to love.
- *The safer sex standard.* If we choose to be sexually active, we should act to prevent unintended pregnancy or disease transmission.

These are not laws or rules, but rather social scripts that have been adopted over time. Sexual standards often shift through the years, and many people choose not to follow them. We are a pluralistic nation, and that pluralism extends to our sexual practices. Rather than making blanket judgments about normal versus abnormal, we might ask the following questions to explore our sexual standards:[47]

- Is a sexual behavior healthy and fulfilling for a particular person?
- Is it safe?
- Does it lead to the exploitation of others?
- Does it take place between responsible, consenting adults?

In this way, we can view behavior along a continuum that takes into account many individual factors. As you read about the options for sexual expression in the pages ahead, use these questions to explore your feelings about what is normal for you.

Options for Sexual Expression

The range of human sexual expression is virtually infinite. What you find enjoyable may not be an option for someone else. The ways you choose to meet your sexual needs today may have been very different two weeks ago or will be different two years from now. Accepting yourself as a sexual person with individual desires and preferences is the first step in achieving sexual satisfaction.

Celibacy **Celibacy** is avoidance of or abstention from sexual activities with others. Some individuals choose celibacy for religious or moral reasons. Others

---

Celibacy State of not being involved in a sexual relationship.

Standing Up for Yourself

myhealthlab

Fill out this assessment online at
www.aw-bc.com/myhealthlab or www.aw-bc.com/donatelle.

You know that sinking feeling. Someone asks you to do something, and your stomach lurches. You don't want to go along, but you can't come up with a good excuse not to do so. It's hard to say no. How often are you caught in the "I can't say no" trap? Read the following situations and assess your response according to the following 5-point scale:

	Never	Seldom	Sometimes	Frequently	Always
1. Friends ask you to ride home with them after they've all been drinking. You know you shouldn't go, but you think one of them is cute and don't want to seem like a prude. You take the ride.	1	2	3	4	5
2. Your decisions can be easily swayed by a strong argument from someone else pushing you in the opposite direction.	1	2	3	4	5
3. You feel strongly about a political issue, but it is the opposite of the opinion your parents hold. You remain silent rather than getting into an argument.	1	2	3	4	5
4. You start out by saying no to something but get talked into doing it after a short time.	1	2	3	4	5
5. You're stressed out with too much to do and too little time, but you can't seem to say no when someone asks for a favor.	1	2	3	4	5
6. Someone says something really nasty about a person you like. You jump to the defense of the person being criticized, even though you are in the minority opinion.	1	2	3	4	5
7. You would describe yourself as assertive and tend to quickly let others know your thoughts about certain issues.	1	2	3	4	5
8. Someone is critical of something you do. You quickly defend your actions by explaining why you did what you did.	1	2	3	4	5

may be celibate for a period of time because of illness, the breakup of a long-term relationship, or lack of an acceptable partner. For some, celibacy is a lonely, agonizing state, but others find it an opportunity for introspection, values assessment, and personal growth.

Autoerotic Behaviors

Autoerotic behaviors involve sexual self-stimulation. The two most common are sexual fantasy and masturbation.

Autoerotic behaviors   Sexual self-stimulation.

Sexual fantasies   Sexually arousing thoughts and dreams.

Masturbation   Self-stimulation of genitals.

Sexual fantasies are sexually arousing thoughts and dreams. Fantasies may reflect real-life experiences, forbidden desires, or the opportunity to practice new or anticipated sexual experiences. The fact that you may fantasize about a particular sexual experience does not mean that you want to, or have to, act that experience out. Sexual fantasies are just that—fantasy.

Masturbation is self-stimulation of the genitals. Although many people feel uncomfortable discussing masturbation, it is a common sexual practice across the life span. Masturbation is a natural, pleasure-seeking behavior in infants and children. It is a valuable and important means for adolescent males and females, as well as adults, to explore sexual feelings and responsiveness.

Kissing and Erotic Touching

Kissing and erotic touching are two very common forms of nonverbal sexual communication. Both males and females

Interpreting Your Score

Think about your responses to each statement. Do your responses indicate an assertive communication style in which you stand up for your feelings or beliefs? What factors cause you to hold back when you should probably speak up? How can you work to improve your communication behaviors in this area? For statements 1 through 5, do you have several "5" responses? If yes, you should consider what skills you could develop to help you communicate more assertively.

Make It Happen!

Assessment: The Assess Yourself activity above gave you the chance to look at how you communicate in certain situations. It is important to be able to communicate assertively and to feel that you can stand up for yourself. Now that you have considered your responses to the statements, you may want to take steps toward becoming a more assertive communicator.

Making a Change: In order to change your behavior, you need to develop a plan. Follow these steps.

1. Evaluate your behavior, and identify patterns. What can you change now? What can you change in the near future?
2. Select one pattern of behavior that you want to change.
3. Fill out the Behavior Change Contract found at the front of your book. It should include your long-term goal for change, your short-term goals, the rewards you'll give yourself for reaching these goals, potential obstacles along the way, and strategies for overcoming these obstacles. For each goal, list the small steps and specific actions that you will take.
4. Chart your progress in a journal. At the end of a week, consider how successful you were in following your plan.

What helped you be successful? What made change more difficult? What will you do differently next week?
5. Revise your plan as needed: Are the short-term goals attainable? Are the rewards satisfying?

Example: When Stacey assessed her responses to the statements about assertiveness, she realized that she tended to say yes when someone asked her for a favor, no matter how busy or stressed out she was. Stacey decided she wanted to learn to say no when necessary. She set a goal of imagining certain situations that she had faced recently and how she would handle them more assertively. The first week, she imagined her older sister asking her to babysit her son at the last minute and her roommates asking her for car rides while she was in the middle of studying. She planned what she would say and how she would explain her reasons for saying no. The second week, when her roommates asked for a ride to the movies, Stacey calmly stated that she was busy and needed two hours more for studying before she could take a break. Her roommates decided to walk to the video store instead and rented a movie they could all watch together when Stacey was ready for a break.

---

have **erogenous zones**, areas of the body that when touched lead to sexual arousal. Erogenous zones may include genital as well as nongenital areas, such as the earlobes, mouth, breasts, and inner thighs. Almost any area of the body can be conditioned to respond erotically to touch. Spending time with your partner to explore and learn about his or her erogenous areas is another pleasurable, safe, and satisfying means of sexual expression.

Oral–Genital Stimulation **Cunnilingus** refers to oral stimulation of a female's genitals and **fellatio** to oral stimulation of a male's genitals. Many partners find oral–genital stimulation intensely pleasurable. For some people, oral sex is not an option because of moral or religious beliefs. Remember, HIV (human immunodeficiency virus) and other sexually transmitted infections (STIs) can be transmitted via unprotected oral–genital sex just as they can through intercourse. Use of an appropriate barrier device is strongly recommended if either partner's health status is in question.

Vaginal Intercourse The term *intercourse* generally refers to **vaginal intercourse** (*coitus,* or insertion of the penis into the vagina), which is the most often practiced form of sexual expression. Coitus can involve a variety of positions, including the missionary position (man on top facing the woman), woman on top, side by

---

Erogenous zones   Areas of the body of both males and females that, when touched, lead to sexual arousal.

Cunnilingus   Oral stimulation of a female's genitals.

Fellatio   Oral stimulation of a male's genitals.

Vaginal intercourse   The insertion of the penis into the vagina.

side, or man behind (rear entry). Many partners enjoy experimenting with different positions. Knowledge of yourself and your body, along with your ability to communicate effectively, will play a large part in determining the enjoyment or meaning of intercourse for you and your partner. Whatever your circumstance, you should practice safer sex to avoid disease and unwanted pregnancy.

Anal Intercourse The anal area is highly sensitive to touch, and some couples find pleasure in the stimulation of this area. **Anal intercourse** is insertion of the penis into the anus. Stimulation of the anus by mouth or with the fingers also is practiced. As with all forms of sexual expression, anal stimulation or intercourse is not for everyone. If you do enjoy this form of sexual expression, remember to use condoms to avoid transmitting disease. Also, anything inserted into the anus should not be then directly inserted into the vagina, since bacteria commonly found in the anus can cause vaginal infections.

Variant Sexual Behavior

Although attitudes toward sexuality have changed radically since the Victorian era, some people still believe that any sexual behavior other than heterosexual intercourse is abnormal or perverted. People who study sexuality prefer the neutral term **variant sexual behavior** to describe sexual activities such as the following that are not engaged in by most people.

- *Group sex.* Sexual activity involving more than two people. Participants in group sex run a higher risk of exposure to HIV and other STIs.

- *Transvestism.* Wearing the clothing of the opposite sex. Most transvestites are male, heterosexual, and married.

- *Fetishism.* Sexual arousal achieved by looking at or touching inanimate objects, such as underclothing or shoes.

Some variant sexual behaviors can be harmful to the individual, to others, or to both. Many of the following activities are illegal in at least some states.

Anal intercourse The insertion of the penis into the anus.

Variant sexual behavior A sexual behavior that is not engaged in by most people.

Sexual dysfunction Problems associated with achieving sexual satisfaction.

Inhibited sexual desire (ISD) Lack of sexual appetite or simply a lack of interest and pleasure in sexual activity.

- *Exhibitionism.* Exposing one's genitals to strangers in public places. Most exhibitionists are seeking a reaction of shock or fear from their victims. Exhibitionism is a minor felony in most states.

- *Voyeurism.* Observing other people for sexual gratification. Most voyeurs are men who attempt to watch women undressing or bathing. Voyeurism is an invasion of privacy and illegal in most states.

- *Sadomasochism.* Sexual activities in which gratification is received by inflicting pain (verbal or physical abuse) on a partner or by being the object of such infliction. A sadist is a person who enjoys inflicting pain, and a masochist is a person who enjoys experiencing it.

- *Pedophilia.* Sexual activity or attraction between an adult and a child. Any sexual activity involving a minor, including possession of child pornography, is illegal.

- *Autoerotic asphyxiation.* The practice of reducing or eliminating oxygen to the brain, usually by tying a cord around one's neck, while masturbating to orgasm. Tragically, some individuals accidentally hang themselves.

What Do You Think? How does our society define "normal" sexual behavior? ■ What behaviors do you consider normal or abnormal? ■ Do you consider your own preferred forms of sexual expression to be normal? Why or why not?

DIFFICULTIES THAT CAN HINDER SEXUAL FUNCTIONING

Research indicates that **sexual dysfunction,** the term used to describe problems that can hinder sexual functioning, is quite common. Don't feel embarrassed if you experience sexual dysfunction at some point in your life. The sexual part of you does not come with a lifetime warranty. You can have breakdowns involving your sexual function just as in any other body system. Sexual dysfunction can be divided into five major classes: disorders of sexual desire, sexual arousal, orgasm, sexual performance, and sexual pain. All of them can be treated successfully.

Sexual Desire Disorders

The most frequent reason why people seek out a sex therapist is **ISD,** or **inhibited sexual desire.**[48] ISD is the lack of a sexual appetite or simply a lack of interest and pleasure in sexual activity. In some instances, it can result from stress or boredom. **Sexual aversion disorder** is another type of desire dysfunction, characterized by sexual phobias (unreasonable fears) and anxiety about sexual contact. The psychological stress of a punitive upbringing, a rigid religious background, or a history of physical or sexual abuse may be sources of these desire disorders.

Sexual Arousal Disorders

The most common disorder in this category is **erectile dysfunction (impotence)**—difficulty in achieving or maintaining a penile erection sufficient for intercourse. At some time in his life, every man experiences impotence. Causes are varied and include underlying diseases, such as diabetes or prostate problems; reactions to some medications (for example, drugs for high blood pressure); depression; fatigue; stress; alcohol; performance anxiety; and guilt over real or imaginary problems (such as when a man compares himself to his partner's past lovers).

Some 30 million men in this country, half of them under age 65, suffer from impotence. Impotence generally becomes more of a problem as men age, affecting one in four men over the age of 65.[49] The FDA has approved the drug Viagra (sildenafil citrate) to treat impotence. Levitra and Cialis, other FDA-approved drug treatments for erectile dysfunction, work in the same way as Viagra. Taken by mouth one hour before sexual activity, Viagra is reported to manage erectile dysfunction successfully in 60 to 80 percent of cases.[50] The medication is not, however, without risk. The most commonly reported side effects include headache, flushing, stomachache, urinary tract infection, diarrhea, dizziness, rash, and mild and temporary visual changes. There have been several deaths in the United States among Viagra users, prompting more caution in prescribing it to patients with known cardiovascular disease and those taking commonly prescribed short- and long-acting nitrates, such as nitroglycerin.[51]

Orgasmic Disorders

Premature ejaculation—ejaculation that occurs prior to or very soon after the insertion of the penis into the vagina—affects up to 50 percent of the male population at some time in their lives. Treatment for premature ejaculation first involves a physical examination to rule out organic causes. If the cause of the problem is not physiological, therapy is available to help a man learn how to control the timing of his ejaculation. Fatigue, stress, performance pressure, and alcohol use can all contribute to orgasm disorders in men.

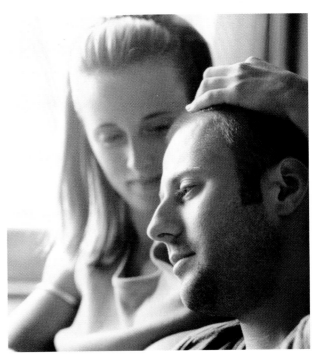

Sexual dysfunction can affect couples of any age. Communication is critical to resolving the problem.

In a woman, the inability to achieve orgasm is termed **female orgasmic disorder.** A woman with this disorder often blames herself and learns to fake orgasm to avoid embarrassment or preserve her partner's ego. Contributing to this response are the messages women have historically been given about sex as a duty rather than a pleasurable act. As with men who experience orgasmic disorders, the first step in treatment is a physical exam to rule out organic causes. However, the problem is often solved by simple self-exploration to learn more about what forms of stimulation are arousing enough to produce orgasm. Through masturbation, a woman can learn how her body responds sexually to various types of touch. Once she has become orgasmic through masturbation, she learns to communicate her needs to her partner.

Sexual aversion disorder   Type of desire dysfunction characterized by sexual phobias and anxiety about sexual contact.

Erectile dysfunction (impotence)   Difficulty in achieving or maintaining a penile erection sufficient for intercourse.

Premature ejaculation   Ejaculation that occurs prior to or almost immediately following penile penetration of the vagina.

Female orgasmic disorder   The inability to achieve orgasm.

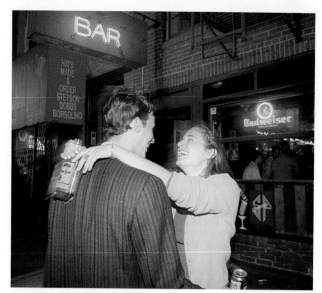

Alcohol and drugs can impair judgment and lead to sexual encounters that are later regretted.

Sexual Performance Anxiety

Both men and women can experience **sexual performance anxiety,** when they anticipate some sort of problem in the sex act. A man may become anxious and unable to maintain an erection, or he may experience premature ejaculation. A woman may be unable to achieve orgasm or to allow penetration because of the involuntary contraction of vaginal muscles. Both can overcome performance anxiety by learning to focus on immediate sensations and pleasures rather than on orgasm.

Sexual Pain Disorders

Two common disorders in this category are dyspareunia and vaginismus. **Dyspareunia** is pain experienced by a female during intercourse. This pain may be caused by diseases such as endometriosis, uterine tumors, chlamydia, gonorrhea, or urinary tract infections. Damage to tissues during childbirth and insufficient lubrication during intercourse may also cause discomfort. Dyspareunia can also be psychological in origin. As with other sexual problems, dyspareunia can be treated with good results.

Sexual performance anxiety   A condition of sexual difficulties caused by anticipating some sort of problem with the sex act.

Dyspareunia   Pain experienced by women during intercourse.

Vaginismus   A state in which the vaginal muscles contract so forcefully that penetration cannot be accomplished.

Vaginismus is the involuntary contraction of vaginal muscles, making penile insertion painful or impossible. Most cases of vaginismus are related to fear of intercourse or to unresolved sexual conflicts. Treatment involves teaching a woman to achieve orgasm through nonvaginal stimulation.

Seeking Help for Sexual Dysfunction

Many theories and treatment models can help people with sexual dysfunction. A first important step is choosing a qualified sex therapist or counselor. A national organization, the American Association of Sex Educators, Counselors, and Therapists (AASECT), has been in the forefront of establishing criteria for certifying sex therapists. These criteria include appropriate degree(s) in the helping professions, specialized coursework in human sexuality, and sufficient hours of practical therapy work under the direct supervision of a certified sex therapist. Lists of certified counselors and sex therapists, as well as clinics that treat sexual dysfunctions, can be obtained by contacting AASECT.

Drugs and Sex

Because psychoactive drugs affect the entire physiology, it is only logical that they affect sexual behavior. Promises of increased pleasure make drugs very tempting to those seeking greater sexual satisfaction. Too often, however, drugs become central to sexual activities and damage the relationship. Drug use can also lead to undesired sexual activity.

Alcohol is notorious for reducing inhibitions and promoting feelings of well-being and desirability. At the same time, alcohol inhibits sexual response; thus, the mind may be willing, but not the body.

Perhaps the greatest danger associated with use of drugs during sex is the tendency to blame the drug for negative behavior. "I can't help what I did last night because I was drunk" is a statement that demonstrates sexual immaturity. A sexually mature person carefully examines risks and benefits and makes decisions accordingly. If drugs are necessary to increase erotic feelings, it is likely that the partners are being dishonest about their feelings for each other. Good sex should not depend on chemical substances.

"Date rape" drugs are a growing concern in recent years. They have become popular among college students and are often used in combination with alcohol.[52] Rohypnol ("roofies," "rope," "forget pill"), gamma-hydroxybutrane or GHB ("Liquid X," "Grievous Bodily Harm," "Easy Lay," "Mickey Finn"), and Ketamine ("K," "Special K," "cat valium") have all been used to facilitate rape. GHB and Rohypnol are difficult-to-detect drugs that depress the central nervous system.

Ketamine can cause dream-like states, hallucinations, delirium, amnesia, and impaired motor function. These drugs are often introduced to unsuspecting women through alcoholic drinks in order to render them unconscious and vulnerable to rape. This problem is so serious that Congress passed the Drug-Induced Rape Prevention and Punishment Act of 1996 to provide increased federal penalties for using drugs to facilitate sexual assault. The dangers of these drugs are discussed in more detail in Chapter 4 (see the Reality Check box).

Taking Charge

Summary

- Intimate relationships have several different characteristics, including behavioral interdependence, need fulfillment, emotional attachment, and emotional availability. These characteristics influence how we interact with others and the types of intimate relationships we form. Family, friends, and partners or lovers provide the most common opportunities for intimacy. Each relationship may include healthy and unhealthy characteristics that affect daily functioning.

- Gender differences in communication include conversation styles as well as differences in sharing feelings and disclosing personal facts and fears. These differences explain why men and women may relate differently in intimate relationships. Understanding these differences and learning how to deal with them are important aspects of healthy relationships.

- Barriers to intimacy often include the different emotional needs of both partners, jealousy, and emotional wounds that could result from being raised in a dysfunctional family.

- For most people, commitment is an important ingredient in successful relationships. The major types of committed relationships are marriage, cohabitation, and gay and lesbian partnerships.

- Success in committed relationships requires understanding the roles of partnering scripts, the importance of self-nurturance, and the elements of a good relationship.

- Life decisions such as whether to marry or have children require serious consideration.

- Remaining single is more common than ever. Most single people lead healthy, happy, and well-adjusted lives. Those who decide to have or not to have children also can lead rewarding, productive lives as long as they have given this decision the utmost thought and weighed the pros and cons of each alternative in the context of their lifestyle.

- Today's family structure may look different from that of previous generations, but love, trust, and commitment to a child's welfare continue to be the cornerstones of successful childrearing.

- Before relationships fail, often many warning signs appear. By recognizing these signs and taking action to change behaviors, partners can save and enhance their relationships.

- Sexual identity is determined by a complex interaction of genetic, physiological, and environmental factors. Biological sex, gender identity, gender roles, and sexual orientation all are blended into our sexual identity.

- Sexual orientation refers to a person's enduring emotional, romantic , sexual, or affectionate attraction to other persons. Irrational hatred or fear of homosexuality or gay and lesbian persons is termed homophobia.

- The major components of the female sexual anatomy include the mons pubis, labia minora and majora, clitoris, urethral and vaginal openings, vagina, cervix, uterine tubes, and ovaries. The major components of the male sexual anatomy are the penis, scrotum, testes, epididymides, ductus deferentia, ejaculatory ducts, and urethra.

- Physiologically, males and females experience four phases of sexual response: excitement/arousal, plateau, orgasm, and resolution.

- Humans can express their sexual selves in a variety of ways, including celibacy, autoerotic behaviors, kissing and erotic touch, oral–genital stimulation, vaginal intercourse, and anal intercourse.

- Sexual dysfunctions can be classified into disorders of sexual desire, sexual arousal, orgasm, sexual performance anxiety, and sexual pain. Drug use also can lead to sexual dysfunction.

Chapter Review

1. Intimate relationships fulfill our psychological need for someone to listen to our worries and concerns. This is known as our need for
   a. dependence.
   b. social integration.
   c. enjoyment.
   d. spontaneity.

2. Lovers tend to pay attention to the other person even when they should be involved in other activities. This is called
   a. inclusion.
   b. exclusivity.
   c. fascination.
   d. authentic intimacy.

3. What percentage of all Americans marry at least once?
   a. 35 percent
   b. 50 percent
   c. 75 percent
   d. 90 percent

4. According to anthropologist Helen Fisher, attraction and falling in love follow a pattern based on
   a. lust, attraction, attachment.
   b. intimacy, passion, and commitment.
   c. imprinting, attraction, attachment, and the production of a cuddle chemical.
   d. fascination, exclusiveness, sexual desire, giving the utmost, and being a champion.

5. Who coined the term *genderlect*?
   a. Helen Fisher
   b. Robert Sternberg
   c. Deborah Tannen
   d. Carol Gilligan

6. After a painful divorce, Rick met a woman he was very interested in but held back his emotions for fear of rejection. This relates to what characteristic of intimate relationships?
   a. behavioral interdependence
   b. need fulfillment
   c. emotional attachment
   d. emotional availability

7. What percentage of people marrying today will get divorced?
   a. 20 percent
   b. 33 percent
   c. 50 percent
   d. 68 percent

8. Predictability, dependability, and faith are three fundamental basic elements of
   a. trust.
   b. friendship.
   c. attraction.
   d. attachment.

9. One important factor in choosing a partner is *proximity,* which refers to
   a. mutual regard.
   b. attitudes and values.
   c. physical attraction.
   d. being in the same place at the same time.

10. Ovulation usually occurs on the:
    a. 7th day of the proliferatory phase.
    b. 14th day of the proliferatory phase.
    c. 21st day of the proliferatory phase.
    d. 28th day of the proliferatory phase.

Answers to these questions can be found on page A-1.

Questions for Discussion and Reflection

1. What are the characteristics of intimate relationships? What are behavioral interdependence, need fulfillment, emotional attachment, and emotional availability, and why is each important in relationship development?

2. Why are relationships with family important? Explain how your family unit was similar to or different from the traditional family unit in early America. Who made up your family of origin? Your nuclear family?

3. How can you tell the difference between a love relationship and one that is based primarily on physical attraction? What characteristics do love relationships share?

4. What problems can form barriers to intimacy? What actions can you take to reduce or remove these barriers?

5. What are the common elements of good relationships? What are some common warning signs of trouble? What actions can you take to improve your own interpersonal relationships?

6. Name some common misconceptions about people who choose to remain single and about couples who choose not to have children. Do you want to have children? Why or why not? What characteristics show that a couple is ready to have children?

7. How have gender roles changed over the past 20 years? Do you view the changes as positive for both men and women?

8. Discuss the cycle of changes that occurs in our bodies in response to various hormones (e.g., sexual differentiation while in the womb, development of secondary sex characteristics at puberty, menopause).

9. What is "normal" sexual behavior? What criteria should we use to determine healthful sexual practice?

10. If scientists ever establish the combination of factors that interact to produce homosexual, heterosexual, or bisexual orientation, will that put an end to antigay prejudice? Why or why not?

11. How can we remove the stigma that surrounds sexual dysfunction so that individuals feel more open to seeking help? Are men and women impacted differently by sexual dysfunction?

Accessing Your Health on the Internet

The following websites explore further topics and issues related to personal health. For links to the websites below, visit the Companion Website for *Health: The Basics,* Seventh Edition at www.aw-bc.com/donatelle.

1. *American Association of Sex Educators, Counselors, and Therapists (AASECT).* Professional organization providing standards of practice for treatment of sexual issues and disorders.

2. *Bacchus and Gamma Peer Education Network.* Student-friendly source of information about sexual and other health issues.

3. *Go Ask Alice.* An interactive question-and-answer resource from the Columbia University Health Services. "Alice" is available to answer questions each week about any health-related issues, including relationships, nutrition and diet, exercise, drugs, sex, alcohol, and stress.

4. *Sexuality Information and Education Council of the United States (SIECUS).* Information, guidelines, and materials for advancement of healthy and proper sex education.

5. *Teen Sexual Health.* Current research and other resources dealing with sexual health for high school and college-age students.

Further Reading

Caron, S. L. *Sex Matters for College Students: Sex FAQ's in Human Sexuality.* Englewood Cliffs, NJ: Prentice Hall, 2002.

This is a brief, easy-to-read, and affordable paperback designed specifically to answer the basic sexual questions of today's young adults in a friendly and age-appropriate way.

Caster, W., R. Bussel, and J. May, *The Lesbian Sex Book: A Guide for Women Who Love Women,* 2nd ed. Los Angeles, CA: Alyson publications, 2003.

A handbook for lesbian sexual practices and health.

Goldstone, S. *The Ins and Outs of Gay Sex: A Medical Handbook for Men.* New York: Dell, 1999.

A comprehensive guide to the sexual and medical concerns of gay men.

Men's Health Books, ed. *The Complete Book of Men's Health: The Definitive, Illustrated Guide to Healthy Living, Exercise, and Sex.* Emmaus, PA: Rodale Press, 2000.

A comprehensive and lushly illustrated guide to information on healthy lifestyles for men.

SIECUS (*Sexuality Information and Education Council of the United States*) *Report.* 130 West 42nd Street, New York, NY 10036.

Highly acclaimed and readable bimonthly journal. Includes timely and thought-provoking articles on human sexuality, sexuality education, and AIDS.

Wingood, G. M., and R. DiClemente, eds. *Handbook of Women's Sexual and Reproductive Health.* Boston: Plenum Publishing, 2002.

Medical researchers, including those in behavioral sciences and health education, summarize in depth the epidemiology, social and behavioral factors, policies, and effective intervention and prevention strategies related to women's sexual and reproductive health.

References

1. MayoClinic.com, "Nurture Relationships: A Healthy Habit for Healthy Aging," 2003, Mayo Foundation for Medical Education and Research (MFMER), www.mayohealth.org; K. Uberg et al., "Supportive Relationships as a Moderator of the Effects of Peer Drinking on Adolescents," *Journal of Research on Adolescents* 15, no.1 (2005): 1–20.

2. C. Snapp and M. Leary, "Hurt Feelings among New Acquaintances: Moderating Effects of Interpersonal Familiarity," *Journal of Social and Personal Relationships* 18, no. 3 (June 2001): 1344–1350.

3. V. Manusov and J. Harvey, eds., *Attribution, Communication Behavior and Close Relationships* (New York: Cambridge University Press, 2001).

4. J. Caputo, H. C. Hazel, and C. McMahon, *Interpersonal Communication* (Boston: Allyn & Bacon, 1994), 224.

5. United States Census Bureau, "Living Arrangements of Children Under 18 Years for All Children" (Washington, DC: United States Census Bureau, 2004).

6. E. Weinstein and E. Rosen, *Teaching about Human Sexuality and Family: A Skills-Based Approach* (Belmont, CA: Thompson Higher Education, 2006).

7. B. Strong et. al., *Human Sexuality: Diversity in Contemporary America,* 5th ed. (New York: NY: McGraw-Hill, 2005), 217–219.

8. L. Lefton and L. Brannon, *Psychology,* 8th ed. (Boston: Allyn & Bacon, 2003), 474.

9. Ibid.

10. J. Holmes, "Healthy Relationships: Their Influence on Physical Health," BC Council for Families, 2004, www.bccf.bc.ca/learn/health_relations.htm.

11. S. Hendrick, *Understanding Close Relationships* (Boston: Allyn & Bacon, 2004).

12. Ibid.

13. E. Hatfield, "Passionate and Companionate Love," in *The Psychology of Love,* eds. R. J. Sternberg and M. L. Barnes. (New Haven, CT: Yale University Press1988), 191–217.

14. R. Sternberg, "Construct Validation of a Triangular Love Scale," *European Journal of Social Psychology* 27 (1997): 313–335.

15. H. Fisher, *Why We Love: The Nature and Chemistry of Romantic Love* (New York: Henry Holt, 2004); H. Fisher, *Anatomy of Love: The Natural History of Monogamy, Adultery, and Divorce* (New York: Norton, 1993).

16. A. Toufexis and P. Gray, "What Is Love? The Right Chemistry," *Time* (1993): 47–52.

17. Ibid.

18. Ibid.

19. C. McLoughlin, "Science of Love—Cupid's Chemistry," 2003, www.thenakedscientist.com/HTML/Columnists/clairemcloughlincolumn1.htm.

20. "I Get a Kick Out of You," *The Economist,* 370 (8367): 73–75.

21. D. Tannen, *You Just Don't Understand: Women and Men in Conversation* (New York: William Morrow, 1990).

22. S. Michaud and R. Warner, "Gender Differences in Self Reported Response in Troubles Talk," *Sex Roles* 37 (1997): 528–540; K. Pasley, J. Kerpelman, and D. Guilbert, "Gender Conflict; Identity Disruption and Marital Instability. Expanding Gottman's Model," *Journal of Social and Personal Relationships* 18, no. 1

(2001): 1107–1114; L. C. Gallo and T. W. Smith, "Attachment Style in Marriage: Adjustments and Responses to Interaction," *Journal of Social and Personal Relationships* 18, no. 2 (2001): 263–289; Manusov eds., *Attribution, Communication Behavior, and Close Relationships.*

23. Ibid.
24. Ibid.
25. Ibid.
26. S. A. Rathus, J. Nevid, and L. Fichner-Rathus, *Human Sexuality in a World of Diversity,* 6th ed. (Boston: Allyn & Bacon, 2005).
27. C. Morris and A. Maisto, *Psychology: An Introduction,* 12th ed. (Upper Saddle River, NJ: Prentice Hall, 2005).
28. Ibid.
29. Brehm et al., *Intimate Relationships,* 3rd ed. (New York: McGraw Hill, 2002), 263.
30. Strong et. al., *Human Sexuality.*
31. The National Marriage Project, Rutgers, the State University of New Jersey, "The State of Our Unions," 2005, http://marriage.rutgers.edu.
32. U.S. Census Bureau, "Estimated Median Age at First Marriage, by Sex: 1890 to Present," June 12, 2003, www.census.gov/population/www/socdemo/hh-fam.html history.
33. Ibid
34. Ibid.
35. U.S. Census Bureau, March Current Population Survey, 2004, www.census.gov/population/www/socdemo/hh-fam.html.
36. U.S. Census Bureau, "Marital Status of People 15 Years and Older, March 2002," June 2003, www.census.gov/population/www.socdemo/hh-fam.html; Centers for Disease Control and Prevention, "Advance Data, First Marriage Dissolution, Divorce, and Remarriage: United States," 2001, www.cdc.gov/nchs/data/ad/ad323.pdf.
37. Ibid.
38. The National Marriage Project, Rutgers, "The State of Our Unions."
39. G. Kelly, *Sexuality Today: The Human Perspective,* 8th ed. (New York: NY, McGraw-Hill, 2006), 271–272.
40. W. K. Halford et al., "Best Practice in Couple Relationship Education," *Journal of Marital and Family Therapy 29,* no. 3 (2003): 385–406.
41. S. Shaw and J. Lee, "Learning Gender in a Diverse Society," in *Women's Voices, Feminist Visions: Classic and Contemporary Readings* (Mountain View, CA: Mayfield Publishing, 2001).
42. G. M. Herek, J. Roy Gillis, and J. C. Cogan, "Psychological Sequelae of Hate-Crime Victimization Among Lesbian, Gay and Bisexual Adults," *Journal of Consulting and Clinical Psychology* 67, no. 6 (1999): 945–951.
43. A. H. Slyper, "Childhood Obesity, Adipose Tissue Distribution, and the Pediatric Practitioner," *Pediatrics* 102 (1998): 4.
44. Writing Group for the Women's Health Initiative Investigators, "Risk and Benefits of Estrogen Plus Progestin in Healthy Postmenopausal Women: Principal Results from the Women's Health Initiative Randomized Controlled Trial," *Journal of the American Medical Association* 288, no. 3 (2002): 321–333.
45. American Academy of Pediatrics, "Just the Facts: Circumcision," 2003, www.aap.org/mrt/factscir.htm.
46. G. F. Kelly, "Sexual Individuality and Sexual Values," in *Sexuality Today: The Human Perspective,* updated 7th ed. (Dubuque, IA: McGraw-Hill, 2004).
47. Ibid.
48. M. E. Guffy, *Business Communication: Process and Products* (Belmont, CA: Wadsworth, 1994), 38.
49. National Kidney and Urological Diseases Information Clearinghouse, "Erectile Dysfunction," 2004, http://kidney.niddk.nih.gov/kudiseases/pubs/impotence/index.htm.
50. B. Handy, "The Potency Pill," *Time,* May 4, 1998, 50–57.
51. Arnot Ogden Medical Center, "Frequently Asked Questions," 1998, www.aomc.org/HOD2/general/ViagraFAQ.html.
52. S. A. Lyman, C. Hughes-McLain, and G. Thompson, "'Date-Rape Drugs': A Growing Concern," *Journal of Health Education* 29, no. 5 (1998): 271–274.

How can I choose the right birth control method for me?

Is emergency contraception the same as abortion?

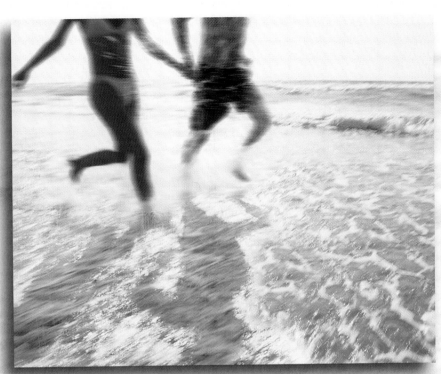

Are home pregnancy testing kits reliable?

What causes infertility?

6 Birth Control, Pregnancy, and Childbirth

Managing Your Fertility

Objectives

- *Describe* the different types of contraceptive methods and their effectiveness in preventing pregnancy and sexually transmitted infections.
- *Summarize* the legal decisions surrounding abortion and the various types of abortion procedures.
- *Discuss* key issues to consider when planning a pregnancy.

- *Explain* the importance of prenatal care and the physical and emotional aspects of pregnancy.
- *Describe* the basic stages of childbirth and complications that can arise during labor and delivery.
- *Explain* primary causes of and possible solutions to infertility.

Today, we not only understand the intimate details of reproduction, but we also possess technologies that can control or enhance our **fertility,** our ability to reproduce. Along with information and technological advances comes choice, and choice goes hand in hand with responsibility. Choosing if and when to have children is one of our greatest responsibilities. A woman and her partner have much to consider before planning or risking a pregnancy. Children, whether planned or unplanned, transform people's lives. They require a lifelong personal commitment of love and nurturing. Are you physically, emotionally, and financially prepared to care for another human being?

One measure of maturity is the ability to discuss reproduction and birth control with one's sexual partner before engaging in sexual activity. Men often assume that their partners are taking care of birth control. Women often feel that bringing up the subject implies they are "easy" or "loose." Both may feel that this discussion interferes with romance and spontaneity. You will find discussion easier and less embarrassing if you understand human reproduction and contraception and honestly consider your attitudes toward these matters before you find yourself in a compromising situation.

METHODS OF FERTILITY MANAGEMENT

Conception refers to the fertilization of an ovum by a sperm. The following conditions are necessary for conception:

1. A viable egg
2. A viable sperm
3. Access to the egg by the sperm

Fertility   A person's ability to reproduce.

Conception   The fertilization of an ovum by a sperm.

Contraception   Methods of preventing conception.

Sexually transmitted infections (STIs)   A variety of infections that can be acquired through sexual contact.

Barrier methods   Contraceptive methods that prevent the egg and sperm from joining by means of a physical barrier (e.g., condom, diaphragm, or cervical cap), a chemical barrier (e.g., spermicide), or both.

Hormonal methods   Contraceptive method that introduces synthetic hormones into the woman's system to prevent ovulation, thicken cervical mucus, or prevent a fertilized egg from implanting.

Male condom   A single-use sheath of strong, thin latex rubber or other material designed to fit over an erect penis and to catch semen upon ejaculation.

The term *contraception* (sometimes called birth control) refers to methods of preventing conception. These methods offer varying degrees of control over when and whether pregnancies occur. Society has searched for a simple, infallible, and risk-free way to prevent pregnancy since people first associated sexual activity with pregnancy; however, we have not yet found one.

To evaluate the effectiveness of a particular contraceptive method, you must be familiar with two concepts: perfect failure rate and typical use failure rate. *Perfect failure rate* refers to the number of pregnancies that are likely to occur in a year (per 100 uses of the method during sexual intercourse) if the method is used absolutely perfectly, that is, without any error. The *typical use failure rate* refers to the number of pregnancies that are likely to occur with typical use—that is, with the normal number of errors, memory lapses, and incorrect or incomplete use. This information is much more practical for people in helping them make informed decisions about contraceptive methods. We'll discuss various contraceptive methods in this chapter.

Many contraceptive methods can also protect, to some degree, against **sexually transmitted infections (STIs)** which you'll learn more about in Chapter 14. This is an important factor to consider in choosing a contraceptive.

Choosing a Method of Contraception

Present methods of contraception fall into several categories. **Barrier methods** use a physical or chemical block to prevent the egg and sperm from joining. **Hormonal methods** introduce synthetic hormones into

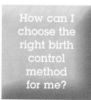
How can I choose the right birth control method for me?

the woman's system that prevent ovulation, thicken cervical mucus, or prevent a fertilized egg from implanting. Surgical methods can prevent pregnancy permanently. Other methods may involve temporary or permanent abstinence or planning intercourse in accordance with fertility patterns.

There are many factors to consider when choosing a method of contraception. Issues to think about range from cost to comfort level of convenience and health risks associated with a particular method. Table 6.1 summarizes the effectiveness of various methods. The Assess Yourself box on page 156 will help you to determine which method is best for you and your partner.

Barrier Methods

The Male Condom   The **male condom** is a thin sheath designed to cover the erect penis and catch semen before it enters the vagina. The majority of male

Table 6.1

Contraceptive Effectiveness and STI Prevention: Number of Unintended Pregnancies per 100 Women during First Year of Use

Method	Typical Use	Perfect Use
Continuous Abstinence*	0.00	0.00
Outercourse†	N/A	N/A
Norplant Implant	0.05	0.05
Sterilization		
Men	0.15	0.1
Women	0.5	0.5
Depo-Provera Injection	0.3	0.3
IUD (Intrauterine Device)		
ParaGard (copper T380A)	0.8	0.6
Mirena	0.1	0.1
Oral Contraceptives (The Pill)	8.0	0.3
Male Condom†	15.0	2.0
Sponge		
Women who have not given birth	16.0	9.0
Women who have given birth	32.0	20.0
Ortho Evra (The Patch)	8.0	0.3
NuvaRing	8.0	0.3
Withdrawal	27.0	4.0
Diaphragm†	20.0	6.0
Cervical Cap†		
Women who have not given birth	16.0	9.0
Women who have given birth	32.0	26.0
Female Condom†	21.0	5.0
Periodic Abstinence	25.0	
Postovulation method		1.0
Symptothermal method		2.0
Cervical mucus (ovulation) method		3.0
Calendar method		9.0
Fertility Awareness Methods	N/A	N/A
Spermicide†	26.0	6.0
No Method	85.0	85.0

Emergency Contraception

Emergency contraception pills: Treatment initiated within 72 hours after unprotected intercourse reduces the risk of pregnancy by 75–89% (with no protection against STIs). Emergency IUD insertion: Treatment initiated within seven days after unprotected intercourse reduces the risk of pregnancy by more than 99 percent (with no protection against STIs).

Note: "Typical Use" refers to failure rates for men and women whose use is not consistent or always correct. "Perfect Use" refers to failure rates for those whose use is consistent and always correct.

N/A means that effectiveness rates are not available.
*indicates complete protection from STIs
†indicates limited protection from STIs
Source: R. Hatcher et al., "Contraceptive Effectiveness Rates," *Contraceptive Technology,* 18th ed. (New York: Ardent Media, 2004). Reprinted by permission of Ardent Media.

condoms are made of latex, although condoms made of polyurethane or lambskin are now available. The condom is the only temporary means of birth control available for men, and latex and polyurethane condoms are the only barrier that effectively prevents the spread of STIs and HIV (human immunodeficiency virus). ("Skin" condoms, made from lamb intestines, are not effective against STIs.)

Condoms come in a wide variety of styles: colored, ribbed for "extra sensation," lubricated, nonlubricated, and with or without reservoirs at the tip. All may be purchased with or without spermicide in pharmacies, supermarkets, public bathrooms, and many health clinics. A new condom must be used for each act of intercourse or oral sex.

In addition to helping to prevent some STIs, including genital herpes and HIV, condoms may also slow or reduce the risk of cervical cancer in women.

A condom must be rolled onto the penis before the penis touches the vagina and held in place when removing the penis from the vagina after ejaculation (Figure 6.1). For greatest efficacy, they should be used with a spermicide containing nonoxynol 9, the same agent found in many contraceptive foams and creams.

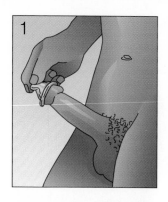
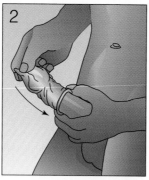
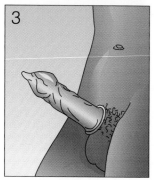
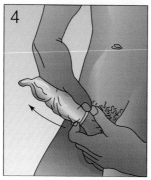

Figure 6.1 ■ How to Use a Condom
The condom should be rolled over the erect penis before any penetration occurs. A small space (about 1/2 inch) should be left at the end of the condom to collect the semen after ejaculation. Hold the tip of the condom, and unroll it all the way to the base of the penis. Hold the base of the condom before withdrawal to avoid spilling any semen.

If desired, users can lubricate their own condoms with contraceptive foams, creams, and jellies or other water-based lubricants (K-Y jelly, ForPlay Lubricants, Astroglide, or Wet or Aqua Lube, etc.). Never use products such as baby oil, cold cream, petroleum jelly, vaginal yeast infection medications, or hand or body lotion with a condom. These products contain mineral oil and will cause the latex to begin to disintegrate within 60 seconds.

Condoms are less effective and more likely to break during intercourse if they are old or poorly stored. To maintain effectiveness, store them in a cool place (not in a wallet or hip pocket), and inspect them for small tears before use.

For some people, a condom ruins the spontaneity of sex because stopping to put it on may break the mood for them. Others report that the condom decreases sensation. These inconveniences and the perception that condoms decrease sensation contribute to improper use or not using them at all. Partners who incorporate

Spermicides   Substances designed to kill sperm.
Female condom   A single-use polyurethane sheath for internal use.

putting a condom on during foreplay are generally more likely to use this form of birth control effectively each time they have sex.

Jellies, Creams, Foams, Suppositories, and Film
Jellies, creams, foam, suppositories, and film, like condoms, do not require a prescription. They are referred to as **spermicides**—substances designed to kill sperm. Recent studies indicate that spermicides containing nonoxynol 9 (N-9) are not effective in preventing certain STIs, including gonorrhea, chlamydia, and HIV. In fact, frequent use of spermicides containing N-9 has been shown to cause irritation and breaks in the mucus layer or skin of the genital tract, creating a point of entry for viruses and bacteria that cause disease.[1] Although they are not recommended as the primary form of contraception, spermicides are often recommended for use with other forms of contraception. They are most effective when used in conjunction with a condom.

Jellies and creams are packaged in tubes, and foams are available in aerosol cans. All are designed for insertion into the vagina. They must be inserted far enough to cover the cervix, thus providing both a chemical barrier that kills sperm and a physical barrier that stops sperm from continuing toward an egg (Figure 6.2).

Suppositories are waxy capsules that are inserted deep in the vagina, where they melt. They must be inserted 10 to 20 minutes before intercourse to have time to melt, but no longer than one hour prior to intercourse or they lose their effectiveness. Additional contraceptive chemicals must be applied for each subsequent act of intercourse.

Vaginal contraceptive film is another method of spermicide delivery. A thin film infused with spermicidal gel is inserted into the vagina, so that it covers the cervix. The film dissolves into a spermicidal gel that is effective for up to three hours. As with other spermicides, a new film must be inserted for each act of intercourse.

The Female Condom
The **female condom** is a single-use, soft, loose-fitting polyurethane sheath meant for internal use. It is designed as one unit with two diaphragm-like rings (see photo). One ring, which lies inside the sheath, serves as an insertion mechanism and internal anchor. The other ring, which remains outside the vagina once the device is inserted, protects the labia and the base of the penis from infection. Many women like the female condom because it gives them more control over reproduction than the male condom. When used correctly, the female condom provides protection against HIV and STIs comparable to that of a latex male condom. The condom's brand name is the Reality Condom. The condom also can be used for male anal sex.

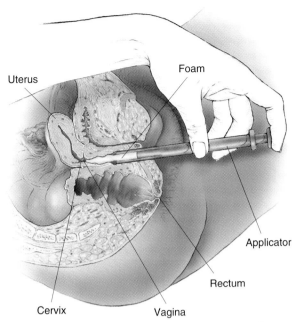

Figure 6.2 ■ The Proper Method of Applying Spermicide within the Vagina

Labels: Uterus, Foam, Applicator, Rectum, Vagina, Cervix

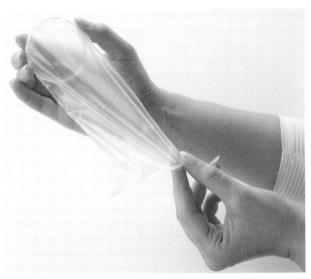

The female condom.

The Diaphragm with Spermicidal Jelly or Cream

Invented in the mid-nineteenth century, the **diaphragm** was the first widely used birth control method for women. The diaphragm is a soft, shallow cup made of thin latex rubber. Its flexible, rubber-coated ring is designed to fit snugly behind the pubic bone in front of the cervix and over the back of the cervix on the other side so it blocks access to the uterus. Diaphragms are manufactured in different sizes and must be fitted to the woman by a trained practitioner. The practitioner also should be certain that the user knows how to insert her diaphragm correctly before she leaves the practitioner's office.

Diaphragms must be used with spermicidal cream or jelly, which is applied to the inside of the diaphragm before insertion. The diaphragm holds the spermicide in place and creates a physical and chemical barrier against sperm. Additional spermicide must be applied before each subsequent act of intercourse; the diaphragm must be left in place for six to eight hours after intercourse to allow the chemical to kill any sperm remaining in the vagina. When used with spermicidal jelly or cream, it offers significant protection against gonorrhea and possibly chlamydia and human papilloma virus (Figure 6.3).

Using the diaphragm during the menstrual period or leaving it in place longer than 24 hours slightly increases the user's risk of **toxic shock syndrome (TSS).** This condition results from the multiplication of bacteria that spread to the bloodstream and cause sudden high fever, rash, nausea, vomiting, diarrhea, and a rapid drop in blood pressure. If not treated, TSS can be fatal.

The diaphragm (as well as wounds or tampons left too long in place) creates conditions conducive to the growth of these bacteria. To reduce the risk of TSS, women should wash their hands carefully with soap and water before inserting or removing a diaphragm.

There are other disadvantages. The diaphragm can put undue pressure on the urethra, which blocks urinary flow and predisposes the user to bladder infections. Inserting the device also can be awkward, especially if the woman is rushed. Diaphragms are much less effective when inserted incorrectly.

The Cervical Cap with Spermicidal Jelly or Cream

The cervical cap is one of the oldest methods used to prevent pregnancy. Early cervical caps were made from beeswax, silver, or copper. Today's **cervical cap** is a small cup made of latex that fits snugly over the entire cervix. It must be fitted by a practitioner and is designed for use with spermicidal jelly or cream. It is somewhat more difficult to insert than a diaphragm because of its smaller size.

The cap keeps sperm out of the uterus. It is held in place by suction created during application. Insertion

---

Diaphragm A latex, saucer-shaped device designed to cover the cervix and block access to the uterus; it should always be used with spermicide.

Toxic shock syndrome (TSS) A potentially fatal disease that occurs when specific bacterial toxins are allowed to multiply unchecked in wounds or through improper use of tampons or diaphragms.

Cervical cap A small cup made of latex that is designed to fit snugly over the entire cervix and used with a spermicide.

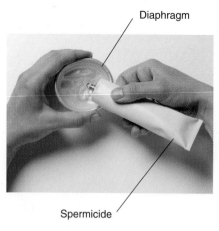
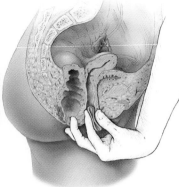
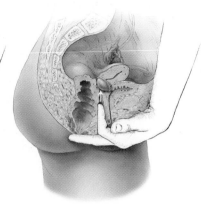

Diaphragm

Spermicide

a. Place spermicide inside and around the rim of the diaphragm.

b. Insertion: squeeze rim together; insert with spermicide-side up.

c. Check placement, making certain cervix is covered.

Figure 6.3 ■ The Proper Use and Placement of a Diaphragm

may take place up to two days prior to intercourse; the device must be left in place for six to eight hours after intercourse. If removed and cleaned, it can be reinserted immediately. The cervical cap may offer protection against some STIs but not HIV.

Some women report unpleasant vaginal odors after use. Because the device can become dislodged during intercourse, placement must be checked frequently. The cap cannot be used during the menstrual period or for longer than 48 hours because of the risk of TSS.

Lea's Shield

Lea's Shield is a one-size-fits-all silicon rubber device that covers the cervix. The device can be inserted anytime prior to intercourse but must remain in place for 8 hours after intercourse; it can remain in place for a maximum of 48 hours. The shield is outfitted with a small loop that aids in both insertion and removal. It must be used with spermicidal jelly or cream, similar to the diaphragm or cervical cap. Approved by the FDA (U.S. Food and Drug Administration) in 2002, it is available by prescription. Because the shield is made of silicon rubber, not latex, it is a suitable alternative for those allergic to latex.

Lea's Shield A one-size-fits-all silicon rubber device that covers the cervix and is available by prescription.

Sponge A contraceptive device, made of polyurethane foam and containing nonoxynol 9, that fits over the cervix to create a barrier against sperm.

Oral contraceptives Pills taken daily for three weeks of the menstrual cycle that prevent ovulation by regulating hormones.

The Sponge The original version of the **sponge,** the Today sponge, was available in the United States from 1983 to 1995, at which time the manufacturer shut down production rather than bring its facility up to FDA standards. In April of 2005, the Today sponge, now produced by a different company, was approved by the FDA but is not yet available in retail stores. The Protectaid sponge is already available in Canada. The sponge is made of polyurethane foam and contains nonoxynol 9. It fits over the cervix, and creates a barrier against sperm. A main advantage is convenience, as it does not require a trip to the doctor for fitting. It can be inserted in advance and remain in place for 24 hours. Some disadvantages of the sponge are limited protection from STIs and only moderate protection against pregnancy.

Hormonal Methods

Oral Contraceptives

Oral contraceptive pills were first marketed in the United States in 1960. Their convenience quickly made them the most widely used reversible method of fertility control. Most oral contraceptives work through the combined effects of synthetic estrogen and progesterone *(combination pills)*. Estrogen in the pill prevents ovulation by inhibiting the production of follicle-stimulating hormone (FSH) (Chapter 5). Progesterone in the pill prevents proper growth of the uterine lining and thickens the cervical mucus, thus forming a barrier against sperm.

Combination pills are taken in 28-day cycles. At the end of each three-week cycle, the user discontinues the drug or takes a placebo pill for one week. The resultant drop in hormones causes the uterine lining to disintegrate, and the user will have a menstrual period, usually within one to three days. Menstrual flow is generally lighter than it is for women who don't use the pill because the hormones in the pill prevent thick endometrial buildup.

A new type of pill available since 2003 is called **Seasonale.** Seasonale is a 91-day, or extended cycle, oral contraceptive. A woman using this type of regimen takes active pills for 12 weeks, followed by one week of placebos. Under this cycle, women can expect to have a menstrual period every three months. Early data indicates that women do have an increased occurrence of spotting or bleeding in the first few cycles.[2] Side effects and risks are similar to 28-day cycle pills.

Because the chemicals in oral contraceptives change the way the body metabolizes certain nutrients, all women using the pill should check with their practitioners to see if dietary supplements are advisable. A nutritious diet that includes whole grains, fresh fruits and vegetables, lean meats, fish and poultry, and nonfat dairy products is important.

Oral contraceptives can interact negatively with other drugs. For example, some antibiotics diminish the pill's effectiveness and may require an adjustment in the antibiotic dosage. Women in doubt should check with their prescribing practitioners or their pharmacists.

Return of fertility may be delayed after discontinuing the pill, but the pill is not known to cause infertility. Women who had irregular menstrual cycles before going on the pill are more likely to have problems conceiving, regardless of pill use.

The pill is convenient and does not interfere with lovemaking. It may lessen menstrual difficulties, such as cramps and premenstrual syndrome. Oral contraceptives also lower the risk of several health conditions, including endometrial and ovarian cancers, noncancerous breast disease, osteoporosis, ovarian cysts, pelvic inflammatory disease (PID), and iron deficiency anemia.[3] Possible serious health problems associated with the pill include blood clots, which can lead to strokes or heart attacks, and an increased risk for high blood pressure (Figure 6.4). The risk is low for most healthy women under 35 who do not smoke; it increases with age and especially with cigarette smoking.

Apart from these risk factors and certain side effects associated with the pill, its greatest disadvantage is that it must be taken every day. If a woman misses one pill, she should use an alternative form of contraception for the remainder of that cycle. Another drawback is that the pill does not protect against STIs. Cost also may be a problem for some women. Some teenagers report that the requirement to have a complete gynecological examination in order to get a prescription for the pill is a huge obstacle. Educating young women about what goes on in a gynecological exam certainly would help ease their anxiety.

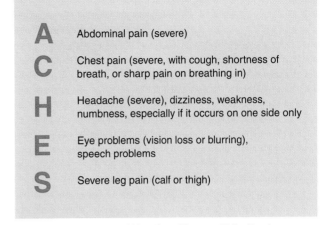

Figure 6.4 ■ Early Warning Signs of Medical Complications for Pill Users

Source: R. A. Hatcher et al., *Contraceptive Technology,* 18th ed. (New York: Ardent Media, 2004).

Progestin-Only Pills Progestin-only pills (or minipills) contain small doses of progesterone. Women who feel uncertain about using estrogen pills, who suffer from side effects related to estrogen, or who are nursing may choose these medications rather than combination pills. There is still some question about how progestin-only pills work. Current thought is that they change the composition of the cervical mucus, thus impeding sperm travel. They also may inhibit ovulation in some women. The effectiveness rate of progestin-only pills is 96 percent, slightly lower than that of estrogen-containing pills. Also, their use usually leads to irregular menstrual bleeding. As with all oral contraceptives, the user has no protection against STIs.

Ortho Evra (The Patch) A hormonal contraceptive patch, **Ortho Evra,** became available by prescription in 2002. A patch is worn for one week and replaced on the same day of the week for three consecutive weeks; the fourth week is patch-free. Ortho Evra is 99 percent effective and works by delivering continuous levels of estrogen and progestin through the skin and into the bloodstream. This patch is easy to apply, barely noticeable, and has adhesive strong enough to withstand even swimming. The patch can be worn on one of four areas of the body: buttocks, abdomen, upper torso (front and back, excluding the breasts), or upper outer arm.

Seasonale   An extended cycle oral contraceptive, where a woman will get her period every three months.

Ortho Evra   A set of patches worn for three weeks at a time that releases hormones similar to those in oral contraceptives.

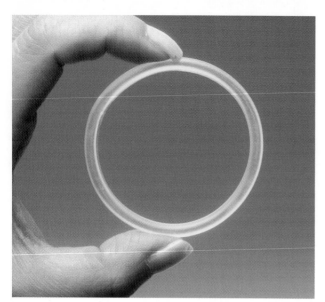
NuvaRing (actual size)

Ortho Evra contains hormones similar to those in birth control pills. Some women report experiencing breast symptoms, headache, application site reaction, nausea, upper respiratory infection, menstrual cramps, and abdominal pain. However, most side effects are not serious. Serious risks, which occur infrequently but can be life threatening, include blood clots, stroke, or heart attacks; tobacco use increases these risks. The contraceptive patch does not protect against STIs.

NuvaRing Introduced in 2002, this effective contraceptive offers protection four weeks at a time when used as prescribed. **NuvaRing** is a soft, flexible ring about 2 inches in diameter that the user inserts into the vagina and leaves in place for three weeks. (The user then removes it for one week for her menstrual period.) Once the ring is inserted, it continuously releases a steady flow of estrogen and progestin.

Advantages to NuvaRing include protection against pregnancy for one month; no pill to take daily; no requirement to be fitted by a clinician; no requirement to use spermicide; and the quick return of the ability to

become pregnant when use is stopped. Possible side effects include increased vaginal discharge and vaginal irritation or infection. Oil-based vaginal medicine to treat yeast infections cannot be used when the ring is in place; and a diaphragm or cervical cap cannot be used as a backup method for contraception.

Depo-Provera and Other Injections

Depo-Provera is a long-acting synthetic progesterone that is injected intramuscularly every three months. Researchers believe that the drug prevents ovulation. There are fewer health problems associated with Depo-Provera than with estrogen-containing pills. The main disadvantage is irregular bleeding, which can be troublesome at first, but within a year, most women are amenorrheic (i.e., they have no menstrual periods). Weight gain (an average of five pounds in the first year) is common. Other possible side effects include dizziness, nervousness, and headache. Some women feel Depo-Provera encourages sexual spontaneity because they do not have to remember to take a pill or insert a device. However, unlike other methods of contraception, this method cannot be stopped immediately if problems arise. Also, women who wish to become pregnant may find that it takes up to a year after their last injection to do so. Lunelle, a monthly injection that contained the time-released synthetic hormones estrogen and progestin, was recalled from the market due to manufacturing problems.

Implants Norplant, an early contraceptive implant, was a set of six silicon capsules containing progestin that were surgically inserted under the skin of a woman's upper arm. The progestin worked in the same way as oral contraceptives to suppress ovulation. Norplant was withdrawn from the market due to legal issues. Two new types of implants, a 2-rod (Jadelle) and a single rod (Implanon) slowly release progestin into the body. They are not on the market in the United States yet but have been approved for sale.

Surgical Methods

Sterilization, permanent fertility control achieved through surgical procedures, has become the second leading method of contraception for women under age 35 in the United States. It is the leading method of contraception for all women over age 35.[4] Although newer surgical techniques make reversal of sterilization theoretically possible, anyone considering sterilization should assume that the operation is not reversible. Before becoming sterilized, people should think through possibilities, such as divorce and remarriage or a future improvement in financial status, that might make a larger family realistic.

NuvaRing A soft, flexible ring inserted into the vagina that releases hormones that prevent pregnancy; it is left in place for three weeks and removed for one week for a menstrual period.

Depo-Provera An injectable method of birth control that lasts for three months.

Sterilization Permanent fertility control achieved through surgical procedures.

Female Sterilization **Tubal ligation** is one method of sterilization for females. In this surgical procedure, the uterine tubes are sealed shut to block sperm's access to released eggs. The operation usually is done in a hospital on an outpatient basis, under some form of anesthesia. First, the abdomen is inflated with carbon dioxide gas through a small incision in the navel. The surgeon then inserts a laparoscope into another incision just above the pubic bone. This specially designed instrument has a fiberoptic light source that enables the physician to see the uterine tubes clearly. The procedure itself usually takes less than an hour, and the patient generally can return home shortly after waking up. Women considering a tubal ligation should discuss all the risks with their physician before the operation. Although rare, possible complications of a tubal ligation can include infection and ectopic pregnancy.[5]

A tubal ligation does not affect ovarian and uterine function. The woman's menstrual cycle continues and released eggs simply disintegrate and are absorbed by the lymphatic system. As soon as her incision heals, the woman may resume sexual intercourse with no fear of pregnancy.

A new sterilization procedure is called **Essure.** Essure involves the placement of small microcoils into the uterine tubes via the vagina by a physician. Once in place, the microcoils expand to the shape of the uterine tubes. The coils promote the growth of scar tissue around the device and leads to blockage of the uterine tubes. Like traditional forms of tubal ligation, Essure is permanent.

A potential advantage to the procedure is that it does not require an incision; the entire procedure takes only 35 minutes and can be performed in the doctor's office. It is recommended for women who definitely do not want more children and especially for those who cannot have a tubal ligation due to chronic health conditions such as obesity or heart disease. Essure is a relatively new technique, and as a result the long-term risks are unknown.

A **hysterectomy,** or removal of the uterus, is a method of sterilization requiring major surgery. It usually is done only when the patient's uterus is diseased or damaged.

Male Sterilization Sterilization in men is less complicated than it is in women. A **vasectomy** is frequently done on an outpatient basis, using a local anesthetic. The surgeon makes an incision on each side of the scrotum, locates the vas deferens on each side, and removes a piece from each. The ends are usually tied or sewn shut.

In a small percentage of cases, serious complications occur, such as formation of a blood clot in the scrotum (which usually disappears without medical treatment), infection, or inflammatory reactions. Because sperm are stored in other areas of the reproductive system besides the vasa deferentia, couples must use alternative methods of birth control for at least one month after the vasectomy. The man must check with his physician (who will do a semen analysis) to determine when unprotected intercourse can take place. The pregnancy rate in women whose partners have had vasectomies after one year is 0.15 percent.[6]

Many men fear that the sterilization will affect sexual performance. However, a vasectomy in no way affects sexual response. Because sperm constitute only a small percentage of semen, the amount of ejaculate does not change significantly. The testes continue to produce sperm, but the sperm can no longer enter the ejaculatory duct. After a time, sperm production may diminish. Any sperm that are manufactured disintegrate and are absorbed into the lymphatic system.

Although a vasectomy should be considered permanent, surgical reversal sometimes can restore fertility. Recent improvements in microsurgery techniques have resulted in annual pregnancy rates of 40 to 60 percent for women whose partners have had reversals. The two major factors influencing the success rate of reversal are the doctor's expertise and the time elapsed since the vasectomy.

Try it ▸NOW

Be prepared. **Any method of contraception can fail. Take steps to protect yourself from unplanned pregnancy and STIs at all times. Whether you are on the pill or rely on condoms, always have a backup plan in mind and supplies available in case the condom tears or you forget to take a pill. An extra pack of condoms and spermicidal jelly, foam, or film are good items to have on hand.**

Tubal ligation   Sterilization of the female that involves the cutting and tying off or cauterizing of the uterine tubes.

Essure   A new, nonsurgical sterilization procedure in which a physician places small microcoils into the uterine tubes in order to block them.

Hysterectomy   The removal of the uterus.

Vasectomy   Sterilization of the male that involves the cutting and tying off of both vasa deferentia.

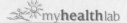

Fill out this assessment online at
www.aw-bc.com/MyHealthLab or www.aw-bc.com/donatelle.

Contraceptive Comfort and Confidence Scale

These questions will help you assess whether the method of contraception you are using now or may consider using in the future will be effective for you. Answering yes to any of these questions predicts potential problems. Most individuals will have a few yes answers. If you have more than a few yes responses, however, you may want to talk to a health care provider, counselor, partner, or friend to decide whether to use this method or how to use it so that it will really be effective. In general, the more yes answers you have, the less likely you are to use this method consistently and correctly with every act of intercourse.

Method of contraception you use now or are considering: _____

Length of time you used this method in the past: _____

Answer yes or no to the following questions:

	Yes	No
1. Have I ever had problems using this method?	❑	❑
2. Have I ever become pregnant while using this method?	❑	❑
3. Am I afraid of using this method?	❑	❑
4. Would I really rather not use this method?	❑	❑
5. Will I have trouble remembering to use this method?	❑	❑
6. Will I have trouble using this method correctly?	❑	❑
7. Do I still have unanswered questions about this method?	❑	❑
8. Does this method make menstrual periods longer or more painful?	❑	❑
9. Does this method cost more than I can afford?	❑	❑
10. Could this method cause serious complications?	❑	❑
11. Am I opposed to this method because of any religious or moral beliefs?	❑	❑
12. Is my partner opposed to this method?	❑	❑
13. Am I using this method without my partner's knowledge?	❑	❑
14. Will using this method embarrass my partner?	❑	❑
15. Will using this method embarrass me?	❑	❑
16. Will I enjoy intercourse less because of this method?	❑	❑
17. If this method interrupts lovemaking, will I avoid using it?	❑	❑
18. Has a nurse or doctor ever told me not to use this method?	❑	❑

Other Methods of Contraception

Intrauterine Devices Women have been using **intrauterine devices (IUDs)** since 1909, but we still are not certain how they work. Although it was once thought that IUDs prevent implantation of a fertilized egg, most experts now believe that they interfere with fertilization.

Two IUDs are currently available. ParaGard is a T-shaped plastic device with copper wrapped around the shaft. It does not contain any hormones and can be left in place for ten years before replacement. A newer IUD, Mirena, is effective for five years and releases small amounts of the progestin levonorgestrel.

A physician must fit and insert an IUD. For insertion, the device is folded and placed into a long, thin plastic applicator. The practitioner measures the depth of the uterus with a special instrument and then uses these measurements to place the IUD accurately so the arms of the T open out across the top of the uterus. One or two strings extend from the IUD into the vagina so the user can check to make sure that her IUD is in place. The device is removed by a practitioner when desired.

> **Intrauterine device (IUD)** A T-shaped device that is implanted in the uterus to prevent pregnancy.

	Yes	No
19. Is there anything about my personality that could lead me to use this method incorrectly?	❑	❑
20. Am I at risk of being exposed to HIV (the human immunodeficiency virus) or other sexually transmitted infections (STIs) if I use this method?	❑	❑

Total number of yes answers: _____

Source: From R. A. Hatcher et al., *Contraceptive Technology,* 17th ed. (New York: Ardent Media, 1998), 238. Reprinted by permission of Ardent Media.

▪■ ▫▪ Make It Happen!

Assessment: The Assess Yourself activity gave you the chance to assess your comfort and confidence with a contraceptive method you are using now or may use in the future. Depending on the results of the assessment, you may consider making a change in your birth control method.

Making a Change: In order to change your behavior, you need to develop a plan. Follow these steps and complete your Behavior Change Contract to take action.

1. Evaluate your behavior, and identify patterns. What can you change now? What can you change in the near future?
2. Select one pattern of behavior that you want to change.
3. Fill out the Behavior Change Contract found at the front of your book. It should include your long-term goal for change, your short-term goals, the rewards you'll give yourself for reaching these goals, potential obstacles along the way, and strategies for overcoming these obstacles. For each goal, list the small steps and specific actions that you will take.
4. Chart your progress in a journal. At the end of a week, consider how successful you were in following your plan. What helped you be successful? What made change more difficult? What will you do differently next week?

5. Revise your plan as needed: Are the short-term goals attainable? Are the rewards satisfying?

Example: Marissa had been using a diaphragm as her form of birth control. When she completed the self-assessment, she discovered that there were several aspects of it that made her uncomfortable. The questions to which she answered "yes" showed that she sometimes forgot to bring her diaphragm when she planned to see her boyfriend Ben, and she disliked using it because it interrupted her sexual activity. She also was embarrassed to use it because she didn't like inserting it in front of Ben. She decided she should investigate other birth control options and discuss them with her boyfriend. Her first step was to visit her student health center and, based on her likes and dislikes, to choose one or two alternatives to the diaphragm. Among the options suggested to her were the contraceptive patch (Ortho Evra) and the vaginal ring (NuvaRing), both of which she would not have to remember to use and would not interrupt sexual activity. Marissa's next step was to talk to her boyfriend about his likes and dislikes and then to make a final decision based on her confidence in the method, its convenience, and its cost.

Disadvantages of IUDs include discomfort, cost of insertion, and potential complications. The device can cause heavy menstrual flow and severe cramps. Women using IUDs have a higher risk of uterine perforation, ectopic pregnancy, pelvic inflammatory disease, infertility, and tubal infections. If a pregnancy occurs while the IUD is in place, the chance of miscarriage is 25 to 50 percent. The device should be removed as soon as possible. Doctors often offer therapeutic abortion to women who become pregnant while using an IUD because of the serious risks (including premature delivery, infection, and congenital abnormalities) associated with continuing the pregnancy.

For a comparison of this and other contraception costs, see Table 6.2.

Withdrawal This birth control method, which is not very effective, is used most commonly by people who have not taken the time to consider alternatives. **Withdrawal,** also called coitus interruptus, involves removing the penis from the vagina just prior to ejaculation. Because there can be up to a half-million sperm in the drop of fluid at the tip of the penis before ejaculation, this method is unreliable. Timing withdrawal is also difficult, and men concentrating on accurate timing may not be able to relax and enjoy intercourse.

> **Withdrawal** A method of contraception that involves removing the penis from the vagina before ejaculation; also called coitus interruptus.

Table 6.2

Costs of Contraceptive Devices and Procedures

Method	Cost
Sterilization	
Tubal ligation: permanently blocks female's uterine tubes where sperm join egg	$1,000–$2,500
Vasectomy: permanently blocks male's vasa deferentia that carry sperm	$240–$520
Depo-Provera	$20–$40/visits to clinician; $30–$75/injection
IUD (intrauterine device)	$175–$400/exam, insertion, and follow-up visit
Oral contraceptives	$15–$35/monthly pill-pack at drugstores, often less at clinics; $35–$125/exam
NuvaRing	$30–$35/monthly supply of rings; $35–$125/exam
Ortho Evra (patch)	$30-$35/monthly supply of patches; $35–$125/exam
Condoms/female condoms and spermicide	50¢ and up/condom—some family planning centers give them away or charge very little; $2.50/female condom; $8/applicator kit of spermicide foam and jelly ($4–$8 refills); similar prices for creams, films, and suppositories
Diaphragm or cervical cap	$13–$25/diaphragm or cap; $50–$125/examination; $4–$8/supplies of spermicide jelly or cream
Fertility awareness methods	$5–$8 and up for temperature kits; free classes often available in health and church centers

Note: Some family planning clinics charge for services on a sliding scale according to income.
Source: Reprinted with permission from Planned Parenthood Federation of America, Inc. © 2001 PPFA. All rights reserved.

Emergency Contraceptive Pills There are more than 2.7 million unintended pregnancies per year in the United States, and nearly half are due to contraceptive failure. According to the Centers for Disease Control and Prevention (CDC), more than 11 million American women report using contraceptive methods associated with high failure rates, including condoms, withdrawal, periodic abstinence, and diaphragms. A recent study in 2004 revealed that approximately 10 percent of sexually active college students reported that they or their partner used emergency contraception in the last school year.[7]

Emergency contraception can be used when a condom breaks, after a sexual assault, or any time unprotected sexual intercourse occurs. **Emergency contraceptive pills (ECPs)** are ordinary birth control pills containing estrogen and progestin. Although the therapy is commonly known as the morning-after pill,

Is emergency contraception the same as abortion?

the term is misleading; ECPs can be used up to 72 hours after intercourse and can reduce the risk of pregnancy by 75 percent. The way that ECPs prevent pregnancy is still unclear; it seems that they prevent ovulation, not implantation of a fertilized egg.

Emergency contraceptives currently require a prescription, although the FDA is considering allowing it to be dispensed over the counter. See the Reality Check box for more on ECP availability. The two FDA-approved products are Preven and Plan B. After a woman determines she is not already pregnant, by using the pregnancy test included in the kit, the first dose of two light blue emergency pills is taken as soon as possible, within 72 hours after intercourse. The second dose is taken 12 hours later.[8] The most common side effects related to ECPs are nausea, vomiting, menstrual irregularities, breast tenderness, headache, abdominal pain and cramps, and dizziness.

Emergency minipills contain progestin only. Like ECPs, minipills can be used immediately after unprotected intercourse and up to 72 hours beyond. Emergency minipills are as effective as ECPs, but nausea and vomiting are far less common. Emergency minipills are an excellent alternative for most women who cannot use ECPs that contain estrogen.

Emergency contraceptive pills (ECPs) Birth control pills containing estrogen and progestin taken within three days after unprotected intercourse to prevent fertilization or implantation.

Emergency minipills Birth control pills containing only progestin that can be taken up to three days after unprotected intercourse.

The Centers for Disease Control and Prevention estimate that 86 percent of college students nationwide have had sexual intercourse and that nearly one-third of college women attending four-year institutions have experienced a pregnancy. The 18- to 24-year-old age group has the highest rate of unwanted pregnancies. Use of emergency contraceptive pills can be a very effective method for dealing with unwanted pregnancy on college campuses. In fact, The Alan Guttmacher Institute estimates that 51,000 abortions were prevented by emergency contraceptive use in 2000 alone. Though no substitute for taking proper precautions (e.g., using latex condoms with a spermicide) before having sex, the potential for emergency contraceptive pills (ECPs) to reduce the rate of unintended pregnancy and ultimately abortion is very strong.

However, access to and knowledge of emergency contraception is limited.

According to an article published in the *Journal of American College Health* in 2002, emergency contraception is available at 52 percent of college or university student health centers nationwide. Advocates would not only like to see this number increase, but would also like to see ECPs available without prescription, as it already is in almost 30 countries, from France and the United Kingdom to much of Africa. Opponents fear easy access to emergency contraception will encourage irresponsible sexual activity among young people. Research indicates otherwise: a recent study of women aged 15 to 20 revealed that providing increased access to ECPs does not increase the likelihood of unprotected sex. Some opponents also identify ECP use with abortion.

Emergency contraceptive effectiveness is reliant on availability. Highest rates of success occur if the pill is taken within 24 to 72 hours after unprotected intercourse. In 2004, an expert advisory panel to the FDA recommended that Plan B, one brand of ECP, be made available without prescription. However, in a controversial move, the FDA rejected its own panel's decision. Currently, the status of ECP availabilty remains in the hands of each individual state.

Source: R. G. Sawyer and E. Thompson, "Knowledge and Attitudes about Emergency Contraception in University Students," *College Student Journal* 4 (December 2003); Alan Guttmacher Institute, "Emergency Contraception Has Tremendous Potential in the Fight to Reduce Unintended Pregnancy," May 2005, www.agi.usa.org; S. K. McCarthy, "Availability of Emergency Contraceptive Pills at University and College Student Health Centers," *Journal of American College Health* 51, no. 1 (2002): 15–22; The American Society for Emergency Contraception, Center for Reproductive Rights, "Governments Worldwide Put Emergency Contraception into Women's Hands," current as of November 7, 2002, www.reproductiverights.org.

Abstinence and "Outercourse"

Strictly defined, *abstinence* means deliberately avoiding intercourse. This strict definition would allow one to engage in such forms of sexual intimacy as massage, kissing, and solitary masturbation. But many people today have broadened the definition of abstinence to include all forms of sexual contact, even those that do not culminate in sexual intercourse.

Couples who go a step further than massage and kissing and engage in activities such as oral–genital sex and mutual masturbation are sometimes said to be engaging in "outercourse." Like abstinence, outercourse can be 100 percent effective for birth control as long as the male does not ejaculate near the vaginal opening. Unlike abstinence, however, outercourse is not 100 percent effective against STIs. Oral–genital contact can transmit disease, although the practice can be made safer by using a condom on the penis or a dental dam on the vaginal opening.

Fertility Awareness Methods

Methods of fertility control that rely upon the alteration of sexual behavior are called **fertility awareness methods (FAMs).**

Proper use of FAMs relies upon a knowledge of basic physiology (Figure 6.5 on page 160). A released ovum can survive up to 48 hours after ovulation. Sperm can live up to five days in the vagina. Natural birth control methods teach women to recognize their fertile times. Changes in cervical mucus prior to and during ovulation and a rise in basal body temperature are two frequently used indicators. Another method involves charting a woman's menstrual cycle and ovulation times on a calendar. Women may use any combination of these methods to determine their fertile times more accurately, although these methods remain far less effective than other methods.

Cervical Mucus Method

The **cervical mucus method** requires women to examine the consistency and color of their normal vaginal secretions to determine

> **Fertility awareness methods (FAMs)** Several types of birth control that require alteration of sexual behavior rather than chemical or physical intervention into the reproductive process.
>
> **Cervical mucus method** A birth control method that relies upon observation of changes in cervical mucus to determine when the woman is fertile.

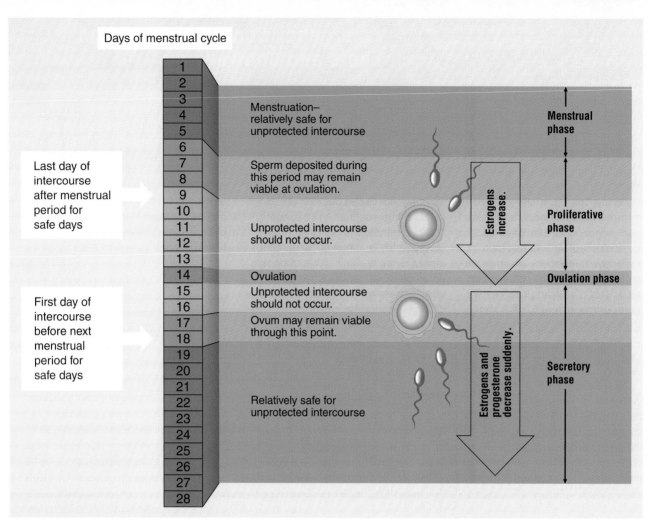

Figure 6.5 ▪ The Fertility Cycle
Fertility awareness methods, or FAMs, can combine the use of a calendar, the cervical mucus method, and body temperature measurements to identify the fertile period. It is important to remember that most women do not have a consistent 28-day cycle.

when they are fertile. Prior to ovulation, vaginal mucus becomes gelatinous and stretchy, and normal vaginal secretions may increase. Sexual activity involving penis–vagina contact must be avoided while this "fertile mucus" is present and for several days afterward.

Body Temperature Method The **body temperature method** relies on the fact that the female's basal body temperature rises 0.4 to 0.8 degree after ovulation. For this method to be effective, the woman

must chart her temperature for several months to learn her body's temperature fluctuations. Abstinence from penis–vagina contact must be observed preceding the temperature rise until several days after the temperature rise is first noted.

The Calendar Method The **calendar method** requires the woman to record the exact number of days in her menstrual cycle. Because few women menstruate with complete regularity, this involves keeping a record of the menstrual cycle for 12 months, during which some other method of birth control must be used. The first day of a woman's period counts as day 1. To determine the first fertile unsafe day of the cycle, she subtracts 18 from the number of days in the shortest cycle. To determine the last unsafe day of the cycle, she subtracts 11 from the number of days in the longest cycle. This method assumes that ovulation occurs during the midpoint of the cycle. The couple must abstain from penis–vagina contact during the fertile time.

Body temperature method A birth control method in which a woman monitors her body temperature for the rise that signals ovulation, the period during which she is fertile.

Calendar method A birth control method in which a woman's menstrual cycle is mapped on a calendar to determine presumed fertile times.

Women interested in fertility awareness methods are advised to take classes in their use. Women who are untrained in these techniques run a high risk of unwanted pregnancy.

ABORTION

In 1973, the landmark U.S. Supreme Court decision in *Roe v. Wade* stated that the "right to privacy… founded on the Fourteenth Amendment's concept of personal liberty… is broad enough to encompass a woman's decision whether or not to terminate her pregnancy."[9] The decision maintained that during the first trimester of pregnancy, a woman and her practitioner have the right to terminate the pregnancy through **abortion** without legal restrictions. It allowed individual states to set conditions for second-trimester abortions. Third-trimester abortions were ruled illegal unless the mother's life or health was in danger.

Prior to the legalization of first- and second-trimester abortions, women wishing to terminate a pregnancy had to travel to a country where the procedure was legal, consult an illegal abortionist, or perform their own abortions. These procedures sometimes led to death from hemorrhage or infection or to infertility from internal scarring. Today, nearly half of all pregnancies that occur each year are unplanned, and 50 percent of these pregnancies are terminated by abortion. The U.S. abortion rate has declined in recent years but is still higher than many of the other industrialized nations. There are several possible factors that influence this difference. Many other nations have fewer unwanted pregnancies, early sex education is strongly emphasized, and contraception is easier and cheaper to obtain.[10]

The political debate surrounding abortion rights is ongoing. Opponents of abortion believe that the embryo or fetus is a human being with rights that must be protected. In recent years, new legislation has given states the right to impose certain restrictions on abortions. Abortions cannot be performed in publicly funded clinics in some states, and other states have laws requiring parental notification before a teenager can obtain an abortion. In 2003 alone, states enacted 45 new antiabortion measures.[11] However, 17 states currently do appropriate public funds to women in poverty who seek an abortion.[12] On the federal level, abortion procedures are not covered by federally funded health care plans. This affects Medicaid recipients, women in the military and military dependents stationed overseas, women in federal prison, Native Americans, federal employees, and even Peace Corps volunteers. *Roe v. Wade* has not been overturned, but it faces many future challenges.

Although many opponents work through the courts and the political process, attacks on abortion clinics and on doctors who perform abortions are not uncommon. Legal protection, such as the Freedom of Access to

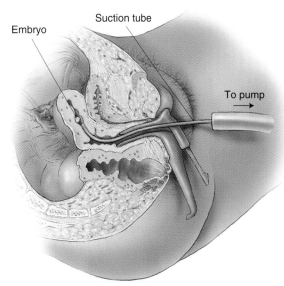

Figure 6.6 ■ Vacuum Aspiration Abortion

Clinic Entrance Act (FACE), offers some relief from the harassment and violence directed at abortion clinics. However, because of such acts, the biggest threat to a woman's access to an abortion now is finding a clinic rather than legal restrictions.

The best birth control methods can fail. Women may be raped. Pregnancies can occur despite every possible precaution. When an unwanted pregnancy does occur, the decision whether to terminate, carry to term and keep the baby, or carry to term and give the baby away must be made. This is a personal decision that each woman must make, based on her personal beliefs, values, and resources after carefully considering all alternatives.

Methods of Abortion

The choice of abortion procedure is determined by how many weeks the woman has been pregnant. Length of pregnancy is calculated from the first day of her last menstrual period.

Surgical Abortions If performed during the first trimester of pregnancy, abortion presents a relatively low risk to the mother. The most commonly used method of first-trimester abortion is **vacuum aspiration** (Figure 6.6). The procedure is usually performed under a local anesthetic. The cervix is dilated with instruments or by placing laminaria, a sterile seaweed product, in the cervical canal. The laminaria is left in place

> **Abortion**   The medical means of terminating a pregnancy.
>
> **Vacuum aspiration**   An abortion technique that uses gentle suction to remove fetal tissue from the uterus.

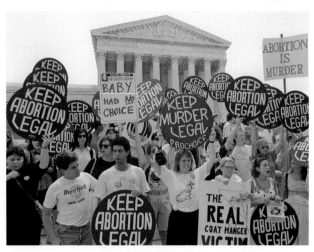

Abortion continues to be a controversial and emotional issue in the United States.

for a few hours or overnight and slowly dilates the cervix. After it is removed, a long tube is inserted into the uterus through the cervix, and gentle suction removes fetal tissue from the uterine walls.

Pregnancies that progress into the second trimester can be terminated through **dilation and evacuation (D&E),** a procedure that combines vacuum aspiration with a technique called **dilation and curettage (D&C),** which involves scraping the uterine lining. Second-trimester abortions frequently are done under general anesthetic. Both procedures can be performed on an outpatient basis (usually in the physician's office), with or without pain medication. Generally, however, the woman is given a mild tranquilizer to help her relax.

Dilation and evacuation (D&E) An abortion technique that combines vacuum aspiration with dilation and curettage; fetal tissue is both sucked and scraped out of the uterus.

Dilation and curettage (D&C) Abortion technique in which the cervix is dilated with laminaria for one to two days, after which the uterine walls are scraped clean.

Induction abortion Abortion technique in which chemicals are injected into the uterus through the uterine wall; labor begins, and the fetus and placenta are expelled from the uterus.

Hysterotomy The surgical removal of the fetus from the uterus.

Intact dilation and extraction (D&X) A late-term abortion procedure in which the body of the fetus is extracted up to the head and then the contents of the cranium are aspirated.

Mifepristone A steroid hormone that induces abortion by blocking the action of progesterone.

Both procedures may cause moderate to severe uterine cramping and blood loss.

Two other methods used in second-trimester abortions, though less common than the D&E, are prostaglandin or saline **induction abortions.** Prostaglandin hormones or saline solution is injected into the uterus, which kills the fetus and initiates labor contractions. After 24 to 48 hours, the fetus and placenta are expelled from the uterus.

A **hysterotomy,** or surgical removal of the fetus from the uterus, may be used during emergencies, when the mother's life is in danger, or when other types of abortions are deemed too dangerous.

The risks associated with abortion include infection, incomplete abortion (when parts of the placenta remain in the uterus), missed abortion (when the fetus is not actually removed), excessive bleeding, and cervical and uterine trauma. Follow-up and attention to danger signs decrease the chances of long-term problems.

The mortality rate for first-trimester abortions averages one death per every 500,000 procedures at eight or fewer weeks. The risk of death increases with the length of pregnancy. At 16 to 20 weeks, the mortality is 1 per 27,000, and at 21 weeks or more it increases to 1 per 8,000.[13] These higher rates are due to the increased risk of uterine perforation, bleeding, infection, and incomplete abortion due to the fact that the uterine wall becomes thinner as the pregnancy progresses.

One surgical method of performing abortion has been the subject of much controversy. **Intact dilation and extraction (D&X),** sometimes referred to by the nonmedical term *partial-birth abortion,* is used only in certain cases, such as when other abortion methods could injure the mother. The procedure involves extraction via vaginal delivery of a dead but otherwise intact fetus.[14] Thirty-one states have passed legislation attempting to ban intact dilation and extraction. However, the wording of the legislation in many states has been so general that it could be used to ban all types of abortion. For this reason, such legislation has often been challenged, and currently only ten states fully enforce the laws as written. Professional organizations such as the American College of Obstetrics and Gynecology and the American Medical Association state that physicians, acting in the best interests of their patients, should choose the safest and most appropriate method of abortion in each individual case.

Medical Abortions Unlike surgical abortions, medical abortions are performed without entering the uterus. **Mifepristone,** formerly known as RU-486, is a steroid hormone that induces abortion by blocking the action of progesterone, a hormone produced by the ovaries and placenta that maintains the lining of the uterus. As a result, the uterine lining and the embryo are expelled from the uterus, which terminates the pregnancy.

Mifepristone's nickname, the "abortion pill," may imply an easy process. However, this treatment actually involves more steps than a surgical abortion, which takes approximately 15 minutes followed by a physical recovery of about one day. With mifepristone, a first visit to the clinic involves a physical exam and a dose of three tablets, which may cause minor side effects such as nausea, headaches, weakness, and fatigue. The patient returns two days later for a dose of prostaglandins (trade name: misoprostol), which causes uterine contractions that expel the fertilized egg. The patient is required to stay under observation at the clinic for four hours and make a follow-up visit 12 days later.[15]

The side effects of this treatment are similar to those reported during heavy menstruation and include cramping, minor pain, and nausea. Approximately 1 in 1,000 women requires a blood transfusion because of severe bleeding. The procedure does not require hospitalization; women may be treated on an outpatient basis.

Another drug that has been used to induce early-term medical abortions is methotrexate, although it is not approved by the FDA for this purpose. Typically a woman receives an injection from her clinician and, during an office visit three to seven days later, receives a prostaglandin dose. The pregnancy usually ends within four hours.

What Do You Think? If you or your partner unexpectedly became pregnant, would you choose to terminate the pregnancy? ■ How might an abortion affect your relationship? ■ What factors would you consider in making your decision? Why?

PLANNING A PREGNANCY

The many methods available to control fertility give you choices that did not exist when your parents—and even you—were born. If you are in the process of deciding whether to have children, take the time to evaluate your emotions, finances, and health.

Emotional Health

First and foremost, consider why you want to have a child: To fulfill an inner need to carry on the family? To escape loneliness? Other reasons? Are you ready to make all the sacrifices necessary to bear and raise a child? Can you care for this new human being in a loving and nurturing manner?

If you feel that you are ready to be a parent, the next step is preparation. You can prepare for this change in your life in several ways: read about parenthood, take classes, talk to parents of children of all ages, and join a support group. If you choose to adopt, you will find many support groups available as well.

Maternal Health

Before becoming pregnant, a woman should have a thorough medical examination. **Preconception care** should include assessment of potential complications that could occur during pregnancy. Medical problems such as diabetes and high blood pressure should be discussed, as well as any genetic disorders that run in the family. Additional suggestions for a healthy pregnancy include:

- Do not smoke or drink alcohol
- Reduce or eliminate caffeine intake
- Exercise
- Eat a healthy diet based on a variety of foods
- Avoid exposure to X rays and environmental chemicals, such as lawn and garden chemicals
- Maintain a normal weight; lose weight if necessary
- Prior to becoming pregnant, get any dental X ray examinations that will be needed for a checkup.[16]

Paternal Health

It is common wisdom that mothers-to-be should steer clear of toxic chemicals that can cause birth defects, eat a healthy diet, and stop smoking and drinking alcohol. Now, similar precautions are recommended for fathers-to-be. New research suggests that a man's exposure to chemicals influences not only his ability to father a child, but also the future health of his child.

Fathers-to-be have been overlooked in past preconception and prenatal studies for several reasons. Researchers assumed that the genetic damage leading to birth defects and other health problems occurred while a child was in the mother's womb or were caused by random errors of nature. However, it now appears that some disorders can be traced to sperm damaged by chemicals. Sperm are naturally vulnerable to toxic assault and genetic damage. Many drugs and ingested chemicals can readily invade the testes from the bloodstream; others ambush sperm after they leave the testes and pass through the epididymides, where they mature and are stored. By one route or another, half of 100 chemicals studied so far (including by-products of cigarette smoke) apparently harm sperm.

Financial Evaluation

Finances are another important consideration. Are you prepared to go out to dinner with friends less often, forego a new pair of shoes, or drive an older car? These

Preconception care Medical care received prior to becoming pregnant that helps a woman assess and address potential maternal health.

are important questions to ask yourself when considering the financial aspects of being a parent. Can you afford to give your child the life you would like him or her to enjoy?

First, check your health insurance: does it provide pregnancy benefits? If not, you can expect to pay $1,500 to $5,000 for medical care during pregnancy and birth—and substantially more if complications arise. Both partners should investigate their employers' policies concerning parental leave, including length of leave available and conditions for returning to work.

The U.S. Department of Agriculture estimates that it can cost as much as $250,000 for a middle class married couple to raise a child to the age of 17. (Housing costs and food are the two largest expenditures.)[17] That figure does not include college, which can now run up to $40,000 per year with room and board at a private institution.

Also consider the cost and availability of quality child care. How much family assistance can you realistically expect with a new baby, and is nonfamily child care available? While you may be aware of the federal tax credit available for child care, you may not realize how little assistance it actually provides. For example, a family with an income of over $28,000 can expect to receive a maximum credit of $480 for one child. A second child doubles the credit, but no further assistance is provided for a third child or more children. Comparatively, the average monthly cost of child care per child can range from $500 to as much as $1,200 or more per month in some regions!

Try it →NOW

Make a budget! **Thinking about starting a family? The financial responsibilities of being a parent go beyond providing basic needs. Make a list of monthly expenses associated with being a parent to a 6-year-old. Consider school supplies and extracurricular activities like piano lessons or Little League. Don't forget basics either, such as food, clothing, and child care. Now look at your monthly income. What types of sacrifices would you have to make to provide the best possible life for a child?**

Contingency Planning

Another consideration is how to provide for the child should something happen to you and your partner. If both of you were to die while the child is young, do you have relatives or close friends who would raise the child? If you have more than one child, would they have to be split up or could they be kept together? Though unpleasant to think about, this sort of contingency planning is crucial. Children who lose their parents are heartbroken and confused. A prearranged plan of action will smooth their transition into new families.

What Do You Think?
Which factors will you consider in deciding whether or when to have children? ■ Is there a certain age at which you feel you will be ready to be a parent? ■ What goals do you hope to achieve first? ■ What are your biggest concerns about parenthood?

PREGNANCY

Pregnancy is an important event in a woman's life. The actions taken before a pregnancy begins, as well as behaviors during pregnancy, can have a significant effect on the health of both infant and mother.

Prenatal Care

A successful pregnancy depends on a mother who takes good care of herself and the fetus. Good nutrition, exercise, avoiding drugs, alcohol, and other harmful substances, and regular medical checkups beginning early in the pregnancy are essential. Early detection of fetal abnormalities, identification of high-risk mothers and infants, and a complication-free pregnancy are the major purposes of prenatal care.

Women should also consider their confidence in their own ability to give birth and the availability of a support system (spouse or partner, family, friends, community groups) willing to give her and her child love and emotional support during and after her pregnancy.

Choosing a Practitioner and Receiving Medical Care
A woman should carefully choose a practitioner to oversee her pregnancy and delivery. If possible, this choice should be made before she becomes pregnant. Recommendations from friends and from one's family physician are a good starting point. Also consider a practitioner's philosophy about pain management during labor, experience handling complications, and if the practitioner will accommodate your personal beliefs on these issues.

Two types of physicians can attend pregnancies and deliveries. The obstetrician-gynecologist (Ob-Gyn) is a medical doctor (MD) who specializes in obstetrics (pregnancy and birth) and gynecology (care of women's reproductive organs). These practitioners are trained to handle all types of pregnancy-related and delivery-related emergencies. A family practitioner is a licensed MD who provides comprehensive care for people of all ages. They may refer a patient to a specialist if necessary. Unlike the Ob-Gyn, the family practitioner can serve as the baby's physician after attending the birth.

Midwives are also experienced practitioners who can assist with both pregnancies and deliveries. *Certified nurse-midwives* are registered nurses with specialized training in pregnancy and delivery. Most midwives work in private practice or in conjunction with physicians. Those who work with physicians have access to traditional medical facilities to which they can turn in an emergency. *Lay midwives* may or may not have extensive training in handling an emergency. They may be self-taught or trained through formal certification procedures. Women should carefully evaluate the credentials of a prospective midwife and be sure they allow access to medical care if needed.

Regular check-ups to measure weight gain and blood pressure and to monitor the size and position of the fetus should continue throughout the pregnancy. Ideally, a woman should begin medical checkups as soon as possible after becoming pregnant (within the first three months). This early care reduces infant mortality and low birth weight. The American College of Obstetricians and Gynecologists recommends seven or eight prenatal visits for women with low-risk pregnancies. Unfortunately, prenatal care is not available to everyone. American Indian and African American women have the lowest rates of prenatal care in the United States.[18]

Nutrition and Exercise

Pregnant women need additional protein, calories, vitamins, and minerals, so their diets should be carefully monitored by a qualified practitioner. Special attention should be paid to getting enough folic acid (found in dark leafy greens), iron (dried fruits, meats, legumes, liver, and egg yolks), calcium (nonfat or low-fat dairy products and some canned fish), and fluids.

Vitamin supplements can correct some deficiencies, but there is no substitute for a well-balanced diet. Babies born to poorly nourished mothers run high risks of substandard mental and physical development. Folic acid, when consumed before and during early pregnancy, reduces the risk of spina bifida, a common disabling birth condition that results from failure of the spinal column to close. Manufacturers of breads, pastas, rice, and other grain products now are required to add folic acid to their products to reduce neural tube defects in newborns.

Weight gain during pregnancy helps nourish a growing baby. For a woman of normal weight before pregnancy, the recommended weight gain during pregnancy is 25 to 35 pounds. For obese or overweight women, 15 to 25 pounds are recommended. Underweight women can gain 28 to 40 pounds, and women carrying twins should gain about 35 to 45 pounds. Gaining too much or too little weight can lead to

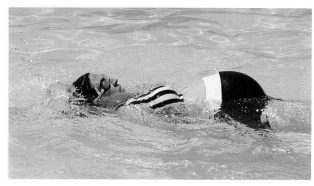

A doctor-approved exercise program during pregnancy can help control weight, make delivery easier, and have a healthy effect on the fetus.

complications. With higher weight gains, women run an increased risk for gestational diabetes, hypertension and other cardiovascular-disease risks, as well as increased risk for delivery complications. Gaining too little weight increases the chance of a low–birth weight baby.

Of the total number of pounds gained during pregnancy, about 6 to 8 are the baby's weight. The baby's birth weight is important because low weight can mean health problems during labor and the baby's first few months. Pregnancy is not the time to think about losing weight—doing so may endanger the fetus.[19]

As in all other stages of life, exercise is an important factor in weight control during pregnancy and in overall maternal health. Pregnant women should consult their physicians before starting any exercise program.

Alcohol and Drugs

A woman should avoid all types of drugs, and alcohol during pregnancy. Even common over-the-counter medications such as aspirin and beverages such as coffee and tea can damage a developing fetus. During the first three months of pregnancy, the fetus is especially subject to the **teratogenic** (birth defect–causing) effects of drugs, environmental chemicals, X rays, or diseases. The fetus also can develop an addiction to or tolerance for drugs that the mother is using. Of particular concern to medical professionals is the use of tobacco and alcohol during pregnancy.

Consumption of alcohol is detrimental to a growing fetus. Symptoms of **fetal alcohol syndrome (FAS)** include mental retardation, slowed nerve reflexes, and small head size. The exact amount of alcohol necessary

---

Midwives   Experienced practitioners who assist with pregnancy and delivery.

Teratogenic   Causing birth defects; may refer to drugs, environmental chemicals, X rays, or diseases.

Fetal alcohol syndrome (FAS)   A collection of symptoms, including mental retardation, that can appear in infants of women who drink alcohol during pregnancy.

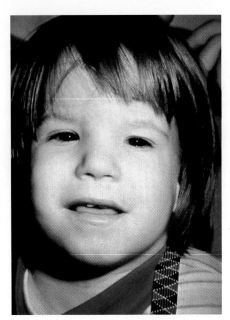

The effects of fetal alcohol syndrome on a child are irreversible.

to cause FAS is not known, but researchers doubt that it is safe to consume any alcohol. Therefore, they recommend total abstinence from alcohol during pregnancy.

Smoking harms every phase of reproduction. Women who smoke have more difficulty becoming pregnant and a higher risk of being infertile. Women who smoke during pregnancy have a greater chance of complications, premature births, low–birth weight infants, stillbirth, and infant mortality.[20] In children, it appears to be a significant factor in the development of cleft lip and palate. Babies with smoker parents can be twice as susceptible to pneumonia, bronchitis, and other illnesses as babies with nonsmoker parents.

Studies are now revealing that secondhand smoke may also be as detrimental to the fetus as to the women who actually smoke during their pregnancy. The exposed fetus is likely to experience low birth weight, increased susceptibility to childhood diseases, and sudden infant death syndrome.[21] Smoking clearly has an influence throughout the pregnancy cycle.

Other Factors A pregnant woman should avoid exposure to X rays, toxic chemicals, heavy metals, pesticides, gases, and other hazardous compounds. She should not clean cat-litter boxes, because cat feces can contain organisms that cause a disease called **toxoplasmosis.** If a pregnant woman contracts this disease, her baby may be stillborn or suffer mental retardation or other birth defects.

If she has never had rubella (German measles), a woman should be immunized for it prior to becoming pregnant. A rubella infection can kill the fetus or cause blindness or hearing disorders in the infant. Sexually transmitted infections such as genital herpes or HIV are also risk factors. A woman should inform her physician of any infectious condition so proper precautions and treatment options can be taken.

A Woman's Reproductive Years

More than half of the average American woman's lifespan is spent between menarche (first menses) and menopause (last menses), a period of approximately 40 years. Deciding whether and when to have children, as well as how to prevent pregnancy when necessary, is a long-term concern.

Many women who wait until their thirties to consider motherhood find themselves wondering, "Am I too old to have a baby?" Today, a woman over 35 who is pregnant has plenty of company. There are some advantages to having a baby later in life. In fact, many doctors note that older mothers tend to be more conscientious about following medical advice during pregnancy and more psychologically mature and ready to include an infant in their family than are some younger women.

However, statistically, the chances of having a baby with birth defects increase after age 35. For example, the incidence of **Down's syndrome,** a condition characterized by mild to severe mental retardation and a variety of physical abnormalities, increases with maternal age.[22] Women who delay motherhood until their late thirties also worry about their physical ability to carry and deliver their babies. A comprehensive exercise program will assist in a healthy pregnancy and delivery.

Pregnancy Testing

Are home pregnancy testing kits reliable?

A woman may suspect she is pregnant before she has any pregnancy tests. A pregnancy test scheduled in a medical office or birth control clinic will confirm the pregnancy. Women who wish to know immediately can purchase home pregnancy test kits sold over the counter in drugstores. A positive test is based on the secretion of **human chorionic**

Toxoplasmosis A disease caused by an organism found in cat feces that, when contracted by a pregnant woman, may result in stillbirth or an infant with mental retardation or birth defects.

Down's syndrome A condition characterized by mental retardation and a variety of physical abnormalities.

Human chorionic gonadotropin (hCG) Hormone detectable in blood or urine samples of a mother within the first few weeks of pregnancy.

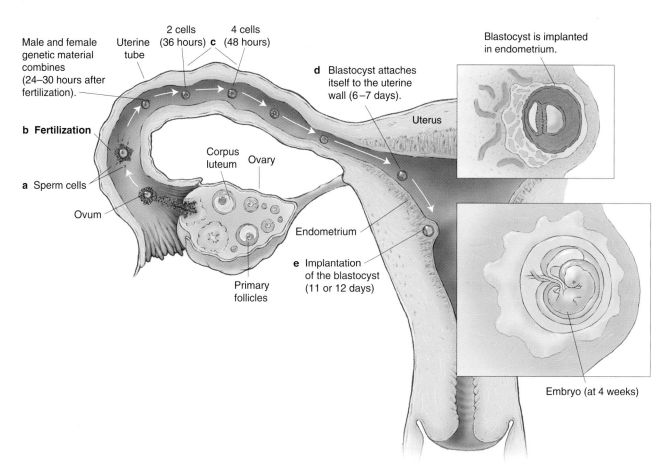

Figure 6.7 ▪ Fertilization

(a) The efforts of hundreds of sperm may allow one sperm to penetrate the ovum's *corona radiata,* an outer layer of cells, and then the *zona pellucida,* a thick inner membrane. **(b)** The sperm nucleus fuses with the egg nucleus at fertilization, which produces a *zygote.* **(c)** The zygote divides first into two cells, then four cells, etc. **(d)** The *blastocyst* attaches itself to the uterine wall. **(e)** The blastocyst implants itself in the endometrium.

gonadotropin (hCG) found in the woman's urine (hCG is also detectable in blood).

Home pregnancy test kits are about 85 to 95 percent reliable. Instructions must be followed carefully. If done too early in the pregnancy, they may show a false negative. Other causes of false negatives are unclean test tubes, ingestion of certain drugs, and vaginal or urinary tract infections. Accuracy also depends on the quality of the test itself and the user's ability to perform it and interpret the results. Blood tests administered and analyzed by a medical laboratory are more accurate.

The Process of Pregnancy

The process of pregnancy begins the moment a sperm fertilizes an ovum in the uterine tubes (Figure 6.7). From there, the single cell multiplies and becomes a sphere-shaped cluster of cells as it travels toward the uterus, a journey that may take three to four days. Upon arrival, the embryo burrows into the thick, spongy endometrium (implantation) and is nourished from this carefully prepared lining. Implantation is the point at which a woman actually becomes pregnant.

Early Signs of Pregnancy The first sign of pregnancy is usually a missed menstrual period (although some women "spot" in early pregnancy, which may be mistaken for a period). Other signs include breast tenderness, emotional upset, extreme fatigue, nausea, sleeplessness, and vomiting (especially in the morning).

Pregnancy typically lasts 40 weeks. The due date is calculated from the expectant mother's last menstrual period. Pregnancy is typically divided into three phases, or **trimesters,** of approximately three months each.

The First Trimester During the first trimester, few noticeable changes occur in the mother's body. She may urinate more frequently and experience morning

> **Trimester**   A three-month segment of pregnancy; used to describe specific developmental changes that occur in the embryo or the fetus.

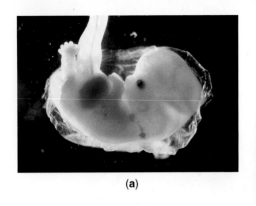
(a)

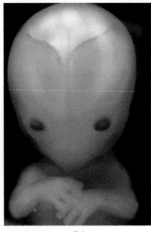
(b)

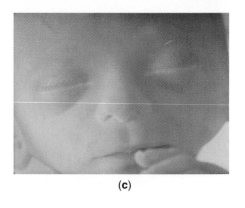
(c)

This series of fetoscopic photographs shows the development of the fetus in the first **(a)**, second **(b)**, and third **(c)** trimesters of pregnancy.

sickness, swollen breasts, or undue fatigue. These symptoms may not be frequent or severe, so she may not even realize she is pregnant unless she has a pregnancy test.

During the first two months after conception, the **embryo** differentiates and develops its various organ systems, beginning with the nervous and circulatory systems. At the start of the third month, the embryo is called a **fetus,** which indicates that all organ systems are in place. For the rest of the pregnancy, growth and refinement occur in each major body system so that they can function independently, yet in coordination, at birth. The photos above illustrate physical changes during fetal development.

The Second Trimester At the beginning of the second trimester, physical changes in the mother become more visible. During this time, the fetus makes greater demands upon the mother's body. In particular, the **placenta,** the network of blood vessels connected to

the umbilical cord that carry nutrients and oxygen to the fetus and fetal waste products to the mother, becomes well established.

The Third Trimester From the end of the sixth month through the ninth is considered the third trimester (Figure 6.8). This is the period of greatest fetal growth, when the fetus gains most of its weight. During the third trimester, the fetus must get large amounts of calcium, iron, and nitrogen from the food the mother eats.

Although the fetus may live if it is born during the seventh month, it needs the layer of fat it acquires during the eighth month, and respiratory and digestive organs have yet to develop to their full potential. Babies born prematurely usually require intensive medical care.

Emotional Changes Of course, the process of pregnancy involves much more than the changes in a woman's body and the developing fetus. Many important emotional changes occur from the time a woman learns she is pregnant through the "**fourth trimester**" (the first six weeks of an infant's life outside the womb). Throughout pregnancy, women may experience fear of pregnancy complications, anxiety over becoming a parent, and wonder and excitement over the developing baby.[23]

Prenatal Testing and Screening

Modern technology enables medical practitioners to detect health defects in a fetus as early as the fourteenth to eighteenth weeks of pregnancy. One common testing procedure, **amniocentesis,** is strongly recommended for women over age 35. It involves inserting a long needle through the mother's abdominal and uterine walls into

Embryo The fertilized egg from conception until the end of two months' development.

Fetus The name given the developing baby from the third month of pregnancy until birth.

Placenta The network of blood vessels connected to the umbilical cord that carries nutrients and oxygen to the developing fetus and carries fetal wastes to the mother.

"Fourth trimester" The first six weeks of an infant's life outside the womb.

Amniocentesis A medical test in which a small amount of fluid is drawn from the amniotic sac to test for Down's syndrome and other genetic abnormalities.

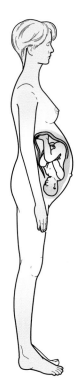

- Heartburn – uterus pushes on *stomach*
- Swelling – especially in *ankles, hands, face*
- Constipation
- Tender *breasts*, size increases, may leak colostrum
- Shortness of breath – uterus is pushing on *diaphragm*
- Navel may protrude

Figure 6.8 ■ The Changes to a Woman's Body during the Third Trimester

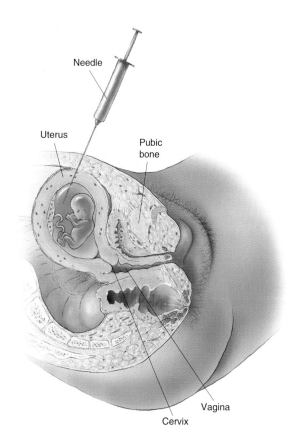

Figure 6.9 ■ Amniocentesis
The process of amniocentesis can detect certain congenital problems as well as the sex of the fetus.

the **amniotic sac,** the protective pouch surrounding the fetus (Figure 6.9), and withdrawing fluid. The fluid is analyzed for genetic information about the baby. This test can reveal the presence of 40 genetic abnormalities, including Down's syndrome, and genetic diseases such as sickle cell disease (a debilitating blood disorder found primarily among blacks). Amniocentesis also can reveal gender, a fact many parents choose not to know until the birth. Although widely used, amniocentesis is not without risk. Chances of fetal damage and miscarriage as a result of testing are 1 in 400.

Another procedure, *ultrasound*, or *sonography*, uses high-frequency sound waves to determine the size and position of the fetus. Ultrasound also can detect fetal defects in the central nervous system and digestive system. Knowing the position of the fetus helps practitioners perform amniocentesis and deliver the infant. New three-dimensional ultrasound techniques clarify images and improve doctors' efforts to detect and treat defects prenatally.

A third procedure called *chorionic villus sampling (CVS)* involves snipping tissue from the developing fetal sac. CVS can be used at 10 to 12 weeks of pregnancy, and results are available in 12 to 48 hours. CVS is an attractive option for couples who are at high risk for having a baby with Down's syndrome or a debilitating hereditary disease.

If any of these tests reveals a serious birth defect, parents are advised to undergo genetic counseling. In the case of a chromosomal abnormality such as Down's

syndrome, the parents usually are offered the option of a therapeutic abortion. Some parents choose this option; others research the disability and decide to go ahead with the birth.

What Do You Think? In looking at your current lifestyle, what behaviors (e.g., nutritional choices, fitness) would you cease or begin in order to promote a healthy pregnancy? ■ What would you look for in selecting a health care provider during your own or your partner's pregnancy? ■ Would you want to know if you were carrying a child with a genetic defect or other abnormality? Why or why not?

CHILDBIRTH

Prospective parents need to make a number of key decisions long before the baby is born. These include where to have the baby, whether to use drugs during labor and

---

Amniotic sac   The protective pouch surrounding the fetus.

delivery, choice of childbirth method, and whether to breast-feed or bottle-feed. Answering these questions will ensure a smoother passage into parenthood.

Choosing Where to Have Your Baby

Prospective mothers have many delivery options, ranging from traditional hospital birth to home birth. Parental values are important. Many couples, for instance, feel that the modern medical establishment has dehumanized the birth process. Thus, they choose to deliver at home or at a *birthing center,* a homelike setting outside a hospital where women can give birth and receive postdelivery care by a team of professional practitioners that includes physicians and registered nurses.

However, hospitals have responded to the desire for a more relaxed, less medically oriented birthing process. Many hospitals now offer labor–delivery–postpartum birthing rooms, which allow patients with noncomplicated deliveries to spend the entire process in one room. "Rooming-in," or keeping the baby in the same room with the mother at all times, is encouraged to facilitate bonding and breast-feeding. Partners are generally encouraged to room-in with mother and baby as well.

Labor and Delivery

The birth process has three stages (Figure 6.10). The exact mechanisms that initiate labor are unknown. During the few weeks preceding delivery, the baby normally shifts to a head-down position, and the cervix begins to dilate (widen). The junction of the pubic bones loosens to permit expansion of the pelvic girdle during birth.

The First Stage of Labor
In the first stage of labor, the amniotic sac breaks, which causes a rush of fluid from the vagina (commonly referred to as "water breaking"). Contractions in the abdomen and lower back also signal the beginning of labor. Early contractions push the baby downward, which puts pressure on the cervix and dilates it further. The first stage of labor may last from a couple of hours to more than a day for a first birth, but it is usually much shorter during subsequent births.

Transition The process during which the cervix becomes nearly fully dilated and the baby's head begins to move into the birth canal.

Episiotomy A straight incision in the mother's perineum.

Afterbirth The placenta expelled from the womb, usually within 30 minutes after delivery.

The end of the first stage of labor, called **transition,** is the process during which the cervix becomes fully dilated and the baby's head begins to move into the vagina (birth canal). Contractions usually come quickly during transition, which generally lasts 30 minutes or less.

The Second Stage of Labor
The second stage of labor (the *expulsion stage*) follows transition when the cervix has become fully dilated. Contractions become rhythmic, strong, and more painful as the uterus pushes the baby through the birth canal. The expulsion stage lasts one to four hours and concludes when the infant is finally pushed out of the mother's body. In some cases, the attending practitioner may perform an **episiotomy,** a straight incision in the mother's perineum (the area between the vulva and the anus), to prevent the baby's head from tearing vaginal tissues and to speed the baby's exit from the vagina. Upon exit, the baby takes its first breath, which is generally accompanied by a loud wail.

After delivery, the attending practitioner assesses the baby's overall condition, cleans the baby's mucus-filled breathing passages, and the umbilical cord is tied and severed.

The Third Stage of Labor
In the meantime, the mother continues into the third stage of labor, during which the placenta, or **afterbirth**, is expelled from the womb. This stage is usually completed within 30 minutes after delivery.

Most mothers prefer to have their new infants next to them following the birth. Together with their spouse or partner, they feel a need to share this time of bonding with their infant.

Managing Labor

It is important to keep a flexible attitude about pain relief during labor because each labor is different. Working in partnership with a health care provider to make the best decision for mother and baby is the best plan. Use of pain-killing medication during a delivery is not a sign of weakness. Remember, pain is to be expected. In fact, many experts say that the pain of labor is the most difficult in the human experience. However, there is no single right answer in managing that pain.

Expectant parents have several options beyond the traditional hospital setting for the process of their infant's birth and their participation in it.

The Lamaze method is the most popular birth alternative in the United States. It discourages the use of drugs; prelabor classes teach the mother to control her pain through special breathing patterns, focusing exercises, and relaxation. Lamaze births usually take place in a hospital or birthing center with a physician or midwife in attendance. The partner (or labor coach) assists

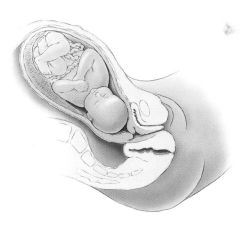

Dilation of the cervix

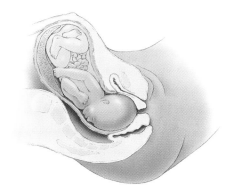

Transition ———————————— **End of Stage I**

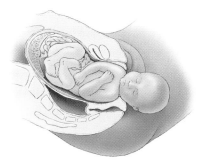

Birth of the baby (Expulsion) ———— **End of Stage II**

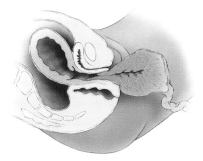

Delivery of the placenta ——————— **End of Stage III**

Figure 6.10 ■ The Birth Process

by giving emotional support, physical comfort, and coaching for proper breath control during contractions.

Other methods prospective parents can research include the Harris method, Childbirth without Fear, the Leboyer method, the Bradley method, and water birth. These vary in their philosophies regarding painkillers, partner participation, and other issues.

The Postpartum Period

The postpartum period typically lasts four to six weeks after delivery. During this period many women experience fluctuating emotions. The physical stress of labor, dehydration and blood loss, and other stresses challenge many new mother's stamina. About 50 to 80 percent of new mothers experience what is called the "baby blues," characterized by periods of sadness, anxiety, headache, sleep disturbances, and irritability. For most women these symptoms disappear. About 10 percent of new mothers experience **postpartum depression,** a more disabling syndrome characterized by mood swings, lack of energy, crying, guilt, and depression. It can happen anytime within the first year after childbirth. Mothers experiencing postpartum depression should be encouraged to seek professional treatment. Counseling and/or medication are two of the most common types of treatment.[24]

Breast-Feeding

Although the new mother's milk will not begin to flow for two or more days, her breasts secrete a thick yellow substance called *colostrum.* Because this fluid contains vital antibodies to help fight infection, the newborn baby should be allowed to suckle.

The American Academy of Pediatrics strongly recommends that infants should be breast-fed for at least six months and ideally for 12 months. Scientific findings indicate there are many advantages to breast-feeding. Breast-fed babies have fewer illnesses and a much lower hospitalization rate because breast milk contains maternal antibodies and immunological cells that stimulate the infant's immune system. When breast-fed babies do get sick, they recover more quickly. They are also less likely to be obese than babies fed on formulas, and they have fewer allergies. They may even be more intelligent: a recent study found that the longer a baby was breast-fed, the higher the IQ in adulthood. Researchers theorize that breast milk contains substances that enhance brain development.[25] Another

> **Postpartum depression** The experience of energy depletion, anxiety, mood swings, and depression that women may feel during the postpartum period four to six weeks after delivery.

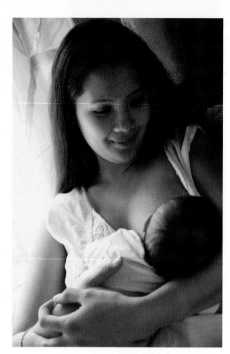
Breast-feeding enhances the development of intimate bonds between mother and child.

study found that women who were able to breast-feed successfully for longer periods of time generally viewed breast-feeding as more positive, had more knowledge about the process, and had higher self-efficacy in their ability to breast-feed.[26]

Some women are unable or unwilling to breast-feed. Prepared formulas can provide nourishment that allows a baby to grow and thrive. When deciding whether to breast- or bottle-feed, mothers need to consider their own desires and preferences too. Both feeding methods can supply the physical and emotional closeness essential to the parent-child relationship.

Preeclampsia A complication in pregnancy characterized by high blood pressure, protein in the urine, and edema.

Eclampsia Untreated preeclampsia can develop into this potentially fatal complication that involves maternal strokes and seizures.

Cesarean section (C-section) A surgical procedure in which a baby is removed through an incision made in the mother's abdominal and uterine walls.

Miscarriage Loss of the fetus before it is viable; also called spontaneous abortion.

Rh factor A blood protein related to the production of antibodies. If an Rh-negative mother is pregnant with an Rh-positive fetus, the mother will manufacture antibodies that can kill the fetus, which causes miscarriage.

Complications

Problems can occur during labor and delivery, even following a successful pregnancy. The possibilities should be discussed prior to labor.

Preeclampsia and Eclampsia

Preeclampsia is a condition that is characterized by high blood pressure, protein in the urine, and edema (fluid retention), which usually causes swelling of the hands and face. It often occurs in the late second or third trimesters. The cause is unknown, but older mothers, very young mothers, and mothers with hypertension or diabetes are at a higher risk. Symptoms may include sudden weight gain, headache, nausea or vomiting, changes in vision, racing pulse, mental confusion, and stomach or right shoulder pain. Treatment for preeclampsia ranges from bed rest and monitoring for those with mild cases to hospitalization and close monitoring for more severe cases, which have the potential to be life-threatening for the woman and her fetus. If preeclampsia is not treated, it can cause strokes and seizures, a condition called **eclampsia.** Potential problems can include liver and kidney damage, internal bleeding, stroke, poor fetal growth, and fetal and maternal death.

Cesarean Section If labor lasts too long or if a baby is about to exit the uterus any way but head first, a **cesarean section (C-section)** may be necessary. This surgical procedure involves making an incision across the mother's abdomen and through the uterus to remove the baby. This operation also is performed if labor is extremely difficult, maternal blood pressure falls rapidly, the placenta separates from the uterus too soon, the mother has diabetes, or other problems occur.

Miscarriage One in ten pregnancies does not end in delivery. Loss of the fetus before it is viable is called a **miscarriage** (also referred to as spontaneous abortion). An estimated 70 to 90 percent of women who miscarry eventually become pregnant again.

Reasons for miscarriage vary. In some cases, the fertilized egg has failed to divide correctly. In others, genetic abnormalities, maternal illness, or infections are responsible. Maternal hormonal imbalance also may cause a miscarriage, as may a weak cervix or toxic chemicals in the environment. In most cases, the cause for miscarriage is not known.

Rh Factor Rh is a blood protein. Problems with **Rh factors** occur when the mother is Rh-negative and the fetus is Rh-positive. During a first birth, some of the baby's blood passes into the mother's bloodstream. An Rh-negative mother may manufacture antibodies to destroy the Rh-positive blood introduced into her bloodstream at the time of birth. Her first baby will be

unaffected, but subsequent babies with positive Rh factor will be at risk for a severe anemia called hemolytic disease because the mother's Rh antibodies will attack the fetus's red blood cells.

Prevention is preferable to treatment. All women with Rh-negative blood should be injected with a medication called RhoGAM within 72 hours of any birth, miscarriage, or abortion. This injection will prevent them from developing the Rh antibodies.

Ectopic Pregnancy The implantation of a fertilized egg outside the uterus, usually in the uterine tube or occasionally in the pelvic cavity, is called an **ectopic pregnancy.** Because these structures are not capable of expanding and nourishing a developing fetus, the pregnancy must be terminated surgically, or a miscarriage will occur. Ectopic pregnancy generally is accompanied by pain in the lower abdomen or aching in the shoulders as the blood flows up toward the diaphragm. If bleeding is significant, blood pressure drops, and the woman can go into shock. If an ectopic pregnancy goes undiagnosed and untreated, the uterine tube will rupture, which puts the woman at great risk of hemorrhage, peritonitis (infection in the abdomen), and even death.

Over the past 12 years, the incidence of ectopic pregnancy has tripled, and no one really understands why. We do know that ectopic pregnancy is a potential side effect of PID, which has become increasingly common in recent years. The scarring or blockage of the uterine tubes that is characteristic of this disease prevents the fertilized egg from passing to the uterus.

Stillbirth One of the most traumatic events a couple can face is a **stillbirth.** A stillborn baby is born dead, often for no apparent reason. The grief experienced following a stillbirth is devastating. Nine months of happy anticipation have been thwarted. Family, friends, and other children may be in a state of shock and need comfort as well. The mother's breasts produce milk, and there is no infant to be fed. A room with a crib and toys is left empty.

Some communities have groups called the Compassionate Friends to help parents and other family members through this grieving process. This nonprofit organization is for parents who have lost a child of any age for any reason.

Sudden Infant Death Syndrome The unexpected death of a child under one year of age, for no apparent reason, is called **sudden infant death syndrome (SIDS).** Though SIDS is the leading cause of death for children aged one month to one year and affects about 1 in 1,000 infants in the United States each year, it is not a disease. Rather, it is ruled the cause of death after all other possibilities are ruled out. A SIDS death is sudden and silent; death occurs quickly, often during sleep, with no signs of suffering.

Research has shown that placing children on their backs or sides to sleep cuts the rate of SIDS by as much as half. The American Academy of Pediatrics sponsors the Back to Sleep educational campaign urging parents to position babies on their backs. Additional precautions against SIDS include having a firm surface for the infant's bed, not allowing the infant to become too warm, maintaining a smoke-free environment, having regular pediatric visits, breast-feeding, and seeking prenatal care.

INFERTILITY

An estimated one in six American couples experiences **infertility,** or difficulties in conceiving. Reasons include the trend toward delaying childbirth (as a woman gets older, she is less likely to conceive), endometriosis, PID, and low sperm count.

Causes in Women

Endometriosis is the leading cause of infertility in women in the United States. With this very painful disorder, parts of the endometrial lining of the uterus implant themselves outside the uterus. This can cause blockage of the uterine tubes. The disorder can be treated surgically or with hormonal therapy.

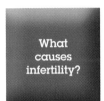
What causes infertility?

Another cause of infertility is **pelvic inflammatory disease (PID),** a serious infection that scars the uterine tubes and blocks sperm migration. PID often results from chlamydia or gonorrheal infections that spread to the uterine tubes or ovaries. (See Chapter 14 for more on PID.)

Ectopic pregnancy Implantation of a fertilized egg outside the uterus, usually in a uterine tube; a medical emergency that can end in the mother's death from hemorrhage or peritonitis.

Stillbirth The birth of a dead baby.

Sudden infant death syndrome (SIDS) The sudden death of a child under one year of age for no apparent reason.

Infertility Difficulties in conceiving.

Endometriosis A disorder in which uterine lining tissue establishes itself outside the uterus; the leading cause of infertility in the United States.

Pelvic inflammatory disease (PID) An infection that causes infertility by scarring the uterine tubes and consequently blocking sperm migration.

Causes in Men

Among men, the single largest fertility problem is **low sperm count.** Although only one viable sperm is needed for fertilization, research has shown that all the other sperm in the ejaculate aid in the fertilization process. There are normally 60 to 80 million sperm per milliliter of semen. When the count drops below 60 million, fertility declines.

Low sperm count may be attributable to environmental factors (such as exposure of the scrotum to intense heat or cold, radiation, or altitude) or even to wearing excessively tight underwear or outerwear. However, other factors, such as the mumps virus, can damage the cells that make sperm. Varicose veins above one or both testicles also can render men infertile.

Treatment

For the couple desperately wishing to conceive, the road to parenthood may be frustrating. Fortunately, medical treatment can identify the cause of infertility in about 90 percent of cases. The chances of becoming pregnant range from 30 to 70 percent, depending on the reason for infertility. Before starting fertility tests, couples should reassess their priorities. Some will choose to undergo counseling to help them clarify their feelings about the fertility process. A good physician or fertility team will take the time to ascertain the couple's level of motivation.

Infertility treatment workups can be expensive, and the costs are not usually covered by insurance companies. Fertility workups for men include a sperm count, a test for sperm motility, and analysis of any disease processes present. Women are thoroughly examined by an obstetrician-gynecologist for the composition of cervical mucus and evidence of problems such as tubal scarring or endometriosis.

Fertility Drugs **Fertility drugs** such as Clomid and Pergonal stimulate ovulation in women who are not ovulating. Fertility drugs can have many side effects, including headaches, irritability, restlessness, depression, fatigue, fluid retention, abnormal uterine bleeding, breast tenderness, hot flashes, and vision problems. Women using fertility drugs are also at increased risk of developing multiple ovarian cysts (fluid-filled growths) and liver damage. The drugs sometimes trigger the release of more than one egg—thus a woman treated with one of these drugs has a 1 in 10 chance of having multiple births. Most such births are twins, but triplets and even quadruplets are not uncommon.

Alternative Insemination Another treatment option is **alternative insemination** of a woman with her partner's sperm. This technique has led to an estimated 250,000 births in the United States, primarily for couples in which the man is infertile. The couple may also choose insemination by an anonymous donor through a sperm bank. The sperm are medically screened, classified according to the physical characteristics of the donor (for example, blonde hair, blue eyes), and then frozen for future use. In the last few years, concern has been expressed about the possibility of transmitting the AIDS virus through alternative insemination. As a result, donors are routinely screened for the disease.

In Vitro Fertilization Often referred to as test tube fertilization, **in vitro fertilization (IVF)** involves collecting a viable ovum from the prospective mother and transferring it to a nutrient medium in a laboratory where it is fertilized with sperm from the woman's partner or a donor. After a few days, the embryo is transplanted into the mother's uterus, where hopefully it will develop normally.

Gamete Intrafallopian Transfer The method known as **gamete intrafallopina transfer (GIFT)** involves harvesting the egg from the woman's ovary and placing it in the uterine tube with the man's sperm. Less expensive and time consuming than in vitro fertilization, GIFT mimics nature by allowing the egg to be fertilized in the uterine tube and migrate to the uterus according to the normal timetable.

Intracytoplasmic Sperm Injection (ICSI) A sperm cell is injected into an egg in **intracytoplasmic sperm injection (ICSI).** This technique can

---

Low sperm count   A sperm count below 60 million sperm per milliliter of semen; the leading cause of infertility in men.

Fertility drugs   Hormones that stimulate ovulation in women who are not ovulating; often responsible for multiple births.

Alternative insemination   Fertilization accomplished by depositing a partner's or a donor's semen into a woman's vagina via a thin tube.

In vitro fertilization (IVF)   Fertilization of an egg in a nutrient medium and subsequent transfer back to the mother's body.

Gamete intrafallopian transfer (GIFT)   Procedure in which an egg harvested from the woman's ovary is placed with her partner's sperm in her uterine tube, where it is fertilized and then migrates to the uterus for implantation.

Intracytoplasmic sperm injection (ICSI) Fertilization accomplished by injecting a sperm cell directly into an egg.

Parents have wanted the ability to choose the gender of their child since prehistoric times. Even in today's high-tech times, people try a variety of avenues, most based on folklore, to conceive a particular sex. Now science may help couples have the baby they want.

Currently, an FDA clinical trial of sophisticated sperm-sorting technology is more than halfway to completion. FDA approval of the technique would add it to the arsenal of couples intent on having a baby of a particular sex. The *MicroSort method* is an experimental technique that separates X (female) from Y (male) chromosomes. Sperm are stained with a fluorescent dye that binds to the chromosomes. The sperm are then zapped with a laser that illuminates the dye. X chromosomes are bigger than Y

and soak up more dye, so they look brighter. Then the dyed sperm pass by an electrode that gives Xs a positive charge and Ys a negative one. Charged plates attract and separate the chromosomes, channeling them into separate receptacles. Separation is not absolutely perfect, but one sample is used to fertilize a woman's eggs, depending upon the requested sex.

Another technique, the *Ericsson method,* has been used for about a decade. In this technique, sperm are poured into a viscous layer of fluid. The heavy head of the sperm makes them swim downward. Sperm carrying the Y (male) chromosome swim faster than those with the X chromosome, reaching the bottom of the tube faster. They can then be extracted and used for insemination. The Ericsson method claims to have a 78 to 85 percent

chance of producing a boy, although critics say the odds are not better than 50:50.

Preimplantation genetic diagnosis, a third technique, was originally used to detect genetic diseases. Doctors remove eggs from the woman and fertilize them with sperm in the lab, creating embryos. After three days, technicians extract a cell from each embryo. They can differentiate male and female embryos by examining their chromosomes. After determining the sex of the embryos, doctors implant the desired ones. While more invasive and costly than other methods, success is virtually guaranteed.

help men with low sperm counts or motility and even those who cannot ejaculate or have no live sperm in their semen as a result of vasectomy, chemotherapy, or a medical disorder. However, recent studies have found that infants conceived with the use of ICSI or in vitro fertilization have twice the risk of a major birth defect as those conceived naturally.[27]

Nonsurgical Embryo Transfer

Another method that involves the fertilization of a donor egg by sperm is **nonsurgical embryo transfer.** The fertilized egg is then implanted in the woman's uterus. This procedure may also be used to transfer an already fertilized ovum into the uterus of another woman. In **embryo transfer,** an ovum from a donor is artificially inseminated by the man's sperm, allowed to stay in the donor's body for a time, and then transplanted into the woman's body.

The ethical and moral questions surrounding experimental infertility treatments are staggering. Before moving forward with any of these treatments, individuals need to ask themselves important questions. Has infertility been absolutely confirmed? Have they explored all possible alternatives and considered potential risks?

Have all parties examined their attitudes, values, and beliefs about conceiving a child in this manner? Finally, they need to consider what and how they will tell the child about their method of conception.

Surrogate Motherhood

Surrogate motherhood is a controversial practice in which an infertile couple enters an agreement as adoptive parents with an agency or surrogate mother. The surrogate mother agrees to be artificially inseminated by the father's sperm or undergo IVF with the couple's embryo, and then carries the baby to term and surren-

---

Nonsurgical embryo transfer In vitro fertilization of a donor egg by the male partner's (or donor's) sperm and subsequent transfer to the female partner's or another woman's uterus.

Embryo transfer Artificial insemination of a donor with the male partner's sperm; after a time, the embryo is transferred from the donor to the female partner's body.

ders it upon birth to the couple. However, many surrogate mothers wrestle with emotional issues of letting a baby go after its birth.

Couples considering surrogate motherhood are advised to consult a lawyer regarding contracts. Most of these legal documents stipulate that the surrogate mother must undergo amniocentesis and that if the fetus is defective, she must consent to an abortion. In that case, or if the surrogate miscarries, she is reimbursed for her time and expenses. The prospective parents also must agree to take the baby if it is carried to term, even if it is unhealthy or has physical abnormalities.

Adoption

For couples who have decided that biological childbirth is not an option, adoption provides an alternative. About 50,000 children are available for adoption in the United States every year. This is far fewer than the number of couples seeking adoptions. By some estimates, only 1 in 30 couples receives the child they want. On average, couples spend two years on the adoption process.

Increasingly, couples are choosing to adopt children from other countries. In 2004, U.S. families adopted 22,884 foreign children.[28] The cost of intercountry adoption varies from approximately $7,000 to $25,000, including agency fees, dossier and immigration processing fees, and court costs. However, it may be a good solution for many couples, especially those who want to adopt an infant.

What Do You Think?
If you or your partner had infertility problems, how much time and money would you be willing to invest in treatment? ■ Do you think that single women and lesbians should have equal access to alternative methods of insemination? Why or why not? ■ Do you think single women, single men, gay males, and lesbians should have equal opportunities to adopt? ■ How do you think society views these types of adoptions?

Taking Charge

Summary

■ Latex condoms and the female condoms, when used correctly for oral sex or intercourse, provide the most effective protection in preventing sexually transmitted infections (STIs). Other contraceptive methods include abstinence, outercourse, oral contraceptives, foams, jellies, implants, suppositories, creams, film, the diaphragm, the cervical cap, Lea's shield, the sponge, skin patches, the vaginal ring, monthly injections, intrauterine devices, withdrawal, and Depo-Provera. Fertility awareness methods rely on altering sexual practices to avoid pregnancy. Whereas all these methods of contraception are reversible, sterilization is permanent.

■ Abortion is currently legal in the United States through the second trimester. Abortion methods include vacuum aspiration, dilation and evacuation (D&E), dilation and curettage (D&C), intact dilation and extraction (D&X), hysterotomy, induction abortion, mifepristone, and methotrexate.

■ Parenting is a demanding job that requires careful planning. Emotional health, maternal health, paternal health, financial evaluation, and contingency planning all need to be taken into account when considering whether to become a parent.

■ Prenatal care includes a complete physical exam within the first trimester and avoidance of those things that could have teratogenic effects on the fetus, such as alcohol and drugs, cigarettes, X rays, and various chemicals. Full-term pregnancy covers three trimesters.

■ Childbirth occurs in three stages. Birth alternatives include the Lamaze method. Partners should jointly choose a labor method early in the pregnancy to be better prepared for labor when it occurs. Complications of pregnancy and childbirth include preeclampsia and eclampsia, miscarriage, ectopic pregnancy, stillbirth, and the need for a C-section.

■ Infertility in women may be caused by pelvic inflammatory disease (PID) or endometriosis. In men, it may be caused by low sperm count. Treatment may include alternative insemination, in vitro fertilization, gamete intrafallopian transfer (GIFT), intracytoplasmic sperm injection (ICSI), nonsurgical embryo transfer, and embryo transfer. Surrogate motherhood involves hiring a fertile woman to be alternatively inseminated by the male partner. International adoptions are an increasingly common option.

Chapter Review

1. What type of contraceptive method involves long-acting synthetic progesterone injected intramuscularly every three months?
   a. Seasonale
   b. Ortho Evra
   c. Depo-Provera
   d. Lea's Shield

2. The calendar method is a
   a. barrier method.
   b. surgical method.
   c. hormonal method.
   d. fertility awareness method.

3. What is the most commonly used method of first-trimester abortion?
   a. vacuum aspiration
   b. dilation and evacuation (D&E)
   c. dilation and curettage (D&C)
   d. induction abortions

4. The surgical procedure in which the female's fallopian tubes are closed or cut and cauterized to prevent access by sperm to released eggs is called
   a. tubal ligation.
   b. vasectomy.
   c. hysterectomy.
   d. abortion.

5. Jane purchased a home pregnancy test kit to find out if she was pregnant. A positive test detects the presence of
   a. HCG.
   b. LH.
   c. FSH.
   d. RU-486.

6. Toxic chemicals, pesticides, X rays, and other hazardous compounds that cause birth defects are referred to as
   a. carcinogens.
   b. teratogens.
   c. mutants.
   d. environmental assaults.

7. For a woman of normal weight before pregnancy, what is the recommended weight gain during pregnancy?
   a. 15 to 20 pounds
   b. 20 to 30 pounds
   c. 25 to 35 pounds
   d. 30 to 45 pounds

8. What prenatal test involves snipping tissue from the developing fetal sac?
   a. fetoscopy
   b. ultrasound
   c. amniocentesis
   d. chorionic villus sampling

9. Rh factor occurs when the mother is _____ and the fetus is _____
   a. Rh positive; Rh positive
   b. Rh positive; Rh negative
   c. Rh negative; Rh positive
   d. Rh negative; Rh negative

10. The number of American couples who experience infertility is
   a. 1 in 6.
   b. 1 in 24.
   c. 1 in 60.
   d. 1 in 100.

Answers to these questions can be found on page A-1.

Questions for Discussion and Reflection

1. List the most effective contraceptive methods. What are their drawbacks? What medical conditions would keep a person from using each one? What are the characteristics of the methods that you think would be most effective for you? Why do you consider them most effective for you personally?

2. What are the various methods of abortion? What are the two opposing viewpoints concerning abortion? What is *Roe v. Wade,* and what impact did it have on the abortion debate?

3. What are the most important considerations in deciding whether the time is right to become a parent? If you choose to have children, what factors will you consider regarding the number of children to have?

4. Discuss the growth of the fetus through the three trimesters. What medical check-ups or tests should be done during each trimester?

5. Discuss the emotional aspects of pregnancy. What types of emotional reactions are common in each trimester and the postpartum period (the "fourth trimester")?

6. If you and you partner are unable to have children, what alternative methods of conception would you consider? Is adoption an option you would consider?

Accessing Your Health on the Internet

The following websites explore further topics and issues related to personal health. For links to the websites below, visit the Companion Website for *Health: The Basics,* Seventh Edition at www.aw-bc.com/donatelle.

1. *The Alan Guttmacher Institute (AGI).* AGI is a nonprofit organization focused on sexual and reproductive health research, policy analysis, and public education.

2. *Dr. Drew.* Provides answers and advice on sex, relationships and many other topics of interest for college students.

3. *Planned Parenthood.* This site offers a range of up-to-date information on sexual health issues, such as birth control, the decision of when and whether to have a child, sexually transmitted infections, and safer sex.

4. *Sexuality Information and Education Council of the United States.* Information, guidelines, and materials for the advancement of sexuality education. The site advocates the right of individuals to make responsible sexual choices.

Further Reading

Boston Women's Health Collective. *Our Bodies, Ourselves : A New Edition for a New Era.* New York: Simon and Schuster, 2005.

Like its earlier editions, this volume contains information about women's health from a decidedly feminist angle. Every aspect of health is covered, including nutrition, emotional health, fitness, relationships, reproduction, contraception, and pregnancy.

Feldt, G. *The War on Choice.* New York: Bantam, 2004.

A history and analysis of threats to women's reproductive rights. Feldt describes political efforts to outlaw abortion and argues that women should mobilize to support pro-choice causes.

Hatcher, R. A. et al. *Contraceptive Technology,* 18th revised edition. New York: Ardent Media, 2004.

Perhaps the best primary reference concerning birth control for physicians, family planning centers, student health services, and educators. Contributors include staff members from the Centers for Disease Control and Prevention.

Kitzinger, S. *The Complete Book of Pregnancy and Childbirth,* 4th edition. New York: Knopf, 2003.

The book provides expectant mothers with new insights into having a healthy pregnancy and what happens in today's birthing rooms. Offers women and their partners an in-depth look at both the baby's and the mother's physical and emotional development during pregnancy.

References

1. World Health Organization, "Nonoxynol-9 Ineffective in Preventing HIV Infection," June 28, 2002, www.who.int/mediacentre/notes/release55/en.

2. U.S. Department of Health and Human Services. "FDA Approves Seasonale Oral Contraceptive," FDA Talk Paper TO3–65, September 5, 2003, www.fda.gov.

3. R. A. Hatcher et al., *Contraceptive Technology,* 18th ed. (New York: Ardent Media, 2004); R. Burkman et al., "Safety Concerns and Health Benefits Associated with Oral Contraception," *American Journal of Obstetrics and Gynecology* 190 (4 Suppl. S) 2004: S5–S22.

4. W. Mosher et al., "Use of Contraception and Use of Family Planning Services in the United States: 1982–2002," *Advance Data from Vital and Health Statistics* 350 (Hyattsville, MD: National Center for Health Statistics, December, 2004); The Allan Guttmacher Institute, "Facts in Brief: Contraceptive Use," 2005, www.agi-usa.org.

5. K. N. Anderson, L. E. Anderson, and W. D. Glanze, eds., *Mosby's Medical, Nursing & Allied Health Dictionary* (Philadelphia: W. B. Saunders, 2002).

6. Ibid; Hatcher, *Contraceptive Technology.*

7. American College Health Association, American College Health Association–National College Health Assessment Web Summary. Updated September 2005. Available at www.acha.org.

8. "FDA Approves Emergency Contraceptive Kit," *College Health Report* 1 (1998): 8.

9. Boston Women's Health Collective, *Our Bodies Ourselves: A New Edition for a New Era* (New York: Simon and Schuster, 2005).

10. Ibid.

11. Ibid.

12. The Alan Guttmacher Institute, "Facts in Brief: Induced Abortion in the United States," 2005, www.agi-usa.org.

13. Ibid.

14. J. G. Epner, H. Jonas, and D. Seckinger, "Late Term Abortion," *Journal of the American Medical Association* 280 (1998): 726.

15. Planned Parenthood, "The Difference between Emergency Contraception Pills and Medication Abortion," July 9, 2005, www.plannedparenthood.org.

16. Mayo Clinic, "Preconception Planning: Take Care of Baby Now for a Healthy Baby Later," June 2004, www.mayoclinic.com.

17. Center for Nutrition Policy and Promotion, "Expenditure on Children by Families, 2003 Annual Report," 2004, www.usda.gov/cnpp/Crc/crc2003.pdf.

18. National Center for Health Statistics, "Births: Preliminary Data for 2003," (PHS 2004-1120) *National Vital Statistics Reports* 53, no. 9, 18 pp.

19. National Center for Health Statistics, "Fertility, Family Planning, and Women's Health, New Data from the 1995 National Survey of Family Growth 23," (19) 7128 pp.

20. U.S. Department of Health and Human Services, "The Health Consequences of Smoking: What It Means to You," in *The 2004 Surgeon General's Report* (Washington, DC: Government Printing Office, 2004).

21. H. Klonoff-Cohen et al., "The Effects of Passive Smoking and Tobacco Exposure Through Breast Milk on Sudden Infant Death Syndrome," *Journal of the American Medical Association* 273 (1995): 795–798.

22. National Institute of Child Health and Human Development, "Facts about Down's Syndrome," 2005, www.nichd.nih.gov/publications/downsyndrome.

23. C. M. Peterson and N. L. Stotland, "Physical and Emotional Changes," *Lamaze Parents Magazine,* 2000 spring/summer issue.

24. National Institute of Mental Health, "Frequently Asked Questions: Depression During and After Pregnancy," April 2005, www.4woman.gov.

25. E. de Lisser, "Breast Feeding Boosts Adult I.Q., Research Suggests," *The Wall Street Journal,* May 2, 2002, D2.

26. M. Avery et al., "Factors Associated with Very Early Weaning among Primiparas Intending to Breastfeed," *Maternal and Child Health Journal* 2 (1998): 167–179.

27. K. Powell, "Fertility Treatments: Seeds of Doubt," *Nature* 422 (2003): 656–658.

28. Bureau of Consular Affairs, "Immigrant Visas Issued to Orphans Coming to the U.S.," 2004, http://travel.state.gov/family/adoption/stats/stats_451.html.

How can I recognize the signs of addiction in a loved one or even myself?

Are there any negative long-term effects from marijuana use?

Should I be concerned about the safety of new prescription drugs?

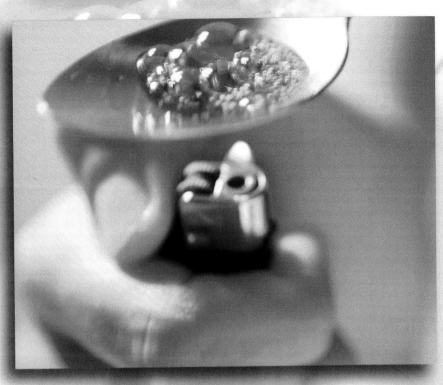

Is it legal for employers to require employees to take a drug test?

7 Licit and Illicit Drugs

Use, Misuse, and Abuse

Objectives

- *Discuss* the six categories of drugs and their routes of administration.
- *Compare* choices in prescription and over-the-counter drugs, and understand proper use and how hazardous drug interactions can occur.
- *Discuss* patterns of illicit drug use in the United States, including who uses illicit

drugs, financial impact, and impact on the workplace.
- *Describe* the use and abuse of controlled substances, including cocaine, amphetamines, marijuana, opiates, hallucinogens, designer drugs, inhalants, and steroids.
- *Describe* the signs of addiction.

Drug misuse and abuse are problems of staggering proportions in our society. Each year, drug and alcohol abuse contributes to the destruction of families and jobs and to the deaths of more than 120,000 Americans. Drug abuse costs taxpayers more than $294 billion in preventable health care costs, extra law enforcement, vehicle crashes, crime, and lost productivity.[1] It's impossible to put a dollar amount on the pain, suffering, and dysfunction that drugs cause in our everyday lives.

While overall use of drugs in the United States has fallen by 50 percent in the last 20 years, the past 10 years have shown an increase in the use of certain drugs by adolescents.[2] Why so many people use drugs and the mechanisms by which drugs cause harm are topics of ongoing research. Human beings appear to have a need to alter their consciousness, or mental state. We like to feel good or escape the normal. Consciousness can be altered in many ways: children spinning until they become dizzy and adults enjoying the rush of thrilling extreme sports are examples. To change our awareness, many of us listen to music, skydive, ski, read, daydream, meditate, pray, or have sexual relations. Others turn to drugs to alter consciousness.

DRUG DYNAMICS

Drugs work because they physically resemble the chemicals produced naturally within the body (Figure 7.1). Most bodily processes result from chemical reactions or from changes in electrical charge. Drugs affect our physical functions by mimicking these natural chemicals in our body. For example, many painkillers resemble the endorphins (the "morphine within") that are manufactured in the body.

One explanation of how drugs work is the receptor site theory, which states that drugs bind to specific **receptor sites** in the body. These sites are specialized cells to which, because of their size, shape, electrical charge, and chemical properties, drugs can attach themselves. Most drugs attach to multiple receptor sites located throughout the body in places such as the heart and circulatory system and the lungs, liver, kidneys, brain, and gonads (testicles or ovaries).

Types of Drugs

Scientists divide drugs into six categories: prescription, over-the-counter, recreational, herbal, illicit, and commercial drugs. These classifications are based primarily on drug action, although some are based on the source of the chemical in question. Each category includes some drugs that stimulate the body and some that depress body functions. Each category also includes **psychoactive drugs,** which have the potential to alter a person's mood or behavior.

- **Prescription drugs** are those substances that can be obtained only with the written prescription of a licensed physician. More than 10,000 types of prescription drugs are sold in the United States, at an annual cost of over $200 billion to consumers.[3]

- **Over-the-counter (OTC) drugs** can be purchased without a prescription. Each year, Americans spend more than $20 billion on OTC products, and the market is increasing at the rate of 20 percent annually. More than 300,000 OTC products are available, and an estimated three out of four people routinely self-medicate with them.

- **Recreational drugs** belong to a somewhat vague category whose boundaries depend on how the term *recreation* is defined. Generally, these drugs contain chemicals used to help people relax or socialize. Most of them are legally sanctioned even though they are psychoactive. Alcohol, tobacco, coffee, tea, and chocolate products are usually included in this category.

- **Herbal preparations** form another vague category. Included among these approximately 750 substances are herbal teas and other products of botanical (plant) origin that are believed to have medicinal properties. (See Chapter 18 for more on herbal preparations.)

- **Illicit (illegal) drugs** are the most notorious type of drug. Although laws governing their use, possession, cultivation, manufacture, and sale differ from state to state, illicit drugs generally are recognized as harmful. All of them are psychoactive.

- **Commercial preparations** are the most universally used yet least commonly recognized chemical

---

Receptor sites   Specialized cells to which drugs can attach themselves.

Psychoactive drugs   Drugs that have the potential to alter mood or behavior.

Prescription drugs   Medications that can be obtained only with the written prescription of a licensed physician.

Over-the-counter (OTC) drugs   Medications that can be purchased without a physician's prescription.

Recreational drugs   Legal drugs that contain chemicals that help people relax or socialize.

Herbal preparations   Substances of plant origin that are believed to have medicinal properties.

Illicit (illegal) drugs   Drugs whose use, possession, cultivation, manufacture, and/or sale are against the law because they generally are recognized as harmful.

Commercial preparations   Commonly used chemical substances including cosmetics, household cleaning products, and industrial by-products.

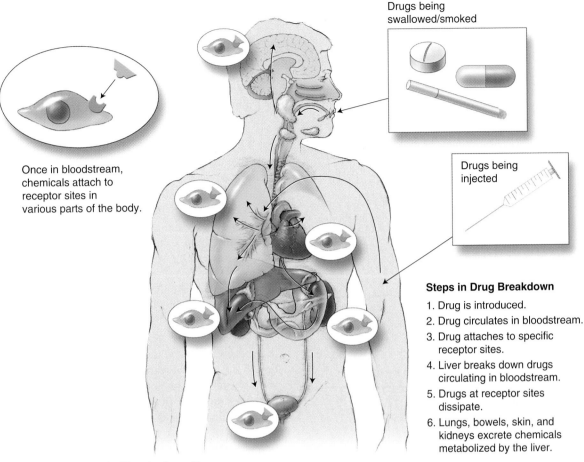

Once in bloodstream, chemicals attach to receptor sites in various parts of the body.

Drugs being swallowed/smoked

Drugs being injected

Steps in Drug Breakdown
1. Drug is introduced.
2. Drug circulates in bloodstream.
3. Drug attaches to specific receptor sites.
4. Liver breaks down drugs circulating in bloodstream.
5. Drugs at receptor sites dissipate.
6. Lungs, bowels, skin, and kidneys excrete chemicals metabolized by the liver.

Figure 7.1 How the Body Metabolizes Drugs

substances that have drug action. More than 1,000 of these substances exist, including seemingly benign items such as perfumes, cosmetics, household cleansers, paints, glues, inks, dyes, gardening chemicals, pesticides, and industrial by-products.

Routes of Administration of Drugs

Route of administration refers to the way in which a given drug is taken into the body. The most common methods include by mouth (**oral ingestion), inhalation** (administration of drugs through the mouth or nostrils via sniffing or smoking), or **injection** into the muscles, bloodstream, or just under the skin. **Intravenous injection,** which involves the insertion of a hypodermic syringe directly into a vein, is the most common method of injection for drug misusers, due to the rapid speed in which a drug's effect is felt. It is also the most dangerous method of administration due to the risk of contracting HIV and damage to blood vessels. Drugs can also be absorbed through the skin (**inunction**)—the nicotine patch is a common example of a drug that is

administered in this manner—or through the vagina or anus (**suppositories**). Suppositories are typically mixed with a waxy medium that melts at body temperature so the drug can be released into the bloodstream. However the drug enters the system, most drugs remain active in the body for several hours.

Route of administration   The manner in which a drug is taken into the body.

Oral ingestion   Intake of drugs through the mouth.

Inhalation   The introduction of drugs through the nostrils or mouth.

Injection   The introduction of drugs into the body via a hypodermic needle.

Intravenous injection   The introduction of drugs directly into a vein.

Inunction   The introduction of drugs through the skin.

Suppositories   Mixtures of drugs and a waxy medium designed to melt at body temperature that are inserted into the anus or vagina.

USING, MISUSING, AND ABUSING DRUGS

Although drug abuse usually is referred to in connection with illicit psychoactive drugs, many people abuse and misuse prescription and OTC medications. **Drug misuse** involves the use of a drug for a purpose for which it was not intended. For example, taking a friend's high-powered prescription painkiller for your headache is a misuse of that drug. This is not too far removed from **drug abuse,** or the excessive use of any drug, and may result in serious harm.

The misuse and abuse of any drug may lead to addiction. Both risks and benefits are involved in the use of any chemical substance. Intelligent decision making requires a clear-headed evaluation of these risks and benefits.

What Do You Think?

What are some situations in which students misuse drugs? ■ Other than alcohol, which drugs (prescription or OTC) do students tend to abuse while they are in college?

Defining Addiction

Addiction is defined by the American Psychiatric Association according to the following traits[4]:

1. Use for the purpose of relieving **withdrawal** symptoms—a series of temporary physical and psychological symptoms that occurs when the addicted person abruptly stops using the drug.

2. Continued use of the substance despite knowledge of the harm it causes yourself and others (deterioration in work performance, relationships, and social interaction).

3. Unsuccessful efforts to cut down or cease using the drug, including **relapse,** the tendency to return to the addictive behavior after a period of abstinence.

4. **Tolerance,** or an acquired reaction to a drug in which continued intake of the same dose has diminished effects. In response to tolerance, drug users must increase the dose in order to achieve the desired effect.

Physiological (physical) dependence, the adaptive state that occurs with regular drug use and results in withdrawal syndrome, is only one indicator of addiction. Psychological dynamics play an important role, which explains why behaviors not related to the use of chemicals—gambling, for example—may also be addictive. In fact, psychological and physiological dependence are so intertwined that it is not really possible to separate the two. For every psychological state, there is a corresponding physiological state. In other words, everything you feel is tied to a chemical process occurring in your body.[5]

To be addictive, a behavior must have the potential to produce a positive mood change and induce a reaction in the brain's reward center. Chemicals are responsible for the most profound addictions, not only because they alter mood dramatically, but also because they cause cellular changes to which the body adapts so well that it eventually requires the chemical in order to function normally. Yet, other behaviors, such as gambling, spending money, working, and engaging in sex, also create changes at the cellular level along with positive mood changes. Although the mechanism is not well understood, all forms of addiction probably reflect dysfunction of certain biochemical systems in the brain.[6]

Until recently, health professionals were unwilling to diagnose an addiction until medical symptoms appeared in the patient. Now we know that although withdrawal, pathological behavior, relapse, and medical symptoms are valid indicators of addiction, they do not characterize all addictive behavior.

Signs of Addiction

How can I recognize the signs of addiction in a loved one or even myself?

Studies show that all animals share the same basic pleasure and reward circuits in the brain that turn on when they come into contact with addictive substances or engage in something pleasurable, such as eating or orgasm. We all engage in potentially addictive behaviors to some extent because some are essential to our survival and are highly reinforcing, such as eating, drinking, and sex. At some point along the continuum, however, some individuals are not able to engage in these behaviors moderately, and they become addicted.

Drug misuse   The use of a drug for a purpose for which it was not intended.

Drug abuse   The excessive use of a drug.

Addiction   Continued involvement with a substance or activity despite ongoing negative consequences.

Withdrawal   A series of temporary physical and biopsychosocial symptoms that occur when the addict abruptly abstains from an addictive chemical or behavior.

Relapse   The tendency to return to the addictive behavior after a period of abstinence.

Tolerance   An acquired reaction to a drug in which continued intake of the same dose has diminished effects.

Physiological (physical) dependence   The adaptive state that occurs with regular drug use and results in withdrawal syndrome.

Addictions are characterized by four common symptoms: (1) **compulsion,** or the excessive need to perform the behavior (characterized by **obsession,** or mental preoccupation with the behavior); (2) **loss of control,** or the inability to predict reliably whether any isolated occurrence of the behavior will be healthy or damaging; (3) **negative consequences,** such as physical damage, legal trouble, financial problems, academic failure, or family dissolution, which do not occur with healthy involvement in any behavior; and (4) **denial,** the inability to perceive that the behavior is self-destructive. These four components are present in all addictions, whether chemical or behavioral.

Try it → NOW

Achieve a drug-free and "natural high." Many people become addicted to drugs because of the positive, short-term effects they can have on your mood. Right now, you can take a walk in a beautiful and sense-stimulating location, lose yourself in a favorite song, or visit an amusement park and ride the roller-coaster to satisfy a craving for an endorphin rush or simply lift your spirits.

PRESCRIPTION DRUGS

Even though prescription drugs are administered under medical supervision, the wise consumer still takes precautions. Hazards and complications arising from the use of prescription drugs are common.

Today, consumers have a variety of resources available to them for determining risks of various prescription medicines and can make educated decisions on whether or not to take a certain drug. One of the best resources currently available is the U.S. Food and Drug Administration's (FDA) Center for Drug Evaluation and Research website (www.fda.gov/cder/drug/). This special consumer section of the FDA provides current information on prescription drug risks and benefits. Being knowledgeable about what you are taking or thinking about taking is a sound strategy to insure safety. (See the Consumer Health box on page 184 for more on prescription drug safety issues.)

Types of Prescription Drugs

Antibiotics are drugs used to fight bacterial infection. Bacterial infections continue to be among the most common serious diseases throughout the world, but the vast majority can be cured with antibiotics. There are close to 100 different antibiotics, which may be dispensed by intramuscular injection or in tablet or capsule form. Some, called broad-spectrum antibiotics, are designed to

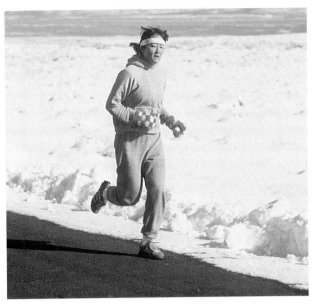

Obsession with a substance or behavior, even a generally positive activity such as exercise, can eventually develop into an addiction.

control disease caused by a number of bacterial species. These medications may also kill off helpful bacteria in the body, thus triggering secondary infections. For example, some vaginal infections are related to long-term use of antibiotics. It is important to follow your health care provider's directions when taking antibiotics, and to use them only when you have a bacterial infection. The misuse of antibiotics has led to a dangerous increase in drug-resistant bacteria in recent years.

Central nervous system depressants are sedative or hypnotic medications commonly used to treat anxiety. The two main types of drugs in this group are

---

Compulsion An overwhelming need to perform a behavior or obtain an addictive object.

Obsession Excessive preoccupation with an addictive object or behavior.

Loss of control Inability to predict reliably whether a particular instance of involvement with the addictive object or behavior will be healthy or damaging.

Negative consequences Physical damage, legal trouble, financial ruin, academic failure, family dissolution, and other severe problems associated with addiction.

Denial Inability to perceive or accurately interpret the self-destructive effects of the addictive behavior.

Antibiotics Prescription drugs designed to fight bacterial infection.

Central nervous system depressents Sedative or hypnotic medications commonly used to treat anxiety.

In 1993, the U.S. Food and Drug Administration (FDA) changed its policies to speed the approval process of new drugs. These changes were made for humanitarian reasons, in response to activists seeking rapid approval of experimental drugs that offered at least a ray of hope to AIDS patients who otherwise faced certain death. The "accelerated development/review" process was seen as a way to offer drugs that could offer a significant improvement over existing treatments or improve the outcome of life-threatening illnesses for which no treatment currently exists.

Hundreds of new drugs have been approved for OTC status since then.

Should I be concerned about the safety of new prescription drugs?

Of that number, a handful have been withdrawn after reports of deaths and severe side effects, risks that do not outweigh the overall benefit the drug may offer. Examples of drugs that have been placed on the pharmacy shelves as a result of the FDA's more lenient approach but have yielded detrimental or fatal results include the COX-2 inhibitor (prescription analgesic) *Bextra* and *Lotronex*. *Bextra* is a widely used drug for treating arthritis pain. In 2004, results of a large scale study unveiled a series of cardiovascular risks associated with the medication,

including heart attack and stroke, and an increased risk for a serious and potentially fatal skin reaction. In April 2005, the FDA requested that the manufacturer of *Bextra* (Pfizer) remove this drug from the market. *Lotronex,* a drug for treating irritable bowel syndrome, was approved despite warnings. It has now been linked to five deaths, the removal of one patient's colon, and other bowel surgeries. *Lotronex* was pulled from the market after only 10 months.

In response to these events and others, the FDA has launched a new drug safety initiative. As part of this initiative, the Drug Safety Oversight Board will be established in order to oversee drug safety issues, consult with medical experts and consumer groups, and provide new information on medication risks and benefits to consumers and health care providers. Also at the core of current changes to the FDA, long considered by public health officials to be the most reliable early warning that a product may be dangerous, will be new and improved communication channels to the general public on drug safety information.

New communication channels include:

- *The Drug Watch Web Page.* This page will include emerging information, for both previously and newly approved drugs, about possible serious side effects or other safety risks and

how risks can be avoided. The agency will enhance access to this information and call for assistance in prioritizing and further evaluating potential adverse health concerns.

- *Healthcare Professional Information Sheets.* One-page information sheets for health care professionals for all drugs on FDA's Drug Watch and all drugs with Medication Guides (FDA-approved patient labeling) containing the most important new information for safe use, including known and potential safety issues based on reports of adverse events, new information that may affect prescribing of the drug, and the approved indications and benefits of the drug.

- *Patient Information Sheets.* One-page information sheets for patients in a consumer friendly format for all products on Drug Watch. Information will include new safety information as well as basic information about how to use the drug.

Sources: "Adverse Event Reporting System (AERS)," U.S. Food and Drug Administration, Center for Drug Evaluation and Research, August 7, 2002, www.fda.gov/cder/aers/default.htm; "Accelerated Development/Review," U.S. Food and Drug Administration, www.fda.gov/cder/handbook/accel.htm; U.S. Department of Health and Human Services, "Reforms Will Improve Oversight and Openness at FDA" (news release), February 15, 2005, www.fda.gov/cder/drugsafety.htm.

benzodiazepines (such as Valium, Ativan, and Xanax), and barbiturates (including Amytal and Seconal). The benzodiazepines are the most widely used drug in this category, most commonly prescribed for tension, muscular strain, sleep problems, anxiety panic attacks, and in treatment of alcohol withdrawal. They differ widely in their mechanism of action, absorption rate, and metabolism, but all produce similar intoxication and withdrawal symptoms. Benzodiazepine sleeping pills have

largely replaced barbiturates, which were used medically in the past for relieving tension and inducing relaxation and sleep.

All sedative or hypnotic drugs can produce physical and psychological dependence in several weeks. A complication specific to sedatives is cross tolerance, which occurs when users develop tolerance for one sedative or become dependent on it and develop tolerance for others as well. Withdrawal from sedative or hypnotic drugs may range from mild discomfort to severe symptoms, depending on the degree of dependence. A major public health issue is whether or not persons using benzodiazepines have an increased risk of cognitive decline and dementia. Ongoing research is investigating this possible link.[7]

Benzodiazepines Central nervous system depressants that relieve anxiety, relax the body, and induce sleep.

Antidepressants are medications typically used to treat major depression, although occasionally they are used for other forms of depression that resist conventional therapy. There are several groups of antidepressant medications approved for use in the United States. Prozac, Zoloft, and Paxil are well-known examples. Antidepressants are among the three most commonly-prescribed classes of drugs. Over the past decade, the use of antidepressant drugs in the United States has increased by 48 percent overall, and by 124 percent in children.[8] For more on antidepressants, see Chapter 2.

Generic Drugs

Generic drugs, medications sold under a chemical name rather than under a brand name, have gained popularity in recent years. They contain the same active ingredients as brand-name drugs but are less expensive. If your doctor prescribes a drug, always ask whether a generic equivalent exists and whether it would be safe and effective for you to try. Not all drugs are available as generics.

Be aware, though, that there is some controversy about the effectiveness of generic drugs because substitutions often are made in minor ingredients that can affect the way the drug is absorbed, which causes discomfort or even allergic reactions in some users. Always note any reactions you have to medications, and tell your doctor about them.

Prescription Drug Costs

Prescription drug costs are an increasing concern for Americans today. Health insurance coverage of prescriptions medications vary (see Chapter 17 for more on insurance plans), but the general trend is for insurance to cover these costs less and less, while consumers must spend more out-of-pocket dollars for drug treatments.[9] To further complicate matters, newer drugs often are patent protected and do not have a generic equivalent, leaving many with no choice but to purchase the high-cost brand-name medication. Figure 7.2 demonstrates the average cost of prescription drugs.

Over-the-Counter Drugs

Over-the-counter drugs are nonprescription substances we use in the course of self-diagnosis and self-medication. More than one-third of the time, people treat their routine health problems with OTC medications. In fact, American consumers spend billions of dollars yearly on OTC preparations for relief of everything from runny noses to ingrown toenails. There are 40,000 OTC drugs and more than 300,000 brand names for them.

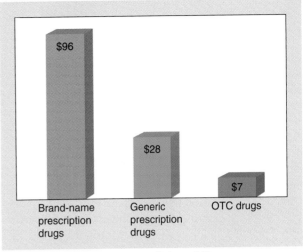

Figure 7.2 ■ The Average Price of Drugs
The cost of brand-name drugs is high now and may only continue to rise. Ask your doctor about generic or OTC options.

Most OTC drugs are manufactured from a basic group of 1,000 chemicals. The many different products available to us are produced by combining as few as two and as many as ten substances.

How Prescription Drugs Become Over-the-Counter Drugs

The FDA regularly reviews prescription drugs to evaluate how suitable they would be as OTC products. For a drug to be switched from prescription to OTC status, it must meet the following criteria.

1. The drug has been marketed as a prescription medication for at least three years.

2. The use of the drug has been relatively high during the time it was available as a prescription drug.

3. Adverse drug reactions are not alarming, and the frequency of side effects has not increased during the time it was available to the public.

Since this policy has been in effect, the FDA has moved hundreds of drugs to OTC status. Some examples are ibuprofen, Claritin, and Prilosec. Many more prescription drugs are currently being considered for OTC status.

Antidepressants Prescription drugs used to treat clinically diagnosed depression.

Generic drugs Medications marketed by chemical name rather than brand name.

Types of Over-the-Counter Drugs

The FDA has categorized 26 types of OTC preparations. Those most commonly used are analgesics, cold/cough/allergy and asthma relievers, sleeping aids, and dieting aids.

Analgesics More than 50 million Americans experience chronic pain. Is it any wonder that we spend more than $2 billion annually on **analgesics** (pain relievers), the largest sales category of OTC drugs in the United States?[10] Although these pain relievers come in several forms, aspirin, acetaminophen (Tylenol, Pamprin, Panadol), ibuprofen (Advil, Motrin, Nuprin), and ibuprofen-like drugs such as naproxen sodium (Aleve, Anaprox) and ketoprofen (Orudis) are the most common.

Most pain relievers work at receptor sites by interrupting pain signals. Some are categorized as NSAIDs (nonsteroidal anti-inflammatory drugs), also called **prostaglandin inhibitors.** Prostaglandins are chemicals released by the body in response to pain. Prostaglandin inhibitors restrain the release of prostaglandins and thus reduce the pain. Common NSAIDs include ibuprofen, naproxen sodium, and aspirin.

Besides relieving pain, aspirin lowers fever by increasing the flow of blood to the skin surface, which causes sweating and cools the body. Aspirin long has been used to reduce the inflammation and swelling associated with arthritis. It is widely accepted that a low dose of aspirin has anticoagulant (interference with blood clotting) effects and can reduce the risk of heart attack and stroke.

Possible side effects of aspirin—and many other NSAIDS—include allergic reactions, ringing in the ears, stomach bleeding, and ulcers. Those taking aspirin regularly to reduce heart disease risk should discontinue use prior to surgery because it inhibits blood's ability to clot. Combining aspirin with alcohol can compound aspirin's gastric irritant properties. As with all drugs, read the labels. Some analgesic labels caution against driving or operating heavy machinery when using the drug, and most warn that analgesics should not be taken with alcohol.

Research has also linked aspirin to a potentially fatal condition called Reye's syndrome. Children, teenagers, and young adults (up to age 25) who are treated with aspirin while recovering from the flu or chickenpox are at risk for developing this syndrome. Aspirin substitutes are recommended for people in these age groups.

Acetaminophen is an aspirin substitute found in Tylenol and related medications. Like aspirin, acetaminophen is an effective analgesic and antipyretic (fever-reducing drug). However, it does not relieve inflamed or swollen joints. The side effects associated with acetaminophen generally are minimal, though overdose can cause liver damage.

Cold, Cough, Allergy, and Asthma Relievers The operative word in this category is *reliever*. Most of these medications are designed to alleviate the discomforting symptoms associated with maladies of the upper respiratory tract. Unfortunately, no drugs exist to cure the actual diseases. The drugs available provide only temporary relief until the sufferer's immune system prevails over the disease. Both aspirin and acetaminophen are on the government's lists of medications that are **Generally Recognized as Safe (GRAS)** and **Generally Recognized as Effective (GRAE).** Table 7.1 describes the basic types of OTC cold, cough, and allergy relievers.

Sleeping Aids A study by the World Health Organization, conducted in 15 health centers around the globe, found that 27 percent of patients reported difficulties with sleeping. A U.S. survey found that 10 percent of American adults experienced chronic insomnia.[11] Many people routinely treat their insomnia with OTC sleep aids (such as Nytol, Sleep-Eze, and Sominex) that are advertised as providing "safe and restful" sleep. These drugs induce the drowsy feelings that precede sleep. The principal ingredient in OTC sleeping aids is an antihistamine called pyrilamine maleate. Chronic reliance on sleeping aids may lead to addiction; people accustomed to using these products may eventually find it impossible to sleep without them.

Dieting Aids In the United States, there is a $200 million market for dieting aids. Some of these drugs (e.g., Acutrim, Dexatrim) are advertised as "appetite suppressants." The FDA has pulled several appetite suppressants off the market because their active ingredient was phenylpropanolamine (PPA), which has been linked to increased risk of stroke.[12] More recently, the FDA has also prohibited the sale of ephedra, a naturally occurring substance often billed as a diet-aid or sports and energy enhancement drug. Ephedra use has been linked to heart attack, stroke, and death.[13]

Analgesics Pain relievers.

Prostaglandin inhibitors Drugs that inhibit the production and release of prostaglandins, hormone-like substances associated with arthritis or menstrual pain.

GRAS list A list of drugs generally recognized as safe, which seldom cause side effects when used properly.

GRAE list A list of drugs generally recognized as effective, which work for their intended purpose when used properly.

Table 7.1
Types of Over-the-Counter Cold, Cough, and Allergy Relievers

- *Expectorants.* These drugs loosen phlegm, which allows the user to cough it up and clear congested respiratory passages. GRAS and GRAE reviewers question the effectiveness of many expectorants. When combined with other medications, particularly among those used by frail or very ill individuals, safety issues may arise.
- *Antitussives.* These OTC drugs calm or curtail the cough reflex. They are most effective when the cough is dry (does not produce phlegm). Oral codeine, dextromethorphan, and diphenhydramine are the most common antitussives that are on both the GRAE and GRAS lists.
- *Antihistamines.* These central nervous system depressants dry runny noses, clear postnasal drip, clear sinus congestion, and reduce tears.
- *Decongestants.* These remedies reduce nasal stuffiness due to colds.
- *Anticholinergics.* These substances often are added to cold preparations to reduce nasal secretions and tears. None of the preparations tested was found to be GRAE or GRAS. Some cold compounds contain alcohol in concentrations that may exceed 40 percent.

Estimates show that, when taken as recommended, even the best OTC dieting aids significantly reduce appetite in less than 30 percent of users, and tolerance occurs in only one to three days of use. Manufacturers of appetite suppressants often include a written 1,200-calorie diet to complement their drug. However, most people who limit themselves to 1,200 calories per day will lose weight—without any help from appetite suppressants. Clearly, these products have no value in treating obesity.

Some people rely on **laxatives** (stool softeners) and **diuretics** (water pills) to lose weight. Frequent use of laxatives disrupts the body's natural elimination patterns and may cause constipation or even obstipation (inability to have a bowel movement). Using laxatives to produce weight loss has unspectacular results and robs the body of needed fluids, salts, and minerals.

Taking diuretics to lose weight is also dangerous. Not only will the user gain the weight back upon drinking fluids, but diuretic use may contribute to dangerous chemical imbalances. The potassium and sodium eliminated by diuretics play important roles in maintaining electrolyte balance. Depletion of these vital minerals can cause weakness, dizziness, fatigue, and sometimes death.

Rules for Proper Use of Over-the-Counter Drugs

Despite a common belief that OTC products are safe and effective, indiscriminate use and abuse can occur with these drugs as with all others. For example, people who frequently drop medication into their eyes to "get the red out" or pop antacids after every meal are likely to become addicted. Many people also experience adverse side effects because they ignore the warnings on the labels or simply do not read them.

The FDA has developed a standard label that appears on most OTC products (see Figure 7.3). It provides directions for use, warnings, and other useful information. (Diet supplements, which are regulated as food products, have their own label that includes a Supplements Facts panel.)

OTC products are far more powerful than ever before, and the science behind them is stronger as well. Therefore, as with any type of medication, do your homework. Observe the following rules when taking nonprescription drugs.

1. Always know what you are taking. Identify the active ingredients in the product.
2. Know the effects, both desired and undesired, of each active ingredient.
3. Read the warnings and cautions.
4. Don't use anything for more than one or two weeks.
5. Be particularly cautious if you are also taking prescription drugs because the drugs may interact.
6. If you have questions, ask your pharmacist.
7. *If you don't need it, don't take it!*

Drug Interactions

Sharing medications, using outdated prescriptions, taking higher doses than recommended, or using medications as a substitute for dealing with personal problems may result in serious health consequences. **Polydrug use,** taking several medications (including vitamins) or illegal drugs simultaneously, also can lead to dangerous health problems associated with drug interactions. The most hazardous interactions are synergism, antagonism, inhibition, intolerance, and cross-tolerance.

Synergism, also known as *potentiation*, is an interaction of two or more drugs in which the effects of the individual drugs are multiplied beyond what normally

---

Laxatives   Medications used to soften stool and relieve constipation.

Diuretics   Drugs that increase the excretion of urine from the body.

Polydrug use   The use of multiple medications or illicit drugs simultaneously.

Synergism   An interaction of two or more drugs that produces more profound effects than would be expected if the drugs were taken separately.

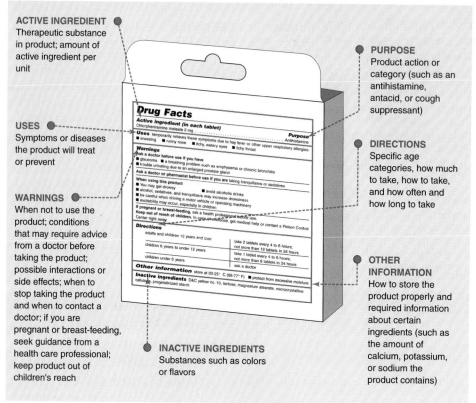

ACTIVE INGREDIENT
Therapeutic substance in product; amount of active ingredient per unit

USES
Symptoms or diseases the product will treat or prevent

WARNINGS
When not to use the product; conditions that may require advice from a doctor before taking the product; possible interactions or side effects; when to stop taking the product and when to contact a doctor; if you are pregnant or breast-feeding, seek guidance from a health care professional; keep product out of children's reach

INACTIVE INGREDIENTS
Substances such as colors or flavors

PURPOSE
Product action or category (such as an antihistamine, antacid, or cough suppressant)

DIRECTIONS
Specific age categories, how much to take, how to take, and how often and how long to take

OTHER INFORMATION
How to store the product properly and required information about certain ingredients (such as the amount of calcium, potassium, or sodium the product contains)

Figure 7.3 ■ The Over-the-Counter Drug Label

Source: Consumer Healthcare Products Association, "The New Over-the-Counter Medicine Label," 2002. Reprinted by permission.

would be expected if they were taken alone. Synergism can be expressed mathematically as $2 + 2 = 10$.

A synergistic reaction can be very dangerous. Prescription and OTC medications carry labels warning the user not to combine them with certain other drugs or with alcohol. You should always verify any possible drug interactions before using a prescribed or OTC drug. Pharmacists, physicians, drug information centers, or community drug education centers can answer your questions. Even if one of the drugs in question is illegal, you still should attempt to determine the dangers involved in combining it with other drugs. Health care professionals are legally bound to maintain confidentiality even when they know that a client is using illegal substances.

Antagonism, although usually less serious than synergism, can also produce unwanted and unpleasant effects. In an antagonistic reaction, drugs work at the same receptor site so that one blocks the action of the other. The blocking drug occupies the receptor site and prevents the other substance from attaching, thus altering its absorption and action.

With **inhibition,** the effects of one drug are eliminated or reduced by the presence of another drug at the receptor site. One common inhibitory reaction occurs between antacid tablets and aspirin. The antacid inhibits the absorption of aspirin and makes it less effective as a pain reliever. Other inhibitory reactions occur between alcohol and antibiotics and between antibiotics and contraceptive pills.

Cross-tolerance occurs when a person develops a physiological tolerance to one drug and shows a similar tolerance to selected other drugs as a result. Taking one drug may actually increase the body's tolerance to another substance. For example, cross-tolerance can develop between alcohol and barbiturates, two depressant drugs.

Antagonism A blocking interaction in which two or more drugs work at the same receptor site.

Inhibition A type of interaction in which the effects of one drug are eliminated or reduced by the presence of another drug at the receptor site.

Cross-tolerance The development of a tolerance to one drug that reduces the effects of another similar drug.

ILLICIT DRUGS

While some people become addicted to prescription drugs and painkillers, others use *illicit drugs*—those drugs that are illegal to possess, produce, or sell. The problem of illicit drug use touches us all. We may use illicit substances ourselves, watch someone we love struggle with drug abuse, or become the victim of a drug-related crime. At the very least, we are forced to pay increasing taxes for law enforcement and drug rehabilitation. An estimated 9.4 percent of full-time employees in the U.S. workforce is under the influence of illicit substances or alcohol on any given day.[14] When our coworkers use drugs, the effectiveness of our own work is diminished. If the car we drive was assembled by drug-using workers at the plant, we are in danger. A drug-using bus driver, train engineer, or pilot jeopardizes our safety.

The good news is that the use of illicit drugs has declined significantly in recent years in most segments of society. Use of most drugs increased from the early 1970s to the late 1970s, peaked between 1979 and 1986, and declined until 1992, from which point it has not changed. In 2003, an estimated 19.2 million Americans were illicit drug users, about three quarters the 1979 peak level of 25 million users. Among youth, however, illicit drug use, notably of marijuana, has been rising in recent years.[15]

Who Uses Illicit Drugs?

While many of us have stereotypes in our minds of who uses illicit drugs, it is difficult to generalize. Illicit drug users span all age groups, ethnicities, occupations, and socioeconomic groups. No matter the group, illicit drug use has a devastating effect on users and their families in the United States and many other countries.

After more than a decade of declining use on U.S. college campuses, illicit drugs have reappeared. The number of college students nationwide who have tried any drug stands at nearly 52 percent; over a third have smoked pot in the past year, and 20 percent have done so in the past month. According to 2003 data, daily use of marijuana was at its highest point since 1989.[16] Cocaine use is down sharply, but LSD use has more than doubled. These figures vary from school to school.

Patterns of drug use vary considerably by age. For example, a nationwide study of college campuses reported that approximately 30.7 percent of students had tried marijuana during the previous year (Table 7.2).[17] In contrast, only 9 percent of all Americans used marijuana during that time. Approximately 4.8 percent of college students surveyed reported using cocaine in the past year, whereas only 2.2 percent of all Americans said they had used cocaine during the previous year.

The pressures to take drugs are often tremendous, and the reasons for using them are complex. However, since most illegal drugs produce physical and psychological dependency, it is unrealistic to think that a person can use them regularly without becoming addicted. Consider whether you are controlled by drugs or a drug user by answering the questions in the Assess Yourself box on page 192.

Table 7.2 Annual Prevalence of Use for Various Types of Drugs, 2003*		
	Full-Time College (%)	Others (%)
Any Illicit Drug	36.5	40.9
Any Illicit Drug Other Than Marijuana	17.9	23.6
Marijuana	33.7	36.0
Inhalants	1.8	1.9
Hallucinogens	7.4	7.4
Cocaine	5.4	8.8
MDMA (Ecstasy)	4.4	6.7
Heroin	0.2	0.6
Other Narcotics	8.7	11.4
OxyContin	2.2	4.5
Vicodin	7.5	11.2
Amphetamines, Adjusted	7.1	9.4
Ritalin	4.7	3.0
Methamphetamine	2.6	4.4
Sedatives (Barbiturates)	4.1	6.2
Tranquilizers	6.9	8.4
Ketamine	1.0	1.9
Alcohol	81.7	76.7
Cigarettes	35.2	47.6
Approximate Weighted N =	1270	880

*Full-time college students vs. respondents 1–4 years beyond high school
Source: Monitoring the Future Study (Ann Arbor, MI: The University of Michigan, 2004).

What Do You Think? What factors do you believe influence illicit drug use in the United States? ■ What is the attitude toward drug use on your campus? ■ Are some substances considered more acceptable than others? ■ Is drug use considered more acceptable at certain times or occasions? Explain your answer.

CONTROLLED SUBSTANCES

Drugs are classified into five schedules (categories) based on their potential for abuse, their medical uses, and accepted standards of safe use (Table 7.3). Schedule I drugs, those with the highest potential for abuse, are considered to have no valid medical uses. Although Schedule II, III, IV, and V drugs have known and accepted medical applications, many of them present serious threats to health when abused or misused. Penalties for illegal use are tied to the drugs' schedule level.

Hundreds of illegal drugs exist. For general purposes, they can be divided into seven representative categories: *stimulants,* such as cocaine; marijuana and its

Table 7.3
How Drugs Are Scheduled

Schedule	Characteristics	Examples
Schedule I	High potential for abuse and addiction; no accepted medical use	Amphetamine (DMA, STP) Heroin LSD Marijuana
Schedule II	High potential for abuse and addiction; restricted medical use	Cocaine Methadone OxyContin Vicodin Ritalin
Schedule III	Some potential for abuse and addiction; currently accepted medical use	Anabolic steroids Nalorphine Noludar Rohypnol
Schedule IV	Low potential for abuse and addiction; currently accepted medical use	Xanax Minor tranquilizers
Schedule V	Lowest potential for abuse; accepted medical use	Robitussin AC OTC preparations

Source: National Institute on Drug Abuse, "Commonly Abused Drugs," 2003, www.drugabuse .gov/DrugPages/DrugsofAbuse.html.

derivatives; *depressants,* such as the opiates; *hallucinogens (psychedelics); designer drugs; inhalants;* and *steroids.*

Stimulants

Cocaine   A white crystalline powder derived from the leaves of the South American coca shrub (not related to cocoa plants), **cocaine** (coke) has been described as one of the most powerful naturally occurring stimulants.

Methods of Cocaine Use   Cocaine can be taken by snorting or injecting. Snorting the powdered form of the drug through the nose is the most common method of use. This can damage mucous membranes in the nose and cause sinusitis; destroy the user's sense of smell; and occasionally even eat a hole through the septum.

Injecting cocaine introduces large amounts into the body rapidly; within seconds, a sense of euphoria sets in. This intense high lasts for 15 to 20 minutes, and then

Cocaine   A powerful stimulant drug made from the leaves of the South American coca shrub.

the user heads into a crash. To prevent the unpleasant effects of the crash, users must shoot up frequently, which can severely damage veins. Injecting users place themselves at risk not only for AIDS and hepatitis, but also for skin infections, inflamed arteries, and infection of the lining of the heart.

Physical Effects of Cocaine   The effects of cocaine are felt rapidly. Snorted cocaine enters the bloodstream through the lungs in less than one minute and reaches the brain in less than three minutes. When cocaine binds at its receptor sites in the central nervous system, it produces intense pleasure. The euphoria quickly abates, however, and the desire to regain the pleasurable feelings makes the user want more cocaine (Figure 7.4).

Cocaine is both an anesthetic and a central nervous system stimulant. In tiny doses, it can slow heart rate. In larger doses, the physical effects are dramatic: increased heart rate and blood pressure, loss of appetite that can lead to dramatic weight loss, convulsions, muscle twitching, irregular heartbeat, and even eventual death due to overdose. Other effects of cocaine include temporary relief of depression, decreased fatigue, talkativeness, increased alertness, and heightened self-confidence. However, as the dose increases, users become irritable and apprehensive, and their behavior may turn paranoid or violent.

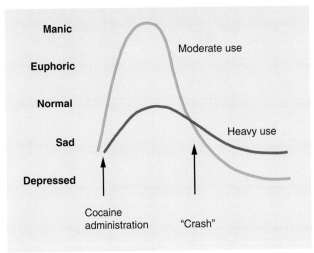

Figure 7.4 ■ Ups and Downs of a Typical Dose of Cocaine

Source: C. Levinthal, *Drugs, Behavior, and Modern Society,* 2nd ed. (Boston: Allyn & Bacon, 1999). © Pearson Education. Reprinted by permission of the publisher.

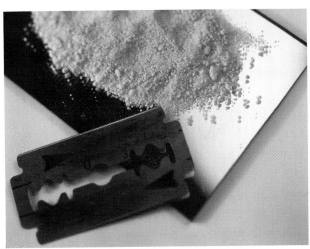

Although cocaine abuse has declined from its peak in the1980s, it continues to be a commonly abused illicit drug today.

Types of Cocaine **Freebase** is a form of cocaine that is more powerful and costly than powder or crack (see next section) and is taken by smoking. Street cocaine (cocaine hydrochloride) is converted to pure base by using ether to remove the hydrochloride salt and many of the "cutting agents" used to dilute the drug. This volatile chemical mixture is very dangerous and can cause severe burns. The end product, freebase, is smoked through a water pipe.

Freebase cocaine reaches the brain within seconds and produces a quick, intense high that disappears quickly, leaving an intense craving for more. Freebasers typically increase the amount and frequency of the dose, often become severely addicted and experience serious health problems.

Side effects of freebasing cocaine include weight loss, increased heart rate and blood pressure, depression, paranoia, and hallucinations. Freebase is an extremely dangerous drug and is responsible for a large number of cocaine-related hospital emergency-room visits and deaths.

The street name **crack** is given to freebase cocaine processed from cocaine hydrochloride by using ammonia or sodium bicarbonate (baking soda), water, and heat to remove the hydrochloride. The mixture (90 percent pure cocaine) is then dried. The soapy-looking substance that results can be broken into "rocks" and smoked. These rocks are approximately five times as strong as cocaine. Crack gets its name from the popping noises it makes when burned. In 2003, 3.1 percent of college students have used crack during their lives.[18]

Because crack is such a pure drug, it takes much less time to achieve the desired high. One puff of a pebble-size rock produces an intense high that lasts for approximately 20 minutes. The user can usually get three or four hits off a rock before it is used up. Crack is typically sold in small vials, folding papers, or heavy tinfoil containing two or three rocks, and costing between $10 and $20.

A crack user can become addicted quickly. Addiction is accelerated by the speed at which crack is absorbed through the lungs (it hits the brain within seconds) and by the intensity of the high. It is not uncommon for crack addicts to spend over $1,000 a day on the habit.

Cocaine-Affected Babies Because cocaine rapidly crosses the placenta (as virtually all drugs do), the fetus is vulnerable when a pregnant woman uses cocaine. Fetuses exposed to cocaine in the womb are more likely to suffer a small head, premature delivery, reduced birthweight, increased irritability, and subtle learning and cognitive deficits. Women who abuse cocaine during pregnancy have an increased risk of miscarriage.

It is estimated that 2.4 to 3.5 percent of pregnant women between the ages of 12 and 34 abuse cocaine. Research suggests that a large number of cocaine-affected babies develop problems with learning and language skills that require remedial attention.[19] It is critical to identify these children early so they can receive immediate intervention. For both financial and humane reasons, prenatal care and education programs for mothers at risk should be a priority for state and local government.[20]

Cocaine Addiction and Society Cocaine addicts often suffer both physiological damage and serious disruption in lifestyle, including loss of employment and self-esteem. It is estimated that the annual cost of

---

Freebase The most powerful distillate of cocaine.

Crack A distillate of powdered cocaine that comes in small, hard chips (rocks).

Recognizing a Drug Problem

Are You Controlled by Drugs?

How do you know whether you are chemically dependent? A dependent person can't stop using drugs. This abuse hurts the user and everyone around him or her. Take the following assessment. The more "yes" checks you make, the more likely you have a problem.

		Yes	No
1.	Do you use drugs to handle stress or escape from life's problems?	☐	☐
2.	Have you unsuccessfully tried to cut down on or quit using your drug?	☐	☐
3.	Have you ever been in trouble with the law or been arrested because of your drug use?	☐	☐
4.	Do you think a party or social gathering isn't fun unless drugs are available?	☐	☐
5.	Do you avoid people or places that do not support your usage?	☐	☐
6.	Do you neglect your responsibilities because you'd rather use your drug?	☐	☐
7.	Have your friends, family, or employer expressed concern about your drug use?	☐	☐
8.	Do you do things under the influence of drugs that you would not normally do?	☐	☐
9.	Have you seriously thought that you might have a chemical dependency problem?	☐	☐

Are You Controlled by a Drug User?

Is your life controlled by a chemical abuser? Your love and care (codependence) may actually be enabling the person to continue the abuse, hurting you and others. Try this assessment; the more "yes" checks you make, the more likely there's a problem.

		Yes	No
1.	Do you often have to lie or cover up for the chemical abuser?	☐	☐
2.	Do you spend time counseling the person about the problem?	☐	☐
3.	Have you taken on additional financial or family responsibilities?	☐	☐
4.	Do you feel that you have to control the chemical abuser's behavior?	☐	☐
5.	At the office, have you done work or attended meetings for the abuser?	☐	☐
6.	Do you often put your own needs and desires after the user's?	☐	☐
7.	Do you spend time each day worrying about your situation?	☐	☐
8.	Do you analyze your behavior to find clues to how it might affect the chemical abuser?	☐	☐
9.	Do you feel powerless and at your wit's end about the abuser's problem?	☐	☐

cocaine addiction in the United States exceeds $3.8 billion. However, there is no way to measure the cost in wasted lives. An estimated 5 million Americans from all socio-economic groups are addicted, and 1,160,000 new users try cocaine or crack every year. National surveys on drug use estimate that 5.9 million people used the drug at least once in the past year. Experts suggest that 10 percent of recreational users will go on to heavy use.[21]

Cocaine has been called unpredictable by drug experts, deadly by coroners, dangerous by former users, and disastrous by the media. Yet to date, there has not been a successful weapon to combat its use in the United States. Apparently, the risks do not override users' desire to experience its effects.

Because cocaine is illegal, a complex underground network has developed to manufacture and sell the drug. Buyers may not always get the product they think they are purchasing. Cocaine marketed for snorting may be only 60 percent pure. Usually, it is mixed, or "cut," with other white powdery substances such as mannitol or sugar, though occasionally it is cut with arsenic or other cocaine-like powders that may themselves be highly dangerous.

What Do You Think?

Have all segments of society been affected by crack use? ■ If not, which segments of the U.S. population experience the greatest impact from crack use? ■ Why might this be the case? ■ Is there a difference in the profile of a person who uses crack rather than cocaine? Explain your answer.

Make It Happen!

Assessment: The Assess Yourself activity describes signs of being controlled by drugs or by a drug user. Depending on your results, you may need to change certain behaviors that may be detrimental to your health.

Making a Change: In order to change your behavior, you need to develop a plan. Follow these steps below and complete your Behavior Change Contract to take action.

1. Evaluate your behavior, and identify patterns and specific things you are doing. What can you change now? What can you change in the near future?
2. Select one pattern of behavior that you want to change.
3. Fill out the Behavior Change Contract found at the front of your book. It should include your long-term goal for change, your short-term goals, the rewards you'll give yourself for reaching these goals, potential obstacles along the way, and strategies for overcoming these obstacles. For each goal, list the small steps and specific actions that you will take.
4. Chart your progress in a journal. At the end of a week, consider how successful you were in following your plan. What helped you be successful? What made change more difficult? What will you do differently next week?
5. Revise your plan as needed. Are the short-term goals attainable? Are the rewards satisfying?

Example: Tranh was surprised to find he had several yes answers to the self-assessment section about being controlled by a drug user. He realized that his girlfriend Kim's drug use was hurting their relationship and negatively affecting his well-being. Kim smoked marijuana almost every day and took club drugs at least twice a month. Tranh often had to lie to Kim's employer if she was too incapacitated to go to work. Recently, she had been in a car accident after smoking pot for several hours, which damaged Tranh's car and increased his insurance rate. And he worried whenever she went out for an evening that she was taking Ecstasy and would find herself in a compromising situation.

These worries, financial consequences, and pressure to lie all made Tranh resolve to take steps to make a change in his responses to Kim's behavior. His first step was to plan what he wanted to say to Kim about her drug use and how it affected both of them. He also started investigating drug counseling resources at school and in the community, both for Kim and for himself to help him cope with the issues raised by Kim's drug use. Finally, he began talking to Kim's friends who, it turned out, also were concerned about her behavior. They worked together to develop strategies to help Kim and provide alternatives to her drug use; Tranh also felt less alone and more supported as soon as he started reaching out to his peers.

Source: Reprinted by permission of Krames Communications, 1100 Grundy Lane, San Bruno, CA 94066-3030. www.krames.com.

Amphetamines The **amphetamines** include a large and varied group of synthetic agents that stimulate the central nervous system. Small doses of amphetamines improve alertness, lessen fatigue, and generally elevate mood. With repeated use, however, physical and psychological dependency develops. Sleep patterns are affected (insomnia); heart rate, breathing rate, and blood pressure increase; restlessness, anxiety, appetite suppression, and vision problems are common. High doses over long time periods can produce hallucinations, delusions, and disorganized behavior.

Certain types of amphetamines are used for medicinal purposes. Drugs such as Ritalin and Adderall are used to treat children with attention deficit hyperactive disorder; however, in recent years these drugs have taken the place of caffeine on college campuses, and many students misuse them to stay awake for all night cramming sessions. In fact, Ritalin is on the Drug Enforcement Agency's Top Ten list of most often stolen prescription drugs. There is a false perception that these drugs improve academic performance. A 2003 study at a large public university found that 3 percent of students had used Ritalin in the past year.

Methamphetamine An increasingly common form of amphetamine, **methamphetamine (meth)** is a

Amphetamines A large and varied group of synthetic agents that stimulate the central nervous system.

Methamphetamine (meth) A powerfully addictive drug that strongly activates certain areas of the brain and affects the central nervous system.

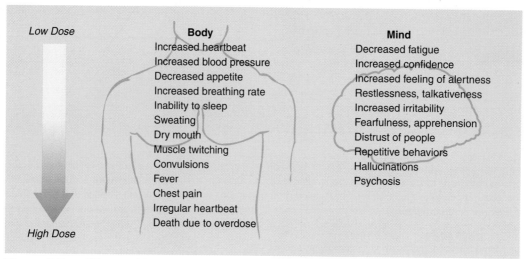

Figure 7.5 ■ Effects of Amphetamines on the Body and Mind

potent, long-acting, addictive drug that strongly activates the brain's reward center by producing a sense of euphoria. Meth can cause brain damage that results in impaired motor skills and cognitive functions, psychosis, and increased risk for heart attack and stroke.

Methods of Methamphetamine Use Methamphetamine can be snorted, smoked, injected, or orally ingested. Depending on the method of use, the drug will affect the user in different ways. Users often experience tolerance immediately, making meth a highly addictive drug from the very first time it is used. When snorted, the effects can be felt in 3 to 5 minutes; if orally ingested, the user will experience effects within 15 to 20 minutes. The pleasurable effects of meth are typically an intense rush lasting only a few minutes when snorted; in contrast, smoking the drug can produce a high lasting over 8 hours.

Physical Effects of Methamphetamine As shown in Figure 7.5, smaller doses of methamphetamine produce increased physical activity, alertness, and a decreased appetite. However, the drug's effects quickly wear off, and the user seeks more. Long-term use of meth can cause severe dependence, psychosis, paranoia, aggression, weight loss, and stroke. Abusers often do not sleep or eat for days, as they continually inject up to 1 gram of the drug every 2 to 3 hours. A high state of irritability and agitation has been associated with violent behavior among some users.

Ice A potent, inexpensive methamphetamine that has long-lasting effects.

Marijuana Chopped leaves and flowers of the *Cannabis indica* or *Cannabis sativa* plant (hemp); a psychoactive stimulant that intensifies reactions to environmental stimuli.

Abuse of meth is an increasingly serious problem, especially in more rural areas of the United States, Hawaii, and the West Coast. In 2004, 6.2 percent of high school seniors reported using meth. Rates among adults are difficult to determine, but it is believed that over 12 million Americans have tried it.[22] A possible contributing factor to the increasing rate of meth use is that it is relatively easy to make. Meth is produced by "cookers" using recipes that often include common over-the-counter ingredients such as ephedrine and pseudoephedrine, found in cold and allergy medication. Many states have taken action by moving all cold and allergy medication behind the pharmacist's counter, so high volume buyers can be carefully monitored. Additionally, laws have strengthened the penalties associated with manufacturing meth.

Ice is a potent form of methamphetamine that is imported primarily from Asia, particularly from South Korea and Taiwan. It is purer and more crystalline than the version manufactured in many large U.S. cities and is odorless when smoked. Ice is usually smoked, and its effects can last for more than 12 hours.

Like other methamphetamines, the "down" side of this drug is devastating. Prolonged use can cause fatal lung and kidney damage, as well as long-lasting psychological damage. In some instances, major psychological dysfunction can persist as long as two and a half years after last use.

Marijuana

Although archaeological evidence documents the use of **marijuana** (grass, weed, pot) as far back as 6,000 years, the drug did not become popular in the United States until the 1960s. Today marijuana is the most commonly used illegal drug in the United States. Nearly one of every three Americans over the age of 12 has tried marijuana at least once. Some 12 million Americans have used it; more than 1 million cannot control their use of it. Its use is also on the rise on college campuses, following the trend of increased use set by the general population.[23]

Physical Effects of Marijuana

Marijuana is derived from either the *Cannabis sativa* or *Cannabis indica* (hemp) plants. Current American-grown marijuana is a turbocharged version of the hippie weed of the late 1960s. Developed using crossbreeding, genetic engineering, and American farming ingenuity, top-grade cannabis packs a punch very similar to that of hashish. **Tetrahydrocannabinol (THC)** is the psychoactive substance in marijuana and the key to determining how powerful a high it will produce. Whereas a marijuana cigarette three decades ago averaged 10 milligrams (mg) of THC, a current cigarette may contain around 150 mg of THC. Thus the modern-day marijuana user may be exposed to doses of THC many times greater than were users in the 1960s and 1970s.[24]

Hashish, a potent cannabis preparation derived mainly from the thick, sticky resin of the plant, contains high concentrations of THC. Hash oil, a substance produced by percolating a solvent such as ether through dried marijuana to extract the THC, is a tarlike liquid that may contain up to 300 mg of THC in a dose.

Most of the time, marijuana is rolled into cigarettes (joints) or smoked in a pipe or water pipe (bong). Effects generally are felt within 10 to 30 minutes and usually wear off within 3 hours.

The most noticeable effect of THC is the dilation of blood vessels that produces the characteristic bloodshot eyes. Smokers of the drug also exhibit coughing, dry mouth and throat ("cotton mouth"), increased thirst and appetite, lowered blood pressure, and mild muscular weakness primarily exhibited in drooping eyelids. Users also can experience severe anxiety, panic, paranoia, and psychosis, as well as intensified reactions to various stimuli. Colors and sounds, as well as the speed at which things move, may seem magnified. High doses of hashish may produce vivid visual hallucinations.

Effects of Chronic Marijuana Use

Because marijuana is illegal in most parts of the United States and has been widely used only since the 1960s, long-term studies of its effects have been difficult to conduct. Also, studies conducted in the 1960s involved marijuana with THC levels constituting only a fraction of today's plant levels, so their results may not apply to the stronger forms available today.

> Are there any negative long-term effects from marijuana use?

Most current information about chronic marijuana use comes from countries such as Jamaica and Costa Rica, where the drug is not illegal. These studies of long-term users (for 10 or more years) indicate that it causes lung damage comparable to that caused by

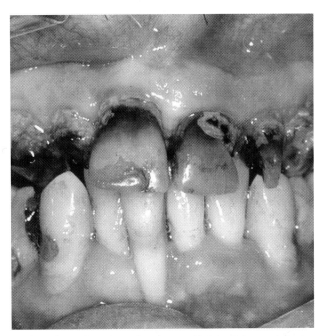

Methamphetamine users often damage their teeth beyond repair, due to the toxic chemicals in the substance. This condition is commonly referred to as "meth" mouth.

tobacco smoking. Indeed, smoking a single joint may be as bad for the lungs as smoking three tobacco cigarettes. Inhalation of marijuana transfers carbon monoxide to the bloodstream. Because the blood has a greater affinity for carbon monoxide than it does for oxygen, this diminishes the oxygen-carrying capacity of the blood. The heart must work harder to pump the vital element to oxygen-starved tissues. Furthermore, the cannabis tar contains higher levels of carcinogens than does tobacco smoke. Smoking marijuana results in three times as much tar inhalation and retention in the respiratory tract than tobacco use.[25]

Other risks associated with marijuana include suppression of the immune system, blood pressure changes, and impaired memory function. Recent studies suggest that pregnant women who smoke marijuana are at a higher risk for stillbirth or miscarriage and for delivering low–birth weight babies and babies with abnormalities of the nervous system. Babies born to marijuana smokers are five times more likely to have features similar to those exhibited by children with fetal alcohol syndrome.[26]

Debates concerning the effects of marijuana on the reproductive system have yet to be resolved. Studies conducted in the mid-1970s suggested that marijuana inhibited testosterone (and thus sperm) production in

---

Tetrahydrocannabinol (THC)   The chemical name for the active ingredient in marijuana.

Hashish   The sticky resin of the cannabis plant, which is high in THC.

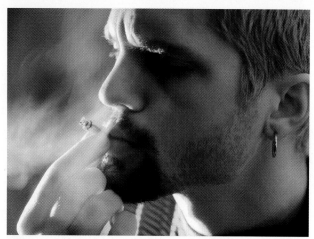

Marijuana is one of the most widely abused illegal substance on college campuses, next to cigarettes and alcohol.

males and caused chromosomal breakage in both ova and sperm. Subsequent research in these areas is inconclusive. The question of whether the high-level THC plants currently available will increase the risks associated with this drug is, as yet, unanswered.[27]

Marijuana and Medicine

Although recognized as a dangerous drug by the U.S. government, marijuana has several medical purposes. It helps control such side effects as the severe nausea and vomiting produced by chemotherapy, the chemical treatment for cancer. It improves appetite and forestalls the loss of lean muscle mass associated with AIDS-wasting syndrome. Marijuana reduces the muscle pain and spasticity caused by diseases such as multiple sclerosis. It also temporarily relieves the eye pressure of glaucoma, although it is unclear whether it is more effective than legal glaucoma drugs.[28] Marijuana's legal status for medicinal purposes continues to be hotly debated.

Marijuana and Driving

Marijuana use presents clear hazards for drivers of motor vehicles as well as others on the road. The drug substantially reduces a driver's ability to react and make quick decisions. Studies reveal that 60 to 80 percent of marijuana users sometimes drive while high.[29] Studies of automobile

accident victims show that 6 to 12 percent of nonfatally injured drivers and 4 to 16 percent of fatally injured drivers had THC in their bloodstreams. Perceptual and other performance deficits resulting from marijuana use may persist for some time after the high subsides. Users who attempt to drive, fly, or operate heavy machinery often fail to recognize their impairment.

What Do You Think?

Why do you think that marijuana is the most popular illicit drug on college campuses? ■ How widespread is marijuana use at your school?

Opiates

Opiates cause drowsiness, relieve pain, and induce euphoria. Also called **narcotics,** they are derived from the parent drug **opium,** a dark, resinous substance made from the milky juice of the opium poppy. Opiates include morphine, codeine, heroin, and black tar heroin.

The word *narcotic* comes from the Greek word for stupor and generally is used to describe sleep-inducing substances. Until the early twentieth century, many patent medicines contained opiates and were advertised as cures for everything from menstrual cramps to teething pains. More powerful than opium, **morphine** (named after Morpheus, the Greek god of sleep) was widely used as a painkiller during the Civil War. **Codeine,** a less powerful analgesic (pain reliever) derived from morphine, also became popular.

As opiates became more common, physicians noted that patients tended to become dependent on them. Growing concern about addiction led to government controls of narcotic use. The Harrison Act of 1914 prohibited the production, dispensation, and sale of opiate products unless prescribed by a physician. Subsequent legislation required physicians prescribing opiates to keep careful records. Physicians are still subject to audits of their prescriptions.

Some opiates are still used today for medical purposes. Morphine is sometimes prescribed for severe pain, and codeine is found in prescription cough syrups and other painkillers. Several prescription drugs, including Percodan, Vicodin, and Dilaudid, contain synthetic opiates. These drugs can be highly addictive and use is strictly regulated. OxyContin, an extremely powerful and long-acting opiate, is commonly abused and is treated as a substitute for heroin by some addicts.

Physical Effects of Opiates

Opiates are powerful depressants of the central nervous system. In addition to relieving pain, these drugs lower heart rate, respiration, and blood pressure. Side effects include weakness, dizziness, nausea, vomiting, euphoria, decreased sex drive, visual disturbances, and lack of

Narcotics   Drugs that induce sleep and relieve pain; primarily the opiates.

Opium   The parent drug of the opiates; made from the milky juice of the opium poppy.

Morphine   A derivative of opium; sometimes used by medical practitioners to relieve pain.

Codeine   A drug derived from morphine; used in cough syrups and certain painkillers.

coordination. Of all the opiates, heroin has the greatest notoriety as an addictive drug. The following section discusses the progression of heroin addiction; addiction to any opiate follows a similar path.

Heroin Addiction

Heroin is a white powder derived from morphine. **Black tar heroin** is a sticky, dark brown, foul-smelling form of heroin that is relatively pure and inexpensive. Once considered a cure for morphine dependency, heroin was later discovered to be even more addictive and potent than morphine. Today, heroin has no medical use.

An estimated 3.7 million people have used heroin at one time in their lives. The highest number of users are young adults, aged 26 or older.[30] Heroin can be snorted, injected, or smoked. Injection remains the most common route of administration; however, the contemporary version of heroin is so potent that users can get high by snorting or smoking the drug. This has attracted a more affluent group of users who may not want to inject, for reasons such as the increased risk of contracting diseases such as HIV.

Heroin is a depressant that produces drowsiness and a dreamy, mentally slow feeling. It can cause drastic mood swings, with euphoric highs followed by depressive lows. Heroin slows respiration and urinary output and constricts the pupils of the eyes. Symptoms of tolerance and withdrawal can appear within three weeks of first use.

The most common route of administration for heroin addicts is "mainlining"—intravenous injection of powdered heroin mixed in a solution. Many users describe the "rush" they feel when injecting themselves as intensely pleasurable, whereas others report unpredictable and unpleasant side effects. The temporary nature of the rush contributes to the drug's high potential for addiction—many addicts shoot up four or five times a day. Mainlining can cause veins to scar and eventually collapse. Once a vein has collapsed, it can no longer be used to introduce heroin into the bloodstream. Addicts become expert at locating new veins to use: in the feet, the legs, the temples, under the tongue, or in the groin.

The physiology of the human body could be said to encourage opiate addiction. Opiate-like substances called **endorphins** are manufactured in the body and have multiple receptor sites, particularly in the central nervous system. When endorphins attach at these points, they create feelings of painless well-being. Medical researchers refer to them as "the body's own opiates." When endorphin levels are high, people feel euphoric. The same euphoria occurs when opiates or related chemicals are active at the endorphin receptor sites.

Treatment for Opiate Addiction

Programs to help heroin addicts and those addicted to other opiates, such as OxyContin or morphine, kick the habit have not been very successful. Some addicts resume drug use even after years of drug-free living because the craving for the injection rush is very strong. It takes a great deal of discipline to seek alternative nondrug highs.

Heroin addicts experience a distinct pattern of withdrawal. Symptoms of withdrawal include intense desire for the drug, sleep disturbance, dilated pupils, loss of appetite, irritability, goose bumps, and muscle tremors. The most difficult time in the withdrawal process occurs 24 to 72 hours following last use. All of the preceding symptoms continue, along with nausea, abdominal cramps, restlessness, insomnia, vomiting, diarrhea, extreme anxiety, hot and cold flashes, elevated blood pressure, and rapid heartbeat and respiration. Once the peak of withdrawal has passed, all these symptoms begin to subside. Still, the recovering addict has many hurdles to jump.

Methadone maintenance is one treatment available for people addicted to heroin or other opiates. Methadone is a synthetic narcotic that blocks the effects of opiate withdrawal. It is chemically similar enough to the opiates to control the tremors, chills, vomiting, diarrhea, and severe abdominal pains of withdrawal. Methadone dosage is decreased over a period of time until the addict is weaned off the drug.

Methadone maintenance is controversial because of the drug's own potential for addiction. Critics contend that the program merely substitutes one addiction for another. Proponents argue that people on methadone maintenance are less likely to engage in criminal activities to support their habits than heroin addicts are. For this reason, many methadone maintenance programs are financed by state or federal government and are available free of charge or at reduced cost.

A number of new drug therapies for opiate dependence are emerging. Most recently, researchers have reported promising results with buprenorphine (Temgesic), a mild, nonaddicting synthetic opiate that, like heroin and methadone, bonds to certain receptors in the brain, blocks pain messages, and persuades the brain that its cravings for heroin have been satisfied. Addicts report that while they are taking buprenorphine, they do not crave heroin anymore.

Heroin   An illegally manufactured derivative of morphine, usually injected into the bloodstream.

Black tar heroin   A dark brown, sticky form of heroin.

Endorphins   Opiate-like hormones that are manufactured in the human body and contribute to natural feelings of well-being.

Methadone maintenance   A treatment for people addicted to opiates that substitutes methadone, a synthetic narcotic, for the opiate of addiction.

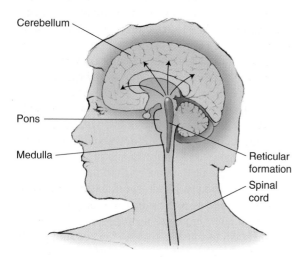

Figure 7.6 ■ Reticular Formation

Hallucinogens (Psychedelics)

Hallucinogens are substances that are capable of creating auditory or visual hallucinations. These drugs are also known as **psychedelics**, a term adapted from the Greek phrase meaning mind-manifesting. Hallucinogens alter a user's feelings, perceptions, and thoughts. The major receptor sites for most of these drugs are located in the brain region that is responsible for interpreting outside stimuli before these signals travel to other parts of the brain. This area, the **reticular formation**, lies in the brain stem at the upper end of the spinal cord (Figure 7.6). When a hallucinogen is present at a reticular formation site, messages become scrambled, and the user may see wavy walls instead of straight ones or may smell colors and hear tastes. This mixing of sensory messages is known as **synesthesia**.

The most widely recognized hallucinogens are LSD, mescaline, psilocybin, and PCP. All are illegal and carry severe penalties for manufacture, possession, transportation, or sale.

Hallucinogens   Substances capable of creating hallucinations.

Psychedelics   Drugs that distort the processing of sensory information in the brain.

Reticular formation   An area in the brain stem that is responsible for relaying messages to other areas in the brain.

Synesthesia   A (usually) drug-created effect in which sensory messages are incorrectly assigned—for example, hearing a taste or smelling a sound.

Lysergic acid diethylamide (LSD)   Psychedelic drug causing sensory disruptions; also called acid.

LSD   Of all the psychedelics, **lysergic acid diethylamide (LSD)** is the most notorious. First synthesized in the late 1930s by Swiss chemist Albert Hoffman, LSD resulted from experiments to derive medically useful drugs from the ergot fungus found on rye and other cereal grains. Because LSD seemed capable of unlocking the secrets of the mind, psychiatrists initially felt it could be beneficial to patients unable to remember suppressed traumas. From 1950 through 1968, the drug was used for such purposes.

Media attention focused on LSD in the 1960s. Young people used the drug to "turn on" and "tune out" the world that gave them the war in Vietnam, race riots, and political assassinations. In 1970, federal authorities, under intense pressure from the public, placed LSD on the list of controlled substances (Schedule I). LSD's popularity peaked in 1972 then tapered off, primarily because of users' inability to control dosages accurately.

Because of the recent wave of nostalgia for the 1960s, this dangerous psychedelic drug, known on the street as "acid," has been making a comeback. Over 11 million Americans, most of them under age 35, have tried LSD at least once. LSD especially attracts younger users. A national survey of college students showed that 2 percent had used the drug in the past year.[31]

The most common and most popular form of LSD is blotter acid—small squares of blotter-like paper that have been impregnated with a liquid LSD mixture. The blotter is swallowed or chewed briefly. LSD also comes in tiny thin squares of gelatin called windowpane and in tablets called microdots, which are less than an eighth of an inch across (it would take 10 or more to add up to the size of an aspirin tablet). As with any illegal drug, purchasers run the risk of buying an impure product.

One of the most powerful drugs known to science, LSD can produce strong effects in doses as low as 20 micrograms. (To give you an idea of how small a dose this is, the average postage stamp weighs approximately 60,000 micrograms.) The potency of the typical dose currently ranges from 20 to 80 micrograms, compared to 150 to 300 micrograms commonly used in the 1960s.

Despite its reputation as primarily a psychedelic, LSD produces a number of physical effects, including increased heart rate, elevated blood pressure and temperature, goose flesh (roughened skin), increased reflex speeds, muscle tremors and twitches, perspiration, increased salivation, chills, headaches, and mild nausea. Since the drug also stimulates uterine muscle contractions, it can lead to premature labor and miscarriage in pregnant women. Research into long-term effects has been inconclusive.

The psychological effects of LSD vary. Euphoria is the common psychological state produced by the drug, but *dysphoria* (a sense of evil and foreboding) may also be experienced. The drug also shortens attention span, causing the mind to wander. Thoughts may be interposed and juxtaposed, so the user experiences several different thoughts simultaneously. Synesthesia occurs occasionally. Users become introspective and suppressed memories may surface, often taking on bizarre symbolism. Many more effects are possible, including decreased aggressiveness and enhanced sensory experiences.

Although LSD rarely produces hallucinations, it can create illusions. These distortions of ordinary perceptions may include movement of stationary objects. "Bad trips," the most publicized risk of LSD, are commonly related to the user's mood. The person, for example, may interpret increased heart rate as a heart attack (a "bad body trip"). Often bad trips result when a user confronts a suppressed emotional experience or memory (a "bad head trip").

While there is no evidence that LSD creates physical dependency, it may well create psychological dependence. Many LSD users become depressed for one or two days following a trip and turn to the drug to relieve this depression. The result is a cycle of LSD use to relieve post-LSD depression, which often leads to psychological addiction.

What Do You Think? Are people today using LSD for the same reasons they did in the 1960s? ▩ What are the perceived attractions and the real dangers of LSD?

Mescaline **Mescaline** is one of hundreds of chemicals derived from the **peyote** cactus, a small cactus that grows in the southwestern United States and parts of Latin America. Natives of these regions have long used dried peyote "buttons" for religious purposes. In fact, members of the Native American Church (a religion practiced by thousands of North American Indians) have been granted special permission to use the drug during religious ceremonies in some states.

Users typically swallow 10 to 12 buttons. They taste bitter and generally induce immediate nausea or vomiting. Long-time users claim that the nausea becomes less noticeable with frequent use. Those who are able to keep the drug down begin to feel the effects within 30 to 90 minutes, when mescaline reaches maximum concentration in the brain. (It may persist for up to 9 or 10 hours.) Unlike LSD, mescaline is a powerful hallucinogen. It is also a central nervous system stimulant.

Products sold on the street as mescaline are likely to be synthetic chemical relatives of the true drug. Street names of these products include DOM, STP, TMA, and MMDA. Any of these can be toxic in small quantities.

Psilocybin **Psilocybin** and *psilocin* are the active chemicals in a group of mushrooms sometimes called magic mushrooms. Psilocybe mushrooms, which grow throughout the world, can be cultivated from spores or harvested wild. Because many mushrooms resemble the psilocybe variety, people who harvest wild mushrooms for any purpose should be certain of what they are doing. Mushroom varieties can be easily misidentified, and mistakes can be fatal. Psilocybin is similar to LSD in its physical effects, which generally wear off in 4 to 6 hours.

PCP **Phencyclidine**, or **PCP**, is a synthetic substance that became a black-market drug in the early 1970s. PCP was originally developed as a dissociative anesthetic, which means that patients administered this drug could keep their eyes open and apparently remain conscious but feel no pain during a medical procedure. Afterward, patients would experience amnesia for the time the drug was in their system. Such a drug had obvious advantages as an anesthetic, but its unpredictability and drastic effects (postoperative delirium, confusion, and agitation) made doctors abandon it, and it was withdrawn from the legal market.

On the illegal market, PCP is a white, crystalline powder that users often sprinkle onto marijuana cigarettes. It is dangerous and unpredictable regardless of the method of administration. Common street names for PCP are "angel dust" for the crystalline powdered form and "peace pill" and "horse tranquilizer" for the tablet form.

The effects of PCP depend on the dosage. A dose as small as 5 mg will produce effects similar to those of strong central nervous system depressants—slurred speech, impaired coordination, reduced sensitivity to pain, and reduced heart and respiratory rate. Doses between 5 and 10 mg cause fever, salivation, nausea, vomiting, and total loss of sensitivity to pain. Doses greater than 10 mg result in a drastic drop in blood pressure, coma, muscular rigidity, violent outbursts, and possible convulsions and death.

Psychologically, PCP may produce either euphoria or dysphoria. It also is known to produce hallucinations as well as delusions and overall delirium. Some users

Mescaline A hallucinogenic drug derived from the peyote cactus.

Peyote A cactus with small "buttons" that, when ingested, produce hallucinogenic effects.

Psilocybin An active chemical found in psilocybe mushrooms; it produces hallucinations.

Phencyclidine (PCP) A hallucinogen commonly called angel dust.

experience a prolonged state of nothingness. The long-term effects of PCP use are unknown.

Designer Drugs (Club Drugs)

Designer drugs are synthetic drugs that produce effects similar to existing illegal drugs. They are manufactured in chemical laboratories and homes and sold illegally. These drugs are easy to produce from available raw materials. The drugs themselves were once technically legal because the law had to specify the exact chemical structure of an illicit substance. However, a law is now in place that bans all chemical cousins of illegal drugs.

Collectively known as **club drugs**, these dangerous substances include Ecstasy, gamma-hydroxybutyrate (GHB), Special K (Ketamine), and Rohypnol. Although users may think them harmless, research has shown that club drugs can produce a range of unwanted effects, including hallucinations, paranoia, amnesia, and in some cases, death. Some club drugs work on the same brain mechanisms as alcohol and can dangerously boost the effects of both substances. Since the drugs are odorless and tasteless, people can easily slip them into drinks. Some of them have been associated with sexual assault and for that reason are referred to as "date rape drugs" (see the Reality Check box in Chapter 4).

Ecstasy (methylene dioxymethamphetamine, or MDMA) use has been reported by almost one of every four students at some universities. Ecstasy creates feelings of openness and warmth, combined with the mind-expanding characteristics of hallucinogens. Effects begin within 30 minutes and can last for 4 to 6 hours. Young people may use Ecstasy initially to improve mood or get energized so they can keep dancing; it also increases heart rate and blood pressure and may raise body temperature to the point of kidney and/or cardio-vascular failure. Chronic use appears to damage the brain's ability to think and regulate emotion, memory, sleep, and pain. Combined with alcohol, Ecstasy can be extremely dangerous and sometimes fatal. Recent studies indicate that Ecstasy may cause long-lasting neurotoxic effects by damaging brain cells that produce serotonin, and it is unknown whether these brain cells will regenerate.[32] For more on the effects of other club drugs, see the Reality Check box.

Inhalants

Inhalants are chemicals that produce vapors that, when inhaled, can cause hallucinations and create intoxicating and euphoric effects. Not commonly recognized as drugs, inhalants are legal to purchase and universally available but dangerous when used incorrectly. They generally appeal to young people who can't afford or obtain illicit substances. Some products often misused as inhalants include rubber cement, model glue, paint thinner, lighter fluid, varnish, wax, spot removers, and gasoline. Most of these substances are sniffed or "huffed" by users in search of a quick, cheap high.

Because they are inhaled, the volatile chemicals in these products reach the bloodstream within seconds. An inhaled substance is not diluted or buffered by stomach acids or other body fluids and thus is more potent than it would be if swallowed. This characteristic, along with the fact that dosages are extremely difficult to control because everyone has unique lung and breathing capacities, makes inhalants particularly dangerous.

The effects of inhalants usually last fewer than 15 minutes and resemble those of central nervous system depressants. Combining inhalants with alcohol produces a synergistic effect and can cause severe liver damage that can be fatal. Users may experience dizziness, disorientation, impaired coordination, reduced judgment, and slowed reaction times.

An overdose of fumes from inhalants can cause unconsciousness. If the user's oxygen intake is reduced during the inhaling process, death can result within five minutes. Whether a user is a first-time or chronic user, sudden sniffing death (SSD) syndrome can be a fatal consequence. This syndrome can occur if a user inhales deeply and then participates in physical activity or is startled.

Amyl Nitrite Sometimes called "poppers" or "rush," **amyl nitrite** is packaged in small, cloth-covered glass capsules that can be crushed to release the active chemical. They tend to be abused by adults, often in an attempt to enhance sexual function. The drug dilates small blood vessels and reduces blood pressure. Dilation of blood vessels in the genital area is thought to enhance sensations or perceptions of orgasm. It also produces fainting, dizziness, warmth, and skin flushing.

Nitrous Oxide **Nitrous oxide** is sometimes used as an adjunct to dental anesthesia or minor surgical anesthesia. It is also a propellant chemical in aerosol

---

Designer drug (club drug) A synthetic analog (a drug that produces similar effects) of an existing illicit drug.

Ecstasy A club drug that creates feelings of openness and warmth but also raises heart rate and blood pressure.

Inhalants Products that are sniffed or inhaled in order to produce highs.

Amyl nitrite A drug that dilates blood vessels and is properly used to relieve chest pain.

Nitrous oxide The chemical name for laughing gas, a substance properly used for surgical or dental anesthesia.

Every era seems to have its hot drug. At one point it was Valium, then LSD, and then crack. Currently the so-called club drugs are popular on college campuses. Three of note include Rohypnol (flunitrazepam), also called "ropies" or "roofies"; GHB (gamma-hydroxybutyrate), or as it is known on the street, "grievous bodily harm"; and Special K (ketamine).

Rohypnol is a potent tranquilizer similar in nature to Valium but many times stronger. The drug produces a sedative effect, amnesia, muscle relaxation, and slowed psychomotor responses. Commonly known as the "date rape" drug, Rohypnol has gained notoriety as a growing problem on college campuses. The drug has been added to punch and other drinks at fraternity parties and college social gatherings, where it is reportedly given to female partiers in hopes of lowering their inhibitions and facilitating potential sexual conquests. The manufacturer changed the formula to give the drug a bright blue color that would make it easy to detect in most drinks, so would-be perpetrators are turning to blue tropical drinks and punches to disguise the drug. While "ropie" fervor has subsided somewhat, it continues to be a concern. See the Reality Check box in Chapter 4 on strategies to protect yourself from being dosed with Rohypnol.

Rohypnol has been joined by a newer, liquid substance called GHB, or gamma-hydroxybutyrate. GHB is used as an aphrodisiac to increase one's sense of touch and sexual prowess, as a muscle builder, and as a tranquilizer. GHB is an odorless, tasteless fluid that can be made easily at home or in a chemistry lab. Like Rohypnol, it has been slipped into drinks without being detected, resulting in loss of memory, unconsciousness, amnesia, and even death. Other side effects of GHB include nausea, vomiting, seizures, memory loss, hallucinations, coma, and respiratory distress. During the 1980s, GHB was available in U.S. health food stores. Concerns about its use led the FDA to ban OTC sales in 1990, and GHB is now a Schedule I controlled substance.

The Special K we're referring to is not the breakfast cereal, but rather ketamine, used as an anesthetic in many hospital and veterinary clinics. On the street, Special K is most often diverted in liquid form from veterinary offices or medical suppliers. Dealers dry the liquid (usually by cooking it) and grind the residue into powder. Special K causes hallucinations by inhibiting the relay of sensory input; the brain fills

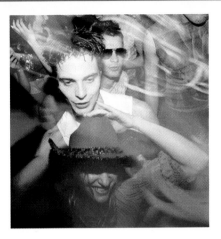

the resulting void with visions, dreams, memories, and sensory distortions. The effects of Special K are not as severe as those of Ecstasy, so it has grown in popularity among people who have to go to work or school after a night of partying.

Sources: U.S. Department of Health and Human Services, "Ketamine: A Fact Sheet," 2004, www.health.org/nongovpubs/ketamine; Office of National Drug Control Policy, "Rohypnol Fact Sheet," February 2003; Office of National Drug Control Policy, "Gamma-Hydroxybutyrate (GHB) Fact Sheet," November 2002; T. Nordenberg, "The Death of the Party: All the Rave, GHB's Hazards Go Unheeded," *FDA Consumer Magazine* (March–April 2000), www.fda.gov/fdac/features/2000/200-ghb.html.

---

products such as whipped toppings. Users experience a state of euphoria, floating sensations, and illusions. Effects also include pain relief and a silly feeling demonstrated by laughing and giggling (hence its nickname, laughing gas). Regulating dosages of this drug can be difficult. Sustained inhalation can lead to unconsciousness, coma, and death.

Steroids

Public awareness of **anabolic steroids** recently has been heightened by media stories about their use by amateur and professional athletes, especially in major league baseball. Anabolic steroids are artificial forms of the male hormone testosterone that promote muscle

growth and strength. These **ergogenic drugs** are used primarily by young men who believe the drugs will increase their strength, power, bulk (weight), speed, and athletic performance.

Most steroids are obtained through the black market. It was once estimated that approximately 17 to 20 percent of college athletes used them. Now that stricter drug-testing policies have been instituted by the

> **Anabolic steroids**   Artificial forms of the hormone testosterone that promote muscle growth and strength.
>
> **Ergogenic drugs**   Substances that enhance athletic performance.

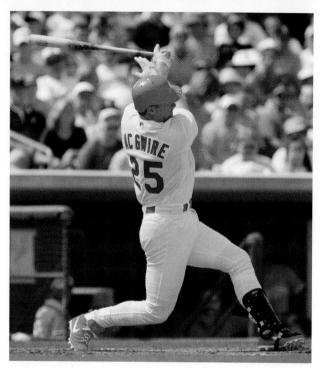

In March 2005, major league baseball players, such as Mark McGwire, were subpoened to testify before Congress on the use of steroids in the sport. McGwire has admitted to the use of the hormonal supplement, andro, in the past.

National Collegiate Athletic Association (NCAA), reported use of anabolic steroids among intercollegiate athletes has dropped to 1.1 percent. However, a recent survey among high school students found a significant increase in the use of anabolic steroids since 1991. Few data exist on the extent of steroid abuse by adults; it has been estimated that hundreds of thousands of people aged 18 and older abuse anabolic steroids at least once a year. Among both adolescents and adults, steroid abuse is higher among males than females. However, steroid abuse is growing most rapidly among young women.[33]

Steroids are available in two forms: injectable solutions and pills. Anabolic steroids produce a state of euphoria, diminished fatigue, and increased bulk and power in both sexes. These qualities give steroids an addictive quality. When users stop, they can experience psychological withdrawal and sometimes severe depression, in some cases leading to suicide attempts. If untreated, depression associated with steroid withdrawal has been known to last for a year or more after steroid use stops.

Men and women who use steroids experience a variety of adverse effects. These drugs cause mood swings (aggression and violence), sometimes known as "roid rage"; acne; liver tumors; elevated cholesterol levels; hypertension; kidney disease; and immune system disturbances. There is also a danger of transmitting AIDS

and hepatitis (a serious liver disease) through shared needles. In women, large doses of anabolic steroids may trigger the development of masculine attributes such as lowered voice, increased facial and body hair, and male pattern baldness; they may also result in an enlarged clitoris, smaller breasts, and changes in or absence of menstruation. When taken by healthy males, anabolic steroids shut down the body's production of testosterone, causing men's breasts to grow and testicles to atrophy.

To combat the growing problem of steroid use, Congress passed the Anabolic Steroids Control Act (ASCA) of 1990. This law makes it a crime to possess, prescribe, or distribute anabolic steroids for any use other than the treatment of specific diseases. Anabolic steroids are now classified as a Schedule III drug. Penalties for their illegal use include up to 5 years' imprisonment and a $250,000 fine for the first offense and up to 10 years' imprisonment and a $500,000 fine for subsequent offenses.

A new and alarming trend is the use of other drugs to achieve the effects of steroids. The two most common steroid alternatives are GHB and clenbuterol. GHB is a deadly, illegal drug that is a primary ingredient in many "performance-enhancing" formulas. GHB does not produce a high but does cause headaches, nausea, vomiting, diarrhea, seizures, and other central nervous system disorders, and possibly death. Clenbuterol is used in some countries for veterinary treatments but is not approved for any use—in animals or humans—in the United States.

New attention was drawn to the issue of steroids and related substances when St. Louis Cardinals slugger Mark McGwire admitted to using a supplement containing androstenedione (andro), an adrenal hormone that is produced naturally in both men and women. Andro raises levels of the male hormone testosterone, which helps build lean muscle mass and promotes quicker recovery after injury. McGwire had done nothing illegal, as the supplement could be purchased over the counter (with sales estimated at up to $800 million a year) and at that time its use was legal in baseball, although banned by the NFL, NCAA, and International Olympic Committee. A recent study found that when men take 100 milligrams of andro three times daily, it increases estrogen levels by up to 80 percent, enlarges the prostate gland, and increases heart disease risk by 10 to 15 percent. Major league baseball banned its use in 2004.

Visits to the locker rooms of many sports teams would disclose large containers of other alleged muscle-building supplements, such as creatine. Although they are legal, questions remain whether enough research has been done concerning the safety of these supplements. Some experts worry that they may bring consequences similar to those of steroids, such as liver damage and heart problems.

ILLEGAL DRUG USE IN THE UNITED STATES

Stories of people who have tried illegal drugs, enjoyed them, and suffered no consequences may tempt you to try them yourself. You may tell yourself it's "just this once," convincing yourself that one-time use is harmless. Given the dangers surrounding these substances, however, you should think twice. The risks associated with drug use extend beyond the personal. The decision to try any illicit substance encourages illicit drug manufacture and transport, thus contributing to the national drug problem. The financial burden of illegal drug use on the U.S. economy is staggering, with an estimated economic cost of around $160 billion.[34] This estimate includes costs associated with substance abuse treatment and prevention, health care, reduced job productivity and lost earnings, and social consequences such as crime and social welfare.

In addition, roughly half of all expenditures to combat crime are related to illegal drugs. The burden of these costs is absorbed primarily by the government (46 percent), followed by those who abuse drugs and members of their households (44 percent). One study found that Americans spend $64 billion on illicit drugs annually. These numbers break down as follows: $35 billion on cocaine, $10 billion each on marijuana and heroin, and $5 billion on methamphetamines. This is eight times what the federal government spends on research for HIV/AIDS, cancer, and heart disease put together.[35]

Drugs in the Workplace

The National Institute of Drug Abuse (NIDA) estimates that 8.5 percent of all U.S. workers use dangerous drugs on the job at some time. With approximately 70 to 75 percent of drug users in the United States employed to some degree, the cost to American business soars into the billions of dollars annually.[36] These costs reflect reduced work performance and efficiency, lost productivity, absenteeism and turnover, increased use of health benefits, accidents, and indirect losses stemming from impaired judgment.

The highest rates of illicit drug use among workers exist in the construction, food preparation, restaurant, transportation, and material-moving industries. Workers who require a considerable amount of public trust, such as police officers, teachers, and child care workers, report the lowest use. In addition, younger employees (18–24 years old) are more likely to report drug use than employees aged 25 and older. Drug users are 1.6 times more likely than nonusers to quit their jobs or be fired and 1.5 times more likely to be disciplined by their supervisor.[37]

Many companies have instituted drug testing for their employees. Mandatory drug urinalysis is controversial. Critics argue that such testing violates Fourth Amendment rights of protection from unreasonable search and seizure. Proponents believe the personal inconvenience entailed in testing pales in comparison to the problems caused by drug use in the workplace. Several court decisions have affirmed the right of employers to test their employees for drug use. They contend that Fourth Amendment rights pertain only to employees of government agencies, not to those of private businesses. Most Americans apparently support drug testing for certain types of jobs.

Is it legal for employers to require employees to take a drug test?

Drug testing is expensive, with costs running as high as $100 per test. Moreover, some critics question the accuracy and reliability of the results. Both false positives and false negatives can occur. As drug testing becomes more common in the work environment, it is gaining greater acceptance by employees, who see testing as a step to improving safety and productivity.

What Do You Think?

What do you believe are the moral and ethical issues surrounding drug testing? ■ Are you in favor of drug testing? ■ Should all employees be subjected to drug tests or just those in high-risk jobs? ■ Is it the employer's right to conduct drug testing at the worksite? Explain your answer.

Solutions to the Problem

Americans are alarmed by the increasing use of illegal drugs. Respondents in public opinion polls feel that the most important strategy for fighting drug abuse is educating young people. They also endorse strategies such as stricter border surveillance to reduce drug trafficking, longer prison sentences for drug dealers, increased government spending on prevention, enforcing antidrug laws, providing treatment assistance and greater cooperation between government agencies and private groups and individuals. All of these approaches will probably help up to a point, but they do not offer a complete solution. Drug abuse has been a part of human behavior for thousands of years and is not likely to disappear in the near future. For this reason, it is necessary to educate ourselves and develop the self-discipline necessary to avoid dangerous drug dependence.

For many years, the most popular antidrug strategies were total prohibition and "scare tactics." Both approaches proved ineffective. Prohibition of alcohol during the 1920s created more problems than it solved, as did prohibition of opiates in 1914. Outlawing other illicit drugs has neither eliminated them nor curtailed their traffic across U.S. borders.

In general, researchers in the field of drug education agree that a multimodal approach is best. Students should be taught the difference between drug use and abuse. Factual information that is free of scare tactics must be presented; lecturing and moralizing do not work. Emphasis should be placed on issues that are important to young people. Telling adolescent males that girls will find them disgusting if their breath stinks of cigarettes or pot will get their attention. Likewise, lecturing on the negative effects of drug use is a much less effective deterrent than teaching young people how to negotiate the social scene. The Drug Abuse Resistance Education, commonly called DARE, is one program intended to educate students but has been largely ineffective. Education efforts need to focus on achieving better outcomes for preventing drug use.

We must also study at-risk groups so we can better understand the circumstances that make them susceptible to drug use. Time, money, and effort by educators, parents, and policy makers are needed to ensure that today's youth receive the love and security essential for building productive and meaningful lives and rejecting drug use.

Taking Charge

Summary

- The six categories of drugs are prescription drugs, over-the-counter (OTC) drugs, recreational drugs, herbal preparations, illicit drugs, and commercial preparations. Administration routes include oral ingestion, injection (intravenous, intramuscular, and subcutaneous), inhalation, inunction, and suppositories.

- Prescription drugs are administered under medical supervision. There are dozens of categories, including antibiotics, sedatives, tranquilizers, and antidepressants. Generic drugs often can be substituted for more expensive brand-name products.

- OTC drug categories include analgesics; cold, cough, allergy, and asthma relievers; stimulants; sleeping aids and relaxants; and dieting aids. Exercise personal responsibility by reading directions for OTC drugs and asking your pharmacist or doctor if any special precautions are advised when taking these substances.

- Addiction is the continued involvement with a substance or activity despite ongoing negative consequences.

- People from all walks of life use illicit drugs, although college students report higher usage rates than does the general population. Drug use has declined since the mid-1980s.

- Controlled substances include cocaine and its derivatives, amphetamines, methamphetamine and ice, marijuana, opiates, hallucinogens/psychedelics , designer drugs, inhalants, and steroids. Users tend to become addicted quickly to such drugs.

- The drug problem reaches everyone through crime and elevated health care costs. Drugs are a major problem in the workplace; workplace drug testing is one proposed solution to this problem.

Chapter Review

1. Which of the following is an example of a recreational drug?
   a. alcohol
   b. Ativan
   c. acetaminophen
   d. analgesics

2. Antacid inhibits the absorption of aspirin and makes it less effective as a pain reliever. This drug interaction is called
   a. antagonism.
   b. inhibition.
   c. intolerance.
   d. cross-tolerance.

3. The nicotine patch is administered by
   a. inunction.
   b. injection.
   c. oral ingestion.
   d. intravenous injection.

4. Cross-tolerance occurs when
   a. drugs work at the same receptor site so that one blocks the action of the other.
   b. the effects of one drug are eliminated or reduced by the presence of another drug at the receptor site.
   c. a person develops a physiological tolerance to one drug and shows a similar tolerance to selected other drugs as a result.
   d. two or more drugs interact and the effects of the individual drugs are multiplied beyond what normally would be expected if they were taken alone.

5. What is the most common method of use for drug misusers?
   a. inunction
   b. injection
   c. oral ingestion
   d. intravenous injection

6. Rebecca takes a number of medications for various medical conditions, including Prinivil (an antihypertensive), insulin (a diabetic medication), and Claritin (an antihistamine). This is an example of
   a. synergism.
   b. illegal drug use.
   c. polydrug use.
   d. antagonism.

7. What drug schedule has the lowest potential for abuse?
   a. Schedule I
   b. Schedule II
   c. Schedule IV
   d. Schedule V

8. Prozac, Zoloft, and Paxil are among the most frequently prescribed
   a. antibiotics.
   b. sedatives.
   c. antidepressants.
   d. tranquilizers.

9. Drugs that are marketed by their chemical names rather than a brand name are called
   a. generic drugs.
   b. OTC drugs.
   c. recreational drugs.
   d. commercial drugs.

10. Rubber cement, model glue, spot removers, and gasoline are examples of
    a. depressants.
    b. inhalants.
    c. stimulants.
    d. psychedelics.

Answers to these questions can be found on page A-1.

Questions for Discussion and Reflection

1. What is the current theory that explains how drugs work in the body? Explain how this theory works.

2. Explain the terms *synergism, antagonism,* and *inhibition.*

3. What are the advantages and disadvantages associated with use of generic drugs?

4. Do you think there is such a thing as responsible use of illicit drugs? Would you change any of the current laws governing drugs? How would you determine what is legitimate use and illegitimate use?

5. Why do you think many people today feel that marijuana use is not dangerous? What are the arguments in favor of legalizing marijuana? What are the arguments against legalization? How common is the use of marijuana on your campus?

6. How do you and your peers feel about illicit drug use? Has your opinion changed in recent years? If so, how and why?

7. Debate the issue of workplace drug testing. Would you apply for a job that had drug testing as an interview requirement? As a continuing requirement?

8. What could you do to help a friend who is fighting a substance abuse problem? What resources on your campus could help you?

9. What types of programs do you think would be effective in preventing drug abuse among high school and college students? How would programs for high school students differ from those for college students?

10. Discuss how addiction affects family and friends. What role do family and friends play in helping the addict get help and maintain recovery?

Accessing Your Health on the Internet

The following websites explore further topics and issues related to personal health. For links to the websites below, visit the Companion Website for *Health: The Basics,* Seventh Edition at www.aw-bc.com/donatelle.

1. *Club Drugs.* A website that disseminates science-based information about club drugs.

2. *U.S. Food and Drug Administration (FDA).* The federal agency responsible for approving prescription and over-the-counter drugs, with information on product approvals, recalls, and more.

3. *Join Together.* An excellent site for the most current information related to substance abuse. Also includes information on gun violence and provides advice on organizing and taking political action.

4. *National Institute on Drug Abuse (NIDA).* The home page of this U.S. government agency has information on the latest statistics and findings in drug research.

5. *Substance Abuse and Mental Health Services Administration (SAMHSA).* Outstanding resource for information about national surveys, ongoing research, and national drug interventions.

Further Reading

Elster, J., ed. *Addiction: Entries and Exits.* New York: Russell Sage Foundation, 2000.

Addresses current addiction controversies from an international perspective, with authors from the United States and Norway. Topics include whether addicts have a choice in their behavior and current addiction theories.

Goldstein, A. *Addiction: From Biology to Drug Policy.* New York: Oxford University Press, 2001.

Discusses how drugs impact the brain, how each drug causes addiction, and how addictive drugs impact society. The author explains what we know about drug addiction, how we know what we know, and what we can and cannot do about the drug problem.

Greenburg, S. *2005 Physician's Desk Reference for Nonprescription Drugs and Dietary Supplements.* Montvale, NJ: Thomson Medical Economics, 2005.

Outlines proper uses, possible dangers, and effective ingredients of nonprescription medications.

Griffith, W. H., and S. Moore. *Complete Guide to Prescription and Nonprescription Drugs 2005.* New York: Perigee, 2004.

This essential guide answers every conceivable question about prescription and nonprescription drugs and contains information about dosages, side effects, precautions, interactions, and more. More than 5,000 brand-name and 800 generic drugs are profiled in an easy-to-use format.

West, J. W. *The Betty Ford Center Book of Answers: Help for Those Struggling with Substance Abuse and the People Who Love Them.* New York: Pocket Books, 1997.

Written by the former director of the Betty Ford Center, one of the leading alcohol and drug treatment centers in the United States. Provides answers to the most frequently asked questions about treatment and recovery; includes comprehensive coverage of drug abuse issues for addicts and their families.

References

1. Substance Abuse and Mental Health Services Administration, "Substance Abuse: A National Health Challenge," October 4, 2001, www.samhsa.gov/oas/oas.html.
2. Ibid.
3. P. Kittenger and D. Herron, "Patient Power: Over-the-Counter Drugs—Brief Analysis," National Center for Policy Analysis, 2005, www.ncpa.org/pub/ba/ba524.
4. M. First et al., *DMM-IV-TR: Handbook of Differential Diagnosis* (Arlington, VA: American Psychiatric Association, 2002).
5. H. F. Doweiko, *Concepts of Chemical Dependency* (Pacific Grove, CA: Brooks/Cole, 1993), 9.
6. C. Nakken, *The Addictive Personality* (Center City, MN: Hazelden, 1996), 24.
7. H. Verdoux et al., "Is Benzodiazepine Use a Risk Factor for Cognitive Decline and Dementia? A Literature Review of Epidemiological Studies," *Psychological Medicine* 35: 307–315.
8. P. Perraglia and R. Stafford, "Trends in Prescribing Selective Serotonin Reuptake Inhibitors and Other Newer Antidepressant Agents in Primary Care," *Journal of Clinical Psychiatry* 4, no. 5 (2003): 153–157.
9. J. Fershein and J. Gapher, "Increases in Prescription Drug Rates," *Health Affairs.*
10. National Institutes of Health, "The Management of Chronic Pain" (program announcement PA-01-115), 2004, www.grants.nih.gov.
11. J. Rowley et al., "Insomnia," June 17, 2004, www.emedicine.com/neuro/topic418.htm.
12. U.S. Food and Drug Administration, "Phenylpropanolamine (PPA) Information Page," 2002, www.fda.gov/cder/drug/infopage/ppa/default.htm.
13. U. S. Food and Drug Administration, "Sales of Supplements Containing Ephedrine Alkaloids Prohibited." April 12, 2004, www.fda.gov.
14. Ibid.
15. Ibid.
16. National Institute on Drug Abuse, "National Survey Results on Drug Use, 1975–2002: College Students and Adults," *Monitoring the Future* (2003), 227.
17. Ibid.
18. Office of National Drug Control Policy, "Drug Facts: Crack," www.whitehousedrugpolicy.gov/drugfact/crack, 2005.
19. M. Fisherman and C. Johanson, "Cocaine," in *Pharmacological Aspects of Drug Dependence: Towards an Integrated Neurobehavior Approach (Handbook of Experimental Pharmacology),* ed. C. Schuster and M. Kuhar (Hamburg: Springer Verlag, 1996): 159–195.
20. Ibid.
21. Substance Abuse and Mental Health Services Administration, *Results from the 2004 National Survey on Drug Use & Health: National Findings* (Rockville, MD: Office of Applied Studies, 2005).
22. L. D. Johnston et al., *Monitoring the Future National Survey Results on Drug Use, 1975–2004* (Bethesda, MD: National Institute on Drug Abuse and Mental Health Services Administration).
23. W. Compton et al., "Prevalence of Marijuana Use Disorders in the United States 2001–2002," *Journal of the American Medical Association,* 291: 2114–2121.
24. H. C. Ashton, "Pharmacology and Effects of Cannabis: A Brief Review," *British Journal of Psychiatry* 178, (2001): 101–106.
25. British Lung Foundation, "A Smoking Gun? The Impact of Cannabis Smoking on Respiratory Health" (London: British Lung Foundation, 2002).
26. American Pregnancy Association, "Using Illegal Drugs During Pregnancy: Marijuana," 2004, www. americanpregnancy.org.
27. Burkman et al., "Marijuana Impacts Sperm Function both in In-Vivo and In-Vitro: Semen Analysis From Men Smoking Marijuana" (conference American Society Reproduction Medicine)(San Antonio, TX: October, 2003), 11–15.
28. American Academy of Ophthalmology, Medical Library, "The Use of Marijuana in the Treatment of Glaucoma," 2003, www.medem.com.
29. R. Mathias, "Marijuana Impairs Driving-Related Skills and Workplace Performance," National Institute on Drug Abuse Notes 11, no. 1 (January/February 1996): 6.
30. National Institute on Drug Abuse, "Research Report Series on Heroin Abuse and Addiction" (Publication No. 05-4165), 2005.
31. Ibid.
32. "National Institute on Drug Abuse (NIDA), Launches Initiative to Combat Club Drugs," *NIDA Notes* 14, no. 2 (2000).
33. National Institute on Drug Abuse, "Anabolic Steroid Abuse," NIDA Research Report Series (Publication No. 00-3721)(Bethesda, MD: National Institute on Drug Abuse, 2000).
34. Office of National Drug Control Strategy, "2002 National Drug Control Strategy" 2002, www.whitehousedrugpolicy.gov.
35. Ibid.
36. National Institute on Drug Abuse, *Worker Drug Use and Workplace Policies and Programs: Results from the 1994 and 1997 National Household Survey on Drug Abuse* (Bethesda, MD: National Institute on Drug Abuse, 1999).
37. Ibid.

Aren't the majority of college students heavy drinkers?

Is secondhand smoke a risk to my health?

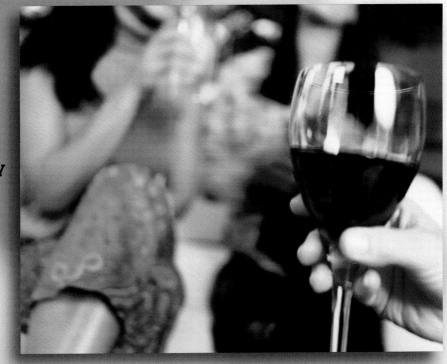

Is there any cure for a hangover?

Is caffeine really addictive?

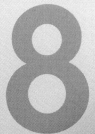

Alcohol, Tobacco, and Caffeine
Daily Pleasures, Daily Challenges

Objectives

- *Discuss* the alcohol use patterns of college students and overall trends in consumption.
- *Explain* the physiological and behavioral effects of alcohol, including blood alcohol concentration, absorption, metabolism, and immediate and long-term effects of alcohol consumption.
- *Explain* the symptoms and causes of alcoholism, its cost to society, effects on the family, and treatment options.

- *Discuss* the social and political issues involved in tobacco use.
- *Discuss* the health risks of smoking, smokeless tobacco, and environmental tobacco smoke, and how the chemicals in tobacco products affect the body.
- *Summarize* the benefits, risks, and long-term health consequences associated with caffeine use.

Usually the word *drug* conjures up images of people abusing illegal substances. We use the term to describe dangerous chemicals such as heroin or cocaine without recognizing that socially accepted substances can be drugs, too—for example, alcohol, tobacco, and caffeine.

ALCOHOL: AN OVERVIEW

Moderate use of alcohol can enhance celebrations and special times. Research shows that very low levels of use may actually decrease some health risks. However, always remember that alcohol is a chemical substance that affects your physical and mental behavior.

An estimated 65 percent of Americans consume alcoholic beverages regularly, though consumption patterns are unevenly distributed throughout the drinking population. Ten percent are heavy drinkers, and they account for half of all the alcohol consumed. The remaining 90 percent of the drinking population are infrequent, light, or moderate drinkers.

Alcohol and College Students

Alcohol is the most widely used (and abused) recreational drug in our society. It is also the most popular drug on college campuses, where approximately 90 percent of students report consuming alcoholic beverages in the last year.[1] About one-third of college students are classified as heavy drinkers, meaning that they consume over four or five drinks per drinking occasion. Therefore, students who might go out and drink only once a week are considered heavy drinkers if they consume a great deal of alcohol. In a new trend on college campuses, women's consumption of alcohol is close to equaling men's.

U.S. colleges and universities have been described as "alcohol-drenched institutions." Nearly 50 percent of all college students nationwide reported consuming four or five drinks during at 00least one occasion every 2 weeks.[2] However, fewer students are drinking alcohol than in the past. In 1980, 9.5 percent of students nationwide said they abstained from alcohol; recently 19 percent of students reported abstaining from alcohol use.[3] According to the University of Michigan's Institute for Social Research, the percentage of students who report drinking daily also has declined (from 6.5 percent in 1980 to 5 percent in 2003).[4]

College is a critical time to become aware of and responsible for drinking. There is little doubt that drinking is a part of campus culture and tradition. Many students may be away from home for the first time and are excited by their newfound independence. For some students, this independence and the rite of passage into the college culture are symbolized by the use of alcohol. It provides the answer to one of the most commonly heard

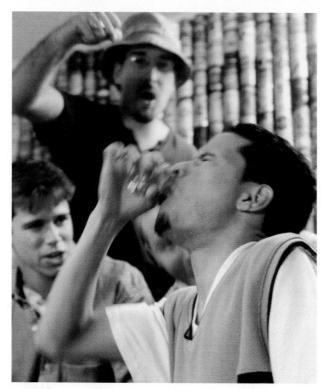

Deciding when and how much to drink is no simple matter. Irresponsible consumption of alcohol can easily result in disaster.

statements on any college campus: "There is nothing to do." Many students say they drink "to have fun," which often means drinking simply to get drunk and may really be a way of coping with stress, boredom, anxiety, or pressures created by academic and social demands.

Statistics about college students' drinking may not always reflect actual consumption. Students consistently report that their friends drink much more than they do and that average drinking within their own social living group is higher than actual self-reports. Such misinformation may promote or be used to excuse excessive drinking practices. In a survey of students at a large midwestern university, 42 percent reported not having a hangover in the past 6 months. Yet that same group of surveyed students believed that only 3 percent of their peers had not had a hangover in the past month.

Aren't the majority of college students heavy drinkers?

Many colleges are working to change misperceptions of normal drinking behavior. An example of such a "social norms" campaign is Oregon State University's Just the Facts program, which publicizes the fact that the majority of the university's students are responsible and moderate drinkers. Students at Oregon State are often surprised to learn that 87 percent of their peers have never driven a car while under the influence of alcohol and 89 percent have never passed out from drinking. Almost 90 percent have never performed poorly on

College Students' Patterns of Alcohol Use, 2001

Category	Total (%)	Men (%)	Women (%)
Abstainer (past year)	19.3	20.1	18.7
Nonbinge drinker	36.3	31.3	40.4
Occasional binge drinker	21.6	23.4	20.0
Frequent binge drinker	22.8	25.2	20.9

Alcohol-Related Problems

Problem Reported	Nonbinge Drinkers (%)	Frequent Binge Drinkers (%)
Did something regrettable	18	62
Missed a class	9	63
Forgot where they were or what they did	10	54
Got behind in schoolwork	10	46
Argued with friends	10	43
Got hurt or injured	4	27
Damaged property	2	23
Engaged in unplanned sexual activities	8	42
Drove after drinking	19	57

Sources: H. Wechsler et al., "Trends in College Binge Drinking during a Period of Increased Prevention Efforts: Findings from Four Harvard School of Public Health College Study Surveys: 1993–2001," *Journal of American College Health* 50, no. 5 (2002): 207; H. Wechsler et al., "College Binge Drinking in the 1990s: A Continuing Problem," *Journal of American College Health* 48 (2002): 207. Reprinted with permission of Helen Dwight Reid Educational Foundation. Published by Heldref Publications, 1319 18th St. NW, Washington, DC 20036. Copyright 2002.

a test or important project due to their alcohol use, and 77 percent have never missed a class because of drinking. Approximately 75 percent consume only zero to four drinks per week, and 60 percent had four or fewer drinks the last time they went to a party. Clearly there are many students who use alcohol responsibly and in moderation.

Binge Drinking and College Students

Binge drinking is defined as five drinks in a row by men and four in a row by women on a single occasion. The stakes of binge drinking are high because of the increased risk for alcohol-related injuries or death. According to a 2005 study, 1,700 college students die each year due to alcohol-related unintentional injuries, including car accidents. Binge drinking is the number one cause of preventable death among undergraduate college students in the United States today.[5]

How bad is the binge drinking problem? A recent study by the Harvard School of Public Health found that 44.8 percent of students were binge drinkers; of those, 22.8 percent were frequent bingers (people who binge drink three times or more in a two-week period).[6] (See Table 8.1.) Compared with nonbingers, frequent binge drinkers are 16 times more likely to miss class, 8 times more likely to get behind in their school work, and more apt to get into trouble with campus or local police.[7]

Although everyone is at some risk for alcohol-related problems, college students seem to be particularly vulnerable for the following reasons:

- Many university customs and traditions encourage dangerous practices and patterns of alcohol use.
- University campuses are heavily targeted by advertising and promotions from the alcoholic beverage industry.
- College students are particularly vulnerable to peer influence and have a strong need to be accepted by their peers.
- There is institutional denial by college administrators that alcohol problems exist on their campuses.

Binge drinking is especially dangerous because it often involves drinking a lot of alcohol in a very short period of time. This type of consumption can quickly lead to extreme intoxication including unconsciousness, alcohol poisoning, and even death. Often, drinking competitions or games, and hazing rituals encourage this type of drinking. See the Reality Check box on page 210 for more facts on campus drinking.

There is also significant evidence that campus rape is linked to binge drinking. Women from colleges with

> **Binge drinking** Drinking for the express purpose of becoming intoxicated; five drinks in a single sitting for men and four drinks in a sitting for women.

Perhaps you have heard conflicting reports in the media about the prevalence and effects of drinking on campus. What are the facts? The following statistics reveal the scope of the problem.

✓ Alcohol kills more people below age 21 than cocaine, marijuana, and heroin combined.

✓ Half a million students aged 15 to 24 are unintentionally injured each year while intoxicated.

✓ One night of heavy drinking can impair the ability to think abstractly for up to 30 days, limiting a student's ability to understand a professor's lecture or think through a football play.

✓ College administrators estimate that alcohol is a factor in 29 percent of dropouts, 38 percent of academic failures, and 64 percent of violent behaviors.

✓ Over the past decade, there has been a threefold increase in the number of college women who report having been drunk on 10 or more occasions in the previous month.

✓ Areas of a college campus offering cheap beer prices have more crime, including trouble between students and police or other campus authorities, arguments, physical fighting, property damage, false fire alarms, and sexual misconduct.

✓ Alcohol is involved in more than two-thirds of suicides among college students, 90 percent of campus rapes and sexual assaults, and 95 percent of violent crime on campus.

✓ The likelihood that a woman will be raped is far greater on campuses with a high rate of binge drinking.

✓ Each year, more than 100,000 students aged 18 to 24 report having been too intoxicated to know if they consented to having sex.

✓ College binge drinking occurs more often among male students, students who reside on campus, intercollegiate athletes, and members of fraternities and sororities. Approximately 40 percent of fraternity and sorority members report being frequent binge drinkers, and college athletes are 50 percent more likely to binge drink than nonathletes.

✓ Rates of binge drinking among high-risk students (younger, white males) are lower on more diverse college campuses. When high-risk students are together to the exclusion of other groups, there are fewer role models for lighter or nondrinking behavior.

✓ College students under the age of 21 are more prone to binge drinking and pay less for their alcohol than their older classmates do. Though underage students drink less often, they consume more per occasion than students aged 21 and older who are allowed to drink legally.

Sources: Data were compiled from the numerous studies cited throughout this chapter and from M. Mohler-Kuo et al., "College Rapes Linked to Binge-Drinking Rates," *Journal of Studies on Alcohol* 65, no. 1 (2004); H. Weschler, "Watering Down the Drinks: The Moderating Effect of College Demographics on Alcohol Use in High Risk Groups," *American Journal of Public Health* 93, no. 11 (2003): 1929–1933; T. F. Nelson et al., "Alcohol and Collegiate Sports Fans," *Addictive Behaviors* 28, no. 1 (2003): 1–11; R. W. Hingson et al., "Magnitude of Alcohol-Related Mortality and Morbidity among U.S. College Students Aged 18–24," *Journal of Studies on Alcohol* 63, no. 2 (2002): 136–144.

medium to high binge-drinking rates are 1.5 times more at risk of being raped than women from those schools with a low binge drinking rate; 72 percent of campus rapes occur when the victim is so intoxicated that she is unable to consent or refuse. For more on rape, see Chapter 4.[8]

Binge drinking also affects those who do not participate in binge drinking behavior. A 2005 study indicates that over 696,000 students aged 18 to 24 are assaulted by another student who has been drinking.[9] Other students report sleep and study disruptions, experiencing sexual abuse and other unwanted sexual advances, and vandalism of personal property.

In an attempt to curb binge drinking and alcohol abuse, many colleges and universities are instituting strong policies against drinking. University presidents have formed a leadership group to help curb the problem of alcohol abuse. Many fraternities have elected to have dry houses. At the same time, schools are making more help available to students with drinking problems. Today, both individual and group counseling are offered on most campuses, and more attention is directed toward the prevention of alcohol abuse. Student organizations such as BACCHUS (Boost Alcohol Consciousness Concerning the Health of University Students) promote responsible drinking and party hosting.

Try it ➤ NOW

Curb your drinking for better health! **Follow these steps today to reduce the amount of alcohol you drink: write down your reasons for cutting back on the amount you drink; choose a limit for the number of drinks you will consume each time you choose to drink; and keep a diary of your drinking habits for one month.**

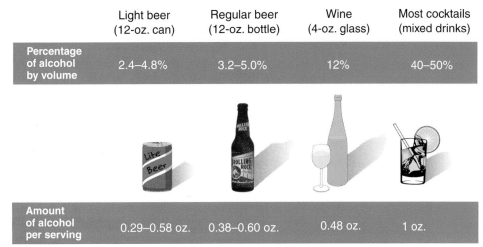

	Light beer (12-oz. can)	Regular beer (12-oz. bottle)	Wine (4-oz. glass)	Most cocktails (mixed drinks)
Percentage of alcohol by volume	2.4–4.8%	3.2–5.0%	12%	40–50%
Amount of alcohol per serving	0.29–0.58 oz.	0.38–0.60 oz.	0.48 oz.	1 oz.

Figure 8.1 ◾ Alcoholic Beverages and Their Alcohol Equivalencies

PHYSIOLOGICAL AND BEHAVIORAL EFFECTS OF ALCOHOL

The Chemical Makeup of Alcohol

The intoxicating substance found in beer, wine, liquor, and liqueurs is **ethyl alcohol,** or **ethanol**. It is produced during a process called **fermentation** in which yeast organisms break down plant sugars, yielding ethanol and carbon dioxide. Fermentation continues until the solution of plant sugars (called mash) reaches a concentration of 14 percent alcohol. For beers, ales, and wines, the process ends with fermentation. Manufacturers then add other ingredients that dilute the alcohol content of the beverage.

Hard liquor is produced through further processing called **distillation,** during which alcohol vapors are released from the mash at high temperatures. The vapors are then condensed and mixed with water to make the final product.

The **proof** of an alcoholic drink is a measure of the percentage of alcohol in the beverage and therefore the strength of the drink. Alcohol percentage is half of the given proof. For example, 80 proof whiskey or scotch is 40 percent alcohol by volume, and 100 proof vodka is 50 percent alcohol by volume. Lower-proof drinks will produce fewer alcohol effects than the same amount of higher-proof drinks will produce. Most wines are between 12 and 15 percent alcohol; ales are between 6 and 8 percent; and beers are between 2 and 6 percent, depending on state laws and type of beer (Figure 8.1).

Absorption and Metabolism

Unlike the molecules found in most foods and drugs, alcohol molecules are sufficiently small and fat-soluble to be absorbed throughout the entire gastrointestinal system. A negligible amount of alcohol is absorbed through the lining of the mouth. Approximately 20 percent of ingested alcohol diffuses through the stomach lining into the bloodstream, and nearly 80 percent passes through the lining of the upper third of the small intestine. Absorption into the bloodstream is rapid and complete.

Several factors influence how quickly your body will absorb alcohol: the alcohol concentration in your drink, the amount of alcohol you consume, the amount of food in your stomach, and pylorospasm. The higher the concentration of alcohol in your drink, the more rapidly it will be absorbed in your digestive tract. As a rule, wine and beer are absorbed more slowly than distilled beverages. Carbonated alcoholic beverages, such as champagne and sparkling wines, are absorbed more rapidly than those containing no sparkling additives, or fizz. Carbonated beverages and drinks served with mixers cause the pyloric valve—the opening from the stomach into the small intestine—to relax (a pylorospasm) thereby emptying the contents of the stomach more rapidly into the small intestine. Because the small intestine is the site of the greatest absorption of alcohol, carbonated beverages increase the rate of absorption. In contrast, if your stomach is full, absorption slows because

---

Ethyl alcohol (ethanol) An addictive drug produced by fermentation and found in many beverages.

Fermentation The process whereby yeast organisms break down plant sugars to yield ethanol and carbon dioxide.

Distillation The process whereby mash is subjected to high temperatures to release alcohol vapors, which are then condensed and mixed with water to make the final product.

Proof A measure of the percentage of alcohol in a beverage.

Table 8.2
Psychological and Physical Effects of Various Blood-Alcohol Concentration Levels*

Number of Drinks†	Blood Alcohol Concentration (%)	Psychological and Physical Effects
2	0.05–0.06	Feeling of relaxation, warmth; slight decrease in reaction time and in fine-muscle coordination
3	0.08–0.09	Balance, speech, vision, and hearing slightly impaired; feelings of euphoria, increased confidence; loss of motor coordination
3–4	0.08–0.10	Legal intoxication in most states; some have lower limits
4	0.11–0.12	Coordination and balance becoming difficult; distinct impairment of mental faculties, judgment
5	0.14–0.15	Major impairment of mental and physical control; slurred speech, blurred vision, lack of motor skills
7	0.20	Loss of motor control—must have assistance in moving about; mental confusion
>10	>0.30	Severe intoxication; minimal conscious control of mind and body
14	0.40	Unconsciousness, coma, death

* For each hour elapsed since the last drink, subtract 0.015 percent blood alcohol concentration, or approximately one drink.
† One drink = one beer (4% alcohol, 12 ounces), one highball (1 ounce whiskey), or one glass table wine (5 ounces).
Source: Modified from data given in Ohio State Police Driver Information Seminars and the National Clearinghouse for Alcohol and Alcoholism Information, Rockville, MD.

the surface area exposed to alcohol is smaller. A full stomach also retards the emptying of alcoholic beverages into the small intestine.

The more alcohol you consume, the longer absorption takes. Alcohol can irritate the digestive system, which causes pylorospasm. When the pyloric valve is closed, nothing can move from the stomach to the upper third of the small intestine, which slows absorption. If the irritation continues, it can cause vomiting.

Alcohol is metabolized in the liver, where it is converted to *acetaldehyde* by the enzyme *alcohol dehydrogenase.* It is then rapidly oxidized to *acetate*, converted to carbon dioxide and water, and eventually excreted from the body. Acetaldehyde is a toxic chemical that can cause immediate symptoms, such as nausea and vomiting, as well as long-term effects, such as liver damage. A very small portion of alcohol is excreted unchanged by the kidneys, lungs, and skin.

Alcohol contains 7 kcal per gram (you will learn more about calories in Chapter 9). This means that the average regular beer contains about 150 calories. Mixed drinks may contain more if they are combined with sugary soda or fruit juice. The body uses the calories in alcohol in the same manner it uses those found in carbohydrates: for immediate energy or for storage as fat if not immediately needed.

When compared to the variable breakdown rates of foods and other beverages, the breakdown of alcohol occurs at a fairly constant rate of 0.5 ounce per hour. This amount of alcohol is equivalent to 12 ounces of 5 percent beer, 5 ounces of 12 percent wine, or 1.5 ounces of 40 percent (80 proof) liquor. Unmetabolized alcohol circulates in the bloodstream until enough time passes for the body to break it down.[10]

Behavioral and Physiological Effects

Blood alcohol concentration (BAC) is the ratio of alcohol to total blood volume. It is the factor used to measure the physiological and behavioral effects of alcohol. Despite individual differences, alcohol produces some general behavioral effects, depending on BAC (see Table 8.2). At a BAC of 0.02, a person feels slightly relaxed and in a good mood. At 0.05, relaxation increases, there is some motor impairment, and a willingness to talk becomes apparent. At a BAC over 0.08, the depressant effects of alcohol become apparent,

Blood alcohol concentration (BAC) The ratio of alcohol to total blood volume; the factor used to measure the physiological and behavioral effects of alcohol.

drowsiness sets in, and motor skills are further impaired, followed by a loss of judgment. At this BAC level, a driver may not be able to estimate distances or speed, and some lose their ability to make value-related decisions and may do things they would not do when sober. As BAC increases, the drinker suffers increased negative physiological and psychological effects. Alcohol ingestion does not enhance any physical skills or mental functions.

A drinker's BAC depends on weight and body fat, the water content in body tissues, the concentration of alcohol in the beverage consumed, the rate of consumption, and the volume of alcohol consumed. Larger people have larger body surfaces through which to diffuse alcohol; therefore, they have lower concentrations of alcohol in their blood than do thin people after drinking the same amount. Because alcohol does not diffuse as rapidly into body fat as into water, alcohol concentration is higher in a person with more body fat. Because a woman is likely to have more body fat and less water in her body tissues than a man of the same weight, she will be more intoxicated than a man will be after drinking the same amount of alcohol.

Both breath analysis (Breathalyzer tests) and urinalysis are used to determine whether an individual is legally intoxicated, but blood tests are more accurate measures of BAC. An increasing number of states are requiring blood tests for people suspected of driving under the influence of alcohol, but legal limits of BAC while driving do vary from one state to another. In some states, refusal to take the breath or urine test results in immediate revocation of the person's driver's license.

People can acquire physical and psychological tolerance to the effects of alcohol through regular use. The nervous system adapts over time, so greater amounts of alcohol are required to produce the same physiological and psychological effects. Though BAC may be quite high, the individual has learned to modify his behavior to appear sober. This ability is called **learned behavioral tolerance.**

Alcohol Poisoning
Alcohol poisoning occurs much more frequently than people realize, and all too often it can be fatal. Drinking large amounts of alcohol in a short period of time can cause the blood alcohol level to reach the lethal range quickly. Alcohol, either used alone or in combination with other drugs, is responsible for more toxic overdose deaths than any other substance.

Death from alcohol poisoning can be caused by either central nervous system (CNS) and respiratory depression or the inhalation of vomit or fluid into the lungs. The amount of alcohol it takes for a person to become unconscious is dangerously close to the lethal dose. Signs of alcohol poisoning include inability to be roused; a weak, rapid pulse; an unusual or irregular breathing pattern; and cool (possibly damp), pale, or bluish skin. If you are with someone who has been drinking heavily and who exhibits these conditions or if you are unsure about the person's condition, call your local emergency number (911 in most areas) for immediate assistance.

Alcohol and Injuries
Alcohol use plays a significant role in the types of injuries people experience. Thirteen percent of emergency room visits by undergraduates are related to alcohol; of this total, 34 percent were the result of acute intoxication. A recent study found that injured patients with a BAC of over 0.08 percent who were treated in emergency rooms were 3.2 times more likely to have a violent injury than an unintentional injury.[11] Men 21 years or older are the most common emergency room admittees, mostly as the result of accidents or fights where alcohol was involved.[12]

Alcohol and Sexual Decision Making
Alcohol has a clear influence on people's abilities to make good decisions about sex because it lowers inhibitions, and you may do things you might not do when sober. Seventy percent of college students admit to having engaged in sexual activity primarily as a result of being under the influence of alcohol. Students who are intoxicated are less likely to use safe sex practices and are more likely to engage in other high-risk sexual activity. The risk of acquiring a sexually transmitted infection (STI, Chapter 14) or an unplanned pregnancy also increase among those who drink more heavily compared to those who drink moderately or not at all.

Women and Alcohol
Body fat is not the only contributor to the differences in alcohol's effects on men and women. Compared to men, women have half as much *alcohol hydrogenase*, the enzyme that breaks down alcohol in the stomach before it has a chance to reach the bloodstream and the brain. Therefore, if a man and a woman drink the same amount of alcohol, the woman's BAC will be approximately 30 percent higher than the man's BAC, leaving her more vulnerable to slurred speech, careless driving, and other drinking-related impairments.

Hormonal differences can also affect a woman's BAC. Specifically, one week prior to menstruating, women maintain the peak level of intoxication for longer periods of time than menstruating or postmenstruating women do. Women who are using oral contraceptives are also likely to maintain peak intoxication for longer periods of time than they would otherwise. This prolonged peak appears to be related to estrogen levels.

Learned behavioral tolerance The ability of heavy drinkers to modify behavior so that they appear to be sober even when they have high BAC levels.

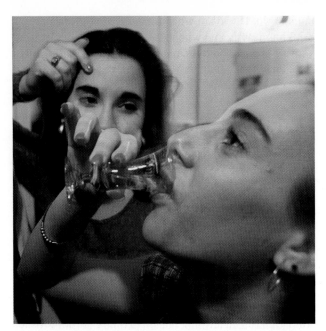

Increasing numbers of women on college campuses are trying to keep up with their male peers when binge drinking. The results can be dangerous; a woman's BAC will be higher than a man's after the same number of drinks.

Immediate Effects of Alcohol

The most dramatic effects produced by ethanol occur within the CNS. The primary action of the drug is to reduce the frequency of nerve transmissions and impulses at synaptic junctions. This depresses CNS functions, which decreases respiratory rate, pulse rate, and blood pressure. As CNS depression deepens, vital functions become noticeably affected. In extreme cases, coma and death can result.

Alcohol is a diuretic that causes increased urinary output. Although this effect might be expected to lead to automatic **dehydration** (loss of water), the body actually retains water, most of it in the muscles or in the cerebral tissues. The reason is that water is usually pulled out of the **cerebrospinal fluid** (fluid within the brain and spinal cord), leading to what is known as mitochondrial dehydration at the cellular level within the nervous system. Mitochondria are miniature organs within cells that are responsible for specific functions,

Dehydration   Loss of water from body tissues.

Cerebrospinal fluid   Fluid within and surrounding the brain and spinal cord tissues.

Hangover   The physiological reaction to excessive drinking, including symptoms such as headache, muscle aches, upset stomach, anxiety, depression, diarrhea, and thirst.

Congeners   Forms of alcohol that are metabolized more slowly than ethanol and produce toxic by-products.

and they rely heavily upon fluid balance. When mitochondrial dehydration occurs, the mitochondria cannot carry out their normal functions. This results in symptoms that include the "morning-after" headaches some drinkers suffer.

Alcohol irritates the gastrointestinal system and may cause indigestion and heartburn if taken on an empty stomach. It damages the mucous membranes and can cause inflammation of the esophagus, chronic stomach irritation, problems with intestinal absorption, and chronic diarrhea.

Hangover   A **hangover** is often experienced the morning after a drinking spree. The symptoms of a hangover are familiar to most people who drink: headache, muscle aches, upset stomach, anxiety, depression, diarrhea, and thirst. **Congeners,** forms of alcohol that are metabolized more slowly than ethanol and are more toxic, are thought to play a role in the development of a hangover. The body metabolizes the congeners after the ethanol is gone from the system, and their toxic by-products may contribute to the hangover. Alcohol also upsets the water balance in the body, which results in excess urination, dehydration, and thirst the next day. Increased production of hydrochloric acid can irritate the stomach lining and cause nausea. It usually takes 12 hours to recover from a hangover. Bed rest, solid food, and aspirin may help relieve its discomforts. The only cure for a hangover is abstaining from excessive alcohol use.

> Is there any cure for a hangover?

Drug Interactions   When you use any drug (and alcohol is a drug), you need to be aware of its possible interactions with any other drugs (Chapter 7), whether prescription or over-the-counter. If you are taking any medication, ask your doctor of pharmacist if alcohol consumption is safe while taking the medication. Avoid using alcohol when taking antihistamines, antibiotics, analgesics, antidepressants, and antianxiety medications due to the potential for hazardous interactions.

Long-Term Effects

Alcohol is distributed throughout most of the body and may affect many organs and tissues. Problems associated with long-term, habitual use of alcohol include diseases of the nervous system, cardiovascular system, and liver, as well as some cancers.

Effects on the Nervous System   The nervous system is especially sensitive to alcohol. Even people who drink moderately experience shrinkage in brain size and weight and a loss of some degree of intellectual ability. The damage that results from alcohol use is localized primarily in the left side of the brain, which is responsible for written and spoken language, logic, and mathematical skills. The degree of shrinkage appears to be directly related to the amount of alcohol consumed. In terms of memory loss, the evidence suggests that having one drink every day is better than saving up for a binge and consuming seven or eight drinks in a night. The amount of alcohol consumed at one time is critical. Alcohol-related brain damage can be partially reversed with good nutrition and staying sober.

Cardiovascular Effects

Alcohol affects the cardiovascular system in a number of ways. Numerous studies have associated light-to-moderate consumption of red wine (no more than two drinks a day) with a reduced risk of coronary artery disease. Several mechanisms have been proposed to explain how this might happen. The strongest evidence favors an increase in high-density lipoprotein (HDL) cholesterol, which is known as "good" cholesterol. Studies have shown that people who consume red wine have higher levels of HDL. Another factor that might help is an *antithrombotic effect*. Alcohol consumption is associated with a decrease in clotting factors that contribute to the development of atherosclerosis.

However, this does not mean that alcohol consumption is recommended as a preventive measure against heart disease—it causes many more cardiovascular health hazards than benefits. Alcohol contributes to high blood pressure and slightly increased heart rate and cardiac output. Those who report drinking three to five drinks a day, regardless of race or sex, have higher blood pressure than those who drink less.

Liver Disease

One result of heavy drinking is that the liver begins to store fat—a condition known as *fatty liver*. If there is insufficient time between drinking episodes, this fat cannot be transported to storage sites, and the fat-filled liver cells stop functioning. Continued drinking can cause a further stage of liver deterioration called *fibrosis,* in which the damaged area of the liver develops fibrous scar tissue. At this stage, cell function can be partially restored with proper nutrition and abstinence from alcohol. If the person continues to drink, **cirrhosis** develops, a condition where liver cells suffer from irreversible liver damage and die. Cirrhosis is one of the top ten causes of death in the United States today, and a common disease related to alcohol abuse.

Alcoholic hepatitis is a serious condition resulting from prolonged use of alcohol. A chronic inflammation of the liver develops, which may be fatal in itself or progress to cirrhosis.

Cancer

Alcohol is considered a carcinogen. The repeated irritation caused by long-term use of alcohol has been linked to cancers of the esophagus, stomach, mouth, tongue, and liver. There is substantial evidence that breast cancer risk is elevated for women consuming high levels of alcohol (more than three drinks per day) compared with abstainers.[13] In a recent study, a team of scientists from the National Institute of Alcohol Abuse and Alcoholism discovered a possible link between acetaldehyde and DNA damage that could help to explain the connection between drinking and certain types of cancer.[14]

Other Effects

Alcohol abuse is a major cause of chronic inflammation of the pancreas, the organ that produces digestive enzymes and insulin. Chronic abuse of alcohol inhibits enzyme production, which further inhibits the absorption of nutrients. Drinking alcohol can block the absorption of calcium, a nutrient that strengthens bones. This should be of particular concern to women because their risk for osteoporosis; bone thinning and calcium loss (Chapter 15) increases with age. Heavy consumption of alcohol worsens this condition.

Evidence also suggests that alcohol impairs the body's ability to recognize and fight foreign bodies such as bacteria and viruses. The relationship between alcohol and AIDS is unclear, especially since some of the populations at risk for AIDS are also at risk for alcohol abuse. But any stressor like alcohol, with a known effect on the immune system, would probably contribute to the development of the disease.

Alcohol and Pregnancy

Recall from Chapter 6 that *teratogenic* substances cause birth defects. Of the 30 known teratogens in the environment, alcohol is one of the most dangerous and common. More than 10 percent of all children have been exposed to high levels of alcohol in utero. All will suffer varying degrees of effects, ranging from mild learning disabilities to major physical, mental, and intellectual impairment. Alcohol consumed during the first trimester poses the greatest threat to organ development; exposure during the last trimester, when the brain is developing rapidly, is most likely to affect CNS development. A disorder called **fetal alcohol syndrome (FAS)** is associated with alcohol consumption during

---

Cirrhosis   The last stage of liver disease associated with chronic heavy use of alcohol during which liver cells die and damage becomes permanent.

Alcoholic hepatitis   Condition resulting from prolonged use of alcohol in which the liver is inflamed; can be death.

Fetal alcohol syndrome (FAS)   A disorder that may affect the fetus when the mother consumes alcohol during pregnancy. Among its effects are mental retardation; small head; tremors; and abnormalities of the face, limbs, heart, and brain.

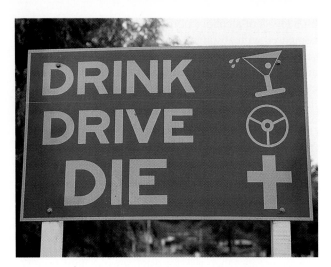

All too often, drinking and driving can be deadly combinations. Approximately 40 percent of U.S. traffic fatalities are alcohol related.

pregnancy. In the United States, it is the third most common birth defect (with an estimated incidence of 1 to 2 of every 1,000 live births) and the second leading cause of mental retardation It is the most common preventable cause of mental impairment in the Western world.

If a woman ingests alcohol while pregnant, it will pass through the placenta and enter the growing fetus's bloodstream. It is recommended that women do not consume any alcohol during pregnancy. Among the symptoms of FAS are mental retardation, small head, tremors, and abnormalities of the face, limbs, heart, and brain. Children with FAS may experience problems such as poor memory and impaired learning, reduced attention span, impulsive behavior, and poor problem solving abilities, among others.[15]

Some children have fewer than the full physical or behavioral symptoms of FAS and can be categorized as having **fetal alcohol effects (FAE)**. FAE is estimated to occur three to four times more often than FAS, although it is much less recognized. The signs of FAE in newborns are low birthweight and irritability, and there may be permanent mental impairment. Infants whose mothers habitually consumed more than three ounces of alcohol (approximately six drinks) in a short time period when pregnant are at high risk for FAS. Risk levels for babies whose mothers consume smaller amounts are uncertain.

Fetal alcohol effects (FAE)   A syndrome describing children with a history of prenatal alcohol exposure but without all the physical or behavioral symptoms of FAS. Among its symptoms are low birth weight, irritability, and possible permanent mental impairment.

Alcohol can also be passed to a nursing baby through breast milk. For this reason, most doctors advise nursing mothers not to drink for at least four hours before nursing their babies and preferably to abstain altogether.

What Do You Think?   Why do we hear so little about FAS in this country when it is the third most common birth defect and second leading cause of mental retardation? ■ Is this a reflection of our society's denial of alcohol as a dangerous drug?

Drinking and Driving

Traffic accidents are the leading cause of death for all age groups from 5 to 45 years old (including college students). Approximately 41 percent of all traffic fatalities in 2002 were alcohol related.[16] Unfortunately, college students are overrepresented in alcohol-related crashes. The College Alcohol Study findings indicated that 20 percent of nonbingers, 43 percent of occasional bingers, and 59 percent of frequent bingers reported driving while intoxicated.[17] Furthermore, it is estimated that three out of every ten Americans will be involved in an alcohol-related accident at some time in their lives.[18] Studies show that those involved in car crashes after drinking have a 40 to 50 percent higher chance of dying than nondrinkers involved in car crashes.

In 2004, there were 16,694 alcohol-related traffic fatalities (ARTFs), a 5 percent reduction from 1982.[19] Over the past 20 years, intoxication rates—BAC of 0.10 percent or greater—decreased for drivers of all age groups involved in fatal crashes (Figure 8.2). This number represents an average of one alcohol-related fatality approximately every 30 minutes.[20] The highest intoxication rates in fatal crashes were recorded for drivers 21 to 24 years old (22 percent), followed by ages 25 to 34 (27 percent) and 35 to 44 (24 percent). In the most current data reported, approximately 1.5 million drivers were arrested in 2002 for driving under the influence of alcohol or drugs. This is an arrest rate of 1 for every 130 licensed drivers in the United States.[21] One possible factor for this reduction in ARTFs is an increased emphasis on zero tolerance (laws prohibiting those under 21 from driving with *any* detectable BAC).

Laboratory and test track research shows that the vast majority of drivers, even experienced drinkers, are impaired at 0.08 percent BAC with regard to critical driving tasks; currently, the federal government is encouraging all 50 states, to implement a BAC limit while driving to 0.08 percent. National groups such as MADD (Mothers Against Drunk Driving), started by a woman whose child was killed by a drunk driver, go as far as tracking drunk driving cases through the court systems to ensure that drunk drivers are punished. Members of the high school group SADD (Students Against Destructive Decisions) educate their peers about the dangers of drinking and driving.

Despite all these measures, the risk of being involved in an alcohol-related automobile crash remains substantial. Researchers have shown a direct relationship between the amount of alcohol in a driver's bloodstream and the likelihood of a crash. A driver with a BAC level of 0.10 percent is approximately 10 times more likely to be involved in a car accident than a driver who has not been drinking.

Fatal crashes involving alcohol are highest between midnight and 3:00 AM (77 percent of all fatal crashes occurring during this window of time involve alcohol), and 9:00 PM to midnight is the next most dangerous time.[22] Risk increases even more on the weekend.

What Do You Think?

What do you think the legal BAC for drivers should be? ■ What should the penalty be for people arrested for driving under the influence of alcohol (DUI) for the first offense? The second offense? The third offense?

ALCOHOL ABUSE AND ALCOHOLISM

Alcohol use becomes **alcohol abuse** when it interferes with work, school, or social and family relationships, or when it entails any violation of the law, including driving under the influence (DUI). **Alcoholism, or alcohol dependency,** results when personal and health problems related to alcohol use are severe, and stopping alcohol use results in withdrawal symptoms. Approximately 6 million Americans can be described as alcoholics.

A recent study shows that 6 percent of college students meet the criteria for a diagnosis of alcoholism, and 31 percent meet the criteria for alcohol abuse. Students who attend colleges that have heavy drinking environments are more likely to be diagnosed with abuse or dependence. Despite the prevalence of alcohol disorders on campus, very few students seek treatment.[23]

Identifying a Problem Drinker

As in other drug addictions, tolerance, psychological dependence, and withdrawal symptoms must be present to qualify a drinker as an addict (see Chapter 7). Addiction results from chronic use over a period of time that varies from person to person. Irresponsible or problem drinkers, such as people who get into fights or embarrass themselves or others when they drink, are not

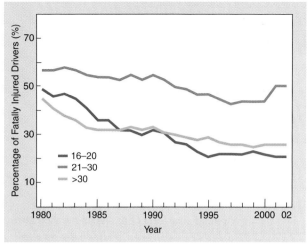

Figure 8.2 ■ Percentage of Fatally Injured Passenger Vehicle Drivers with BACs > 0.10 Percent, by Driver Age

Source: Insurance Institute for Highway Safety, "Fatality Facts: Alcohol 2002," 2003, www.iihs.org.

necessarily alcoholics. The stereotype of the alcoholic on skid row applies to only 5 percent of the alcoholic population. The remaining 95 percent live in some type of extended family unit. Alcoholics can be found at all socioeconomic levels and in all professions, ethnic groups, geographical locations, religions, and races.

Studies suggest that the lifetime risk of alcoholism in the United States is about 10 percent for men and 3 percent for women. Moreover, almost 25 percent of the American population (50 million people) is affected by the alcoholism of a friend or family member. The 2003 National Survey on Drug Use and Health found that 6.7 percent of Americans were heavy drinkers and 22.9 percent were binge drinkers.[24]

Recognizing and admitting the existence of an alcohol problem are often extremely difficult. Alcoholics themselves deny their problem, often making statements such as "I can stop any time I want to. I just don't want to right now." Their families also tend to deny the problem, saying things like "He really has been under a lot of stress lately. Besides, he only drinks beer." The fear of being labeled a "problem drinker" often prevents people from seeking help.

Alcoholics tend to have a number of symptoms in common. The Assess Yourself box lists several. People

Alcohol abuse Use of alcohol that interferes with work, school, or personal relationships or that entails violations of the law.

Alcoholism (alcohol dependency) Condition when personal and health problems related to alcohol use are severe, and stopping alcohol use results in withdrawal symptoms.

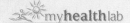

Alcohol Abuse and Alcoholism: Common Questions

Although many people think that they have a clear understanding of alcoholism, much remains in question. Answering the following questions will indicate your own level of knowledge about the disease. For further information about alcohol use on college campuses, check out the National Institute of Alcohol Abuse and Alcoholism's website (www.niaaa.nih.gov).

1. Alcoholism is a disease characterized by what four symptoms?
   a.
   b.
   c.
   d.
2. Is alcoholism an inherited trait?
   Yes
   Probably
   No
3. Do you have to be an alcoholic to experience alcohol-related problems?
   Yes
   No
4. What groups of individuals tend to have the most problems with alcoholism?

ANSWERS

1. The four symptoms of alcoholism include
   a. craving (a strong need or urge to drink alcohol)
   b. loss of control (not being able to stop drinking once drinking begins)
   c. physical dependence (withdrawal symptoms, such as nausea, sweating, shakiness, and anxiety after stopping drinking)
   d. tolerance (the need to drink greater amounts of alcohol for the same effect)
   For more information, see the *Diagnostic and Statistical Manual of Mental Disorders (DSM-IV)*, 4th ed., published by the American Psychiatric Association.
2. Probably yes. The risk for developing alcoholism does indeed run in families; however, lifestyle is also a major factor. Currently, researchers are trying to locate the actual genes that put people at risk. Your friends, the amount of stress in your life, and how readily available alcohol is are also factors that increase risk. Remember that risk is not destiny. A child of an alcoholic won't automatically become an alcoholic, while others develop alcoholism even though no one in their family is an alcoholic. If you know you are at risk, you can take steps to protect yourself.
3. No. Alcoholism is only one type of alcohol problem. Alcohol abuse can be just as harmful. A person can abuse alcohol without being an alcoholic—that is, he or she may drink too much and/or too often and still not be dependent on alcohol. Some of the problems of alcohol abuse include: not being able to meet work, school, or family responsibilities; drunk driving arrests and car crashes; and drinking-related medical conditions. Under some circumstances, even social or moderate drinking is dangerous—for example, when driving, during pregnancy, or when taking certain medications.

who recognize one or more of these behaviors in themselves may wish to seek professional help to determine whether alcohol has become a controlling factor in their lives. You may also feel that you wish to moderate the amount of alcohol that you drink. See the Try it Now boxes in this chapter for some tips to accomplish this.

Women are the fastest-growing population of alcohol abusers. They tend to become alcoholic at a later age and after fewer years of heavy drinking than do male alcoholics. Women at highest risk for alcohol-related problems are those who are unmarried but living with a partner, are in their twenties or early thirties, or have a husband or partner who drinks heavily.

The Causes of Alcohol Abuse and Alcoholism

We know that alcoholism is a disease with biological and social/environmental components, but we do not know what role each component plays in the disease.

Biological and Family Factors
Research into the hereditary and environmental causes of alcoholism has found higher rates of alcoholism among children of alcoholics than in the general population. In fact, alcoholism is four to five times more common among children of alcoholics. These children may be strongly influenced by their parents' behavior.

4. Alcohol abuse and alcoholism cut across gender, race, and nationality. Nearly 1 in 3 adults abuse alcohol in the United States today. In general, more men than women are alcohol dependent or have alcohol prob-lems. Alcohol problems are highest among young adults, aged 18–29, and lowest among adults aged 65 and older. We also know that the younger you start, the more likely that you will have a problem.

Source: National Institute on Alcohol Abuse and Alcoholism, "College Drinking: FAQs on Alcohol Abuse and Alcoholism," 2004, www.collegedrinkingprevention.gov/facts/faq.aspx.

Make It Happen!

Assessment: The Assess Yourself activity gave you the chance to test your knowledge about alcoholism. If you couldn't answer some of the questions or were surprised by some of the answers, you may want to take steps to learn more or to change your behavior.

Making a Change: In order to change your behavior, you need to develop a plan. Follow these steps below and complete your Behavior Change Contract to take action.

1. Evaluate your behavior, and identify patterns and specific things you are doing. What can you change now? What can you change in the near future?
2. Select one pattern of behavior that you want to change.
3. Fill out the Behavior Change Contract found at the front of your book. It should include your long-term goal for change, your short-term goals, the rewards you'll give yourself for reaching these goals, potential obstacles along the way, and strategies for overcoming these obstacles. For each goal, list the small steps and specific actions that you will take.
4. Chart your progress in a journal. At the end of a week, consider how successful you were in following your plan. What helped you be successful? What made change more difficult? What will you do differently next week?
5. Revise your plan as needed. Are the short-term goals attainable? Are the rewards satisfying?

Example: After completing the Assess Yourself activity, Mark was surprised to discover that he had several misper-ceptions about alcohol abuse. In particular, he was surprised to realize that he exhibited one of the symptoms that char-acterize alcoholism. During his three years in college, he had developed a tolerance to alcohol that caused him to drink more to achieve the same effect. He decided to address his concerns about his alcohol use in several steps.

First, Mark kept a log of his alcohol consumption over two weeks. He saw that he was drinking almost every night of the week. Mark decided he wanted to reduce his drinking and set two goals: taking a "break" from drinking altogether for three weeks, and after that, drinking only on Friday and Saturday nights for the rest of the semester. Mark explained to his friends that he was taking a break and invited them to go with him on hikes, to the movies, and to other alco-hol-free environments. After successfully taking this break, Mark decided to set some goals and limits for himself on the alcohol he would consume in the future. He went to a fraternity party on a Friday night and drank two beers, his predetermined limit. He was happy to realize when he woke up the next morning that he felt refreshed, not hung over. When he went out for dinner with his friends Saturday night, they wanted to go barhopping afterwards. He volunteered to be the designated driver, and the bar gave him free sodas for the night. The next weekend, Mark found he had extra money that he hadn't spent on beer during the week and bought himself a new DVD.

Despite evidence of heredity's role in alcoholism, scientists do not yet understand the precise role of genes and increased risk for alcoholism and have not identified a specific "alcoholism" gene. Studies of identical twins (twins who share the same genes) and frater-nal twins (twins who share about half of their genes, like other siblings) suggest that heredity accounts for two-thirds of the risk for becoming alcoholic in both men and women.

Social and Cultural Factors Although a family history of alcoholism may predispose a person to problems, numerous other factors may mitigate or exac-erbate that tendency. Social and cultural factors may trigger the affliction for many people who are not genet-ically predisposed to alcoholism.

Some people begin drinking as a way to dull the pain of an acute loss or an emotional or social problem. For example, college students may drink to escape the stress of college life; disappointment over unfulfilled expectations; difficulties in forming relationships; or loss of the security of home, loved ones, and close friends. Involvement in a painful relationship, death of a family member, and other problems may trigger a search for an anesthetic. Unfortunately, the emotional discomfort that causes many people to turn to alcohol also ultimately causes them to become even more un-comfortable as the depressant effect of the drug begins to take its toll. Thus, the person who is already depressed may become even more depressed, antagonizing friends and other social supports. Eventually, the drinker becomes physically dependent on the drug.

Family attitudes toward alcohol also seem to influence whether a person will develop a drinking problem. It has been clearly demonstrated that people who are raised in cultures in which drinking is a part of religious or ceremonial activities or in which alcohol is a traditional part of the family meal are less prone to alcoholism. In contrast, in societies in which alcohol purchase is carefully controlled and drinking is regarded as a rite of passage to adulthood, the tendency for abuse appears to be greater.

Certain social factors have been linked with alcoholism, including urbanization, increased mobility, the weakening of links to the extended family and a general loosening of kinship ties, and changing religious and philosophical values. Apparently, then, some combination of heredity and environment plays a decisive role in the development of alcoholism. Some ethnic and racial groups also have special alcohol abuse problems.

Try it ►NOW_____

Make a conscious effort to alter your drinking habits. Take these measures to be sure you do not become extremely intoxicated the next time you go out: switch to light beers or other beverages with a lower alcohol content; don't drink fast—be sure to space your drinks farther apart; eat a meal if you plan on drinking to slow down the rate of alcohol absorption.

Effects of Alcoholism on the Family

Only recently have people begun to recognize that it is the alcoholic *and* the alcoholic's entire family that suffer. Although most research focuses on family effects during the late stages of alcoholism, the family unit actually begins to react early on as the person starts to show symptoms of the disease.

An estimated 76 million Americans (about 43 percent of the U.S. adult population) have been exposed to alcoholism in the family.[25] Twenty-two million members of alcoholic families are age 18 or older, and many have carried childhood emotional scars into adulthood. Approximately one in four children under age 18 lives in an atmosphere of anxiety, tension, confusion, and denial.[26]

In dysfunctional families, children learn certain rules from an early age: don't talk, don't trust, and don't feel. These unspoken rules allow the family to avoid dealing with real problems and issues as family members unconsciously adapt to the alcoholic's behavior by adjusting their own behavior. Unfortunately, these behaviors enable the alcoholic to keep drinking. Children in such dysfunctional families generally assume at least one of the following roles:

- *Family hero.* Tries to divert attention from the problem by being too good to be true.
- *Scapegoat.* Draws attention away from the family's primary problem through delinquency or misbehavior.
- *Lost child.* Becomes passive and quietly withdraws from upsetting situations.
- *Mascot.* Disrupts tense situations by providing comic relief.

For children in alcoholic homes, life is a struggle. They have to deal with constant stress, anxiety, and embarrassment. Because the alcoholic is the center of attention, the children's wants and needs are often ignored. It is not uncommon for these children to be victims of violence, abuse, neglect, or incest. As we have seen, when such children grow up, they are much more prone to alcoholic behaviors themselves than are children from nonalcoholic families.

In the past decade, we have come to recognize the unique problems of adult children of alcoholics whose difficulties in life stem from a lack of parental nurturing during childhood. Among these problems are difficulty in developing social attachments, a need to be in control of all emotions and situations, low self-esteem, and depression. Fortunately, not all individuals who have grown up in alcoholic families are doomed to have lifelong problems. As many of these people mature, they develop a resiliency in response to their families' problems. They thus enter adulthood armed with positive strengths and valuable career-oriented skills, such as the ability to assume responsibility, strong organizational skills, and realistic expectations of their jobs and others.

Women and Alcoholism

In the past, women have consumed less alcohol and have had fewer alcohol-related problems than have men. But now, greater percentages of women, especially college-age women, are choosing to drink and are drinking more heavily.

Studies indicate that there are now almost as many female as male alcoholics. Risk factors for drinking problems among *all women* include a family history of drinking problems, peer or spousal pressure to drink, depression, and stress.

Young women have a unique set of risk factors including college attendance (women in college drink more), low-status or part-time jobs and unemployment, and being single, divorced, or separated. Unique risk factors among middle-aged and older women include loss of a social role or network (children leave home, divorce) or a spouse who is a heavy or problem drinker.

Drinking patterns among different age groups also differ in these ways.

- Younger women drink more overall, drink more often, and experience more alcohol-related problems, such as drinking and driving, assaults, suicide attempts, and difficulties at work.
- Middle-aged women are more likely to develop drinking problems in response to a traumatic or life-changing event, such as divorce, surgery, or death of a significant other.
- Older women are more likely to develop or show alcohol problems later in life when compared to men.[27]

It is estimated that only 14 percent of women who need treatment get it. In one study, women cite potential loss of income, not wanting others to know they may have a problem, inability to pay for treatment, and fear that treatment would not be confidential as reasons for not seeking treatment.[28] Another major obstacle is child care. Most residential treatment centers do not allow women to bring their children with them.

Alcohol and Ethnic or Racial Differences

Different ethnic and racial minority groups have their own patterns of alcohol consumption and abuse. Among Native American Indian populations, alcohol is the most widely used drug; the rate of alcoholism in this population is two to three times higher than the national average, and the death rate from alcohol related causes is eight times higher than the national average. Some possible factors for the alcoholism problem in the Native American Indian population are poor economic conditions and the cultural belief that alcoholism is a spiritual problem, not an actual disease.

African American and Latino populations also exhibit distinct patterns of abuse. As a group African Americans drink less than the average white American; however, those who do drink tend to be heavy drinkers. Among Latinos, males have a higher than average rate of alcohol abuse and alcohol-related health problems. Cirrhosis and drunk driving are the most common causes of alcohol-related death or injury for Latino men. Latino women often abstain. Many researchers agree that a major factor for alcohol problems in this ethnic group is the key role drinking plays in Latino culture.

Asian Americans have a very low rate of alcoholism. Social and cultural influences, such as strong kinship ties, are thought to discourage heavy drinking. A very high percentage of Asians have a defect in the gene that manufactures aldehyde dehydrogenase, a key enzyme in alcohol metabolism, which makes drinking a less pleasurable experience due to unpleasant side effects.[29]

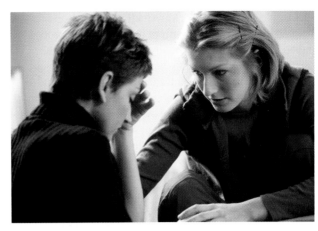

Often, family members or friends have to confront alcohol dependent individuals to help them take the first step toward recovery.

Despite growing recognition of our national alcohol problem, fewer than 10 percent of alcoholics in the United States receive any care. Factors contributing to this low figure include an inability or unwillingness to admit to an alcohol problem; the social stigma attached to alcoholism; breakdowns in referral and delivery systems (failure of physicians or psychotherapists to follow up on referrals, client failure to follow through with recommended treatments, or failure of rehabilitation facilities to give quality care); and failure of the professional medical establishment to recognize and diagnose alcoholic symptoms among patients.

What Do You Think? Why do women appear to be drinking more heavily today than they did in the past? ■ Does society look at men's and women's drinking habits in the same way? ■ Can you think of ways to increase support for women in their recovery process?

RECOVERY

Most problem drinkers who seek help have experienced a turning point: a spouse walks out, taking children and possessions; the boss issues an ultimatum to dry out or ship out. Devoid of hope, physically depleted, and spiritually despairing, the alcoholic finally recognizes that alcohol controls his or her life. The first steps on the road to recovery are to regain that control and to assume responsibility for personal actions.

The Family's Role

Members of an alcoholic's family sometimes take action before the alcoholic does. They may go to an organization or a treatment facility to seek help for themselves and their relative. An effective method of helping an alcoholic to confront the disease is a process called **intervention.** Essentially, an intervention is a planned confrontation with the alcoholic that involves several family members and friends plus professional counselors. Family members express their love and concern, telling the alcoholic that they will no longer refrain from acknowledging the problem and affirming their support for appropriate treatment. A family intervention is the turning point for a growing number of alcoholics.

Treatment Programs

The alcoholic who is ready for help has several avenues of treatment: psychologists and psychiatrists specializing in the treatment of alcoholism, private treatment centers, hospitals specifically designed to treat alcoholics, community mental health facilities, and support groups such as **Alcoholics Anonymous (AA).**

Private Treatment Facilities Private treatment facilities have been making concerted efforts to attract patients through advertising. On admission to the treatment facility, the patient receives a complete physical exam to determine whether underlying medical problems will interfere with treatment. Alcoholics who decide to quit drinking will experience a variety of withdrawal symptoms, ranging from confusion and depression to sleep disorders and hand tremors.

For a small percentage of people, alcohol withdrawal results in a severe syndrome known as **delirium tremens (DTs).** The DT syndrome is characterized by confusion, delusions, agitated behavior, and hallucinations.

For any long-term addict, medical supervision is usually necessary. *Detoxification,* the process by which addicts end their dependence on a drug, is commonly carried out in a medical facility, where patients can be monitored to prevent fatal reactions. Withdrawal takes 7 to 21 days. Shortly after detoxification, alcoholics begin their treatment for psychological addiction. Most treatment facilities keep their patients three to six weeks. Treatment at private treatment centers costs several thousand dollars, but some insurance programs or employers will assume most of this expense.

Family Therapy, Individual Therapy, and Group Therapy In family therapy, the person and family members gradually examine the psychological reasons underlying the addiction. In individual and group therapy with fellow addicts, alcoholics learn positive coping skills for situations that have regularly caused them to turn to alcohol.

On some college campuses, the problems associated with alcohol abuse are so great that student health centers are opening their own treatment programs. At the University of Texas, a new support service is being offered called Complete Recovery 101, and at other schools, students in recovery live together in special housing. Because it can be difficult to recover from an alcohol abuse problem in college, support programs such as these hope to offer the support and comfortable environment recovering students need.

Relapse

Success in recovery from alcoholism varies with the individual. A return to alcoholic habits often follows what appears to be a successful recovery. Some alcoholics never recover. Some partially recover and improve other parts of their lives but remain dependent on alcohol. Many alcoholics refer to themselves as "recovering" throughout their lifetime; they never use the word *cured.*

Roughly 60 percent of alcoholics relapse (resume drinking) within the first three months of treatment. Why is the relapse rate so high? Treating an addiction requires more than getting the addict to stop using a substance; it also requires getting the person to break a pattern of behavior that has dominated his or her life.

People who are seeking to regain a healthy lifestyle must not only confront their addiction, but also must guard against the tendency to relapse. Drinkers with compulsive personalities need to learn to understand themselves and take control. Others need to view treatment as a long-term process that takes a lot of effort beyond attending a weekly self-help group meeting. In order to work, a recovery program must offer the alcoholic ways to increase self-esteem and resume personal growth.

OUR SMOKING SOCIETY

Tobacco use is the single most preventable cause of death in the United States.[30] While tobacco companies continue to publish full-page advertisements refuting the dangers of smoking, nearly 440,000 Americans die each year of tobacco-related diseases[31] (see Figure 8.3 on page 225). This is 50 times as many as will die from all illegal drugs combined, and another 10 million people will suffer from disorders caused by tobacco. To date, tobacco is known to cause about 25 diseases, and one in every five deaths in the United States is related to smoking. About half of all regular smokers die of

---

Intervention A planned confrontation with an alcoholic in which family members, friends, and professional counselors express their concern about the alcoholic's drinking.

Alcoholics Anonymous (AA) An organization whose goal is to help alcoholics stop drinking; includes auxiliary branches such as Al-Anon and Alateen.

Delirium tremens (DTs) A state of confusion brought on by withdrawal from alcohol. Symptoms include hallucinations, anxiety, and trembling.

smoking-related diseases. Therefore, any contention by the tobacco industry that tobacco use is not dangerous is irresponsible and ignores the scientific evidence.

In 1991, the Youth Risk Assessment Survey, which includes students in grades 9 through 12, indicated that 27.5 percent of teenagers smoked; by 2003, 21.9 percent were current smokers. This survey indicates a downward trend among adolescent smokers. Currently, the percentage of teenage males and females who smoke is equal, at approximately 21.8 percent. Table 8.3 shows how many Americans smoke in various groups.[32] Every day another 6,000 teens under the age of 18 smoke their first cigarette and more than 3,000 others become daily smokers. Cigarette use among teens is attributed in part to marketing campaigns designed to appeal to young people.

Tobacco and Social Issues

The production and distribution of tobacco products in the United States and abroad involve many political and economic issues. Tobacco-growing states derive substantial income from tobacco production, and federal, state, and local governments benefit enormously from cigarette taxes. More recently, nationwide health awareness has led to a decrease in the use of tobacco products among U.S. adults.

Advertising The tobacco industry spends an estimated $18 million per day on advertising and promotional materials. With the number of smokers declining by about 1 million each year, the industry must actively recruit new smokers. Campaigns are directed at all age, social, and ethnic groups, but because children and teenagers constitute 90 percent of all new smokers, much of the advertising has been directed toward them. Evidence of product recognition among underage smokers is clear: 86 percent of underage smokers prefer one of the three most heavily advertised brands—Marlboro, Newport, or Camel. One of the most blatant campaigns aimed at young adults was the popular Joe Camel ad campaign. After R. J. Reynolds introduced the cartoon figure, Camel's market share among underage smokers jumped from 3 to 13.3 percent in 3 years.

Advertisements in women's magazines imply that smoking is the key to financial success, independence, and social acceptance. Many brands also have thin spokeswomen pushing "slim" and "light" cigarettes to cash in on women's fear of gaining weight. These ads have apparently been working. From the mid-1970s through early 2000s, cigarette sales to women increased dramatically. Not coincidentally, by 1987 cigarette-induced lung cancer had surpassed breast cancer as the leading cancer killer among women.

Women are not the only targets of gender-based cigarette advertisements. Males are depicted in locker rooms, charging over rugged terrain in off-road vehicles, or riding stallions into the sunset in blatant appeals

Table 8.3

Percentage of Population that Smokes (aged 18 and older) among Select Groups in the United States

	Percentage
United States overall	22.5
Race	
American Indian/Alaska Native	40.8
Asian/Pacific Islander	13.3
Black	22.4
Hispanic	16.7
White	23.6
Age	
18–24	28.5
25–44	25.7
45–64	22.7
>64	9.3
Sex	
Male	25.2
Female	20.0
Education	
>12 years	12.1
12 years	25.6
<12 years	31.0
Income Level	
Below poverty level	32.9
At or above poverty level	22.2

Source: Centers for Disease Control, "Cigarette Smoking Among Adults—United States 2002," *Morbidity and Mortality Weekly Report* 53, no. 20 (2004): 427–431.

to a need to feel and appear masculine. Minorities are often targeted.

Apparently, 18- to 24-year-olds have become the latest target for tobacco advertisers. The tobacco industry has set up aggressive marketing promotions at bars, music festivals, and the like, specifically targeted to this age group. Modeling and peer influence have an impact on smoking initiation. This potential impact is heightened by the fact that, although over half of campuses are considered smoke-free, they do permit smoking in residence hall rooms, student centers, and cafeterias, and many sell tobacco products in campus stores and student lounges.

Financial Costs to Society The use of tobacco products is costly to all of us in terms of lost productivity and lost lives. Estimates show that tobacco use caused over $167 billion in annual health-related economic losses from 1997 to 2001. The economic burden of tobacco use totaled more than $75.5 billion in medical expenditures (costs include hospital, physician, and nursing home expenditures; prescription drugs; and home health care expenditures) and $92 billion in indirect costs (absenteeism, added cost of fire insurance, training costs to replace employees who die prematurely, disability payments, and so on). The economic costs of smoking are estimated to be about $3,391 per smoker per year.[33]

College Students and Smoking

College students are especially vulnerable when placed in a new, often stressful social and academic environment. For many, the college years are their initial taste of freedom from parental supervision. Smoking may begin earlier, but most college students are a part of the significant age group in which people initiate smoking and become hooked.

Cigarette smoking among U.S. college students increased by 32 percent between 1991 and 1999. Researchers surveyed more than 14,000 students from 119 U.S. colleges and took into account all types of tobacco use, including cigars, smokeless tobacco, pipe smoking, and cigarettes. Researchers found that more than 60 percent of college students had tried some tobacco product. One-third of students had used tobacco in the month before the study, and just under half had used tobacco in the past year—but they did not consider themselves "smokers." The survey found a wide range of smoking behaviors among current smokers: 32 percent smoked less than a cigarette a day, while 13 percent smoked a pack or more per day. The study also found students who used tobacco products were more likely to smoke marijuana, binge drink, have multiple sex partners, earn lower grades, rate parties as more important than academic activities, and spend more time socializing with friends.[34]

A common perception is that students do not want to stop smoking. However, a recent study reported that 70 percent of cigarette smokers had tried to quit smoking, but three out of four were still smokers.[35] Colleges and universities should engage in antismoking efforts, strictly control tobacco advertising, provide smoke-free residence halls, and offer greater access to smoking cessation programs.

Nicotine The stimulant chemical in tobacco products.

Tar A thick, brownish substance condensed from particulate matter in smoked tobacco.

Carbon monoxide A gas found in cigarette smoke that binds at oxygen receptor sites in the blood, blocking oxygen transport.

What Do You Think? Have you noticed an increase in the number of your friends who have become regular smokers or occasional smokers? ■ How many of them smoked prior to coming to college, and how many picked up the habit at college? ■ What are their reasons for smoking? ■ What barriers keep your friends from quitting?

TOBACCO AND ITS EFFECTS

The chemical stimulant **nicotine** is the major psychoactive substance in all tobacco products. In its natural form, it is a colorless liquid that turns brown upon exposure to air. When tobacco leaves are burned in a cigarette, pipe, or cigar, nicotine is released and inhaled into the lungs. Sucking or chewing a quid (a pinch of snuff typically tucked between the gum and lower lip) of tobacco releases nicotine into the saliva, and the nicotine is then absorbed through the mucous membranes in the mouth.

Particulate matter condenses in the lungs to form a thick, brownish sludge called **tar.** Tar contains various carcinogenic (cancer-causing) agents such as benzo[a]pyrene and chemical irritants such as phenol. Phenol has the potential to combine with other chemicals to contribute to the development of lung cancer.

In healthy lungs, millions of tiny hairlike projections (cilia) on the cell surfaces lining the upper respiratory passages sweep away foreign matter, which is expelled from the lungs by coughing. Nicotine impairs the cleansing function of the cilia by paralyzing them for up to one hour following the smoking of a single cigarette. This allows tars and other solids in tobacco smoke to accumulate and irritate sensitive lung tissue.

Smoking is the most common form of tobacco use. Smoking delivers a strong dose of nicotine to the user, along with an additional 4,700 chemical substances such as arsenic, formaldehyde, and ammonia. In fact, tars account for only 8 percent of tobacco smoke. The remaining 92 percent consists of various gases and vapors that carry particulate matter in concentrations that are 500,000 times greater than those of the most air-polluted cities in the world.[36] The most dangerous of the gases is **carbon monoxide.** In tobacco smoke, the concentration of carbon monoxide is 800 times higher than the level considered safe by the U.S. Environmental Protection Agency (EPA). In the human body, carbon monoxide reduces the oxygen-carrying capacity of the red blood cells by binding with the receptor sites for oxygen, causing oxygen deprivation in many body tissues.

The heat from tobacco smoke, which can reach 1,616°F, is also harmful. Inhaling hot gases exposes sensitive mucous membranes to irritating chemicals that weaken the tissues and contribute to cancers of the mouth, larynx, and throat.

Tobacco Products

Tobacco comes in several forms. Cigarettes, cigars, pipes, and bidis are used for burning and inhaling tobacco. Smokeless tobacco is inhaled or placed in the mouth.

Cigarettes *Filtered cigarettes* designed to reduce levels of gases such as hydrogen cyanide and carbon monoxide may actually deliver more hazardous gases to the user than nonfiltered brands. Some smokers use low-tar and low-nicotine products as an excuse to smoke more cigarettes. This practice is self-defeating because they wind up exposing themselves to more harmful substances than they would with regular-strength cigarettes.

Clove cigarettes contain about 40 percent ground cloves (a spice) and about 60 percent tobacco. Many users mistakenly believe that these products are made entirely of ground cloves and that smoking them eliminates the risks associated with tobacco. In fact, clove cigarettes contain higher levels of tar, nicotine, and carbon monoxide than do regular cigarettes—and the numbing effect of eugenol, the active ingredient in cloves, allows smokers to inhale the smoke more deeply.

Cigars Those big stogies that we see celebrities and government figures puffing on these days are nothing more than tobacco fillers wrapped in more tobacco. Since 1991, cigar sales in the United States have increased dramatically. The fad, especially popular among young men and women, is fueled in part by the willingness of celebrities to be photographed puffing on one. Among some women, cigar smoking symbolizes an impulse to be slightly outrageous and liberated.

Many people believe that cigars are safer than cigarettes, when in fact nothing could be further from the truth.[37] Cigar smoke contains 23 poisons and 43 carcinogens. Smoking as little as one cigar per day can increase the risk of several cancers, including cancer of the oral cavity (lip, tongue, mouth, and throat), esophagus, larynx, and lungs. Daily cigar smoking, especially for people who inhale, also increases the risk of heart disease (cigar smokers double their risk of heart attack and stroke) and a lung disease known as chronic obstructive pulmonary disease (COPD). Former president Bill Clinton, a regular cigar smoker, recently underwent quadruple bypass heart surgery necessitated in part due to his habit. Smoking one or two cigars daily doubles the risk for oral cancers and esophageal cancer, compared with the risk for someone who has never smoked. The risks increase with the number of cigars smoked per day.

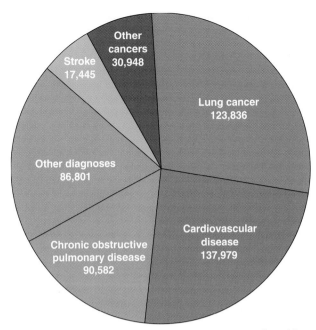

Figure 8.3 ■ Annual Deaths Attributable to Smoking in the United States

Source: Centers for Disease Control, "Annual Smoking-Attributable Mortality, Years of Potential Life Lost, and Economic Costs," *Morbidity and Mortality Weekly Report* 51, no. 14 (2002): 300–303.

A common question is whether cigars are addictive. Most cigars contain as much nicotine as several cigarettes; nicotine is highly addictive. When cigar smokers inhale, nicotine is absorbed as rapidly as it is with cigarettes. For those who don't inhale, nicotine is still absorbed through the mucous membranes in the mouth.

Bidis Generally made in India or Southeast Asia, **bidis** are small, hand-rolled, flavored cigarettes. They come in a variety of flavors, such as vanilla, chocolate, and cherry. Bidis resemble a marijuana joint or a clove cigarette and have become increasingly popular with college students, who view them as safer, cheaper, and easier to obtain than cigarettes. However, they are far more toxic than cigarettes. A study by the Massachusetts Department of Health found that bidis produced three times more carbon monoxide and nicotine and five times more tar than cigarettes during an identical testing process. The tendu leaf wrappers are nonporous, which means that smokers have to pull harder to inhale and inhale more to keep the bidi lit. During testing, it took an average of 28 puffs to smoke a bidi, compared to only 9 puffs for a regular cigarette. This results in much more exposure to the higher amounts of tar, nicotine, and carbon monoxide, and bidis lack any sort of filter to lower these levels. Bidi smokers are at the same, if not higher, risk for coronary heart disease and cancer due to smoking.[38]

Bidis Handrolled flavored cigarettes.

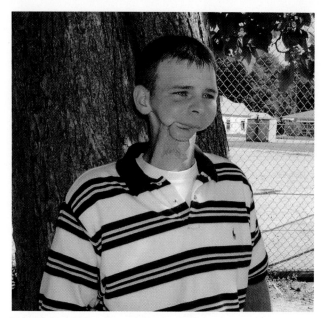

This 25-year-old cancer survivor has undergone surgery to remove neck muscles, lymph nodes, and his tongue. He began using smokeless tobacco at age 13; by age 17, he was diagnosed with squamous cell carcinoma. He now speaks out about the dangers of chewing tobacco.

Smokeless Tobacco Approximately 5 million U.S. adults use smokeless tobacco. Most of them are teenage (20 percent of male high school students) and young adult males, who are often emulating a professional sports figure or family member. There are two types of smokeless tobacco: chewing tobacco and snuff.

Chewing tobacco is placed between the gums and teeth for sucking or chewing. It comes in three forms: loose leaf, plug, or twist. Chewing tobacco contains tobacco leaves treated with molasses and other flavorings. The user places a quid of tobacco in the mouth between the teeth and gums and then sucks or chews the quid to release the nicotine. Once the quid becomes ineffective, the user spits it out and inserts another. **Dipping** is another method of using chewing tobacco. The dipper places a small amount of tobacco between the lower lip and teeth to stimulate the flow of saliva and release the nicotine. Dipping rapidly releases nicotine into the bloodstream.

Chewing tobacco A stringy type of tobacco that is placed in the mouth and then sucked or chewed.

Dipping Placing a small amount of chewing tobacco between the front lip and teeth for rapid nicotine absorption.

Snuff A powdered form of tobacco that is sniffed and absorbed through the mucous membranes in the nose or placed inside the cheek and sucked or chewed.

Leukoplakia A condition characterized by leathery white patches inside the mouth; produced by contact with irritants in tobacco juice.

Snuff is a finely ground form of tobacco that can be inhaled, chewed, or placed against the gums. It comes in dry or moist powdered form or sachets (tea bag–like pouches). Usually snuff is placed inside the cheek.

Smokeless tobacco is just as addictive as cigarettes because of its nicotine content. There is nicotine in all tobacco products, but smokeless tobacco contains even more than cigarettes. Holding an average-sized dip or chew in the mouth for 30 minutes delivers as much nicotine as smoking four cigarettes. A two-can-a-week snuff dipper gets as much nicotine as a one-and-a-half-pack-a-day smoker. Smokeless tobacco contains 10 times the amount of cancer-producing substances found in cigarettes and 100 times more than the U.S. Food and Drug Administration (FDA) allows in foods and other substances used by the public.

A major risk of chewing tobacco is **leukoplakia,** a condition characterized by leathery white patches inside the mouth produced by contact with irritants in tobacco juice. Between 3 and 17 percent of diagnosed leukoplakia cases develop into oral cancer.

An estimated 75 percent of the 29,370 oral cancer cases in 2004 resulted from either smokeless tobacco or cigarettes.[39] Users of smokeless tobacco are 50 times more likely to develop oral cancers than are nonusers. Warning signs include lumps in the jaw or neck; color changes or lumps inside the lips; white, smooth, or scaly patches in the mouth or on the neck, lips, or tongue; a red spot or sore on the lips or gums or inside the mouth that does not heal in two weeks; repeated bleeding in the mouth; and difficulty or abnormality in speaking or swallowing.

The lag time between first use and contracting cancer is shorter for smokeless tobacco users than for smokers because absorption through the gums is the most efficient route of nicotine administration. A growing body of evidence suggests that long-term use of smokeless tobacco also increases the risk of cancer of the larynx, esophagus, nasal cavity, pancreas, kidney, and bladder. Moreover, many smokeless tobacco users eventually "graduate" to cigarettes.

The stimulant effects of nicotine may create the same circulatory and respiratory problems for chewers as for smokers. Chronic smokeless tobacco use also delays wound healing and promotes peptic ulcer disease.

Like smoked tobacco, smokeless tobacco impairs the senses of taste and smell, causing the user to add salt and sugar to food, which may contribute to high blood pressure and obesity. Some smokeless tobacco products contain high levels of sodium (salt), which also promotes high blood pressure. Dental problems also are common among users of smokeless tobacco. Contact with tobacco juice causes receding gums, tooth decay, bad breath, and discolored teeth. Damage to the teeth and jawbone can contribute to early loss of teeth. Users of any tobacco products may not be able to absorb vitamins and other nutrients in food effectively.

Physiological Effects of Nicotine

Nicotine is a powerful CNS stimulant that produces a variety of physiological effects. Its stimulant action in the cerebral cortex produces an aroused, alert mental state. Nicotine also stimulates the adrenal glands, which increases the production of adrenaline. The physical effects of nicotine stimulation include increased heart and respiratory rate, constricted blood vessels, and subsequent increased blood pressure because the heart must work harder to pump blood through the narrowed vessels.

Nicotine decreases blood sugar levels and the stomach contractions that signal hunger. These factors, along with decreased sensation in the taste buds, reduce appetite. For this reason, many smokers eat less than nonsmokers do and weigh, on average, seven pounds less than nonsmokers.

Beginning smokers usually feel the effects of nicotine with their first puff. These symptoms, called **nicotine poisoning,** include dizziness, lightheadedness, rapid and erratic pulse, clammy skin, nausea, vomiting, and diarrhea. The effects of nicotine poisoning cease as tolerance to the chemical develops. Tolerance develops almost immediately in new users, perhaps after the second or third cigarette. In contrast, tolerance to most other drugs, such as alcohol, develops over a period of months or years. Regular smokers often do not experience the "buzz" of smoking. They continue to smoke simply because stopping is too difficult.

HEALTH HAZARDS OF SMOKING

Cigarette smoking adversely affects the health of every person who smokes, as well as the health of everyone nearby. Each day, cigarettes contribute to more than 1,000 deaths from cancer, cardiovascular disease, and respiratory disorders.

Cancer

The American Cancer Society estimates that tobacco smoking causes 85 to 90 percent of all cases of lung cancer—fewer than 10 percent of cases occur among nonsmokers.[40] Lung cancer is the leading cause of cancer deaths in the United States. There were an estimated 172,570 *new* cases of lung cancer in the United States in 2004 alone, and an estimated 163,510 Americans died of the disease in 2004.[41] Figure 8.4 on the next page illustrates how tobacco smoke damages the lungs.

Lung cancer can take 10 to 30 years to develop, and the outlook for its victims is poor. Most lung cancer is not diagnosed until it is fairly widespread in the body; at that point, the five-year survival rate is only 13 percent. When a malignancy is diagnosed and recognized while still localized, the five-year survival rate rises to 47 percent.

If you are a smoker, your risk of developing lung cancer depends on several factors. First, the number of cigarettes you smoke per day is important. Someone who smokes two packs a day is 15 to 25 times more likely to develop lung cancer than a nonsmoker. If you started smoking in your teens or if you inhale deeply when you smoke, you have a greater chance of developing lung cancer than people who started later. Occupational or domestic exposure to other irritants, such as asbestos and radon, will also increase your likelihood of developing lung cancer.

Tobacco is linked to other cancers as well. The rate of pancreatic cancer is more than twice as high for smokers as nonsmokers. Typically, people diagnosed with pancreatic cancer live about three months after their diagnosis. Smokers can reduce those odds by 30 percent if they quit for 11 years or more.[42] Cancers of the lip, tongue, salivary glands, and esophagus are five times more likely to occur among smokers than among nonsmokers. Smokers are also more likely to develop kidney, bladder, and larynx cancers.

Cardiovascular Disease

Half of all tobacco-related deaths occur from some form of heart disease.[43] Smokers have a 70 percent higher death rate from heart disease than nonsmokers do, and heavy smokers have a 200 percent higher death rate than moderate smokers do. In fact, smoking cigarettes poses as great a risk for developing heart disease as high blood pressure and high cholesterol levels do.

Smoking contributes to heart disease by encouraging the buildup of fatty deposits in the heart and major blood vessels (atherosclerosis).[44] For unknown reasons, smoking decreases blood levels of HDLs, the "good cholesterol" that helps protect against heart attacks.

Nicotine poisoning Symptoms often experienced by beginning smokers, including dizziness, diarrhea, lightheadedness, rapid and erratic pulse, clammy skin, nausea, and vomiting.

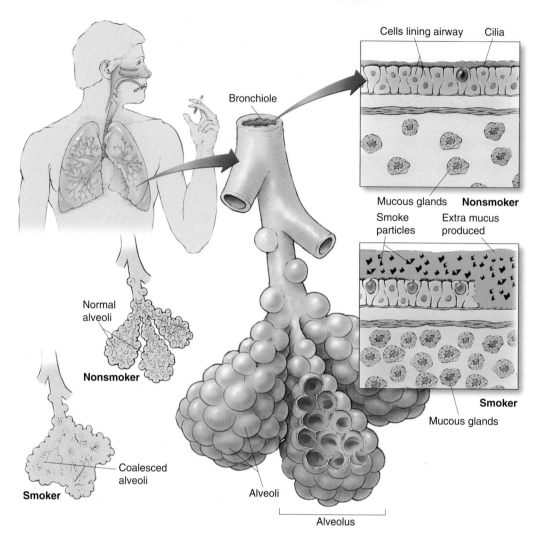

Figure 8.4 ■ How Cigarette Smoking Damages the Lungs
Smoke particles irritate the lung pathways, which causes excess mucus production. They also indirectly destroy the walls of the lungs' alveoli, which coalesce. Both factors reduce lung efficiency. Tar in tobacco smoke also has a direct cancer-causing action.

Smoking also contributes to **platelet adhesiveness,** which is the sticking together of red blood cells that is associated with blood clots. The oxygen deprivation associated with smoking decreases the oxygen supplied to the heart and can weaken tissues. Smoking also contributes to irregular heart rhythms, which can trigger a heart attack. Both carbon monoxide and nicotine in cigarette smoke can precipitate angina attacks (pain spasms in the chest when the heart muscle does not get the blood supply it needs).

The number of years a person has smoked does not seem to bear much relation to cardiovascular risk. If a person quits smoking, the risk of dying from a heart attack is reduced by half after only one year without smoking and declines steadily thereafter. After about 15 years without smoking, the ex-smoker's risk of car-

diovascular disease is similar to that of people who have never smoked.[45]

Stroke Smokers are twice as likely to suffer strokes as nonsmokers are.[46] A stroke occurs when a small blood vessel in the brain bursts or is blocked by a blood clot, which denies oxygen and nourishment to vital portions of the brain. Depending on the area of the brain affected, stroke can result in paralysis, loss of mental functioning, or death. Smoking contributes to strokes by raising blood pressure, which thereby increases the stress on vessel walls. Platelet adhesiveness contributes to clotting. Five to 15 years after they stop smoking, the risk of stroke for ex-smokers is the same as that for people who have never smoked.[47]

Respiratory Disorders

Smoking quickly impairs the respiratory system. Smokers can feel its impact in a relatively short period of

Platelet adhesiveness Stickiness of red blood cells associated with blood clots.

time—they are more prone to breathlessness, chronic cough, and excess phlegm production than are non-smokers their age. Smokers tend to miss work one-third more often than nonsmokers do, primarily because of respiratory problems, and they are up to 18 times more likely to die of lung disease.[48]

Chronic bronchitis is the presence of a productive cough that persists or recurs frequently. It may develop in smokers because their inflamed lungs produce more mucus and constantly try to rid themselves of this mucus and foreign particles. The effort to do so results in "smoker's hack," the persistent cough most smokers experience. Smokers are more prone than are nonsmokers to respiratory ailments such as influenza, pneumonia, and colds.

Emphysema is a chronic disease in which the alveoli (the tiny air sacs in the lungs) are destroyed, which impairs the lungs' ability to obtain oxygen and remove carbon dioxide. As a result, breathing becomes difficult. Whereas healthy people expend only about 5 percent of their energy in breathing, people with advanced emphysema spend nearly 80 percent of their energy. A simple movement such as rising from a seated position becomes painful and difficult for the emphysema patient. Because the heart has to work harder to do even the simplest tasks, it may become enlarged, and the person may die from heart damage. There is no known cure for emphysema and once the damage is done, it is irreversable. Approximately 80 percent of all cases are related to cigarette smoking.

Sexual Dysfunction

Despite attempts by tobacco advertisers to make smoking appear sexy, research shows just the opposite: it can cause impotence in men. A number of recent studies have found that male smokers are about two times more likely than are nonsmokers to suffer from some form of impotence. Toxins in cigarette smoke damage blood vessels, which reduces blood flow to the penis and leads to an inadequate erection. It is thought that impotence could indicate oncoming cardiovascular disease.

Other Health Effects of Smoking

Gum disease is three times more common among smokers than among nonsmokers, and smokers lose significantly more teeth.[49] Smokers are also likely to use more medications. Nicotine and the other ingredients in cigarettes interfere with the metabolism of drugs. Nicotine speeds up the process by which the body uses and eliminates drugs, so that medications become less effective. The smoker may therefore have to take a larger dose of a drug or take it more frequently.

What Do You Think? Most people are very aware of the long-term hazards associated with tobacco use yet, despite prevention efforts, continue to smoke. Why do you think this is so? ■ What strategies might be effective at reducing the number of people who begin smoking?

ENVIRONMENTAL TOBACCO SMOKE

Although fewer than 30 percent of Americans smoke, air pollution from smoking in public places continues to be a problem. **Environmental tobacco smoke (ETS)** is divided into two categories: mainstream and sidestream smoke (commonly called secondhand smoke). **Mainstream smoke** refers to smoke drawn through tobacco while inhaling; **secondhand smoke** refers to smoke from the burning end of a cigarette or smoke exhaled by a smoker. People who breathe smoke from someone else's smoking product are said to be involuntary or passive smokers. Nearly nine out of ten nonsmoking Americans are exposed to environmental tobacco smoke. In fact, measurable levels of nicotine were found in the blood of 88 percent of all nontobacco users.

Risks from Environmental Tobacco Smoke

Although involuntary smokers breathe less tobacco than active smokers do, they still face risks from exposure to tobacco smoke. Secondhand smoke actually contains more carcinogenic substances than the smoke that a smoker inhales. According to the American Lung Association, secondhand smoke has about 2 times more tar and nicotine, 5 times more carbon monoxide, and 50 times more ammonia than mainstream smoke. Every year, ETS is estimated to be

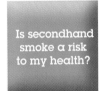 Is secondhand smoke a risk to my health?

Emphysema   A chronic lung disease in which the tiny air sacs in the lungs are destroyed, which makes breathing difficult.

Environmental tobacco smoke (ETS)   Smoke from tobacco products, including secondhand and mainstream smoke.

Mainstream smoke   Smoke that is drawn through tobacco while inhaling.

Secondhand smoke (sidestream smoke)   The cigarette, pipe, or cigar smoke breathed by nonsmokers.

responsible for approximately 3,000 lung cancer deaths, 35,000 cardiovascular disease deaths, and 13,000 deaths from other cancers.[50] The Environmental Protection Agency (EPA) has designated secondhand tobacco smoke a *group A cancer-causing agent* that is even worse than other group A threats such as benzene, arsenic, and radon. There is also evidence that secondhand smoke poses an even greater risk for death due to heart disease than for death due to lung cancer.[51]

Secondhand smoke is estimated to cause more deaths per year than any other environmental pollutant. The risk of dying because of exposure to passive smoking is 100 times greater than the risk that requires the EPA to label a pollutant as carcinogenic and 10,000 times greater than the risk that requires the labeling of a food as carcinogenic.[52]

Lung cancer and heart disease are not the only dangers involuntary smokers face. Exposure to ETS among children increases their risk of infections of the lower respiratory tract. An estimated 300,000 children are at greater risk of pneumonia and bronchitis as a result.[53] Children exposed to secondhand smoke have a greater chance of developing other respiratory problems such as coughing, wheezing, asthma, and chest colds, along with a decrease in lung function. The greatest effects of secondhand smoke are seen in children under the age of five. Children exposed to secondhand smoke daily in the home miss 33 percent more school days and have 10 percent more colds and acute respiratory infections than those not exposed. Secondhand smoke also impacts children's cognitive abilities and academic success. A recent study discovered that children exposed to high levels of secondhand smoke had lower standardized test scores in reading, math, and problem solving.[54] Children exposed to secondhand smoke are also twice as likely to become smokers during adolescence than children who are not exposed to secondhand smoke.[55]

Cigarette, cigar, and pipe smoke in enclosed areas presents other hazards. Ten to 15 percent of nonsmokers are extremely sensitive (hypersensitive) to cigarette smoke. These people experience itchy eyes, difficulty in breathing, painful headaches, nausea, and dizziness in response to minute amounts of smoke. The level of carbon monoxide in cigarette smoke contained in enclosed places is 4,000 times higher than that allowed in the clean air standard recommended by the EPA.

Efforts to reduce the hazards associated with passive smoking have gained momentum in recent years. Groups such as GASP (Group Against Smokers' Pollution) and ASH (Action on Smoking and Health) have been working since the early 1970s to reduce smoking in public places. In response to their efforts, some 44 states have enacted laws restricting smoking in public places such as restaurants, theaters, and airports. The federal government has restricted smoking in all government buildings. Hotels and motels now set aside rooms for nonsmokers, and car rental agencies designate certain vehicles for nonsmokers. Since 1990, smoking has been banned on all domestic and many international flights.

What Do You Think?   What rights, if any, should smokers have with regard to smoking in public places? ■ Does your campus allow smoking in residence halls? ■ Does your community have nonsmoking restaurants, or does it only have nonsmoking sections? ■ Do you think your community would support nonsmoking restaurants and bars? Why or why not?

TOBACCO AND POLITICS

It has been nearly 40 years since the government began warning that tobacco use was hazardous to the health of the nation. Public health care spending associated with smoking is over $150 billion each year.[56] In response, 46 states have sued to recover health care costs related to treating smokers.

In 1998, the tobacco industry reached a Master's Settlement Agreement with 39 of the states. This agreement requires tobacco companies to pay approximately $206 billion, over 25 years nationwide. The agreement also includes a variety of measures to support antismoking education and advertising and for funding for research to determine effective smoking cessation strategies. The agreement also curbs tobacco industry billboard advertising and promotions and advertising that appeal to youth (including merchandise samples and use of cartoon characters in ads).

Unfortunately, the majority of the money designated for tobacco control and prevention at the state level has not been used for this purpose. Facing budget woes, many states have drastically cut spending on antismoking programs.[57]

Many states and communities are advocating stricter tobacco control. A number of states have imposed extra taxes on cigarette sales in an effort to discourage use. The monies are then used for various purposes, including prevention and cessation programs and school health programs. Two community-based programs, ASSIST (American Stop Smoking Intervention Study) and IMPACT (Initiatives to Mobilize for the Prevention and Control of Tobacco Use), are tobacco control initiatives focused on creating legislation to prohibit the sale of tobacco to minors and assist with enforcement.

QUITTING

Quitting smoking isn't easy. Smokers must break both the physical addiction to nicotine and the habit of lighting up at certain times of day. From what we know about successful quitters, quitting is often a lengthy process involving several unsuccessful attempts before success is finally achieved. Even successful quitters suffer occasional slips, which emphasizes the fact that stopping smoking is a dynamic process that occurs over time.

Approximately one-third of all smokers attempt to quit each year. Unfortunately, 90 percent or more of those attempts fail. The person who wishes to quit smoking has several options. Most try to quit "cold turkey"—that is, they decide simply not to smoke again. Over 90 percent of former smokers report that they quit by stopping or slowly decreasing the amount they smoked.[58] Others resort to short-term quitting programs, such as those offered by the American Cancer Society, which are based on behavior modification and a system of self-rewards. Still others turn to treatment centers that are part of large franchises or part of a local medical clinic's community outreach plan. Finally, some people work privately with their physicians to reach their goal.

Prospective quitters must decide which method or combination of methods will work best for them. Programs that combine several approaches have shown the most promise. Financial considerations, personality characteristics, and level of addiction are all factors to consider.

Breaking the Nicotine Addiction

Nicotine addiction may be one of the toughest addictions to overcome. Symptoms of **nicotine withdrawal** include irritability, restlessness, nausea, vomiting, and intense cravings for tobacco.

Nicotine Replacement Products

Nontobacco products that replace depleted levels of nicotine in the bloodstream have helped some people stop using tobacco. The two most common are nicotine chewing gum and the nicotine patch, both of which are available over the counter. The FDA has also approved a nicotine nasal spray and a nicotine inhaler.

Some patients use Nicorette, a prescription chewing gum containing nicotine, to reduce nicotine consumption over time. Under the guidance of a physician, the user chews 12 to 24 pieces of gum per day for up to six months. Nicorette delivers about as much nicotine as a cigarette does, but because it is absorbed through the mucous membrane of the mouth, it doesn't produce the same rush. Users experience no withdrawal symptoms and fewer cravings for nicotine as the dosage is reduced until they are completely weaned.

Some controversy surrounds the use of nicotine replacement gum. Opponents believe that it substitutes one addiction for another. Successful users counter that it is a valid way to help break a deadly habit without suffering the unpleasant cravings that often lead to relapse.

The nicotine patch, first marketed in 1991, is generally used in conjunction with a comprehensive smoking-behavior cessation program. A small, thin, 24-hour patch placed on the smoker's upper body delivers a continuous flow of nicotine through the skin, helping to relieve cravings. The patch is worn for 8 to 12 weeks under the guidance of a clinician. During this time, the dose of nicotine is gradually reduced until the smoker is fully weaned from the drug. Occasional side effects include mild skin irritation, insomnia, dry mouth, and nervousness. The patch costs less than a pack of cigarettes—about four dollars—and some insurance plans will pay for it.

The nasal spray, which requires a prescription, is much more powerful and delivers nicotine to the bloodstream faster than gum or the patch. Patients are warned to be careful not to overdose; as little as 40 milligrams of nicotine taken at once could be lethal. The spray is somewhat unpleasant to use. The FDA has advised that it should be used for no more than three months and never for more than six months, so that smokers don't find themselves as dependent on nicotine in spray form as they were on cigarettes. The FDA also advises that no one who experiences nasal or sinus problems, allergies, or asthma should use it.

The nicotine inhaler, which also requires a prescription, consists of a mouthpiece and cartridge. By puffing on the mouthpiece, the smoker inhales air saturated with nicotine, which is absorbed through the lining of the mouth, not the lungs. This nicotine enters the body much more slowly than the nicotine in cigarettes does. Using the inhaler mimics the hand-to-mouth actions used in smoking and causes the back of the throat to feel as it would when inhaling tobacco smoke. Each cartridge lasts for 80 long puffs, and each cartridge is designed for 20 minutes of use.

Approved in 1997 by the FDA, Zyban, the smoking cessation pill, offers hope to many who thought they could never quit. Zyban is thought to work on dopamine and norepinephrine receptors in the brain to decrease craving and withdrawal symptoms. Because of the way this prescription medication works, it is important to start the pills one to two weeks before the targeted quit date; it requires planning ahead.

How effective are these therapies? The evidence is strong that consistent pharmacological treatments can help a smoker quit, with estimated abstinence after use ranging from 17 to 30 percent.[59]

Nicotine withdrawal Symptoms, including nausea, headaches, and irritability, suffered by smokers who cease using tobacco.

There is no magic cure that can help you stop. Take the first step by answering this question: Why do I want to stop smoking? Write your reasons in the space below. Once you have prepared your list, carry a copy of it with you. Memorize it. Every time you are tempted to smoke, go over your reasons for stopping.

My Reasons for Stopping

1. _____
2. _____
3. _____
4. _____
5. _____

Develop a Plan; Change Some Habits

Over time, smoking becomes a strong habit. Daily events such as finishing a meal, talking on the phone, drinking coffee, and chatting with friends trigger the urge to smoke. Breaking the link between the trigger and the smoking will help you stop. Think about the times and places you usually smoke. What could you do instead of smoking at those times?

Things to Do Instead of Smoking

1. _____
2. _____
3. _____

The Bottom Line: Commit Yourself

There comes a time when you have to say good-bye to your cigarettes.

- Pick a day to stop smoking.
- Fill out the Behavior Change Contract.
- Have a family member or friend sign the contract.

THEN

- Throw away all your cigarettes, lighters, and ashtrays at home and at work. You will not need them again.
- Be prepared to feel the urge to smoke. The urge will pass whether or not you smoke. Use the four Ds to fight the urge: Delay, Deep breathing, Drink water, and Do something else.

- Keep "mouth toys" handy: lifesavers, gum, straws, and carrot sticks can help.
- If you've had trouble stopping before, ask your doctor about nicotine chewing gum, patches, nasal sprays, inhalers, or pills.
- Tell your family and friends that you've stopped smoking.
- Put "no smoking" signs in your car, work area, and house.
- Give yourself a treat for stopping. Go to a movie, go out to dinner, or buy yourself a gift.

Focus on the Positives

Now that you have stopped smoking, your mind and your body will begin to feel better. Think of the good things that have happened since you stopped. Can you breathe more easily? Do you have more energy? Do you feel good about what you've done?

Make a list of the good things about not smoking. Carry a copy with you, and look at it when you have the urge to smoke.

Breaking the Habit For some smokers, the road to quitting includes antismoking therapy. Two common techniques are operant conditioning and self-control therapy. Pairing the act of smoking with an external stimulus is a typical example of an operant strategy. For example, one technique requires smokers to carry a timer that sounds a buzzer at different intervals. When the buzzer sounds, the patient is required to smoke a cigarette. Once the smoker is conditioned to associate the buzzer with smoking, the buzzer is eliminated, and, one hopes, so is the smoking. Self-control strategies view smoking as a learned habit associated with specific situations. Therapy is aimed at identifying these situations and teaching smokers the skills necessary to resist smoking.

The Skills for Behavior Change box presents one of the American Cancer Society's approaches.

Benefits of Quitting According to the American Cancer Society, many tissues damaged by smoking can repair themselves. As soon as smokers stop, the body begins the repair process (Figure 8.5). Within eight hours, carbon monoxide and oxygen levels return to normal, and "smoker's breath" disappears. Often, within a month of quitting, the mucus that clogs airways is broken up and eliminated. Circulation and the senses of taste and smell improve within weeks. Many ex-smokers say they have more energy, sleep better, and feel more alert. By the end of one year, the risk for lung cancer and stroke decreases. Ex-smokers considerably reduce their risks of developing cancers of the mouth, throat, esophagus, larynx, pancreas, bladder, and cervix. They also cut their risk of peripheral artery disease, chronic obstructive lung disease, coronary heart disease, and ulcers. Women are less likely to bear babies with low birth weight. Within two years, the risk

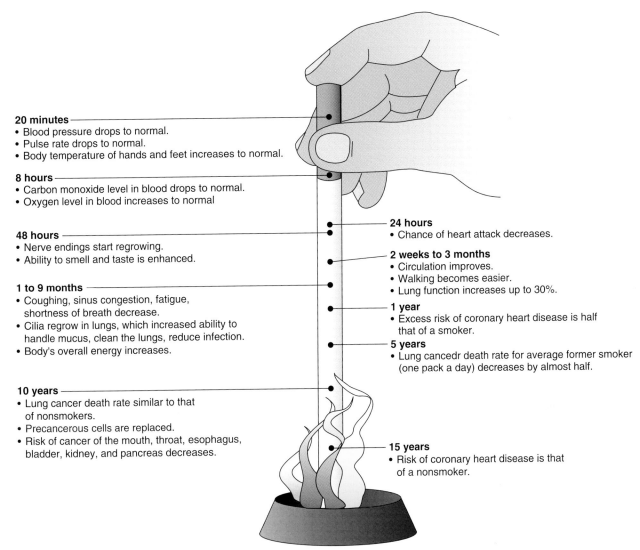

20 minutes
- Blood pressure drops to normal.
- Pulse rate drops to normal.
- Body temperature of hands and feet increases to normal.

8 hours
- Carbon monoxide level in blood drops to normal.
- Oxygen level in blood increases to normal

48 hours
- Nerve endings start regrowing.
- Ability to smell and taste is enhanced.

1 to 9 months
- Coughing, sinus congestion, fatigue, shortness of breath decrease.
- Cilia regrow in lungs, which increased ability to handle mucus, clean the lungs, reduce infection.
- Body's overall energy increases.

10 years
- Lung cancer death rate similar to that of nonsmokers.
- Precancerous cells are replaced.
- Risk of cancer of the mouth, throat, esophagus, bladder, kidney, and pancreas decreases.

24 hours
- Chance of heart attack decreases.

2 weeks to 3 months
- Circulation improves.
- Walking becomes easier.
- Lung function increases up to 30%.

1 year
- Excess risk of coronary heart disease is half that of a smoker.

5 years
- Lung cancedr death rate for average former smoker (one pack a day) decreases by almost half.

15 years
- Risk of coronary heart disease is that of a nonsmoker.

Figure 8.5 ■ When Smokers Quit
Within 20 minutes of smoking that last cigarette, the body begins a series of changes that continues for years. However, by smoking just one cigarette a day, the smoker loses all these benefits, according to the American Cancer Society.
Source: G. Hanson and P. Venturelli, *Drugs and Society*, 5th ed. (Sudbury, MA: Jones and Bartlett, 1998), 320. © Jones and Bartlett, www.jbpub.com. Reprinted with permission.

for heart attack drops to near normal. At the end of ten smoke-free years, the ex-smoker can expect to live out his or her normal life span.

What Do You Think? Do you know

people who have tried to quit smoking? ■ What was this experience like for them? ■ Were they successful? If not, what factors contributed to relapse?

CAFFEINE

Caffeine is the most popular and widely consumed drug in the United States. Almost half of all Americans drink coffee every day, and many others consume caffeine in some other form, mainly for its well-known "wake-up" effect. Drinking coffee is legal, even

socially encouraged. Many people believe caffeine is not a drug and not really addictive. Coffee and other caffeine-containing products seem harmless. If you share these attitudes, think again; research in the past decade has linked caffeine to certain health problems.

Caffeine is a drug derived from the chemical family called **xanthines.** Two related chemicals, *theophylline* and *theobromine,* are found in tea and chocolate, respectively. The xanthines are mild CNS stimulants that enhance mental alertness and reduce feelings of

Caffeine A stimulant found in coffee, tea, chocolate, and some soft drinks.

Xanthines The chemical family of stimulants to which caffeine belongs.

fatigue. Other stimulant effects include increases in heart muscle contractions, oxygen consumption, metabolism, and urinary output. These effects are felt within 15 to 45 minutes of ingesting a product that contains caffeine.

Side effects of the xanthines include wakefulness, insomnia, irregular heartbeat, dizziness, nausea, indigestion, and sometimes mild delirium. Some people also experience heartburn. As with some other drugs, the user's psychological outlook and expectations will influence the effects.

Different products contain different concentrations of caffeine. A 5-ounce cup of coffee contains 65 to 115 milligrams. Caffeine concentrations vary with the brand of the beverage and the strength of the brew. Small chocolate bars contain up to 15 milligrams of caffeine and theobromine. Table 8.4 compares various caffeine-containing products.

Caffeine Addiction

As the effects of caffeine wear off, users may feel let down—mentally or physically depressed, exhausted, and weak. To counteract this, people commonly choose to drink another cup of coffee. Habitually engaging in this practice leads to tolerance and psychological dependency. Until the mid-1970s, caffeine was not medically recognized as addictive. Chronic caffeine use and its attendant behaviors were called "coffee nerves." This syndrome is now recognized as *caffeine intoxication*, or **caffeinism.**

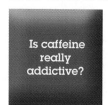

Is caffeine really addictive?

Symptoms of caffeinism include chronic insomnia, jitters, irritability, nervousness, anxiety, and involuntary muscle twitches. Withdrawing the caffeine may compound the effects and produce severe headaches. (Some physicians ask their patients to take a simple test for caffeine addiction: don't consume anything containing caffeine, and if you get a severe headache within four hours, you are addicted.) Because caffeine meets the requirements for addiction—tolerance, psychological dependency, and withdrawal symptoms—it can be classified as addictive.

Although you would have to drink 67 to 100 cups of coffee in a day to produce a fatal overdose of caffeine, you may experience sensory disturbances after consuming only 10 cups of coffee within a 24-hour period. These symptoms include tinnitus (ringing in the ears), spots before the eyes, numbness in arms and legs, poor circulation, and visual hallucinations. Because ten cups of coffee is not an extraordinary amount to drink in one day, caffeine use clearly poses health threats.

Caffeinism   Caffeine intoxication brought on by excessive caffeine use; symptoms include chronic insomnia, irritability, anxiety, muscle twitches, and headaches.

Table 8.4
Caffeine Content of Various Products

Product	Caffeine Content (Average mg per Serving)
Coffee (5-oz. cup)	
Regular brewed	65–115
Decaffeinated brewed	3
Decaffeinated instant	2
Tea (6-oz. cup)	
Hot steeped	36
Iced	31
Bottled (12 oz.)	15
Soft Drinks (12-oz. servings)	
Jolt Cola	100
Dr. Pepper	61
Mountain Dew	54
Coca-Cola	46
Pepsi	36–38
Chocolate	
1 oz. baking chocolate	25
1 oz. chocolate candy bar	15
1/2 cup chocolate pudding	4–12
Over-the-Counter Drugs	
No Doz (2 tablets)	200
Excedrin (2 tablets)	130
Midol (2 tablets)	65
Anacin (2 tablets)	64

Source: Office of Department of Health and Welfare, October 2001.

The Health Consequences of Long-Term Caffeine Use

Long-term caffeine use has been suspected of being linked to a number of serious health problems, ranging from heart disease and cancer to mental dysfunction and birth defects. However, no strong evidence exists to suggest that moderate caffeine use (less than 300 milligrams daily, approximately three cups of coffee) produces harmful effects in healthy, nonpregnant people.

It appears that caffeine does not cause long-term high blood pressure and it has not been linked to strokes, nor is there any evidence of a relationship between coffee and heart disease.[60] However, people who suffer from irregular heartbeat are cautioned against using caffeine because the resultant increase in heart rate might be life-threatening. Both decaffeinated and caffeinated coffee products contain ingredients that can irritate the stomach lining and be harmful to people with stomach ulcers.

For years, caffeine consumption was linked with fibrocystic breast disease, a condition characterized by painful, noncancerous lumps in the breast. Although these conclusions have been challenged, many clinicians advise patients with mammillary cysts to avoid caffeine. In addition, some reports indicate that very high doses of caffeine given to pregnant laboratory animals can cause stillbirths or offspring with low birth weights or limb deformations. Studies have found that moderate consumption of caffeine (less than 300 milligrams per day) did not significantly affect human fetal development.[61] However, women are usually advised to avoid or at least reduce caffeine use during pregnancy.

What Do You Think? How much caffeine do you consume, and why? ▪ What is your pattern of caffeine consumption for the day? ▪ Have you ever experienced any ill effects after going without caffeine for a period of time?

▪ Taking Charge

Summary

- Alcohol is a central nervous system (CNS) depressant used by 70 percent of all Americans and 83 percent of all college students; over 44 percent of college students are binge drinkers. While consumption trends are slowly creeping downward, college students are under extreme pressure to consume alcohol.

- Alcohol's effect on the body is measured by the blood alcohol concentration (BAC), the ratio of alcohol to total blood volume. The higher the BAC, the greater the drowsiness and impaired judgment and coordination.

- Negative consequences associated with alcohol use and college students include lower grade point averages, academic problems, traffic accidents, dropping out of school, unplanned sex, hangovers, and injury. Long-term alcohol overuse includes damage to the nervous system, cardiovascular damage, liver disease, and increased risk for cancer. Use during pregnancy can cause fetal alcohol effects (FAE) or fetal alcohol syndrome (FAS). Alcohol is also a causative factor in traffic accidents.

- Alcohol use becomes alcoholism when it interferes with school, work, or social and family relationships, or entails violations of the law. Causes of alcoholism include biological, family, social, and cultural factors. Alcoholism has far-reaching effects on families, especially on children.

- Treatment options for alcoholism include detoxification at private medical facilities, therapy (family, individual, or group), and programs such as Alcoholics Anonymous.

- The use of tobacco involves many social and political issues, including advertising targeted at youth and women, the largest growing populations of smokers. Health care and lost productivity resulting from smoking cost the nation as much as $157 billion per year.

- Tobacco is available in smoking and smokeless forms, both containing addictive nicotine (a psychoactive substance). Smoking also delivers 4,000 other chemicals to the lungs of smokers.

- Health hazards of smoking include markedly higher rates of cancer, heart, and circulatory disorders, respiratory diseases, and gum diseases. Smoking while pregnant presents risks for the fetus, including miscarriage and low birth weight. Smokeless tobacco dramatically increases risks for oral cancer and other oral problems.

- Environmental tobacco smoke (secondhand smoke) puts nonsmokers at risk for cancer and heart disease.

- Nicotine replacement products or Zyban can help wean smokers off nicotine. Several therapy methods can help smokers break the habit.

- Caffeine is a widely used CNS stimulant. No long-term ill-health effects have been proven, although chronic users who try to quit may experience withdrawal.

Chapter Review

1. What percentage of Americans consume alcoholic beverages regularly?
   a. 30%
   b. 48%
   c. 65%
   d. 83%

2. If a man and a woman drink the same amount of alcohol, the woman's BAC will be approximately
   a. the same as the man's BAC.
   b. 60% higher than the man's BAC.
   c. 30% higher than the man's BAC.
   d. 30% lower than the man's BAC.

3. What is the lifetime risk of alcoholism in the United States?
   a. 3% for both men and women
   b. 3% for men and 10% for women
   c. 10% for men and 3% for women
   d. 10% for both men and women

4. The fastest-growing population of alcohol abusers are
   a. the elderly.
   b. adolescents.
   c. women.
   d. immigrants.

5. Children in dysfunctional families generally assume a specific role. Which role draws attention away from the family's primary problem through delinquency or misbehavior?
   a. family hero
   b. scapegoat
   c. lost child
   d. mascot

6. Blood alcohol concentration (BAC) is the
   a. concentration of plant sugars in the blood stream.
   b. percentage of alcohol in a beverage.
   c. level of alcohol content in the blood before becoming drunk.
   d. ratio of alcohol to the total blood volume.

7. Paul's doctor prescribed him Zyban to help
   a. quit smoking cigarettes.
   b. alleviate heartburn.
   c. quit drinking coffee.
   d. him stay awake to study.

8. How many years must an ex-smoker be smoke-free to expect to live out his or her normal life span?
   a. 2 years
   b. 5 years
   c. 10 years
   d. 15 years

9. The symptoms of chronic insomnia, jitters, irritability, anxiety, muscle twitches, and headaches describe
   a. caffeine overload.
   b. caffeine poisoning.
   c. theobromine syndrome.
   d. caffeinism.

10. A derivative of the chemical family of stimulants called xanthines is found in
    a. snuff.
    b. nicotine.
    c. tobacco.
    d. coffee.

Answers to these questions can be found on page A-1.

Questions for Discussion and Reflection

1. When it comes to drinking alcohol, how much is too much? How can you avoid drinking amounts that will affect your judgment? When you see a friend having too many drinks at a party, what actions do you normally take? What actions could you take?

2. What are some of the most common negative consequences college students experience as a result of drinking? What are secondhand effects of binge drinking? Why do students tolerate negative behaviors of students who have been drinking?

3. What physiological effects could you expect to feel after four 12-ounce beers? Would a person of similar weight show greater effects after having four gin and tonics instead of beer? Why or why not? At what point in your life should you start worrying about the long-term effects of alcohol abuse?

4. Describe the difference between a problem drinker and an alcoholic. What factors can cause someone to slide from responsibly consuming alcohol to becoming an alcoholic? What effect does alcoholism have on an alcoholic's family?

5. Does anyone ever recover from alcoholism? Why or why not? Do you think society's views on drinking have changed over the years? Explain your answer.

6. New research suggests that genetic factors might be more influential than environmental factors in smoking initiation and nicotine dependence. How might this information change current prevention efforts? How would you design smoking prevention strategies targeted at adolescents?

7. Discuss short-term and long-term health hazards associated with tobacco. How will increased tobacco use among adolescents and college students impact the medical system in the future? Who should be responsible for the medical expenses of smokers? Insurance companies? Smokers themselves?

8. Restrictions on smoking are increasing in our society. Do you think these restrictions are fair? Do they infringe on people's rights? Are the restrictions too strict or not strict enough?

9. Describe the pros and cons of each method of tobacco cessation. Which would be most effective for you? Explain why.

10. Discuss problems related to the ingestion of caffeine. How much caffeine do you consume? Why?

Accessing Your Health on the Internet

The following websites explore further topics and issues related to personal health. For links to the websites below, visit the Companion Website for *Health: The Basics,* Seventh Edition at www.aw-bc.com/donatelle.

1. *American Lung Association.* This site offers a wealth of information regarding smoking trends, environmental smoke, and advice on smoking cessation.

2. *ASH (Action on Smoking and Health).* The nation's oldest and largest antismoking organization, ASH regularly takes hard-hitting legal actions and does other work to fight smoking and protect the rights of nonsmokers.

3. *College Drinking: Changing the Culture.* This online resource center is based on a series of reports published by the Task Force of the National Advisory Council on Alcohol Abuse and Alcoholism. It targets three audiences: the student population as a whole, the college and its surrounding environment, and the individual at-risk or alcohol-dependent drinker.

4. *Had Enough.* This entertaining site is designed for college students who have suffered the secondhand effects (baby-sitting a roommate who has been drinking, having sleep interrupted, etc.) of other students' drinking. It offers suggestions for taking action and being proactive about policy issues on your campus.

5. *Higher Education Center for Alcohol and Other Drug Prevention.* This site is funded through the U.S. Department of Education and provides information relevant to colleges and universities. A specific site exists for students who are seeking information regarding alcohol.

6. *TIPS (Tobacco Information and Prevention Source).* This site provides access to a variety of information regarding tobacco use in the United States, with specific information for and about young people.

Further Reading

Glantz, S. A. and E. D. Balbach. *The Tobacco War: Inside the California Battles.* Berkeley: University of California Press, 2000.

Charts the dramatic and complex history of tobacco politics in California over the past quarter century. Shows how the accomplishments of tobacco-control advocates have changed and how people view the tobacco industry and its behavior.

Jersild, D. *Happy Hours: Alcohol in a Woman's Life.* New York: HarperCollins, 2001.

This book, a combination of cutting-edge research and personal stories of women who have struggled with alcohol problems, examines the role that alcohol plays in women's lives.

Kluger, R. *Ashes to Ashes: America's Hundred-Year Cigarette War, the Public Health, and the Unabashed Triumph of Philip Morris.* New York: Vintage Books, 1997.

A definitive history of America's controversial tobacco industry, focusing on Philip Morris. Traces the development of the cigarette, revelations of its toxicity, and the impact of political and corporate shenanigans on the battle over smoking.

Kuhn, C., S. Swartzwelder, W. Wilson, J. Foster, and L. Wilson. *Buzzed: The Straight Facts,* National Institute on Alcohol Abuse and Alcoholism (NIAAA), *Research Monographs.* Washington, DC: U.S. Department of Health and Human Services.

A series of publications containing the results of a number of studies conducted by research scientists under the auspices of NIAAA through 2002. These monographs address issues such as alcohol use among older adults, occupational alcoholism, social drinking, and the relationship between heredity and alcoholism.

Nuwer, H. *Wrongs of Passage: Fraternities, Sororities, Hazing, and Binge Drinking.* Bloomington: Indiana University Press, 1999.

A comprehensive exposé on the continuing crisis of death and injury among fraternity and sorority pledges. The book provides an overview of Greek customs and demands that encouraged hazing as well as the recent deaths of students at some of the nation's most prestigious universities. The author argues that we need to control the Greek system as well as other organizations that employ similar, sometimes deadly, hazing practices.

Sperber, M. *Beer and Circus: How Big Time College Sports Is Crippling Undergraduate Education.* New York: Henry Holt, 2000.

Sperber's book is an indictment of the attraction of undergraduates to schools based on the school's sports success and party reputations. He links student drinking behaviors to sports programs and argues that such an atmosphere shortchanges undergraduates of their education.

Wechsler, H. and B. Wuethrich. *Dying to Drink: Confronting Binge Drinking on College Campuses.* Emmaus, PA: Rodale, 2002.

A report of the widespread alcohol culture that is on many campuses.

Whelan, E. *Cigarettes: What the Warning Label Doesn't Tell You—The First Comprehensive Guide to the Health Consequences of Smoking.* New York: Prometheus Books, 1997.

From impotence to diabetes, cataracts to psoriasis, the proven dangers of smoking go well beyond heart and lung disease. This book details all the known health threats of smoking. Twenty-one experts explain how smoking can affect the body.

Zailckas, K. *Smashed: A Story of a Drunken Girlhood.* New York: Viking, 2005.

A 24-year-old woman writes about her own experiences of drinking through high school and college.

References

1. L. D. Johnson, P. M. O'Malley, and J. G. Bachman, *The Monitoring the Future Study, 1975–2004,* vol. 2 (Rockville, MD: *National Institute of Drug Abuse,* 2005).
2. H. Weschler et al., "Trends in College Binge Drinking during a Period of Increased Prevention Efforts: Findings from Four Harvard School of Public Health College Study Surveys: 1993–2001," *Journal of American College Health* 50, no. 5 (2002): 207.
3. Ibid.
4. Johnson, *The Monitoring the Future Study.*

5. R. Hingson et al., "Magnitude of Alcohol-Related Mortality and Morbidity Among U.S. College Students Ages 18–24: Changes from 1998 to 2001," *Annual Review of Public Health* 26 (2005): 259–79.

6. Ibid.

7. H. Weschler et al., "College Binge Drinking in the 1990s: A Continuing Problem," *Journal of American College Health* 48, no. 10 (2000): 199–210.

8. M. Mohler-Kuo et al., "Correlates of Rape while Intoxicated in a National Sample of College Women," *Journal of Studies on Alcohol* 65, no.1 (2004): 37.

9. R. Hingson et al., "Magnitude of Alcohol-Related Mortality and Morbidity."

10. J. Kinney et al., *Loosening the Grip,* 8th ed., (New York: McGraw-Hill, 2005).

11. S. MacDonald, "The Criteria for Causation of Alcohol in Violent Injuries in Six Countries," *Addictive Behaviors* 30, no. 1 (2005): 103–113.

12. J. Turner et al., "Serious Health Consequences Associated with Alcohol Use Among College Students: Demographic and Clinical Characteristics of Patients Seen in the Emergency Department," *Journal of Studies on Alcohol* 65, no. 2 (2004): 179.

13. C. Ikonomidou et al., "Ethanol-Induced Apoptotic Neurodegeneration and the Fetal Alcohol Syndrome," *Science* 287 (2000): 1056–1060.

14. J. Theruvathu et al., "Polyamines Stimulate the Formation of Mutagenic 1, N2-Propanodeoxyguanosine Adducts from Acetaldehyde," *Nucleic Acids Research* 33, no. 11 (2005): 3513–3520.

15. National Organization on Fetal Alcohol Syndrome, 2005, www.nofas.org.

16. National Highway Traffic Safety Administration, "Traffic Safety Facts 2003," www.nhtsa.dot.gov.

17. H. Wechsler et al., "Changes in Binge Drinking and Related Problems among American College Students between 1993 and 1997," *Journal of American College Health* 47, no. 2 (1998): 57–68.

18. National Highway Traffic Safety Administration, "Traffic Safety Facts 2003," www.nhtsa.dot.gov.

19. National Highway Traffic Safety Administration, "Crash Stats: Alcohol Related Fatalities by State, 2004," www. nhtsa.dot.gov.

20. Ibid.

21. National Highway Traffic Safety Administration, "Traffic Safety Facts 2003."

22. National Highway Traffic Safety Administration, "Fatality Analysis Reporting System: Alcohol," 2004, www.nhtsa.dot.gov.

23. J. Knight et al., "Alcohol Abuse and Dependence among U.S. College Students," *Journal of Studies on Alcohol* 63, no. 3 (2002): 263–270.

24. Substance Abuse and Mental Health Services Administration, "Results from the 2003 National Survey on Drug Use and Health: National Findings" (Office of Applied Studies, NHSDA Series H-24, DHHS Publication No. SMA 04–3963), (U.S. Department of Health and Human Services, Rockville, MD: 2004).

25. "Adult Children of Alcoholics," *Alcohol Issues and Solutions* 6, no. 2 (2000): 6.

26. B. F. Grant, "Estimates of U.S. Children Exposed to Alcohol Abuse and Dependence in the Family," *American Journal of Public Health* 90, no. 1 (2000): 112–115.

27. U.S. Department of Health and Human Services, "Alcohol: A Women's Issue," National Institute on Alcohol Abuse and Alcoholism, January 2005.

28. National Institute on Drug Abuse, "Info Facts: Treatment Methods for Women," August 30, 2004, www.nida.nih.gov/Infofax/treatwomen.html.

29. T. Wall and C. Ehlers, "Genetic Influences Affecting Alcohol Use Among Asians," *Alcohol Health and Research World* 19, no. 3: 184–189.

30. W. Max, "The Financial Impact of Smoking on Health-Related Costs: A Review of the Literature," *American Journal of Health Promotion* 15 (2001): 321–331.

31. Centers for Disease Control and Prevention, "Annual Smoking-Attributable Mortality, Years of Potential Life Lost, and Economic Costs—United States," *Morbidity and Mortality Report* 51, no. 14 (2002): 300–303.

32. Centers for Disease Control and Prevention, "Trends in Cigarette Smoking Among High School Students—United States, 1991–2001," *Morbidity and Mortality Weekly Report* 51, no. 19 (2002): 409–412; Centers for Disease Control and Prevention, "Cigarette Use Among High School Students—United States, 1991–2003," *Morbidity and Mortality Weekly Report* 53, no. 23 (2004): 499–502.

33. Centers for Disease Control and Prevention, Annual Smoking-Attributable Mortality, Years of Potential Life Lost, and Productivity Losses—United States, 1997-2001. *Morbidity and Mortality Weekly Reports Highlights* 54, no. 25: 625–628.

34. N. Rigotti, J. Lee, and H. Wechsler, "U.S. College Students' Use of Tobacco Products," *Journal of the American Medical Association* 284 (2000): 699–705.

35. S. A. Everett et al., "Smoking Initiation and Smoking Patterns among U. S. College Students," *Journal of American College Health* 48 (1999): 55.

36. American Cancer Society, "The Facts About Secondhand Smoke," 2004, www.cancer.org

37. American Lung Association, "Trends in Cigarette Smoking," March 1999, www.lungusa.org

38. S. Hansen, "Bidis," University of Iowa's Student Health Service/Health Iowa. www.uiowa.edu/~shs.

39. American Cancer Society, "Cancer Facts and Figures 2004," (Atlanta: American Cancer Society), 2005, www.cancer.org.

40. Ibid.

41. Ibid.

42. Ibid.

43. Ibid.

44. American Cancer Society, "Cancer Facts and Figures," 2004, www.acs.org.

45. American Lung Association, "Quit Smoking: Benefits," www.lungusa.org.

46. American Heart Association, "Risk Factors for a Stroke," www.americanheart.org.

47. Ibid.

48. American Cancer Society, "Cancer Facts- 2005," www.acs.org.

49. American Academy of Periodontology, "Tobacco Use and Periodontal Disease," 2004, www.perio.org.

50. American Lung Association National Cancer Institute, "Health Effects of Exposure to Environmental Tobacco Smoke," *Smoking and Tobacco Control Monograph* No. 10, (February 2004).

51. Centers for Disease Control and Prevention, "Second National Report on Human Exposure to Environmental Chemicals: Tobacco Smoke," (USDHHS Publication No. 03-0022) (Bethesda, MD: U.S. Department of Health and Human Services, 2003).

52. P. Hilts, "Wide Peril Is Seen in Passive Smoking," *New York Times*, (May 9, 1990), A25.

53. American Lung Association, "Secondhand Smoke," 2004, http://ala.org.

54. K. Yolton et al., "Exposure to Environmental Tobacco Smoke and Cognitive Abilities among U.S. Children and Adolescents," *Environmental Health Perspectives* 113, no.1 (2005): 9–103.

55. M. R. Becklake et al., "Childhood Predictors of Smoking in Adolescence: A Follow-Up Study of Montreal School Children," *Canadian Medical Association Journal,* 173 no. 4 (2005): 377–379.

56. Centers for Disease Control and Prevention, "Annual Smoking-Attributable Mortality."

57. M. Fogarty, "Public Health and Smoking Cessation," *The Scientist*, 17, no. 6 (2003), 23; Tobacco Control Research Center, (Tobacco Litigation Documents), "Multistate Settlement with Tobacco Industry" 2004, www.library.ucsf.edu/tobacco/litigation.

58. American Cancer Society, "Cancer Facts and Figures" 2004, 25.

59. Ibid.

60. Your Nutrition and Food Safety Resource, "Questions and Answers about Caffeine and Health," January 2003, http://ific.org.

61. Ibid.

Will energy bars or drinks improve my athletic performance?

Is there really a way to make a meal from McDonald's healthy?

Can I get enough protein in my diet if I'm a vegetarian?

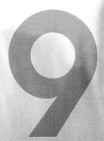

Can I substitute dietary supplements for a balanced diet?

Nutrition
Eating for Optimum Health

Objectives

- *Examine* the factors that influence dietary choices.
- *Discuss* how to change old eating habits, improve behaviors, and use the new USDA MyPyramid Plan appropriately.
- *Summarize* the major essential nutrients and their roles in maintaining health.
- *Explain* the role of nutrition in disease prevention and the facts related to new

trends in nutrition, including food supplements and fad diets.
- *Discuss* issues surrounding gender and nutrition.
- *Discuss* the unique challenges that college students face when trying to eat healthy foods, and strategies to eat healthfully.
- *Explain* food safety concerns facing Americans and people in other regions of the world.

When was the last time you ate something without thinking about how much fat or carbohydrates it contained? Clearly, Americans are trying to heed expert advice about how to have a healthy diet. In survey after survey, 60 to 80 percent of food shoppers say they read food labels before selecting products, yet these same surveys reveal frequent misunderstandings and confusion.[1] Nutritionists, fad diet advocates, and media reports of research studies offer an array of claims and warnings. Although the U.S. Food and Drug Administration (FDA) does a remarkable job in helping to protect us, it can't possibly regulate every dietary claim or new food product that comes into the market. That means that the responsibility for making wise dietary decisions is largely your own. The good news is that, according to the American Dietetic Association, more Americans are seeking information on food and nutrition and taking action to improve their habits than ever before.[2]

Just how important is sound nutrition? A review of over 4,500 research studies concluded that widespread consumption of 5 to 6 servings of fruits and vegetables daily would lower cancer rates by over 20 percent in the global population.[3] Subsequent research has emphasized the impact of diet and nutrition on cardiovascular disease, diabetes, and a host of other chronic and disabling conditions.[4]

The next three chapters focus on fundamental principles designed to help you eat more healthy foods, avoid the problems that so many people face with their weight, and improve your general fitness. In this chapter, we will discuss basic nutrition science and apply sound principles to lifestyle behaviors. You will also gain an appreciation for why you eat as you do, the role of your family of origin and basic biology in determining your eating patterns and choices, and the resources that can help you change negative patterns while building on the healthy choices you are already making.

ASSESSING EATING BEHAVIORS

True **hunger** is a basic physiological drive to find food when there is a lack or shortage of basic foods needed to provide the energy and nutrients necessary to support health. Few Americans have experienced the type of hunger that continues for days and threatens survival. Most of us eat because of our **appetite,** a learned psychological desire to consume certain foods, whether or

Hunger   The feeling associated with the physiological need to eat.

Appetite   The desire to eat; normally accompanies hunger but is more psychological than physiological.

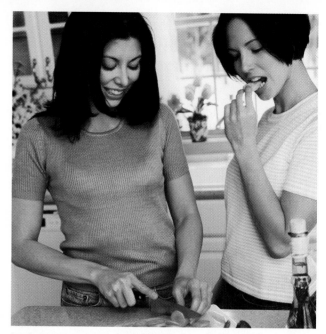

It takes information and planning to make healthy food choices, whether you are eating out, in the dining hall, or cooking your meals at home.

not you are hungry. Appetite can be triggered by smells, tastes, and other triggers such as certain times of day, special occasions, or proximity to a favorite food, such as freshly baked bread.

Hunger sensations are driven by a small region of the brain known as the *hypothalamus.* When the stomach is empty, it sends chemical messages to the hypothalamus, which in turn, triggers hunger sensations. Hunger and appetite are not the only forces involved in our physiological drive to eat; other factors that influence when, how, and what we eat include:

- *Cultural and social meanings attached to food.* Cultural traditions and food choices give us many of our *food preferences.* We learn to like the tastes of certain foods, especially the foods we grew up eating. A yearning for sweet, salty, or high-fat foods can evolve from our earliest days.
- *Convenience and advertising.* That juicy burger on TV looked really good. You've got to have it.
- *Habit or custom.* Often we select foods because they are familiar and fit religious, political, or spiritual views.
- *Emotional comfort.* Eating it makes you feel better— a form of reward and security. We derive pleasure or sensory delight from eating the foods.
- *Nutritional value.* You think the food is good or bad for you or may help you achieve a weight maintenance goal.
- *Social interaction.* Eating out or having company over for a meal is an enjoyable social event.

In addition to physiological need or psychological desire to eat, the type of food you eat has a direct effect on hunger. Foods high in sugar or other refined carbohydrates can cause blood sugar levels to skyrocket. In response, hormones such as *insulin* are produced to lower blood glucose. When this happens you might feel sluggish or even slightly sick. You will often feel hungry again soon after consuming high sugar foods, causing you to seek out food and return your blood sugar levels to normal. Choosing high fat foods, high protein foods, and those with high levels of dietary fiber can help us feel full longer. For example, eating a whole orange, which has more fiber, will help you feel full for a longer period than drinking a glass of orange juice. Eating a piece of cheese (high protein and fat) with that orange will help you stay full even longer.

EATING FOR HEALTH

Nutrition is the science that investigates the relationships between physiological function, health, and the foods we eat. If we eat to maintain and improve our health, we should be healthier. Conversely, if we eat unhealthy foods, consume far more nutrients than we need, or short-change our bodies in basic nutrient needs, we will have more health problems. Today, Americans have a wide range of nutritional problems, even though they live in a country where the majority of people have sufficient means to obtain the foods they need. Consequently, we suffer from many diseases that could be preventable with proper nutrition in the United States. Our "diets of affluence" contribute to soaring rates of heart disease, high blood pressure, bone and joint problems, flat feet, varicose veins, sleep apnea, cirrhosis of the liver, gout, gallbladder diseases, and general problems with activities of daily living (ADLs).[5] Most notably, epidemic increases in type 2 diabetes and obesity are largely due to poor diet, excess weight, and lack of exercise (see Chapters 10 and 11). Most of us want to be in better physical shape, have strong bodies, and look good, but finding the right recipe for optimal diet and exercise is a challenge for many.

Characteristics of a Healthy Diet

Generally, a healthful diet provides the proper combination of energy and nutrients. It is sufficient to keep us functioning well in our daily activities. A healthful diet should be:[6]

- *Adequate.* It provides enough of the energy, nutrients, and fiber to maintain health and essential body functions. Everyone's needs differ (Table 9.1): A small woman who has a sedentary lifestyle may only need 1,800 kilocalories of energy to support her body's functions. A professional biker, such as Lance Armstrong,

Table 9.1
Estimated Daily Calorie Needs

	Calorie Range		
	Sedentary[a]	→	Active[b]
Children			
2–3 years	1,000	→	1,400
Females			
4–8 years	1,200	→	1,800
9–13	1,600	→	2,200
14–18	1,800	→	2,400
19–30	2,000	→	2,400
31–50	1,800	→	2,200
51+	1,600	→	2,200
Males			
4–8 years	1,400	→	2,000
9–13	1,800	→	2,600
14–18	2,200	→	3,200
19–30	2,400	→	3,000
31–50	2,200	→	3,000
51+	2,000	→	2,800

a. A lifestyle that includes only the light physical activity associated with typical day-to-day life.
b. A lifestyle that includes physical activity equivalent to walking more than 3 miles per day at 3 to 4 miles per hour, in addition to the light physical activity associated with typical day-to-day life.
Source: Department of Agriculture Center for Nutrition Policy & Promotion, April 2005, www.MyPyramid.gov.

may need several thousand kilocalories of energy to be up for his competition.

- *Moderate.* The quantity of food you consume can cause you to gain weight. A **calorie** is the unit of measurement used to quantify the amount of energy we obtain from a particular food. Moderate caloric consumption, portion control, and awareness of the total amount of nutrients in the foods you eat is a key aspect of dietary health.

Nutrition   The science that investigates the relationship between physiological function and the essential elements of foods eaten.

Calorie   A unit of measure that indicates the amount of energy obtained from a particular food.

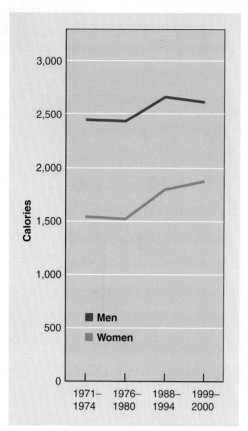

Figure 9.1 ■ Trends in Caloric Intake

Source: J. D. Wright et al., "Trends in Intake of Energy and Macronutrients, United States: 1971–2000," *Morbidity and Mortality Weekly Report* (February 6, 2004).

■ *Balanced.* Your diet should contain the proper combination of foods from different groups. Following the recommendations for the new MyPyramid Plan (page 258) should help you achieve balance.

■ *Varied.* Eat a lot of different foods each day. Variety helps you avoid boredom and can make it easier to keep your diet interesting and in control.

Our habits are important: the quantity and quality (nutritional content) of food eaten and the amount of physical exercise performed all affect our body weights. In a 30-year study of changes in consumption, women's overall caloric intake increased by 22 percent and men's by 7 percent (Figure 9.1).[7] Americans typically get

---

Nutrients The constituents of food that sustain us physiologically: proteins, carbohydrates, fats, vitamins, minerals, and water.

Digestive process The sequence of functions by which the body breaks down foods and either absorbs or excretes them.

Dehydration Abnormal depletion of body fluids; a result of lack of water.

---

approximately 38 percent of their calories from fat, 15 percent from proteins, 22 percent from complex carbohydrates, and 24 percent from simple sugars—and nearly one-third of the calories we consume come from junk foods.[8] Sweets and desserts, soft drinks, and alcoholic beverages make up 25 percent of those calories, and another 5 percent come from salty snacks and fruit-flavored drinks. In sharp contrast, healthy foods such as vegetables and fruit make up only 10 percent of our total calories.[9] When this trend is combined with our increasingly sedentary lifestyle, it is not surprising that we have seen a dramatic rise in obesity. How much do you know about nutrition and healthy eating? Find out by completing the quiz in the Assess Yourself box on page 244.

OBTAINING ESSENTIAL NUTRIENTS

The Digestive Process

Food provides the chemicals we need for activity and body maintenance. Because our bodies cannot synthesize or produce certain essential nutrients, we must obtain them from the foods we eat. **Nutrients** are the elements of food that physiologically sustain us, and include proteins, carbohydrates, fats, vitamins, minerals, and water. Before foods can be used properly, the digestive system must break down the larger food particles into smaller, more usable forms. The sequence of functions by which the body breaks down foods and either absorbs or excretes them is known as the **digestive process** (Figure 9.2).

Water: A Crucial Nutrient

You may be surprised to learn that you could survive much longer without food than you could without water. Even in severe conditions, the average person can go for weeks without certain vitamins and minerals before experiencing serious deficiency symptoms. However, **dehydration** (abnormal depletion of body fluids) can cause serious problems within a matter of hours and death after a few days without water.

The total human body weight consists of 50 to 60 percent water. The water in our bodies bathes cells, aids in fluid and electrolyte balance, maintains pH balance, and transports molecules and cells throughout the body. Water is the major component of our blood, which carries oxygen and nutrients to the tissues and is responsible for maintaining cells in working order.

Individual needs for water vary drastically according to dietary factors, age, size, overall health, environmental temperature and humidity levels, and exercise. Certain diseases, such as diabetes or cystic fibrosis,

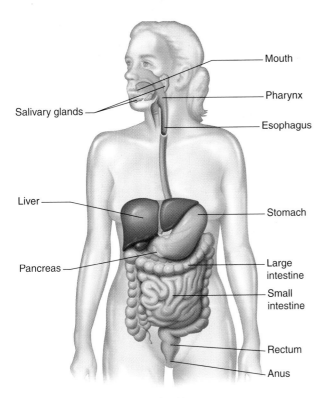

Salivary glands

Liver

Pancreas

Mouth

Pharynx

Esophagus

Stomach

Large intestine

Small intestine

Rectum

Anus

Figure 9.2 ■ **The Digestive Process**
Your mouth prepares for food by increasing production of saliva, which contains enzymes that begin the digestive process. From the mouth, food passes down the esophagus to the stomach. Here, food is mixed by muscular contractions and is broken down by enzymes and stomach acids. Further digestive activity and absorption of nutrients takes place in the small intestine, aided by enzymes from the liver and the pancreas. Next, water and salts are absorbed by the large intestine, and then solid waste moves into the rectum and is passed out through the anus. The entire digestive process takes approximately 24 hours.
Source: Adapted from M. Johnson, *Human Biology: Concepts and Current Issues,* 3rd ed. (San Francisco: Benjamin Cummings, 2006), 314.

cause people to lose fluids at a rate necessitating a higher volume of fluid intake.

Is bottled water healthier than tap water? In most instances, when you buy expensive "spring" water and bottled water, you are actually purchasing chlorinated city water from another area of the country, and the water may not be any better than your own city's tap water. Some of the better bottled waters go through a process to remove chemicals. Is it worth the extra cost? Most experts think not. If you are concerned about your current water source, have it tested. Otherwise, spend your slim student budget another way.

Proteins

Next to water, **proteins** are the most abundant substances in the human body. Proteins are major components of nearly every cell and have been called the "body builders" because of their role in developing and

repairing bone, muscle, skin, and blood cells. They are the key elements of the antibodies that protect us from disease, of enzymes that control chemical activities in the body, and of hormones that regulate body functions. Proteins help transport iron, oxygen, and nutrients to all body cells and supply another source of energy to cells when fats and carbohydrates are not readily available. In short, adequate amounts of protein in the diet are vital to many body functions and ultimately to survival.

Whenever you consume proteins, your body breaks them down into smaller molecules known as **amino acids,** the building blocks of protein, which link together like beads in a necklace to form 20 different combinations. Nine of these combinations are termed **essential amino acids,** which means the body must obtain them from the diet; the other 11 are produced by the body.

Dietary protein that supplies all of the essential amino acids is called **complete (high-quality) protein.** Typically, protein from animal products is complete. When we consume foods that are deficient in some of the essential amino acids, the total amount of protein that can be synthesized from the other amino acids is decreased. For proteins to be complete, they also must be present in digestible form and in amounts proportional to body requirements.

What about plant sources of protein? Proteins from plant sources are often **incomplete proteins** in that they are missing one or two of the essential amino acids. Nevertheless, it is relatively easy for the non–meat eater to combine plant foods effectively and eat complementary sources of plant protein (Figure 9.3 on page 247). An excellent example of this mutual supplementation process is eating peanut butter on whole-grain bread. Although each of these foods lacks certain essential amino acids, eating them together provides complete protein.

Plant sources of protein fall into three general categories: *legumes* (beans, peas, peanuts, and soy products), *grains* (whole grains, corn, and pasta products), and *nuts and seeds.* Certain vegetables, such as leafy

Proteins   The essential constituents of nearly all body cells; necessary for the development and repair of bone, muscle, skin, and blood; the key elements of antibodies, enzymes, and hormones.

Amino acids   The building blocks of protein.

Essential amino acids   Nine of the basic nitrogen-containing building blocks of protein that must be obtained from foods to ensure health.

Complete (high-quality) proteins   Proteins that contain all nine essential amino acids.

Incomplete proteins   Proteins that are lacking in one or more of the essential amino acids.

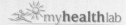

Fill out this assessment online at
www.aw-bc.com/myhealthlab or www.aw-bc.com/donatelle.

What's Your EQ (Eating Quotient)?

Keeping up with the latest on what to eat—or not eat—isn't easy. If you think a few facts might have slipped past you, this quiz should help. There's only one correct answer for each question.

		True	False
1.	Fresh fruits and vegetables contain more nutrients than canned or frozen varieties.	❑	❑
2.	While you are shopping, it makes a difference what area of the store you start in, in terms of keeping your foods safe.	❑	❑
3.	Fruit drinks count as a serving from the fruit group in the MyPyramid Plan.	❑	❑
4.	Baked potatoes have a higher glycemic index (carbohydrate's ability to raise blood sugar levels quickly) than sweet potatoes or apples.	❑	❑
5.	A late dinner is more likely to cause weight gain than eating the same meal earlier in the day.	❑	❑
6.	Nuts are okay to eat if you are trying to stick to a low-fat diet.	❑	❑
7.	Certain foods, like grapefruit, celery, or cabbage soup, can burn fat and make you lose weight.	❑	❑

8. Which of the following has the most fiber?
   a. chuck roast
   b. dark meat chicken with skin
   c. skinless chicken wing
   d. they are all about the same

9. Which of the following is the strongest predictor of obesity in America today?
   a. region of the country you live in
   b. ethnicity/culture
   c. lack of exercise
   d. socioeconomic status

10. When you eat a meal, how long does it take for your brain to get the message that you are full?
    a. 10 minutes
    b. 20 minutes
    c. at least an hour
    d. 2 hours or more

11. Which of the following are at the *top* of the list in bacterial levels among domestically grown vegetables?
    a. green onions, cantaloupe, and cilantro
    b. beets, potatoes, and summer squash
    c. celery, leaf lettuce, and parsley
    d. strawberries, apples, and tomatoes

12. Which of the following foods contains the most grams of fiber per serving?
    a. ½ cup of strawberries
    b. ½ cup of kidney beans
    c. 1 cup popcorn
    d. 1 medium banana

13. To insure that you are getting your antioxidants each day, which tip below would be most helpful?
    a. Eat several dark green vegetables and orange, red, and yellow fruits and vegetables.
    b. Eat at least 2 servings of lean red meat per day.
    c. Eat whole grain foods with at least 2 grams of fiber per serving.
    d. Eat several servings of tuna and salmon per week.

14. Olive oil, one of the heart-healthy monounsaturated fats, is a great source for antioxidants. To reap the most benefits from olive oil, which recommendation should you follow?
    a. Buy it only in amounts that you will use relatively quickly. Nutrients are lost quickly after 12 months sitting on the shelf.
    b. If you buy larger bottles, separate it into smaller bottles and keep the lid on tightly to reduce oxidation from air contact. Refrigerate if possible. Refrigeration causes cloudiness but doesn't affect quality.
    c. Store it in opaque airtight glass bottles or metal tins away from heat and light.
    d. All of the above.

15. Which strategy will help you identify high fiber breads to maximize your quality carbohydrate intake?
    a. Choose a whole-grain bread that lists a whole grain as the first ingredient.
    b. Try to purchase breads with 1 to 2 grams of fiber per slice.
    c. Look for bread that is dark colored. The darker it is, the greater the chance that it has lots of good quality fiber in its recipe.
    d. All of the above.

ANSWERS

1. *False:* There is usually little difference, depending on how produce is handled and how quickly it reaches your supermarket. Canned and frozen produce is typically picked at its peak and may contain more nutrients than fresh produce that was picked over-ripe or too early, sat in a warehouse, spent days in transit, or sat at improper temperatures for prolonged periods. However, canned or frozen fruits and vegetables may have added salt or sugar, so check labels carefully. Whenever possible, buy local produce fresh from the fields or neighboring areas.

2. *True:* As a general rule, milk, meat and other perishables that have been left at room temperature for more than 2 hours have a significant risk of conveying a foodborne illness. Be sure to factor in the time that you spend driving home from the store or running other errands. Start your shopping in the canned and non-refrigerated sections of the store and save your meat and dairy products and frozen foods until last. Run your other errands before you shop for food, and, if you know it will take time to get home, bring a cooler with ice.

3. *False:* Even if fruit juice is an actual ingredient (often it is not), most fruit drinks are primarily water and high fructose corn syrup or other sweeteners, colorings, and fruit flavoring. It is always better to eat the whole fruit, as you will get added fiber, more nutrients, and other benefits. Next best are 100 percent fruit juices, preferably with added vitamin C. Lowest on the nutrient quality list are the sweetened, flavored fruit drinks.

4. *True:* Unfortunately we'd probably be better off with a sweet potato or apple instead of substituting baked potatoes for fries if we are trying to keep our blood sugar levels down or control diabetes. For more information, check the glycemic index reference books available at most bookstores or use the handy guide found at www.diabetesnet.com/diabetes_food_diet/glycemic_index.php.

5. *False:* It's not when you eat but what you eat that makes a difference in weight gain. If you ate a 500 calorie salad at 10 PM and it was your only meal, you wouldn't gain weight. However, a 5,000 calorie pizza for breakfast, followed by a big lunch and dinner would provide enough total calories to thicken a person's waist.

6. *True:* Although they are high in fat, nuts contain mostly unsaturated (good) fat and are good sources of protein, magnesium, and the antioxidants vitamin E and selenium. Moderation is the key. Be mindful of how many calories you are eating.

7. *False:* No foods can burn fat. Some foods with caffeine may speed up your metabolism for a short time but do not cause weight loss.

8. *D:* There is no fiber in animal foods. Fiber is found only in plants and plant-based foods such as fruits, beans, whole grains, and vegetables.

9. *E:* Although the other responses are all contributors to obesity, the greatest single predictor of obesity is low socioeconomic status. Although related factors such as education play a role, the poor nutritional quality of foods commonly eaten when people are forced to stretch their food budget—high-fat meats, hot dogs, inexpensive white breads and pastries, and other high-calorie, low-fiber foods—often increases the risk of obesity.

10. *B:* It takes about 20 minutes for your brain to get the message that you are full. To make sure you don't gorge yourself, eat slowly, talk with others, put your fork down after taking a bite, take a drink of water, or do other things to delay your meal. Let your brain catch up to your fork, and slow it down!

11. *A:* The bad news is that in a recent government study of bacterial levels found in domestic produce, green onions, cantaloupe, and cilantro scored the highest in positive tests for two common bacteria: *Salmonella* or *Shigella*. The good news is that out of nearly 1,100 samples, only 2 to 3 percent were contaminated, but washing your produce is still a must; run a heavy stream of water over the produce while rubbing the outside under the water.

12. *B:* One-half cup of kidney beans provides 4.5 grams of fiber; the medium banana has 2 grams of fiber; strawberries and popcorn each have 1 gram of fiber per serving.

13. *A:* Antioxidants, particularly vitamins C and E, the mineral selenium, and plant pigments known as carotenoids (which include beta-carotene) are found in green leafy vegetables and orange, yellow, and red vegetables and fruit. Eating several servings of these per day helps avoid risks from several health problems.

14. *D:* Olive oil does lose nutrients over time, with one year being the general guesstimate of "use by" time. If the oil smells rancid or if you note mold or other discoloration, discard the bottle.

15. *A:* A true whole-grain bread clearly says so on the label (e.g., "100 percent whole wheat" or "100 percent stone ground whole wheat"). If all the ingredients aren't whole grain, then it's not a true whole-grain bread. The more fiber in each slice the better; look for a minimum of 3 grams. Color is not a good indicator of nutrient value. Dyes and coloring may make even the whitest white bread brown.

Scoring

If you answered all of the above correctly, congratulations! You clearly have a good sense of some of the current issues and facts surrounding dietary choices. If you missed one or more questions, read the corresponding section of this chapter to find out more. Don't despair. Nutrition information changes rapidly, and there is a wealth of information available. Check with your instructor for courses you can take to increase your nutritional knowledge. Review the resources that are recommended, and work hard to stay current.

(continues)

(continued)

Make It Happen!

Assessment: The Assess Yourself activity gave you the chance to test your knowledge of some of the health effects of various foods. Now that you have considered these results, you can decide whether you need to do more to keep up on what to eat and what to avoid for long-term health.

Making a Change: In order to change your behavior, you need to develop a plan. Follow these steps below and complete your Behavior Change Contract to take action.

1. Evaluate your behavior, and identify patterns and specific things you are doing. What can you change now? What can you change in the near future?
2. Select one pattern of behavior that you want to change.
3. Fill out the Behavior Change Contract found at the front of your book. It should include your long-term goal for change, your short-term goals, the rewards you'll give yourself for reaching these goals, potential obstacles along the way, and strategies for overcoming these obstacles. For each goal, list the small steps and specific actions that you will take.
4. Chart your progress in a journal. At the end of a week, consider how successful you were in following your plan. What helped you be successful? What made change more difficult? What will you do differently next week?
5. Revise your plan as needed. Are the short-term goals attainable? Are the rewards satisfying?

Example: Tara discovered that she had very little idea about what foods to eat and to avoid for long-term health. She decided to keep track of her normal diet for a week and then to evaluate it in light of some of the guidelines in this chapter. She considered her diet fairly balanced and was surprised to find that she was eating less than 2 servings of vegetables a day, instead of the recommended 3 to 5. Tara looked at her eating patterns and identified several times when she snacked on foods that could be replaced with healthier snacks. She decided to cut carrots up into sticks that she could toss into her backpack. They stayed fresh all day and made a good snack between classes instead of a candy bar from the vending machine. She also found that her favorite Mexican restaurant offered a vegetarian burrito full of black beans (not refried), squash, tomatoes, and other vegetables that was even tastier than her usual pork burrito. At the end of the first week, Tara and her friends decided to order pizza after a late night of studying. Instead of getting pepperoni or sausage, Tara suggested a pizza with green peppers, spinach, and onions as toppings. Tara did have a setback when she went to a baseball game and ate peanuts and hot dogs all day, but the next day she had a salad for lunch and saw that her vegetable consumption was almost at her goal.

Tara's goal for the next week is to continue to substitute healthy snacks and to look for healthy alternatives when she is eating out. When she is consistently eating the recommended servings of vegetables each week, she will start focusing on other parts of her diet that could use improvement. She is already thinking about how to replace some of the white bread and sugary breakfast cereals she eats now with more whole wheat and whole grains.

---

green vegetables and broccoli, also contribute valuable plant proteins. Mixing two or more foods from each of these categories during the same meal will provide all of the essential amino acids necessary to ensure adequate protein absorption. People who are not interested in obtaining all of their protein from plants can combine incomplete plant proteins with complete low-fat animal proteins, such as chicken, fish, turkey, and lean red meat. Low-fat or nonfat cottage cheese, skim milk, egg whites, and nonfat dry milk all provide complete proteins and have few calories and little dietary fat.

Recently, several low-calorie diets that practically eliminate carbohydrates and focus on eating large quantities of protein have reemerged in the popular press. Diets that deviate from a balanced nutritional approach are almost certainly flawed. Eating too much protein, particularly animal protein, can place added stress on the liver and kidneys. It also may increase calcium excretion in urine, which can elevate the risk of osteoporosis and bone fractures.[10] People who have kidney or liver problems or suffer from fluid imbalances should avoid such diets. For more information, see the following section on carbohydrates and Chapter 10 on weight management.

Although protein deficiency continues to pose a threat to the global population, few Americans suffer from protein deficiencies. In fact, the average American consumes more than 100 grams of protein daily, and about 70 percent of this comes from high-fat animal flesh and dairy products.[11] The recommended protein intake for the average man is only 63 grams, and the average woman needs only 50 grams. (As an example, a 6-ounce broiled sirloin steak contains about 53 grams of protein.) For a 2,000-calorie diet, about 10 percent of calories should come from protein. When we eat more than these recommended amounts, the extra calories contribute to weight gain. See Figure 9.4 to determine your protein requirement.

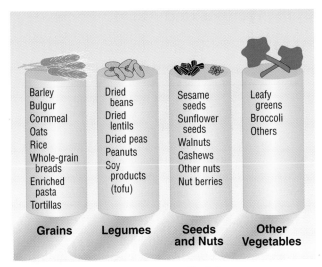

Figure 9.3 ■ Complementary Proteins

Source: Adapted from J. Thompson and M. Manore, *Nutrition: An Applied Approach,* (San Francisco: Benjamin Cummings, 2005).

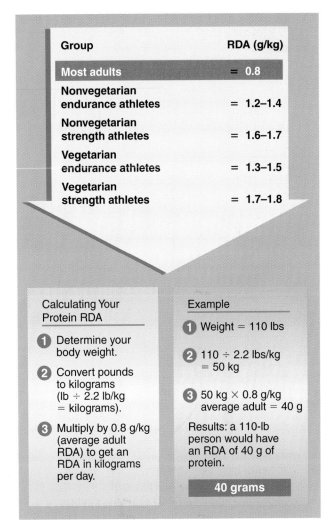

Figure 9.4 ■ Calculating Your Protein RDA (Recommended Dietary Allowance)

Source: Adapted from J. Thompson and M. Manore, *Nutrition: An Applied Approach,* (San Francisco: Benjamin Cummings, 2005).

Carbohydrates

Although the importance of proteins in the body cannot be underestimated, it is **carbohydrates** that supply us with the energy needed to sustain normal daily activity. Carbohydrates can actually be metabolized more quickly and efficiently than proteins and are a quick source of energy for the body, being easily converted to glucose, the fuel for the body's cells. These foods also play an important role in the functioning of internal organs, the nervous system, and the muscles. They are the best fuel for endurance athletics because they provide both an immediate and a time-released energy source as they are digested easily and then consistently metabolized in the bloodstream.

Not all carbohydrates are the same. There are two major types of carbohydrates: **simple sugars,** which are found primarily in fruits, and **complex carbohydrates,** which are found in grains, cereals, dark green leafy vegetables, yellow fruits and vegetables (carrots, yams), *cruciferous* vegetables (such as broccoli, cabbage, and cauliflower), and certain root vegetables, such as potatoes. Most of us do not get enough complex carbohydrates in our daily diets.

A typical American diet contains large amounts of simple sugars. The most common form is *glucose.* Eventually, the human body converts all types of simple sugars to glucose to provide energy to cells. In its natural form, glucose is sweet and is obtained from substances such as corn syrup, honey, molasses, vegetables, and fruits. *Fructose* is another simple sugar found in fruits and berries. Glucose and fructose are **monosaccharides**—they contain only one molecule of sugar.

Disaccharides are simple sugars that contain two molecules of sugar. Perhaps the best-known example is granulated table sugar (*sucrose*). *Lactose* (milk sugar), found in milk and milk products, and *maltose* (malt

sugar) are other examples of common disaccharides. Disaccharides must be broken down into simple sugars before they can be used by the body.

Controlling the amount of simple sugar in your diet can be difficult because it is often present in food products that you might not expect to contain it. Such diverse items

---

Carbohydrates   Basic nutrients that supply the body with the energy needed to sustain normal activity.

Simple sugar   A major type of carbohydrate; provides short-term energy.

Complex carbohydrates   A major type of carbohydrate; provides sustained energy.

Monosaccharide   A simple sugar that contains only one molecule of sugar.

Disaccharide   A combination of two monosaccharides.

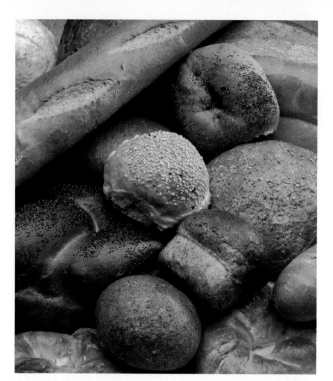

Understanding the role of carbohydrates in your body and the differences between simple carbohydrates and complex carbohydrates will help you make wise decisions about your eating patterns.

as ketchup, salad dressing, flavored coffee creamer, crackers, and yogurt have extremely high sugar content. Read food labels carefully before purchasing.

Complex carbohydrates, or **polysaccharides,** are formed by long chains of sugar molecules. Like disaccharides, they must be broken down into simple sugars before the body can use them. There are two major forms of complex carbohydrates: *starches* and *fiber,* or **cellulose.**

Starches make up the majority of the complex carbohydrate group. Starches in our diets come from flours, breads, pasta, potatoes, and related foods. The body breaks these complex carbohydrates down into glucose, which can be easily absorbed by cells to use as energy. Polysaccharides can also be stored in body muscles and the liver as **glycogen.** When the body requires a sudden burst of energy, it breaks down glycogen into glucose.

Polysaccharide   A complex carbohydrate formed by the combination of long chains of saccharides.

Cellulose   Fiber; a major form of complex carbohydrates.

Glycogen   The polysaccharide form in which glucose is stored in the liver and muscles.

Carbohydrates and Athletic Performance

In the past decade, carbohydrates have become the "health food" of many athletes. Some fitness enthusiasts consume concentrated sugary foods or drinks before or during athletic activity because they think that the sugars provide extra energy. High-sugar, high-calorie sports bars are part of this growing market. However, if you eat a balanced diet and stay well hydrated, these types of concentrated energy foods and drinks aren't necessary—and can be counterproductive.

Will energy bars or drinks improve my athletic performance?

One possible problem involves the gastrointestinal tract. If your intestines react to activity (or the nervousness before competition) by moving material through the small intestine more rapidly than usual, undigested disaccharides and/or unabsorbed monosaccharides will reach the colon, which can result in a very inopportune bout of diarrhea.

Consuming large amounts of sugar during exercise also can have a negative effect on hydration. Concentrations exceeding 24 grams of sugar per 8 ounces of fluid can delay stomach emptying and hence absorption of water. Some fruit juices, fruit drinks, and other sugar-sweetened beverages have more than this amount of sugar. If you use these products, dilute them with ice cubes or water.

Marathon runners and other people who require reserves of energy for demanding tasks often attempt to increase stores of glycogen in the body by *carbohydrate loading.* This process involves modifying the nature of both workouts and diet, usually during the week or so before competition. The athletes train very hard early in the week while eating small amounts of carbohydrates. Right before competition, they dramatically increase their intake of carbohydrates to force the body to store more glycogen to be used during endurance activities (such as the last miles of a marathon).

Is Sugar Addictive?

Although some media reports have suggested that sugar might be addictive, recent research has essentially debunked this myth.[12] Our taste for sweetness is acquired early on in life, based on learned eating patterns and a preference for sweet foods. Culture, genetics, and other factors appear to be reasons for why some of us love sugar far too much. The keys are to monitor sugar intake and eat sweet foods in moderation.

Carbohydrates and Weight Loss

Throughout the 1990s and the low-fat diet craze, a plate of pasta served as a healthy alternative to many who were trying to cut down on high-fat meats. More recently, carbohydrates captured the national attention of millions of would-be-dieters who started dumping their carbohydrates for programs such as the Atkin's Diet,

Protein Power, The Zone, South Beach Diet, and other diet plans. As Americans bought into the low-carb diet trend, sales of items such as white bread and pasta slumped, while an entire low-carb/no-carb industry emerged. Though the interest in extreme carb reduction plans seems to be waning, one positive legacy of these diet plans is that they educated consumers and the food industry on the importance of whole grains, high fiber, and low-sugar food choices.

Fiber

Fiber, often referred to as "bulk" or "roughage," is the indigestible portion of plant foods that helps move foods through the digestive system, delays absorption of cholesterol and other nutrients, and softens stools by absorbing water. Fiber also helps to control weight by creating a feeling of fullness without adding extra calories and appears to reduce risk from heart disease.[13] In spite of all the fiber advocates, the average American consumes between 12 and 17 grams of fiber a day, about half the recommended daily amount of 20 and 35 grams.[14]

Insoluble fiber, which is found in bran, whole-grain breads and cereals, and most fruits and vegetables, is associated with these gastrointestinal benefits and has been found to reduce the risk for several forms of cancer. *Soluble fiber* appears to be a factor in lowering blood cholesterol levels and reducing risk for cardiovascular disease. Major sources of soluble fiber in the diet include oat bran, dried beans (such as kidney, garbanzo, pinto, and navy beans), and some fruits and vegetables.

What's the best way to increase your intake of dietary fiber? Eat more complex carbohydrates, such as whole grains, fruits, vegetables, dried peas and beans, nuts, and seeds. As with most nutritional advice, however, too much of a good thing can pose problems. Sudden increases in dietary fiber may cause flatulence (intestinal gas), cramping, or a bloated feeling. Consume plenty of water or other liquids to reduce such side effects.

A few years ago, fiber was thought to be the remedy for just about everything. Much of this hope was probably unrealistic, although research does support many benefits of fiber, such as:[15]

- *Protection against colon and rectal cancer.* One of the leading causes of cancer deaths in the United States, colorectal cancer is much rarer in countries having diets high in fiber and low in animal fat. Several studies contributed to the theory that fiber-rich diets, particularly those including insoluble fiber, prevent the development of precancerous growths. Whether this was because more fiber helps to move foods through the colon faster (thereby reducing the colon's contact time with cancer-causing substances)

or because insoluble fiber reduces bile acids and certain bacterial enzymes that may promote cancer remained in question. Although research continues, controversy continues over the mechanics and potential health benefits of fiber alone.

- *Protection against breast cancer.* Research into the effects of fiber on breast cancer risk is inconclusive. However, some studies indicate that wheat bran (rich in insoluble fiber) reduces blood-estrogen levels, which may affect the risk for breast cancer. Another theory is that people who eat more fiber have proportionally less fat in their diets and this is what reduces overall risk.

- *Protection against constipation.* Insoluble fiber, consumed with adequate fluids, is the safest, most effective way to prevent or treat constipation. The fiber acts like a sponge, absorbing moisture and producing softer, bulkier stools that are easily passed. Fiber also helps produce gas, which in turn may initiate a bowel movement.

- *Protection against diverticulosis.* About one in ten Americans over the age of 40 and at least one in three over age 50 suffers from *diverticulosis,* a condition in which tiny bulges or pouches form on the large intestinal wall. These bulges can become irritated and cause chronic pain if under strain from constipation. Insoluble fiber helps to reduce constipation and discomfort.

- *Protection against heart disease.* Many studies have indicated that soluble fiber (as in oat bran, barley, and fruit pectin) helps reduce blood cholesterol, primarily by lowering low-density lipoprotein (LDL or "bad") cholesterol. Whether this reduction is a direct effect or occurs through the displacement of fat calories by fiber calories or through intake of other nutrients (such as iron) remains in question.[16]

- *Protection against diabetes.* Some studies suggest that soluble fiber improves control of blood sugar and can reduce the need for insulin or medication in people with diabetes. Soluble fiber seems to delay the emptying of the stomach and slow the absorption of glucose by the intestine. Whether fiber protects against diabetes or not, it is clear that fiber plays a vital role in controlling blood glucose levels.[17]

- *Protection against obesity.* Because most high-fiber foods are high in carbohydrates and low in fat, they help control *caloric* intake. Many take longer to chew, which slows you down at the table and makes you feel full sooner.

> **Fiber** The indigestible portion of plant foods that moves food through the digestive system and absorbs water.

Most experts believe that Americans should double their current consumption of dietary fiber—to 20 to 35 grams per day for most people and perhaps to 40 to 50 grams for others. (A large bowl of high-fiber cereal with a banana provides close to 20 grams.)

Fats

Fats (a type of *lipid*), another group of basic nutrients, are perhaps the most misunderstood of the body's required energy sources. Fats play a vital role in maintaining healthy skin and hair, insulating body organs against shock, maintaining body temperature, and promoting healthy cell function. Fats make foods taste better and carry the fat-soluble vitamins A, D, E, and K to the cells. They also provide a concentrated form of energy in the absence of sufficient amounts of carbohydrates and make you feel full after eating. Some even suggest that the variety of fat-free promotions and products available have made us fatter because we feel less satiated and want more food. If fats perform all these functions, why are we constantly urged to cut back on them?

Although moderate consumption of fats is essential to health, overconsumption can be dangerous. **Triglycerides,** which make up about 95 percent of total body fat, are the most common form of fat circulating in the blood. When we consume too many calories, the liver converts the excess into triglycerides, which are stored throughout our bodies.

The remaining 5 percent of body fat is composed of substances such as **cholesterol,** which can accumulate on the inner walls of arteries and narrow the channel through which blood flows. This buildup, called **plaque,** is a major cause of *atherosclerosis* (hardening of the arteries). At one time, the amount of circulating cholesterol in the blood was thought to be crucial. Current thinking is that the actual amount of circulating cholesterol itself is not as important as is the ratio of total cholesterol to a group of compounds called **high-density lipoproteins (HDLs).** Lipoproteins are the transport facilitators for cholesterol in the blood. High-density lipoproteins are capable of transporting more cholesterol than are **low-density lipoproteins (LDLs).** Whereas LDLs transport cholesterol to the body's cells, HDLs apparently transport circulating cholesterol to the liver for metabolism and elimination from the body. People with a high percentage of HDLs therefore appear to be at lower risk for developing cholesterol-clogged arteries. Regular vigorous exercise plays a part in reducing cholesterol by increasing HDLs.

MUFAs and PUFAs: Unsaturated "Good Guys"

Fat cells consist of chains of carbon and hydrogen atoms. Those that are unable to hold any more hydrogen in their chemical structure are labeled **saturated fats.** They generally come from animal sources, such as meat, poultry, and dairy products, and are solid at room temperature. **Unsaturated fats,** which come from plants and include most vegetable oils, are generally liquid at room temperature and have room for additional hydrogen atoms in their chemical structure. The terms *monounsaturated fat* (MUFA) and *polyunsaturated fat* (PUFA) refer to the relative number of hydrogen atoms that are missing. Peanut and olive oils are high in monounsaturated fats, whereas corn, sunflower, and safflower oils are high in polyunsaturated fats.

There is currently a great deal of controversy about which type of unsaturated fat is most beneficial. Today, many nutritional researchers believe that PUFAs may decrease beneficial HDL levels while reducing LDL levels. PUFAs come in two forms: omega-3 fatty acids and omega-6 fatty acids. MUFAs, such as olive oil, seem to lower LDL levels and increase HDL levels and thus are currently the preferred, or least harmful, fats. Nevertheless, a tablespoon of olive oil gives you a hefty 10 grams of MUFAs. MUFAs are also resistant to oxidation, a process that leads to cell and tissue damage. For a breakdown of the types of fats in common vegetable oils, see Figure 9.5.

Fats   Basic nutrients composed of carbon and hydrogen atoms; needed for the proper functioning of cells, insulation of body organs against shock, maintenance of body temperature, and healthy skin and hair.

Triglycerides   The most common form of fat in the body; excess calories consumed are converted into triglycerides and stored as body fat.

Cholesterol   A form of fat circulating in the blood that can accumulate on the inner walls of arteries.

Plaque   Cholesterol buildup on the inner walls of arteries, which causes a narrowing of the channel through which blood flows; a major cause of atherosclerosis.

High-density lipoproteins (HDLs)   Compounds that facilitate the transport of cholesterol in the blood to the liver for metabolism and elimination from the body.

Low-density lipoproteins (LDLs)   Compounds that facilitate the transport of cholesterol in the blood to the body's cells.

Saturated fats   Fats that are unable to hold anymore hydrogen in their chemical structure; derived mostly from animal sources; solid at room temperature.

Unsaturated fats   Fats that do have room for more hydrogen in their chemical structure; derived mostly from plants; liquid at room temperature.

Reducing Fat in Your Diet
Want to cut the fat? These guidelines offer a good place to start.

- *Know what you are putting in your mouth.* Read food labels. Remember that no more than 7 to 10 percent of your total calories should come from saturated fat, and no more than 30 percent should come from all forms of fat.

- *Use olive oil or canola oil for baking and sautéing.* Animal studies have shown that they don't raise cholesterol or promote the growth of tumors.

- *Whenever possible, use liquid, diet, or whipped margarine.* Choose products that do not have any *trans* fatty acids.

- *Choose lean meats, fish, or poultry.* Remove skin. Broil or bake whenever possible. In general, the more well-done the meat, the fewer the calories. Drain off fat after cooking.

- *Choose fewer cold cuts, bacon, sausages, hot dogs, and organ meats.* Be careful of those products claiming to be "95 percent fat-free"—they may still have high levels of fat.

- *Select nonfat dairy products whenever possible.* Part-skim-milk cheeses, such as mozzarella, farmer's, lappi, and ricotta are good choices.

- *When cooking, use substitutes for butter, margarine, oils, sour cream, mayonnaise, and salad dressings.* Chicken broths, wine, vinegar, and low-calorie dressings provide flavor with less fat.

- *Think of your food intake as an average over a day or a couple of days.* If you have a high-fat breakfast or lunch, balance it with a low-fat dinner.

Trans Fatty Acids: Still Bad?
Since 1961, Americans have decreased their intake of butter by over 43 percent. Instead, they have substituted margarine, which became known as the "better butter" after reports labeled unsaturated fats the "heart-healthy" alternative. In 1990, a widely publicized landmark study questioned the benefits of margarine, indicating that margarine contains fats that raise blood cholesterol at least as much as the saturated fat in butter does.[18] The culprits? **Trans fatty acids (*trans* fats)** (fatty acids having unusual shapes) are produced when polyunsaturated oils are *hydrogenated,* a process in which hydrogen is added to unsaturated fats to make them more solid and resistant to chemical change.[19] Besides raising cholesterol levels, *trans* fatty acids have been implicated in certain types of cancer, increased risk for diseases such as Alzheimer's, and inflammatory processes that increase the risk of cardiovascular disease.[20]

Keep in mind that *trans* fatty acids, even monounsaturated acids, alter blood cholesterol the same way as some saturated fats; they raise LDL and lower HDL cholesterol. The bottom line? Moderation in all fat intake is

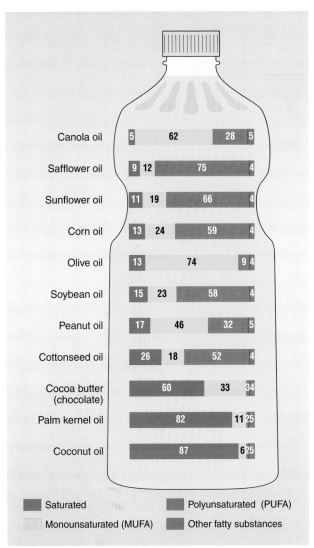

Figure 9.5 ■ Percentages of Saturated, Polyunsaturated, and Monounsaturated Fats in Common Vegetable Oils

the best rule of thumb. Whenever possible, opt for other condiments on your bread, using jams, fat-free cream cheese, garlic, or other toppings. Some experts advocate using low-fat salad dressings as toppings for bread and pasta or using olive oil in moderation to add a bit of flavor. If you have high cholesterol, reducing all types of fat and cholesterol in the diet is still sound advice.

New Fat Advice: Is More Fat Ever Better?
Although most of this chapter has promoted the age-old recommendation to reduce saturated fat, avoid *trans* fatty acids, and eat more monounsaturated

---

Trans fatty acids (*trans* fats)   Fatty acids that are produced when polyunsaturated oils are hydrogenated to make them more solid.

fats, some experts worry that we have gone too far and that our zeal to eat no fat or low-fat foods may be one of the greatest causes of obesity in America today.[21] According to the American Heart Association, eating fewer than 15 percent of our calories as fat (less than 34 grams a day on a 2,000 calorie diet) can actually increase blood triglycerides to levels that promote heart disease, while lowering levels of protective HDLs ("good" cholesterol). There is also a concern that very low-fat diets may lead to shortages of *essential fatty acid* (EFA) in the diet.[22]

Not all fat is bad. In addition to the benefits already mentioned, dietary fat supplies the two EFAs that we must receive from our diets, *linolenic acid* and *alpha-linolenic acid*. These two fats are needed to make hormone-like compounds that control immune function, pain perception, and inflammation, to name a few key benefits.[23]

Although linoleic acid and alpha-linolenic acid are both polyunsaturated fats, they are actually quite different in what they do. Linoleic acid, a member of the *omega-6* family of fats (found in soybeans, peanuts, corn, and sunflower seeds), reduces blood levels of total cholesterol and LDL ("bad" cholesterol) when consumed in reasonable amounts. Alpha-linolenic acid is part of the *omega-3* fats, and is found in flax, canola oil, sardines, spinach, kale, green leafy vegetables, walnuts, wheat germ, and cold water fish such as salmon and tuna.

While both of these essential fats are important, too much linoleic acid may promote blood clots and constrict arteries, which leads to inflammation and damaged blood vessels. Recent research indicates that a form of linoleic acid known as *conjugated linoleic acid (CLA)* seems to be effective in inhibiting breast cancer and, in fact, may moderate the negative effects of high-fat diets. CLA is found in minute quantities in meat and dairy products, so eating small portions of these foods as part of a mostly plant-based diet may provide the health benefits of CLA without the risks of consuming too much fat.[24] Consuming more alpha-linolenic acid reduces risks for blood clots and abnormal heart rhythms and may improve immune function. The best rule of thumb is to balance, following these recommendations.[25]

- Eat fatty fish (bluefish, herring, mackerel, salmon, sardines, or tuna) at least twice weekly.
- Substitute soy and canola oils for corn, safflower, and sunflower oils. Keep using olive oil.

Vitamins Essential organic compounds that promote growth and reproduction and help maintain life and health.

Hypervitaminosis A toxic condition caused by overuse of vitamin supplements.

Minerals Inorganic, indestructible elements that aid physiological processes.

- Add healthy doses of green leafy vegetables, walnuts, walnut oil, and ground flaxseed to your diet to increase intake of alpha-linolenic acid.
- Limit processed and convenience foods, because they often contain harmful saturated and *trans* fats.
- Pick the MUFA or PUFA with the fewest calories and most nutrients.

Although Americans are eating more omega-3 fats than ever before, there is still much research to be done on the benefits versus the risks of consuming large amounts of omega-3s. A new epidemiological study indicates that high levels of omega-3s could increase the risk for neurological disorders. Despite this concern, consuming a moderate amount of foods high in omega-3s can be beneficial to your health.[26]

Vitamins

Vitamins are potent and essential organic compounds that promote growth and help maintain life and health. Every minute of every day, vitamins help maintain nerves and skin, produce blood cells, build bones and teeth, heal wounds, and convert food energy to body energy—they do all of this without adding any calories to your diet.

Age, heat, and other environmental conditions can destroy vitamins in food. Vitamins can be classified as either *fat soluble,* which means they are absorbed through the intestinal tract with the help of fats, or *water soluble,* which means they are dissolved easily in water. Vitamins A, D, E, and K are fat soluble; B-complex and C vitamins are water soluble. Fat-soluble vitamins tend to be stored in the body, and toxic accumulations in the liver may cause cirrhosis-like symptoms. Water-soluble vitamins generally are excreted and cause few toxicity problems (Table 9.2, page 254).

Despite many media suggestions to the contrary, few Americans suffer from true vitamin deficiencies if they eat a diet containing all of the food groups at least part of the time. Nevertheless, Americans continue to purchase large quantities of vitamin supplements. For the most part, vitamin supplements are unnecessary and, in certain instances, may even be harmful. Overusing them can lead to a toxic condition known as **hypervitaminosis.**

Minerals

Minerals are the inorganic, indestructible elements that aid physiological processes within the body. Without minerals, vitamins could not be absorbed. Minerals are readily excreted and are usually not toxic. **Macrominerals** are those minerals that the body needs in fairly large amounts: sodium, calcium, phosphorus, magnesium, potassium, sulfur, and chloride. **Trace minerals** include iron, zinc, manganese, copper, iodine, and cobalt. Only very small amounts of these minerals are needed, and serious problems may result if excesses or deficiencies occur (Table 9.3, page 256). Americans tend to overuse or underuse certain minerals.

Sodium Sodium is necessary for the regulation of blood and body fluids, transmission of nerve impulses, heart activity, and certain metabolic functions. However, we consume much more than we need. It is estimated that the average adult needs only 500 milligrams of sodium (about ¼ teaspoon) per day; yet the average American consumes 6,000 to 12,000 milligrams. Most professional groups recommend restricting sodium to 1,100 to 2,300 milligrams per day; less is better.[27]

The most common form of sodium in the American diet comes from table salt. However, table salt accounts for only 15 percent of sodium intake; the remainder comes from water and from highly processed foods that are infused with sodium to enhance flavor. Pickles, salty snack foods, processed cheeses, many breads and bakery products, and smoked meats and sausages often contain several hundred milligrams of sodium per serving. Many fast-food and convenience entrées pack 500 to 1,000 milligrams of sodium per serving.

Many experts believe that there is a link between excessive sodium intake and hypertension (high blood pressure). Though controversial, it is recommended that hypertensive Americans cut back on sodium to reduce their risk for cardiovascular disorders.[28] Osteoporosis researchers confirm that high sodium intake may increase calcium loss in urine, raising your risk for debilitating fractures as you age.

Try it ▸NOW

Reduce your sodium intake! **Extra salt can be found in almost everything from cereal to bread to snack foods. Take simple steps today to reduce your overall sodium intake: read food labels, and be sure to choose low sodium products. The next time you season food try using either fresh or pre-packaged herb blends instead of salt. Once you cut your sodium intake, you'll taste the difference the next time you eat a sodium-packed product.**

Calcium The issue of calcizum consumption has gained national attention with the rising incidence of osteoporosis among elderly women. Although calcium plays a vital role in building strong bones and teeth, muscle contraction, blood clotting, nerve impulse transmission, regulating heartbeat, and fluid balance within cells, most Americans do not consume the 1,200 mg of calcium per day established by the RDA.

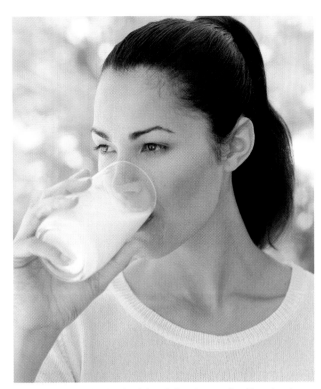

Consuming your RDA of calcium is key to your health not only now, but in the future.

It is critical to consume the minimum required amount each day. More than half of our calcium intake usually comes from milk, one of the richest sources of dietary calcium. Calcium-fortified orange juice and soy milk provide a good way to get calcium if you do not drink dairy milk. Many green leafy vegetables are good sources of calcium, but some contain oxalic acid, which makes their calcium harder to absorb. Spinach, chard, and beet greens are not particularly good sources of calcium, whereas broccoli, cauliflower, and many peas and beans offer good supplies (pinto beans and soybeans are among the best). Other good sources include nuts, seeds, molasses, citrus fruits, and raisins. Bone meal is not a recommended calcium source because of possible contamination.

Do you consume carbonated soft drinks? Be aware that the added phosphoric acid (phosphate) in these drinks can cause you to excrete extra calcium, which may result in calcium loss from your bones. Calcium-phosphorus imbalance may lead to kidney stones and other calcification problems and to increased atherosclerotic plaque.

Macrominerals Minerals that the body needs in fairly large amounts.

Trace minerals Minerals that the body needs in only very small amounts.

Table 9.2
A Guide to Vitamins

Vitamin	Best Sources	Chief Functions in the Body
Water-Soluble Vitamins		
Vitamin B_1 (thiamin) 1.5 mg (RDA + RDI)	Meat, pork, liver, fish, poultry, whole-grain and enriched breads, cereals, pasta, nuts, legumes, wheat germ, oats	Helps carbohydrate convert to energy; supports normal appetite and nervous system function
Vitamin B_2 (riboflavin) 1.7 mg (RDA + RDI)	Milk, dark green vegetables, yogurt, cottage cheese, liver, meat, whole-grain or enriched breads and cereals	Helps carbohydrates, fat, and protein convert to energy; promotes healthy skin and normal vision
Niacin 20 mg NE (RDA + RDI)	Meat, eggs, poultry, fish, milk, whole-grain and enriched breads and cereals, nuts, legumes, peanuts, nutritional yeast, all protein foods	Helps convert nutrients to energy; promotes health of skin, nerves, and digestive system
Vitamin B_6 (pyridoxine) 2.0 mg (RDA + RDI)	Meat, poultry, fish, shellfish, legumes, whole-grain products, green leafy vegetables, bananas	Protein and fat metabolism, formation of antibodies and red blood cells; helps convert tryptophan to niacin
Folate 400 µg (DFE + RDA)	Green leafy vegetables, liver, legumes, seeds	Red blood cell formation; protein metabolism; new cell division; prevents neural tube defects
Vitamin B_{12} (cobalamin) 2.4 mg (RDA)	Meat, fish, poultry, shellfish, milk, cheese, eggs, nutritional yeast	Maintainance of nerve cells; red blood cell formation; synthesis of genetic material
Pantothenic acid 5–7 mg (AI)	Widespread in foods	Coenzyme in energy metabolism
Biotin 30 µg (AI)	Widespread in foods	Coenzyme in energy metabolism; fat synthesis; glycogen formation
Vitamin C (ascorbic acid) (RDI + RDA) 60 mg	Citrus fruits, cabbage-type vegetables, tomatoes, potatoes, dark green vegetables, peppers, lettuce, cantaloupe, strawberries	Heals wounds, maintain bone and teeth, strengthen blood vessels; antioxidant; strengthens resistance to infection; aids iron absorption
Fat-Soluble Vitamins		
Vitamin A 5,000 IU	Fortified milk and margarine, cream, cheese, butter, eggs, liver, spinach, and other dark leafy greens, broccoli, deep orange fruits and vegetables (carrots, sweet potatoes, peaches)	Vision; growth and repair of body tissues; reproduction; bone and tooth formation; immunity; cancer protection; hormone synthesis
Vitamin D 400–600 IU (RDA + RDI)	Self-synthesis with sunlight, fortified milk, fortified margarine, eggs, liver, fish	Calcium and phosphorus metabolism (bone and tooth formation); aids body's absorption of calcium
Vitamin E 30 IU (RDA + RDI)	Vegetable oils, green leafy vegetables, wheat germ, whole-grain products, butter, liver, egg yolk, milk fat, nuts, seeds	Protects red blood cells; antioxidant; stabilization of cell membranes
Vitamin K 70–140 µg	Liver; green leafy, and cabbage-type vegetables; milk	Bacterial synthesis in digestive tract. Synthesis of blood-clotting proteins and a blood protein that regulates blood calcium

Table 9.2

A Guide to Vitamins (continued)

Deficiency Symptoms	Toxicity Symptoms
Beriberi, edema, heart irregularity, mental confusion, muscle weakness, low morale, impaired growth	Rapid pulse, weakness, headaches, insomnia, irritability
Eye problems, skin disorders around nose and mouth	None reported, but an excess of any of the B vitamins can cause a deficiency of the others
Pellagra: skin rash on parts exposed to sun, loss of appetite, dizziness, weakness, irritability, fatigue, mental confusion, indigestion	Flushing, nausea, headaches, cramps, ulcer irritation, heartburn, abnormal liver function, low blood pressure
Nervous disorders, skin rash, muscle weakness, anemia, convulsions, kidney stones	Depression, fatigue, irritability, headaches, numbness, damage to nerves, difficulty walking
Anemia, heartburn, diarrhea, smooth tongue depression, poor growth	Diarrhea, insomnia, irritability, may mask a vitamin B_{12} deficiency
Anemia, smooth tongue, fatigue, nerve degeneration progressing to paralysis	None reported
Rare; sleep disturbances, nausea, fatigue	Occasional diarrhea
Loss of appetite, nausea, depression, muscle pain, weakness, fatigue, rash	None reported
Scurvy, anemia, depression, frequent infections, bleeding gums, loosened teeth, muscle degeneration, rough skin, bone fragility, poor wound healing	Nausea, abdominal cramps, diarrhea, breakdown of red blood cells in persons with certain genetic disorders; deficiency symptoms may appear at first on withdrawal of high doses
Night blindness, rough skin, susceptibility to infection, impaired bone growth, vision problems	Nosebleeds, abdominal cramps, nausea, diarrhea, weight loss, blurred vision, irritability, bone pain, rashes, cessation of menstruation, growth retardation
Rickets in children; osteomalacia in adults; abnormal growth, joint pain, soft bones	Raised blood calcium, constipation, weight loss, irritability, weakness, nausea, kidney stones, mental and physical retardation
Muscle wasting, weakness, red blood cell breakage, anemia, hemorrhaging, fibrocystic breast disease	Interference with anticlotting medication, general discomfort
Hemorrhaging	Interference with anticlotting medication; may cause jaundice

Note: Values increase among women who are pregnant or lactating.
Source: From *An Applied Approach,* by J. Thompson and M. Manore. (San Francisco: Benjamin Cummings, 2005). Reprinted by permission of Pearson Education, Inc.

Table 9.3

A Guide to Minerals

Mineral	Significant Sources	Chief Functions in the Body
Calcium AI: 1,000 mg/day (men and women aged 19 to 50); 1,200 mg/day (men and women over 50)	Milk and milk products, small fish (with bones), tofu, greens, legumes	Principal mineral of bones and teeth; involved in muscle contraction and relaxation, nerve function, blood clotting, blood pressure
Phosphorus RDA = 700 mg/day	All animal tissues	Part of every cell; involved in acid-base balance
Magnesium RDA = 400 mg/day (men); 310 mg/day (women)	Nuts, legumes, whole grains, dark green vegetables, seafood, chocolate, cocoa	Involved in bone mineralization, protein synthesis, enzyme action, normal muscular contraction, nerve transmission
Sodium AI: 1.5 g/day	Salt, soy sauce; processed foods; cured, canned, and pickled foods	Helps maintain normal fluid and acid-base balance
Chloride AI: 2.3 g/day	Salt, soy sauce; processed foods	Part of stomach acid, necessary for proper digestion, fluid balance
Potassium AI: 4.7 g/day	All whole foods: meats, milk, fruits, vegetables, grains, legumes	Facilitates many reactions including protein synthesis, fluid balance, nerve transmission, and contraction of muscles
Iodine RDA = 150 µg	Iodized salt, seafood	Part of thyroxine, which regulates metabolism
Iron RDA = 8 mg/day (men; women over 51); 18 mg/day (women aged 19 to 50)	Beef, fish, poultry, shellfish, eggs, legumes, dried fruits	Hemoglobin formation; part of myoglobin; energy use
Zinc RDA = 11 mg/day (men); 8 mg/day (women)	Protein-containing foods: meats, fish, poultry, grains, vegetables	Part of many enzymes; present in insulin; involved in making genetic material and proteins, immunity, vitamin A transport, taste, wound healing, sperm creation, normal fetal development
Fluoride AI: 3 to 4 mg/day	Drinking water (if naturally fluoride-containing or fluoridated), tea, seafood	Formation of bones and teeth; helps make teeth resistant to decay and bones resistant to mineral loss
Selenium RDA = 55 µg	Seafood, meats, grains	Helps protect body compounds from oxidation

It is generally best to take calcium throughout the day; consume it with foods containing protein, vitamin D, and vitamin C for optimum absorption. Advice varies on which type of supplemental calcium is absorbed most readily and efficiently, although aspartate and citrate salts of calcium often are recommended. The best way to obtain calcium, like all nutrients, is to consume it as part of a balanced diet.

Iron Worldwide, iron deficiency is the most common nutrient deficiency, affecting more than 1 billion people. How much iron do adults need? Females aged 19 to 50

Anemia Iron deficiency disease that results from the body's inability to produce hemoglobin.

need about 18 mg per day, and males aged 19 to 50 need about 10 mg. In developing countries, more than one-third of the children and women of childbearing age suffer from *iron-deficiency anemia.*[29] **Anemia** is a problem resulting from the body's inability to produce hemoglobin, the bright red, oxygen-carrying component of the blood. In the United States, iron-deficiency anemia is less prevalent but still affects 10 percent of toddlers, adolescent girls, and women of childbearing age, which makes prevention a high priority.[30]

When iron deficiency occurs, body cells receive less oxygen, and carbon dioxide wastes are removed less efficiently. As a result, the iron-deficient person feels tired and run down. Although iron deficiency in the diet is a common cause of anemia, anemia also can result from blood loss, cancers, ulcers, and other

Table 9.3

A Guide to Minerals (continued)

Deficiency Symptoms	Toxicity Symptoms
Stunted growth in children; bone loss (osteoporosis) in adults	Excess calcium is excreted except in hormonal imbalance states
Unknown	Can create relative deficiency of calcium
Weakness, confusion, depressed pancreatic hormone secretion, growth failure, behavioral disturbances, muscle spasms	Pharmacological overuse can cause nausea, cramps, dehydration
Muscle cramps, mental apathy, loss of appetite	Hypertension (in salt-sensitive persons)
Growth failure in children, muscle cramps, mental apathy, loss of appetite	Normally harmless (different from poisonous chlorine gas); disturbed acid-base balance; vomiting
Muscle weakness, paralysis, confusion; can cause death, accompanies dehydration	Causes muscular weakness; triggers vomiting; if given into a vein, can stop the heart
Goiter, cretinism	Very high intakes depress thyroid activity
Anemia: weakness, pallor, headaches, reduced resistance to infection, inability to concentrate	Nausea, vomitting, dizziness, damage to organs, death
Growth failure in children, delayed development of sexual organs, loss of taste, poor wound healing	Fever, nausea, vomiting, diarrhea
Susceptibility to tooth decay and bone loss	Fluorosis (discoloration of teeth)
Impared immune function, depression, muscle pain	Vomiting, nausea, rash, brittle hair and nails

Note: RDA = Recommended Daily Allowance; AI = Adequate Intakes. Values are for all adutls aged 19 and older, except as noted.
Source: From *Nutrition: An Applied Approach,* by J. Thompson and M. Manore. (San Francisco: Benjamin Cummings, 2005). Reprinted by permission of Pearson Education, Inc.

conditions. Generally, women are more likely to develop iron-deficiency problems because they typically eat less than men do and their diets contain less iron. Women having heavy menstrual flow may be at greater risk.[31]

Iron overload (known as **hemochromatosis**), or iron toxicity due to ingesting too many iron-containing supplements, remains the leading cause of accidental poisoning in small children in the United States. Symptoms of iron toxicity include nausea, vomiting, diarrhea, rapid heartbeat, weak pulse, dizziness, shock, and confusion. Overdoses of as few as five iron tablets containing as little as 200 mg of iron have killed dozens of children.

Determining Your Nutritional Needs

Historically, dietary guidelines were developed to reduce the public's risk of diseases from nutrient deficiency. Known as the **Recommended Dietary Allowances (RDAs)**, these guidelines have provided

Hemochromatosis   Iron toxicity due to excess consumption.

Recommended Dietary Allowances (RDAs)   The average daily intakes of energy and nutrients considered adequate to meet the needs of most healthy people in the United States under usual conditions.

Americans and Canadians with recommended intake levels necessary to meet the nutritional needs for about 97 percent of healthy individuals. More recently, the U.S. Food and Nutrition Board replaced and expanded upon the RDAs by creating new **Dietary Reference Intakes (DRIs),** a list of 26 nutrients essential to maintaining health. The DRIs identify recommended and maximum safe intake levels for healthy people and establish the amount of a nutrient needed to prevent deficiencies or to reduce the risk of chronic disease. These DRIs are considered the umbrella guidelines under which the following categories fall:

- **United States Recommended Daily Allowances (USRDAs)**—The reference standard for intake levels necessary to meet the nutritional needs of 97 to 98 percent of healthy individuals.

- **Adequate Intake (AI)**—The recommended average daily nutrient intake level of a nutrient by healthy people when there is not enough research to determine the full RDA.

- **Tolerable Upper Intake Level (UL)**—The highest amount of a nutrient an individual can consume daily without the risk of adverse health effects.

Reading Labels for Health In order to help consumers determine the nutritional values of foods, the FDA and the U.S. Department of Agriculture (USDA) developed the **Reference Daily Intakes (RDIs)** and **Daily Reference Values (DRVs).** RDIs are the recommended amounts of 19 vitamins and minerals, also known as micronutrients, and DRVs are the recommended amounts for macronutrients, such as total fat,

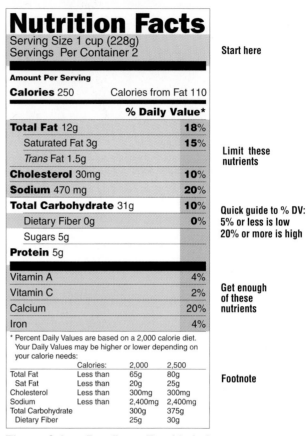

Sample Label for Macaroni and Cheese

Figure 9.6 ■ Reading a Food Label

Source: Center for Food Safety and Applied Nutrition, "Questions and Answers about *Trans* Fat Nutrition Labeling," 2003, www.cfsan.fda.gov/~dms/qatrans2.html.

Dietary Reference Intake (DRI) A set of nutritional values, new combined listing, including more than 26 essential vitamins and minerals, that apply to healthy people.

U.S. Recommended Daily Allowances (USRDAs) Dietary guidelines developed by the FDA and the USDA.

Adequate Intake (AI) Best estimates of nutritional needs.

Tolerable Upper Intake Level (UL) The highest amount of a nutrient that an individual can safely consume every day without risking adverse health effects.

Reference Daily Intakes (RDIs) Recommended amounts of 19 vitamins and minerals, also known as micronutrients.

Daily Reference Values (DRVs) Recommended amounts for macronutrients such as total fat, saturated fat, and cholesterol.

Daily Values (DVs) The RDIs and DRVs together make up the Daily Values seen on food and supplement labels.

---

saturated fat, cholesterol, total carbohydrates, dietary fiber, sodium, potassium, and protein.

Together, RDIs and DRVs make up the **Daily Values (DVs)** that you will find on food and supplement labels listed as a percentage (% DV; Figure 9.6). In addition to the percentage of nutrients found in a serving of food, labels also include information on the serving size, calories and calories from fat per serving, and percentage of *trans* fats in a food.

THE NEW FOOD GUIDE PYRAMID

Early in 2005, the Food Guide Pyramid underwent a landmark overhaul in order to better account for the variety of different nutritional needs throughout the United States population (Figure 9.7). This new pyramid, called the MyPyramid Plan, replaces the former Food Guide Pyramid that had been promoted since 1993 by the USDA and incorporates the *2005 Dietary Guidelines for Americans,* released in January 2005.[32]

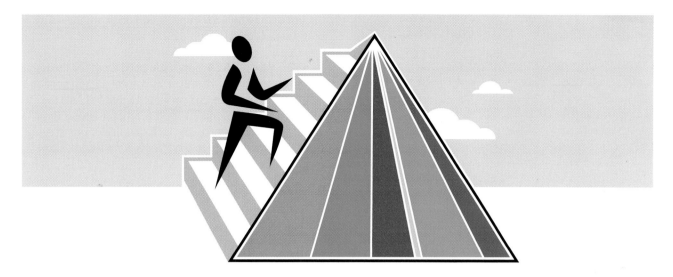

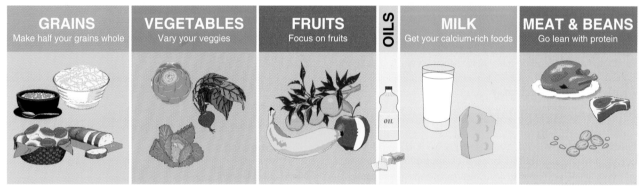

Figure 9.7 ■ MyPyramid Plan

The USDA MyPyramid Plan takes a new approach to dietary and exercise recommendations. Each colored section of the pyramid represents a food group, with the specific needs of individuals in mind. Figure 9.8 on page 261 can help you determine the right number of servings from each food group for you.

Source: United States Department of Agriculture, 2005, www.MyPyramid.gov.

Although the former pyramid emphasized variety in daily intake, it did not reflect what we now know about restricting fats, eating more fruits and vegetables, and consuming whole grains. The new pyramid is also significantly improved in that it takes into consideration activity levels and the various dietary and caloric needs for a variety of individuals (those over 65, children, active adults, etc.). Table 9.1 can help you determine the appropriate level of calorie intake for you.

Goals of the MyPyramid Plan

The MyPyramid Plan is meant to promote personalized dietary and exercise recommendations based upon individual need and to encourage consumers to make healthier food choices and to be active every day.[33] MyPyramid strives to illustrate the following:

■ *Personalization,* demonstrated by the MyPyramid website, www.MyPyramid.gov. The website offers personalized recommendation of the kinds and amounts of food to eat each day, tips and ideas for achieving a

healthy diet, and interactive assessments based on an individual's gender, age, and activity level.

■ *Gradual improvement* encourages individuals to take small steps to improve their diet and lifestyle each day.

■ *Physical activity,* represented by the person climbing steps, reminds individuals about the importance of daily physical activity in maintaining a healthy weight and improving overall health and disease prevention.

■ *Variety* is represented by the six color bands. It is important to eat foods from each group every day in order to receive the proper nutrients for overall health.

■ *Moderation* of food intake is represented by the narrowing of each color band from bottom to top. You should select foods with little or no fat or sugar more often to get the most from the foods you eat.

■ *Proportionality* is symbolized by the varying width of each color band. A wider band generally suggests you should choose more foods from that group, while a narrow band suggests you limit your intake of foods from the corresponding group.

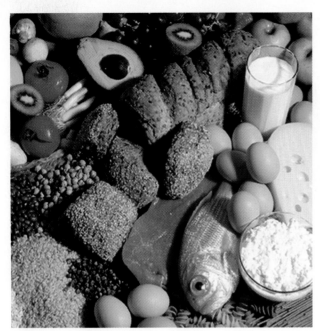

Eating a variety of foods is a key goal of the new MyPyramid Plan.

Using the New MyPyramid Plan

Understanding serving sizes, daily physical activity, and eating a nutritionally balanced diet are key components to using the MyPyramid Plan recommendations successfully. Though these elements are not new to the 2005 Pyramid, they have been updated to reflect the latest in nutritional science.

Understanding Serving Sizes How much is one serving? Is it different than a portion? While these two terms are often used interchangeably, they actually mean very different things, and it is important to understand the difference to be able to use the Pyramid and other nutrition guidelines effectively. A *serving* is the recommended amount you should consume, while a *portion* is the amount you choose to eat at any one time and may be more or less than a serving. Most of us select portions that are much bigger than servings. According to a survey conducted by the American Institute for Cancer Research (AICR), respondents were asked to estimate the standard servings defined by the old USDA Food Guide Pyramid for eight different foods. Only 1 percent of those surveyed correctly answered all serving size questions, and nearly 65 percent answered five or more of them incorrectly.[34] See the Skills for Behavior Change box on page 263 for tips on recognizing serving sizes.

Unfortunately, we don't always get a clear picture from food producers and advertisers about what a serving really is. Consider a bottle of soda: the food label may list one serving size as 8 fluid ounces and 100 calories. However, note the size of the entire bottle; the bottle may hold 20 ounces, and drinking the entire bottle serves up a whopping 250 calories.

Be sure to eat at least the lowest number of servings from the major food groups; you need them for the nutrients they provide. However, if you eat a large portion, count it as more than one serving. Figure 9.8 lists the suggested daily amount of food from each group for a variety of calorie intake levels. Examples of one serving from each food group in MyPyramid are listed below.

Grains
- 1 slice of bread or ½ English muffin
- ½ cup cooked rice, pasta, or hot cereal
- 1 cup ready-to-eat cereal

Fruits
- 1 small apple or 1 large banana
- 1 cup of raw, cooked, or canned fruit
- 1 cup of fruit juice
- ½ cup dried fruit

Vegetables
- 1 cup raw greens or 2 cups cooked greens
- 1 cup beans, peas, or carrots (raw or cooked)
- 1 medium baked potato

Meat and Beans
- 1 ounce lean meat, poultry, or fish
- 1 tablespoon peanut butter
- ¼ cup tofu or cooked beans
- 1 egg

Milk
- 1 cup milk or yogurt
- 1½ ounces natural cheese or ⅓ cup shredded cheese
- 2 ounces processed cheese

Oil
- 1 tablespoon margarine or mayonnaise equals 2½ teaspoons of oil
- ½ avocado equals 3 teaspoons of oil
- 2 tablespoons Italian dressing equals 2 teaspoons oil

Discretionary Calories Every day you must consume a certain number of nutrient-rich foods in order to maintain health. *Discretionary calories* are those obtained from food that do not provide a significant course of nutritional value. Most of us have a very small discretionary caloric allowance at the end of the day. For example, suppose you are on a 2000-calorie diet, and you've eaten wisely all day, choosing whole grains, low-fat, and low-sugar food items, and your calorie balance for the day is at 1,800. This means you

	1,200	1,400	1,600	1,800	2,000	2,200	2,400	2,600	2,800	3,000
Fruits	1 cup	1.5 cups	1.5 cups	1.5 cups	2 cups	2 cups	2 cups	2 cups	2.5 cups	2.5 cups
Vegetables	1.5 cups	1.5 cups	2 cups	2.5 cups	2.5 cups	3 cups	3 cups	3.5 cups	3.5 cups	4 cups
Grains	4 oz.-eq.	5 oz.-eq.	5 oz.-eq.	6 oz.-eq.	6 oz.-eq.	7 oz.-eq.	8 oz.-eq.	9 oz.-eq.	10 oz.-eq.	10 oz.-eq.
Meat and Beans	3 oz.-eq.	4 oz.-eq.	5 oz.-eq.	5 oz.-eq.	5.5 oz.-eq.	6 oz.-eq.	6.5 oz.-eq.	6.5 oz.-eq.	7 oz.-eq.	7 oz.-eq.
Milk	2 cups	2 cups	3 cups	3 cups	3 cups	3 cups	3 cups	3 cups	3 cup	3 cups
Oils	4 tsp.	4 tsp.	5 tsp.	5 tsp.	6 tsp.	6 tsp.	7 tsp.	8 tsp.	8 tsp.	10 tsp.
Discretionary calorie allowance	171	171	132	195	267	290	362	410	426	512

Figure 9.8 ■ Nutritional Needs for Different Groups
Once you've determined your daily caloric requirements (Table 9.1), use this chart to determine how many servings of each food group you need per day to maintain good health.

can spend the remaining 200 calories on what might be considered luxury indulgences. This might include a soda, a small serving of ice cream, or a higher fat cheese or meat than you would normally consume.

Physical Activity Strive to be physically active for at least 30 minutes daily, preferably with moderate to vigorous activity levels on most days. Physical activity does not mean you have to go to the gym, jog 3 miles a day, or hire a personal trainer. Any activity that gets your heart pumping (such as gardening, playing basketball, heavy yard work, and dancing the night away) are all examples of ways to get moving. For more on physical fitness see Chapter 11.

Eating Nutrient-Dense Foods Although eating the proper number of servings from MyPyramid is important, it is also important to recognize that there are large caloric, fat, and energy differences between foods within a given food group. For example, fish and hot dogs provide vastly different fat and energy levels per ounce, with fish providing better energy and caloric value per serving. Nutrient density is even more important for someone who is ill and unable to keep food down. It is important to eat foods that have a high nutritional value for their caloric content. Avoid empty calories, or high-calorie foods that have little nutritional value.

VEGETARIANISM: EATING FOR HEALTH

For aesthetic, animal rights, economic, personal, health, cultural, or religious reasons, some people choose specialized diets. Between 5 and 15 percent of all Americans today claim to be vegetarians. Normally, vegetarianism provides a superb alternative to our high-fat, high-calorie, meat-based cuisine. But without proper information and food choices, vegetarians can also develop dietary problems.

The term *vegetarian* means different things to different people. Strict vegetarians, or *vegans,* avoid all foods of animal origin, including dairy products and eggs. Vegans must be careful to obtain all of the necessary nutrients. Far more common are *lacto-vegetarians,* who eat dairy products but avoid flesh foods. Their diet can be low in fat and cholesterol, but only if they consume skim milk and other low-fat or nonfat products. *Ovo-vegetarians* add eggs to their diet, while *lacto-ovo-vegetarians* eat both dairy products and eggs. *Pesco-vegetarians* eat fish, dairy products, and eggs, while *semivegetarians* eat chicken, fish, dairy products, and eggs. Some people in the semivegetarian category prefer to call themselves "non–red meat eaters."

What Do You Think? Which food groups from the MyPyramid Plan are you most likely to eat enough of during a typical day? ■ Which ones are you most likely to skimp on? ■ What are some simple changes that you could make right now in your diet to help meet MyPyramid recommendations?

Vegetarian A term with a variety of meanings: vegans avoid all foods of animal origin; lacto-vegetarians do not eat meat or eggs but eat dairy products; ovo-vegetarians avoid flesh foods but eat eggs; lacto-ovo-vegetarians do not eat meat but eat both dairy products and eggs; pesco-vegetarians eat fish, dairy products, and eggs; semivegetarians eat chicken, fish, dairy products, and eggs.

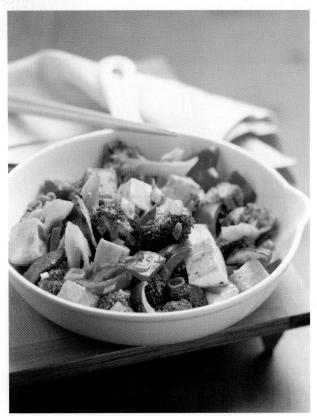

Meals like this tofu and vegetable stir-fry provide the vegetarian with essential vitamins and protein. Adding a whole grain, such as brown-rice, would further enhance this meal by making use of complementary plant proteins.

Generally, people who follow a balanced vegetarian diet weigh less and have better cholesterol levels, fewer problems with irregular bowel movements (constipation and diarrhea), and a lower risk of heart disease than do nonvegetarians. The benefits of vegetarianism also include a reduced risk of some cancers, particularly colon, and a reduced risk of kidney disease.[35]

Although in the past vegetarians often suffered from vitamin deficiencies, the vegetarian of the new millennium is usually extremely adept at combining the right

> Can I get enough protein in my diet if I'm a vegetarian?

types of foods to ensure proper nutrient intake. In fact, while vegans (individuals who do not eat any animal products) typically get 50 to 60 grams of protein per day, lacto-ovo-vegetarians (those who eat dairy and eggs) normally consume between 70 and 90 grams per day, well beyond the RDA. Vegan diets may be deficient in vitamins B_2 (riboflavin), B_{12}, and D. Vitamin B_2 is found mainly in meat, eggs, and dairy products; but broccoli, asparagus, almonds, and fortified cereals are also good sources. Vitamins B_{12} and D are found only in dairy products and fortified products such as soy milk. Vegans are also at risk for deficiencies of calcium, iron, zinc, and other minerals but can obtain these nutrients from supplements. Strict vegans and vegetarians have to pay much more attention to what they eat than the average person does, but by eating complementary combinations of plant products, they can receive adequate amounts of essential amino acids. Examples of complementary combinations are corn with beans and peanut butter with whole-grain bread. Eating a full variety of grains, legumes, fruits, vegetables, and seeds each day will keep even the strictest vegetarian in excellent health. For more information on plant source of protein, see the proteins section on page 243. Pregnant women, the elderly, the sick, and children who are vegans need to take special care to ensure that their diets are adequate. People who take part in heavy aerobic exercise programs (over three hours per week) may need to increase their protein consumption. In all cases, seek advice from a health care professional if you have questions.

Adapting MyPyramid for Vegatarians

Vegetarian diets can easily meet all of the recommendations for nutrient needs. By focusing on nonmeat sources of protein, iron, calcium, zinc, and vitamin B_{12} while paying attention to personalized serving size and physical activity guidelines, vegetarians can be just as healthy as omnivores.

CAN FOOD HAVE MEDICINAL VALUE?

Over the last two decades, interest in the importance of nutrients in preventing and treating various diseases has increased dramatically as research points to promising new benefits and certain risks to health from various foods. The old adage "you are what you eat" is gaining credibility among those in the scientific community.

Functional foods are foods that may be biologically active and may provide health benefits beyond basic nutrition. Exciting new findings about the potential benefits of dark chocolate, soy, nuts, and cranberries encourage experts to investigate just how much of these foods it takes to improve health outcomes.

Antioxidants and Your Health

Many people today believe that **antioxidants** are wonder nutrients that will prevent just about anything. Antioxidants produce enzymes that destroy excess free

---

Functional foods Foods believed to be beneficial and/or to prevent disease.

Antioxidants Substances believed to protect active people from oxidative stress and resultant tissue damage at the cellular level.

One of the challenges of following a healthy diet is judging how big a portion size should be and how many servings you are really eating each time you put your hand in the potato chip bag or scoop some ice cream into a dish. The American Dietetic Association and other experts have developed some tips for getting a grip.

Serving Sizes

- A deck of playing cards = 1 serving (3 ounces) of meat, poultry, or fish. The palm of a woman's hand or a computer mouse can also be used, but these can vary in size.

- Half a baseball (not a softball!) = 1 serving (½ cup) of fruit, vegetables, pasta, or rice

- Your thumb = 1 serving (1 ounce) of cheese

- A small hand holding a tennis ball = 1 cup serving of yogurt or fresh greens

Managing Your Portions

- Before eating, visualize the serving sizes recommended above. Putting one of these servings onto a smaller plate may help it look bigger.

- Don't eat out of a bag or a carton. There can be a lot hidden in there, and it's very difficult to compare it to a serving size.

- Use measuring cups or a small scale at home until you can accurately assess the size of a serving.

- Buffets and meals served family style make it difficult to gauge servings. Try to avoid these situations unless you can really pay attention to how much food ends up on your plate.

---

radicals and protect tissues from the damage incurred by free radicals. *Free radicals* are molecules produced in excess when the body is overly stressed through exposure to toxic substances or events; they damage or kill healthy cells, cell proteins, or genetic material in the cells. Among the more commonly cited nutrients touted as providing a protective effect are vitamin C, vitamin E, beta-carotene and other carotenoids, and the mineral selenium.

How valid is the theory? To date, many claims about the benefits of antioxidants in reducing the risk of heart disease, improving vision, and slowing the aging process have not been fully investigated. Some studies do indicate that when people's diets include foods rich in vitamin C, they seem to develop fewer cancers, but other studies detect no effect from dietary vitamin C.[36]

The role of vitamin E is even more controversial. It has long been hypothesized that because many cancers result from DNA damage and vitamin E appears to protect against DNA damage, vitamin E would also reduce cancer risk. Surprisingly, the great majority of studies demonstrate no effect.[37] Certain minerals, including selenium, copper, zinc, iron, and magnesium, also have shown promising results in trials where they are linked to a variety of health benefits. Like their vitamin cousins, much of this research continues to be controversial. The American Heart Association cautions people to get their antioxidants from a balanced diet rather than from supplements in pill form.

Carotenoids are part of the red, orange, and yellow pigments found in fruits and vegetables. They are fat soluble, transported in the blood by lipoproteins, and stored in the fatty tissues of the body. Beta-carotene, the most researched carotenoid, is a precursor of vitamin A. This means that vitamin A can be produced in the body from beta-carotene; like vitamin A, beta-carotene has antioxidant properties.[38]

Although there are over 600 carotenoids in nature, two that receive the most attention are *lycopene* (found in tomatoes, papaya, pink grapefruit, and guava) and *lutein* (found in green leafy vegetables such as spinach, broccoli, kale, and brussels sprouts). Both are believed to be more beneficial than beta-carotene in preventing disease.

The National Cancer Institute and the American Cancer Society have endorsed lycopene as a possible factor in reducing the risk of cancer. A landmark study assessing the effects of tomato-based foods reported that men who ate 10 or more servings of lycopene-rich foods per week had a 45 percent reduced risk of prostate cancer.[39] Subsequent research has indicated positive benefits of lycopene on other cancers and on heart disease.[40]

Lutein is most often touted as a means of protecting the eyes, particularly from age-related macular degeneration (ARMD), a leading cause of blindness for people aged 65 and over. Researchers speculate that oxidative damage may contribute to ARMD; and thus, antioxidants may be a means of prevention.[41] Researchers at the National Eye Institute found that individuals with the highest blood levels of lutein and other antioxidants found in foods were 70 percent less likely to develop ARMD than those with the lowest levels. Researchers

Carotenoids Fat-soluble pigment compounds with antioxidant properties.

in the Nurses' Health Study found that eating spinach more than five days a week lowered risk by 47 percent and also lowered risk of cataracts.[42]

"Antioxidants should always be taken as part of a well-balanced mixture, either as a diet or as a supplement, and not singly," says Dr. John R. Smythies, a researcher at the University of California–San Diego and author of *Every Person's Guide to Antioxidants*.[43] Smythies, like many other experts, advocates balance in intake and advises that adults take 500 mg of daily vitamin C and 400 to 800 IU of vitamin E, plus 10 mg of beta-carotene. Researchers agree that intake should vary based on physical activity levels and overall health. Dr. Balz Frei at the Linus Pauling Institute indicates that the "200 rule" might be the best option. This recommendation calls for fruits and vegetables in the diet and a supplement of 200 mg of vitamin C, 200 IU of vitamin E, and 200 μg of selenium, along with 400 μg of folate and 3 mg of vitamin B_6.[44] Until research conclusively proves the benefit or harm, a moderate intake as part of a vegetable- and fruit-rich diet is desirable.

Probiotics are currently receiving much attention as a natural healer. Probiotics are live microorganisms found in or added to fermented foods; they optimize the bacterial environment in our intestines. Commonly, they are found in fermented milk products such as yogurt, and you will see them labeled as *Lactobacillus* or *Bifidobacterium* in a products list of ingredients. Although thousands of studies of various supplements and functional foods have been done, no single supplement has been proven effective in a compelling way.[45] Probiotics do not typically pose harm to healthy humans; however, someone with a compromised immune system could have complications over time.

Folate

In 1998, the FDA began requiring *folate* fortification of all bread, cereal, rice, and macaroni products sold in the United States. This practice, which boosts folate intake by an average of 100 micrograms daily, is expected to decrease the number of infants born with spina bifida and other neural tube defects.

Folate is a form of vitamin B believed to decrease blood levels of *homocysteine,* an amino acid that has

been linked to vascular diseases, and to protect against cardiovascular disease.[46] See Chapter 12 for more on homocysteine.

Although the amount of folate needed to protect the heart has not been determined, many people have jumped on the folate bandwagon and take daily folate supplements of up to 800 micrograms. Recently, a new *dietary folate equivalent (DFE)* was established to distinguish folate in food from its synthetic counterpart, *folic acid.* As a food additive or a supplement, folic acid is absorbed about twice as efficiently as folate. The DFE for folate in women aged 19 or older is approximately 400 micrograms, with higher levels for pregnant or lactating women. (See Table 9.2 for daily recommended amounts of other B vitamins.) Potential dangers of taking too much folate include masking of vitamin B_{12} deficiencies and resulting problems, ranging from nerve damage, immunodeficiency problems, anemia, fatigue, and headache, to constipation, diarrhea, weight loss, gastrointestinal disturbances, and a host of neurological symptoms.[47]

GENDER AND NUTRITION

Men and women differ in body size, body composition, and overall metabolic rates. They therefore have differing needs for most nutrients throughout the life cycle (see Tables 9.2 and 9.3 on vitamin and mineral requirements) and face unique difficulties in keeping on track with their dietary goals. Some of these differences have already been discussed, but some factors need further consideration.

Different Cycles, Different Needs

Women have many landmark times in life when their nutritional requirements vary significantly from requirements at other times. From menarche to menopause, women undergo cyclical physiological changes that can exert dramatic effects on metabolism and nutritional needs. For example, during pregnancy and lactation, women's nutritional requirements increase substantially. Those who are unable to follow the strict dietary recommendations of their doctors may find themselves gaining much more weight during pregnancy and retaining it afterward. During the menstrual cycle, many women report significant food cravings. Later in life, with the advent of menopause, nutritional needs again change rather dramatically. With depletion of the hormone estrogen, the body's need for calcium to ward off bone deterioration becomes pronounced. Women must pay closer attention to exercise and to getting enough calcium through diet or dietary supplements, or they run the risk of osteoporosis.

Probiotics   Live microorganisms found in or added to fermented foods; optimize the bacterial environment in our intestines.

Folate   A type of vitamin B believed to decrease levels of homocysteine, an amino acid that has been linked to vascular diseases.

Changing the "Meat-and-Potatoes" American

Since our earliest agrarian years, many Americans, especially men, have relied on a "meat-and-potatoes" diet. What's wrong with all those hamburgers and french fries? Heart disease, stroke, and cancer are probably the greatest threats. Add increased risks for colon and prostate cancer, and the rationale for dietary change becomes even more compelling. Consider the following points.

- Heavy red meat eaters are more than twice as likely to get prostate cancer and nearly five times more likely to develop colon cancer.

- For every three servings of fruits or vegetables they consume per day, men can expect a 22 percent lower risk of stroke.

- Diets high in fruit and vegetables may lower the risk of lung cancer in smokers from 20 times the risk of nonsmokers to "only" 10 times the risk. They may also protect against oral, throat, pancreatic, and bladder cancers, all of which are more common among smokers.

- The fastest-rising malignancy in the United States is cancer of the lower esophagus, particularly among white men. Though obesity seems to be a factor, fruits and vegetables are the protectors. (The average American male eats fewer than three servings per day, although five to nine servings are recommended. Women average three to seven servings per day.)

Does something in meat make it inherently bad? The fat content of meat and fried potatoes and the potential carcinogenic substances produced through cooking have been implicated. Probably something more basic is also involved. By eating so much protein, a person fills up sooner and never gets around to the fruits and vegetables. Thus, the potential protective value of consuming these foods is lost.

IMPROVED EATING FOR THE COLLEGE STUDENT

College students often face a challenge when trying to eat healthy foods. Some students live in dorms and do not have their own cooking or refrigeration facilities. Others live in crowded apartments where everyone forages in the refrigerator for everyone else's food. Still others eat at university food services where food choices may be limited. Nearly all have financial and time constraints that make buying, preparing, and eating healthy food a difficult task. What's a student to do?

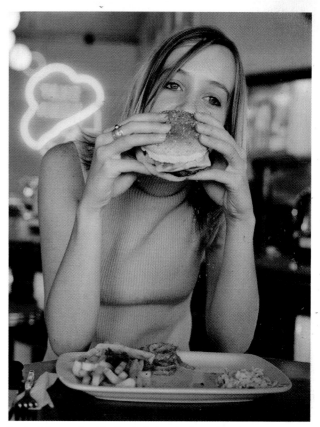

Lack of time or healthy food choices in the cafeteria can be an obstacle to healthy eating. What types of changes could make this meal more healthful?

When Time Is Short: Eating on the Run

Many college students may find it hard to fit a well-balanced meal into the day, but eating breakfast and lunch are important in order to keep energy levels up and get the most out of your classes. If your campus is like many others, you've probably noticed a distinct move toward fast-food restaurants in your student unions in order to fit students' needs for a fast bite of food at a reasonable price between classes. Eating a complete breakfast that includes complex carbohydrates and protein and bringing a small healthy snack (such as carrots, an apple, or even a small sandwich on whole-grain bread) to class are ways to ensure you fit meals into your day. If you must eat fast food, follow the tips below (see the Consumer Health box for more ideas about how to eat healthily while eating out).

- Ask for nutritional analyses of items. Most fast-food chains now have them.

- Order salads, and be careful how much dressing you add. Many people think they are being health-smart by eating salad, only to load it with calorie- and fat-rich dressing. Try the vinegar and oil or low-fat alternative dressings. Stay away from eggs and other high-fat add-ons such as bacon bits.

While some restaurants offer hints for health-conscious diners, you're on your own most of the time. To help you order wisely, here are lighter options and high-fat pitfalls. "Best" choices contain fewer than 30 grams of fat, a generous meal's worth for an active, medium-size woman. "Worst" choices have up to 100 grams of fat.

Fast Food

Best Grilled chicken sandwich; roast beef sandwich; single hamburger; salad with light vinaigrette

Worst Bacon burger; double cheeseburger; french fries; onion rings

Tips Order sandwiches without mayo or special sauce. Avoid deep-fried items like fish fillets, chicken nuggets, and french fries.

Italian

Best Pasta with red or white clam sauce; spaghetti with marinara or tomato-and-meat sauce

Worst Eggplant parmigiana; fettuccine alfredo; fried calamari; lasagna

Tips Stick with plain bread instead of garlic bread made with butter or oil. Ask for the waiter's help in avoiding cream- or egg-based sauces. Try vegetarian pizza, and don't ask for extra cheese.

Mexican

Best Bean burrito (no cheese); chicken fajitas

Worst Beef chimichanga; chile relleno; quesadilla; refried beans

Tips Choose soft tortillas (not fried) with fresh salsa, not guacamole. Special-order grilled shrimp, fish, or chicken. Ask for beans made without lard or fat and for cheeses and sour cream provided on the side or left out altogether.

Chinese

Best Hot-and-sour soup; stir-fried vegetables; shrimp with garlic sauce; Szechuan shrimp; wonton soup

Worst Crispy chicken; kung pao chicken; moo shu pork; sweet-and-sour pork

Tips Share a stir-fry; help yourself to steamed rice. Ask for vegetables steamed or stir-fried with less oil. Order moo shu vegetables instead of pork. Avoid fried rice, breaded dishes, egg rolls, spring rolls, and items loaded with nuts. Avoid high-sodium sauces.

Japanese

Best Steamed rice and vegetables; tofu as a substitute for meat; broiled or steamed chicken and fish

Worst Fried rice dishes; miso (very high in sodium); tempura

Tips Avoid soy sauces. Use caution in eating sashimi and sushi (raw fish) dishes to avoid possible bacteria or parasites.

Thai

Best Clear broth soups; stir-fried chicken and vegetables; grilled meats

Worst Coconut milk; peanut sauces; deep-fried dishes

Tips Avoid coconut-based curries. Ask for steamed, not fried, rice.

Breakfast

Best Hot or cold cereal with 2 percent milk; pancakes or French toast with syrup; scrambled eggs with hash browns and plain toast

Worst Belgian waffle with sausage; sausage and eggs with biscuits and gravy; ham-and-cheese omelette with hash browns and toast

Tips Ask for whole-grain cereal or shredded wheat with 1 percent milk or whole-wheat toast without butter or margarine. Order omelettes without cheese, fried eggs without bacon or sausage.

Sandwiches

Best Ham and Swiss cheese; roast beef; turkey

Worst Tuna salad; Reuben; submarine

Tips Ask for mustard; hold the mayo and cheese. See if turkey-ham is available.

Seafood

Best Broiled bass, halibut, or snapper; grilled scallops; steamed crab or lobster

Worst Fried seafood platter; blackened catfish;

Tips Order fish broiled, baked, grilled, or steamed—not pan-fried or sauteed. Ask for fresh lemon instead of tartar sauce. Avoid creamy and buttery sauces.

Sources: American Dietetic Association, 2002, www.eatright.org; *Health* 10 (November/December 1996): 79.

- If you must have fries, check to see what type of oil is used to cook them. Avoid lard-based or other saturated fat products.
- Avoid giant sizes and refrain from ordering extra sauce, bacon, and other extras that add additional calories and fat.

When Funds Are Short

Maintaining a nutritious diet within the confines of student life can be challenging. However, if you take the time to plan healthy meals, you will find that you are eating better, enjoying your food more, and actually saving money. Follow these steps to ensure a healthy but affordable diet, and see Table 9.4 for ideas on how to eat healthy in the dining hall.

> Is there really a way to make a meal from McDonald's healthy?

- Buy fruits and vegetables in season whenever possible for their lower cost, higher nutrient quality, and greater variety.
- Use coupons and specials to get price reductions.
- Shop at discount warehouse food chains; capitalize on volume discounts and no-frills products.
- Plan ahead to get the most for your dollar and avoid extra trips to the store; extra trips usually mean extra purchases. Make a list and stick to it.
- Purchase meats and other products in volume; freeze portions for future needs. Or purchase small amounts of meats and other expensive proteins and combine them with beans and plant proteins for lower cost, calories, and fat.
- Drain off extra fat after cooking. Save juices to use in soups and other dishes.
- If you find that you have no money for food, talk to staff at your county or city health department. They may know of ways for you to get assistance.

Try it →NOW_____

Eating for health and convenience. **Eating while you are short on time shouldn't mean you have to compromise on nutrition. Make it a habit to purchase items like small bags of carrots and salad-in-a-bag. If you have to eat at McDonald's, order a Happy Meal or get a grilled chicken sandwich and toss half the bun. Choose one day of the week to prepare a quick, big, healthy meal with your roommates. Make enough for leftovers, and you'll be eating well for lunch the next day too!**

Table 9.4
Eating Well in the Dining Hall

- Choose lean meats, grilled chicken, fish, or vegetable dishes. Avoid fried chicken, fatty cuts of red meat, or meat dishes smothered in creamy or oily sauce.
- Hit the salad bar and load up on leafy greens, beans, tuna, or tofu. Choose items such as avocado or nuts for a little "good" fat, and go easy on the dressing.
- Get creative: Choose items such as a baked potato with salsa, or add a grilled chicken breast to your salad. Toast some bread, and top it with veggies, hummus, or grilled chicken or tuna.
- When choosing foods from a made-to-order food station, ask the preparer to hold the butter or oil, mayonnaise, sour cream, or a cheese or cream-based sauce. Do ask for extra servings of veggies and lean meat or white-meat chicken.
- Avoid going back for seconds and consuming large portions. Many colleges limit the number of visits you make each day to the dining hall, but don't view this as a reason to overeat.
- If there is something you'd like, but you don't see it in your dining hall or are vegetarian and feel like your food choices are limited, speak to your food services manager and provide suggestions.
- Pass on high-calorie, low-nutrient rich foods such as sugary cereals, soft-serve ice cream, waffles, and other sweet treats. Choose fruit or low-fat yogurt to satisfy your sweet tooth.

Supplements: New Research on the Daily Dose

In 2002, sales of dietary supplements increased to nearly $20 billion, with projections for rapid increases over the next decade.[48] **Dietary supplements** are usually vitamins and minerals taken by mouth and are intended to supplement existing diets. Ingredients range from vitamins and minerals to enzymes and organ tissues. They can come in tablet, capsule, liquid, or other forms. An important thing to remember about all dietary supplements is that they are regulated differently than other food and drug products. Currently, there are no formal guidelines for their sale and safety, and supplement manufacturers are responsible for self-monitoring their activities. The FDA is developing guidelines for their sale. Nevertheless, consumers are using them for a wide variety of health promoting reasons, from improving performance and energy, to preventing colds and flu.

For years, health experts touted the benefits of eating a balanced diet over popping a vitamin-mineral supplement so eyebrows were raised when an article in the esteemed *Journal of the American Medical Association*

> **Dietary supplements** Vitamins and minerals taken by mouth that are intended to supplement existing diets.

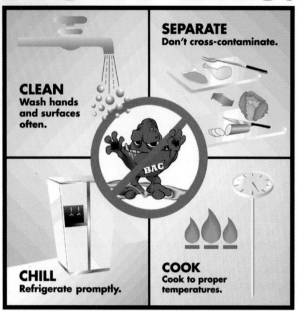

FIGHT BAC!

SEPARATE
Don't cross-contaminate.

CLEAN
Wash hands and surfaces often.

CHILL
Refrigerate promptly.

COOK
Cook to proper temperatures.

Keep Food Safe From Bacteria™

Figure 9.9 ■ The USDA's Fight BAC!
This logo reminds consumers how to prevent foodborne illness.

> **Can I substitute dietary supplements for a balanced diet?**

(JAMA) recommended that "a vitamin/mineral supplement a day just might be important in keeping the doctor away, particularly for some groups of people."[49] The article indicated that elderly people, vegans, alcohol-dependent individuals, and patients with malabsorption problems may be at particular risk of deficiency of several vitamins. Although it acknowledged a possible risk of overdosing on fat-soluble vitamins, it noted that preliminary research has linked inadequate amounts of nutrients such as vitamins B_6, B_{12}, D, E, and lycopene to chronic diseases, including coronary heart disease, cancer, and osteoporosis. As a result of this study, *JAMA* advised that all adults should take a basic multivitamin. It is important to note that supplements should be just that; there is no substitute for a well-balanced diet consisting of healthy meals.

If you are in doubt about which supplements might be best for you, make sure you eat from the major food groups. If you are facing extreme stressors on the body from physical endurance events, illness, or other nutrient-depleting events, supplements might be beneficial; in general, a multivitamin added to a balanced diet is likely to do more good than harm. In all cases, beware of megadoses, overdosing on ultravitamin supplements, and possible interactions with any drugs you may be taking.

FOOD SAFETY: A GROWING CONCERN

Foodborne Illnesses

Are you concerned that the chicken you are buying doesn't look pleasingly pink or that your "fresh" fish smells a little *too* fishy? Are you *sure* that your apple juice is free of animal waste? You may have good reason to be worried. In increasing numbers, Americans are becoming sick from what they eat, and many of these illnesses are life threatening. Scientists estimate, based on several studies conducted over the past 10 years, that foodborne pathogens sicken over 76 million people and cause some 325,000 hospitalizations and 5,200 deaths in the United States annually.[50] Because most of us don't go to the doctor every time we feel ill, we may not make a connection between what we eat and later symptoms.

Signs of foodborne illnesses vary tremendously and usually include one or several symptoms: diarrhea, nausea, cramping, and vomiting. Depending on the amount and virulence of the pathogen, symptoms may appear as early as 30 minutes after eating contaminated food or as long as several days or weeks later. Most of the time, symptoms occur 5 to 8 hours after eating and last only a day or two. For certain populations, however, such as the very young, the elderly, or people with severe illnesses such as cancer, diabetes, kidney disease, or AIDS, foodborne diseases can be fatal.

Several factors may be contributing to the increase in foodborne illnesses. According to Michael T. Osterholm, PhD, state epidemiologist in Minneapolis, the movement away from a traditional meat-and-potato American diet to "heart-healthy" eating—increased consumption of fruits, vegetables, and grains—has spurred demand for fresh foods that are not in season most of the year.[51] This means that we must import fresh fruits and vegetables, thus putting ourselves at risk for ingesting exotic pathogens. Depending on the season, up to 70 percent of the fruits and vegetables consumed in the United States come from Mexico alone.[52] Although we are told when we travel to developing countries, "boil it, peel it, or don't eat it," we bring these foods into our kitchens and eat them, often without even washing them.[53] Food can become contaminated by being watered with contaminated water, fertilized with "organic" fertilizers (animal manure), or not subjected to the same rigorous pesticide regulations as American-raised produce. To give you an idea of the implications, studies have shown that *Escherichia coli* (a lethal bacterial pathogen) can survive in cow manure for up to 70 days and can multiply in foods grown with manure unless heat or additives such as salt or preservatives are used to kill the microbes.[54] There are essentially no regulations that prohibit farmers from using animal manure to fertilize crops. Additionally, *E. coli*

O157:H7 actually increases in summer months as cows await slaughter in crowded, overheated pens. This increases the chances of meat coming to market already contaminated.[55] See Figure 9.9 for the USDA's food safety recommendation.

Other key factors associated with the increasing spread of foodborne diseases include inadvertent introduction of pathogens into new geographic regions and insufficient education about food safety.[56]

Responsible Use: Avoiding Risks in the Home

Part of the responsibility for preventing foodborne illness lies with consumers—more than 30 percent of such illnesses result from unsafe handling of food at home.

■ When shopping for fish, buy from markets that get their supplies from state-approved sources. Check for cleanliness at the salad bar and meat and fish counters.

■ Most cuts of meat, fish, and poultry should be kept in the refrigerator no more than one or two days. Check the shelf life of all products before buying.

■ Eat leftovers within three days.

■ Keep hot foods hot and cold foods cold.

■ Use a meat thermometer to ensure that meats are completely cooked. Beef and lamb steaks and roasts should be cooked to at least 145°F; ground meat, pork chops, ribs, and egg dishes to 160°F; ground poultry and hot dogs to 165°F; chicken and turkey breasts to 170°F; and chicken and turkey legs, thighs, and whole birds to 180°F.

■ Fish is done when the thickest part becomes opaque and the fish flakes easily when poked with a fork.

■ Never leave cooked food standing on the stove or table for more than two hours.

■ Never thaw frozen foods at room temperature.

■ Wash your hands and countertop with soap and water when preparing food, particularly after handling meat, fish, or poultry.

■ When freezing foods like chicken, make sure juices can't spill over into ice cubes or into other areas of the refrigerator.

Food Irradiation: How Safe Is It?

Food irradiation is a process that involves treating foods with gamma radiation from radioactive cobalt, cesium, or other sources of X rays. When foods are irradiated, they are exposed to low doses of radiation (ionizing energy) which breaks chemical bonds of harmful bacteria

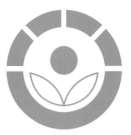

Figure 9.10 ■ Label for Irradiated Foods

Source: Center for Food Safety and Applied Nutrition, "Food Safety A to Z Reference Guide," 2004, www.cfsan.fda.gov/~dms/a2z-i.html.

in the DNA, destroys the pathogens, and keeps them from replicating. The rays essentially pass through the food without leaving any radioactive residue.[57]

Irradiation lengthens food products' shelf life and prevents the spread of deadly microorganisms, particularly in high-risk foods such as ground beef and pork. Thus, the minimal costs of irradiation should result in lower overall costs to consumers and reduce the need for toxic chemicals now used to preserve foods and prevent contamination from external pathogens. Foods that are irradiated include fruits, vegetables, dried spices, meat and poultry, and some prepackaged foods. Look for the food irradiation symbol (Figure 9.10) to know if food has undergone this process. Some environmentalists and consumer groups have raised concerns, so irradiated products are not common fare; however, the facts appear to support the use of irradiation.

Food Additives

Additives generally reduce the risk of foodborne illness (e.g., nitrates added to cured meats), prevent spoilage, and enhance the ways foods look and taste. Additives can also enhance nutrient value, especially to benefit the general public. Good examples include the fortification of milk with vitamin D and of grain products with folate. Although the FDA regulates additives according to effectiveness, safety, and ability to detect them in foods, questions have been raised about those additives put into foods intentionally and those that get in unintentionally before or after processing. Whenever these substances are added, consumers should take the time to determine what they are and if there are alternatives. As a general rule, the fewer chemicals, colorants, and preservatives, the better. Also, it should be noted that certain foods and additives can interact with medications. To be a smart consumer, be aware of these potential dietary interactions. Examples of common additives include the following.

> **Food irradiation** A process that involves treating foods with gamma radiation from radioactive cobalt, cesium, or other sources of X rays.

- *Antimicrobial agents.* Substances such as salt, sugar, nitrates, and others that tend to make foods less hospitable for microbes.
- *Antioxidants.* Substances that preserve color and flavor by reducing loss due to exposure to oxygen. Vitamins C and E are among those antioxidants believed to play a role in reduced cancer and cardiovascular disease. The additives BHA and BHT are also antioxidants.
- *Artificial colors, nutrient additives and flavor enhancers such as MSG (monosodium glutamate).*
- *Sulfites.* Used to preserve vegetable color; some people have severe allergic reactions to them.
- *Dioxins.* Found in coffee filters, milk containers, and frozen foods.
- *Methylene chloride.* Found in decaffeinated coffee.
- *Hormones.* Bovine growth hormone (BGH) found in animal meat.

Food Allergy or Food Intolerance?

At some point, a *food allergy* or *food intolerance* will affect nearly everyone. You eat something, develop gas or have an unpleasant visit to the bathroom, and assume that it is a food allergy. One out of every three people today either say they have a food allergy or avoid something in their diet because they think they are allergic to it; in fact, only 3 percent of all children and 1 percent of all adults experience genuine allergic reactions to what they eat.[58] Surprised? Most people are when they hear this.

A **food allergy,** or hypersensitivity, is an abnormal response to a food that is triggered by the immune system. Reactions range from minor rashes to severe swelling in the mouth, tongue, and throat, to violent vomiting and diarrhea and occasionally death. In adults, the most common foods to cause true allergic reactions are shellfish (such as shrimp, crayfish, lobster, and crab); peanuts, which can cause severe anaphylaxis (a sudden drop in blood pressure that can be fatal if not

treated promptly); tree nuts such as walnuts; fish; and eggs. In children, food allergens that cause the most problems are eggs, milk, and peanuts.[59]

In contrast to allergies, in cases of **food intolerance** you may have symptoms of gastric upset, but they are not the result of an immune system response. Probably the best example of a food intolerance is *lactose intolerance,* a problem that affects about one in every ten adults. Lactase is an enzyme in the lining of the gut that degrades lactose, which is in dairy products. If you don't have enough lactase, lactose cannot be digested and remains in the gut to be used by bacteria. Gas is formed, and you experience bloating, abdominal pain, and sometimes diarrhea. Food intolerance also occurs in response to some food additives, such as the flavor enhancer MSG, certain dyes, sulfites, gluten, and other substances. In some cases, the food intolerance may have psychological triggers.

If you suspect that you have an actual allergic reaction to food, see an allergist to be tested. Because there are several diseases that share symptoms with food allergies (ulcers and cancers of the gastrointestinal tract can cause vomiting, bloating, diarrhea, nausea, and pain), you should have persistent symptoms checked out as soon as possible. If particular foods seem to bother you consistently, look for alternatives or modify your diet. With true allergies, you may not be able to consume even the smallest amount safely. For example, people have experienced severe allergic reactions to peanuts from ingesting as little as a crumb.

Is Organic for You?

Due to mounting concerns about food safety, many people refuse to buy processed foods and mass-produced agricultural products. Instead, they purchase foods that are **organically grown**—foods reported to be pesticide- and chemical-free. Less than a decade ago, buying organic foods meant going to a specialty store and paying premium prices for produce that was likely to be wilted, wormy, and smaller than its nonorganic alternative. These products also came with no guarantee that they were really grown in organic environments. People who bought these foods did so out of a desire to eat healthier produce and avoid the chemicals that they were increasingly being told caused cancer, immune system problems, and a host of other ailments.

Enter the organics of the twenty-first century—larger, more attractive, and fresher looking but still carrying a hefty price tag. Is buying organic really better for you? Perhaps if we could put a group of people in a pristine environment and ensure that they never ate, drank, or were exposed to chemicals, we could test this hypothesis. In real life, however, it is almost impossible to assess the health impact of organic versus nonorganic. Nevertheless, the market for organics has been

---

Food allergies   Overreaction by the body to normally harmless substances, which are perceived as allergens. In response, the body produces antibodies, triggering allergic symptoms.

Food intolerance   Adverse effects resulting when people who lack the digestive chemicals needed to break down certain substances eat those substances.

Organically grown   Foods that are grown without use of pesticides or chemicals.

increasing by 15 to 20 percent per year—5 times faster than food sales in general.

As of 2002, any food sold as organic has to meet criteria set by the USDA under the National Organic Rule and can carry a new USDA seal verifying products as "certified organic" (Figure 9.11). Under this rule, something that is certified may carry one of the following terms: 100 percent Organic (100 percent compliance with organic criteria), Organic (must contain at least 95 percent organic materials), Made with Organic Ingredients (must contain at least 70 percent organic ingredients), or Some Organic Ingredients (contains less than 70 percent organic ingredients—usually listed individually). In order to use any of the above terms, the foods must be produced without hormones, antibiotics, herbicides, insecticides, chemical fertilizers, genetic modification, or germ-killing radiation.

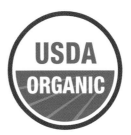

Figure 9.11 ■ Label for Certified Organic Foods
This seal indicates that the product is at least 95 percent organic according to USDA guidelines.

Source: USDA Agriculture Marketing Program, The National Organic Program, "Organic Food Standards and Labels: The Facts," 2002, www.ams.usda.gov/nop.

Taking Charge

Summary

- Recognizing that we eat for more reasons than just survival is the first step toward changing our health.

- The major nutrients that are essential for life and health include water, proteins, carbohydrates, fiber, fats, vitamins, and minerals. MyPyramid provides guidelines for healthy eating.

- Vegetarianism can provide a healthy alternative for those wishing to cut fat from their diets or to reduce animal consumption. The MyPyramid Plan may be adapted to help vegetarians obtain needed nutrients.

- Men and women have differing needs for most nutrients throughout the life cycle because of different body size and composition.

- Experts are interested in the role of food as medicine and in the benefits of functional foods. These foods may play an important role in improving certain conditions, such as hypertension.

- College students face unique challenges in eating healthfully. Learning to make better choices at fast-food restaurants, eat healthfully when funds are short, and eat nutritionally in the dorm are all possible when you use the information contained in this chapter.

- Foodborne illnesses, food allergies, and other food safety and health concerns are becoming increasingly important to health-wise consumers. Recognizing potential risks and taking steps to prevent problems are part of a sound nutritional plan.

Chapter Review

1. What type of carbohydrates is found primarily in fruits?
   a. glucose
   b. dextrose
   c. simple carbohydrates
   d. complex carbohydrates

2. What percentage of our total body weight is water?
   a. 15 to 20 percent
   b. 30 to 40 percent
   c. 50 to 60 percent
   d. 70 to 75 percent

3. What is the most crucial nutrient?
   a. water
   b. fiber
   c. minerals
   d. starch

4. Which of the following nutrients moves food through the digestive tract?
   a. fat
   b. fiber
   c. minerals
   d. starch

5. Which of the following is an example of one serving of grains?
   a. ½ cup ready-to-eat cereal
   b. 1 cup cooked rice
   c. 1 bagel
   d. 1 slice of bread

6. How long does the entire digestive process take?
   a. 8 hours
   b. 12 hours
   c. 24 hours
   d. 48 hours

7. What substance supplies us with the energy needed to sustain normal daily activity?
   a. fats
   b. fibers
   c. proteins
   d. carbohydrates

8. What is the most common nutrient deficiency worldwide?
   a. fat deficiency
   b. iron deficiency
   c. fiber deficiency
   d. calcium deficiency

9. Carrie eats fish, dairy products, and eggs, but does not eat red meat. Carrie is considered a(n)
   a. vegan.
   b. lacto-vegetarian.
   c. ovo-vegetarian.
   d. pesco-vegetarian.

10. What substance plays a vital role in maintaining healthy skin and hair, insulating body organs against shock, maintaining body temperature, and promoting healthy cell function?
    a. fats
    b. fibers
    c. proteins
    d. carbohydrates

Answers to these questions can be found on page A-1.

Questions for Discussion and Reflection

1. Which factors influence the dietary patterns and behaviors of the typical college student? What factors have been the greatest influences on your eating behaviors? Why is it important to recognize influences on your diet as you think about changing eating behaviors?

2. What are the six major food groups in MyPyramid? From which groups do you eat too few servings? What can you do to increase or decrease your intake of selected food groups? How can you remember the six groups?

3. What are the major types of nutrients that you need to obtain from the foods you eat? What happens if you fail to get enough of some of them? Are there significant differences between the sexes in particular areas of nutrition?

4. Distinguish between the different types of vegetarianism. Which types are most likely to lead to nutrient deficiencies? What can be done to ensure that even the most strict vegetarian receives enough of the major nutrients?

5. What are functional foods? What are the major functional foods discussed in this chapter? What are their reported benefits, if any?

6. What are the major problems that many college students face when trying to eat the right foods? List five actions that you and your classmates could take immediately to improve your eating.

7. What are the major risks for foodborne illnesses, and what can you do to protect yourself? How do food illnesses differ from food allergies?

Accessing Your Health on the Internet

The following websites explore further topics and issues related to personal health. For links to the websites below, visit the Companion Website for *Health: The Basics,* Seventh Edition at www.aw-bc.com/donatelle.

1. *American Dietetic Association (ADA).* Provides information on a full range of dietary topics, including sports nutrition, healthful cooking, and nutritional eating. Links to scientific publications and information on scholarships and public meetings.

2. *American Heart Association (AHA).* Includes information about a heart-healthy eating plan and an easy-to-follow guide to healthy eating.

3. *U.S. Food and Drug Administration (FDA).* Provides information for consumers and professionals in the areas of food safety, supplements, and medical devices. Links to other sources of information about nutrition and food.

4. *Food and Nutrition Information Center.* Offers a wide variety of information related to food and nutrition.

5. *National Institutes of Health: Office of Dietary Supplements.* Site of the International Bibliographic Database Information on Dietary Supplements (IBIDS), updated quarterly.

6. *U.S. Department of Agriculture (USDA).* Offers a full discussion of the USDA Dietary Guidelines for Americans.

7. *National Center for Complementary and Alternative Medicine (NCCAM).* Includes information on new research results for supplements and functional foods.

Further Reading

Center for Science in the Public Interest. *Nutrition Action Healthletter,* Washington, DC: Author.

This newsletter, published ten times a year, contains up-to-date information on diet and nutritional claims and current research issues. The newsletter can be obtained by writing to the Center for Science in the Public Interest, 1501 16th St. NW, Washington, DC 20036.

Nutrition Today.

> An excellent magazine for the interested nonspecialist. Covers controversial issues and provides a forum for conflicting opinions. Six issues per year. Order from Williams and Wilkins, 351 West Camden Street, Baltimore, MD 21201-2436.

Schlosser, E. *Fast Food Nation.* Boston: Houghton Mifflin, 2001.

> Overview of the influence of the fast-food industry and its effect on health and well-being in America.

Tufts University Health and Nutrition Letter.

> An excellent source for quick "fixes" on current nutritional topics. Reputable sources and information. E-mail tufts@tiac.net or phone (800) 274-7581. The Tufts Nutrition Navigator website (http://navigator.tufts.edu) rates nutrition-related websites for information and accuracy.

U.S. Department of Agriculture (USDA)

> For information on the proper handling of meat and poultry and other information, call the USDA's Meat and Poultry Hot Line at (800) 535-4555 between 10:00 AM and 4:00 PM on weekdays. Write to the Meat and Poultry Hot Line, USDA-FSIS, Room 1165-S, Washington, DC, 20250 for a new booklet, A Quick Consumer's Guide to Safe Food Handling.

References

1. Centers for Disease Control and Prevention, "Behavioral Risk Factor Surveillance System," 2004, (July 27, 2005), www.cdc.gov/brfss.
2. Ibid.
3. American Institute of Cancer Research, "Food, Nutrition, and the Prevention of Cancer: A Global Perspective" (Washington, DC: American Institute of Cancer Research, 1997).
4. K. Flegal et al., "Excess Death Associated with Underweight, Overweight, and Obesity," *Journal of the American Medical Association* 293, (2005): 1861–1867.
5. National Center for Health Statistics, "Prevalence of Overweight and Obesity Among Adults: United States," 1999, www.cdc.gov/nchs/products/pubs/pubd/hestats/obese/obse99/htm.
6. J. Thompson and M. Manore, *Nutrition: An Applied Approach* (San Francisco: Benjamin Cummings, 2005), 36–38.
7. J. D. Wright et al., "Trends in Intake of Energy and Macronutrients—United States 1971–2000," *Morbidity and Mortality Weekly Report* 53, no. 4 (February 6, 2004): 80.
8. D. Ludwig, "Obesity: A New Dietary Treatment for a Major Public Health Threat" (paper presented at the Linus Pauling Institute International Conference on Diet and Optimum Health, Portland, OR: May 2001).
9. G. Block, "Foods Contributing to Energy Intake in the U.S.: Data from NHANES III and NHANES 1999–2000," *Journal of Food Composition and Analysis* 17, no. 3–4 (2004): 439–447.
10. "Proteins," *Harvard Women's Health Watch* 5 (1998): 4.
11. FAO Global and Regional Food Trends and Consumption Patterns, 2003, www.fao.org/documents/show_cdr.asp?url_file=/DOCREP/005/AC911E/ac911e05.htm12.
12. "Is Sugar Really Addictive?" *Tufts University Health and Nutrition Letter: Special Report* 20, no. 8 (2002): 1–4.
13. M. Pereira et al., "Dietary Fiber and Risk of Coronary Heart Disease: A Pooled Analysis of Cohort Studies," *Archives of Internal Medicine* 164, no. 4 (2004): 370–376.
14. Ibid.
15. Ibid.
16. Ibid.
17. M. Schulz and F. Hu, "Primary Prevention of Diabetes: What Can Be Done and How Much Can Be Prevented?" *Annual Review of Public Health* 26, (2005): 445–67.
18. R. Mensink and M. Katan, "Effect of Dietary *Trans*-Fatty Acids on High-Density and Low-Density Lipoprotein and Cholesterol Levels in Healthy Subject," *New England Journal of Medicine* 323, no. 7: 339–343.
19. G. Ruoff, "Reducing Fat Intake with Fat Substitutes," *American Family Physician* 43, (1991): 1235–1242.
20. R. Maddox and S. Maddox, "Reducing the Risk of Alzheimer's Disease," *U.S. Pharmacist* 30, no. 3 (2005): 34–36; American Cancer Society (July 18, 2005), www.asc.com; National Women's Health Resource Center, "Women and Alzheimer's Disease," *National Women's Health Report* 26, no. 6 (2004): 1–8; R. Mensink, "Metabolic and Health Effects of Fatty Acids," *Current Opinions in Epidemiology* 16, no. 1 (2005): 27–30.
21. L. Lowrey, "Dietary Fat and Sports Nutrition: A Primer," *Journal of Sports Science and Medicine* 3, (2004): 106–107; S. Weinberg, "The Diet Heart Hypothesis: A Critique," *Journal of the American College of Cardiology* 43, no. 5 (2004): 731–733.
22. E. Ward, "Balancing Essential Dietary Fats: When More Might Be Better," *Environmental Nutrition* 24, no. 12 (2002): 1–6.
23. B. McKevith, "Review: Nutritional Aspects of Oilseeds," *Nutrition Bulletin* 30, no. 1 (2005): 13–14.
24. "The CLA Paradox," *American Institute for Cancer Research Newsletter,* 78 (Winter 2003): 8–9.
25. "MUFAs and PUFAs," *Food and Fitness Advisor,* September 2002, www.foodandfitnessadvisor.com.
26. G. Young and J. Conquer, "Omega-3 Fatty Acids and Neuropsychiatric Disorders," *Reproduction Nutrition Development* 45, (2005): 1–28.
27. Institute of Medicine, "Dietary Reference Intake for Water, Potassium, Sodium, Chloride, and Sulfate," March 4, 2004, www.nap.edu.
28. "American Heart Association Position Statement," 2005, www.americanheart.org.
29. World Health Organization, "Micronutrient Deficiencies: Battling Iron Deficiency Anemia, 2003," August 2005, www.who.int.
30. E. Kennedy and L. Meyers, "Dietary Reference Intakes: Development and Uses for Assessment of Micronutrient Status of Women—A Global Perspective," (Special Supplements: Women and Macronutrients, Addressing the Gap Throughout the Life Cycle), *American Journal of Clinical Nutrition* 81, no. 5: 11945–11975.
31. Ibid.
32. Department of Health and Human Services and the Department of Agriculture, "Dietary Guidelines for American Government 2005" (Washington DC: Government Printing Office).
33. United States Department of Agriculture, "Johanns Reveals USDA's Steps to a Healthier You," Press Release, April 19, 2005.
34. B. Black, "Healthgate: Just How Much Food IS on that Plate? Understanding Portion Control," 2004, http://community.healthgate.com/getcontent.asp?siteid=contentupdate&docid=/healthy.
35. Thompson et al., *Nutrition: An Applied Approach.*
36. Ibid.
37. C. M. Hasler et al., "Position Statement of the American Dietetic Association: Functional Foods," *Journal of the American Dietetic Association* 104, no. 5 (2004): 814–818.
38. M. Manore and J. Thompson, *Sport Nutrition for Health and Performance,* (Champaign, IL: Human Kinetics Publishing, 2000), 283.
39. J. Chan and E. Giovannucci, "Vegetables, Fruits, Associated Micronutrients and Risk of Prostate Cancer" *Epidemiology Review* 23, no. 1 (2001): 82–86.
40. E. Giovannucci et al., "A Prospective Study of Tomato Products, Lycopene, and Prostate Cancer Risk," *Journal of the National Cancer Institute* 94, no. 5 (2002): 391–398.
41. "Kale, Collards, and Spinach Beat Carrots for Protecting Aging Eyes," *Environmental Nutrition* 24, no. 4 (2001).
42. Ibid.

43. J. Smythies, *Every Person's Guide to Antioxidants* (Newark, NJ: Rutgers University Press, 1998).

44. B. Frie, "Linus Pauling Institute Seminar Series" (Portland, OR: 2000).

45. Ibid.

46. A. Chait et al., "Increased Dietary Micronutrients Decrease Serum Homocystienal Concentrations in Patients at High Risk of Cardiovascular Disease," *The American Journal of Clinical Nutrition* 70, no. 5: 881–887.

47. R. Malinow, "Homocysteine, Folic Acid, and CVD" (guest lecturer for Diet and Seminar, Oregon State University, Corvallis, OR, 2001).

48. National Institute of Health, NCCAM Backgrounder, "Biologically-Based Practices: An Overview, 2004," July 16, 2005, http://nccam.nih.gov/health/backgrounds/biobasedprac.htm.

49. K. M. Fairfield and R. H. Fletcher, "Vitamins for Chronic Disease Prevention in Adults: Scientific Review," *Journal of the American Medical Association* 287, no. 23 (2001): 3116–3126.

50. Centers for Disease Control and Prevention, "Food Borne Illnesses," 2002, www.cdc.gov; American Medical Association, "Diagnosis and Management of Foodborne Illness: A Primer for Physicians and Other Health Care Professionals," 2004, www.ama-assn.org/ama/org.

51. Ibid.

52. Ibid.

53. Ibid.

54. Ibid.

55. L. Hughes, "Don't Let Unexpected Visitors 'Spoil' Summer Meals," *Environmental Nutrition* 25, no. 6 (June 2002): 2.

56. P. Morris, Y. Motarjemi, and F. Kaferstein, "Emerging Food-Borne Diseases," *World Health* 50 (1997): 16–22; Centers for Disease Control and Prevention "Food Borne Illnesses," www.cdc.gov.

57. "Special Report: Irradiation Plants Geared to 'Zap' Meat and Poultry—Is It Safe?" *Tufts University Health and Nutrition Letter* 18, no. 1 (2000): 4–7.

58. National Institute of Allergy and Infectious Diseases, "Fact Sheet: Food Allergy and Intolerances," 2002, www.niaid.nih.gov/factsheets/food.htm.

59. Ibid.

How can I determine my ideal body weight?

What's the best way to lose weight or maintain my current weight?

I exercise and eat right, but I can't seem to lose any more weight. Why?

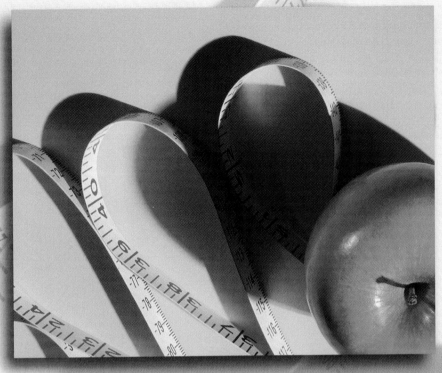

Do men ever have eating disorders?

10 Managing Your Weight
Finding a Healthy Balance

Objectives

- **Define** obesity, describe the current epidemic of obesity in the United States, and understand risk factors associated with obesity.
- **Explain** why so many people are obsessed with thinness and how to determine the right weight for you.
- **Discuss** reliable options for determining body fat content.

- **Discuss** the roles of exercise, dieting, nutrition, lifestyle, fad diets, and other strategies of weight control, and which methods are most effective.
- **Describe** major eating disorders, explain the health risks related to these conditions, and indicate the factors that make people susceptible to them.

Over the past 20 years, the United States has become known as one of the fattest nations on earth. From young children to seniors, virtually no segment of the populace is immune to the epidemic of overweight and obesity (Figure 10.1). Just how serious is the problem?

The National Health and Nutrition Examination Survey (NHANES) reports that 34 percent of American adults are overweight and an additional 31 percent are obese.[1] The trend does not seem to be reversing: according to a report released in 2005, obesity rates continued to rise dramatically in nearly every state in 2004. Mississippi ranked as the heaviest and Colorado as the least heavy state. The heaviest states tended to be in the southeastern United States.[2] Experts predict that, at the current pace, 50 percent of Americans will be obese by the year 2025.[3]

What does all of this excess weight really mean to the health of our population? Recent studies indicate that obesity is one of the top underlying preventable causes of death in the United States. Like tobacco, obesity and inactivity increase the risks from three of our leading killers: heart disease, cancer, and cerebrovascular ailments, including strokes.[4] Other associated health risks (Table 10.1) include diabetes, gallstones, sleep apnea, osteoarthritis, and several cancers. For example, some experts predict that the numbers of Americans diagnosed with diabetes, a major obesity-associated problem, will increase by a whopping 165 percent, from 11 million in 2000 to 29 million in 2050; since 1990, we have seen a 49 percent increase in the number of Americans who have diabetes.[5] The relationship between obesity and psychosocial development, including self-esteem, also is believed to be significant.

Short- and long-term health consequences of obesity are not our only concern: the estimated annual cost of obesity in the United States is between $117 and $123 billion in medical expenses and lost productivity.[6] Of course, it is impossible to place a dollar value on a life lost prematurely due to diabetes, stroke, or heart attack or to assess the cost of social isolation and discrimination against overweight individuals. Of growing importance is the recognition that obese individuals suffer significant disability during their lives, both in terms of mobility and activities of daily living.[7]

This chapter will help you understand why we have such a weight problem in America today and provide simple strategies to help you manage your weight. (See the Assess Yourself box on page 286 to obtain a better understanding of your own dietary habits.) It will also help you understand what *underweight, normal weight, overweight,* and *obesity* really mean, and why managing your weight is essential to overall health and well-being.

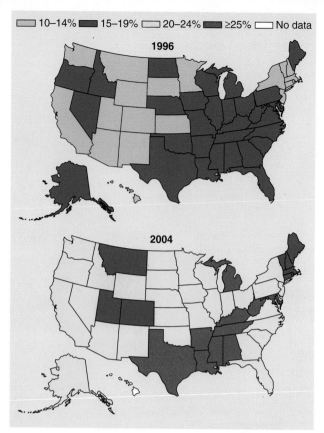

Figure 10.1 ■ Obesity Trends Among U.S. Adults, 1996 and 2004

Source: Centers for Disease Control and Prevention, "Behavioral Risk Factor Surveillance Survey," and www.cdc.gov/nccdphp/dnpa/obesity/trend

DETERMINING THE RIGHT WEIGHT FOR YOU

What weight is right for you? This depends on a wide range of variables, including your body structure, height, weight distribution, and the ratio of fat to lean tissue. In fact, weight can be a deceptive indicator. Many extremely muscular athletes would be considered overweight based on traditional height–weight charts. Many young women think that they are the right weight based on charts but are shocked to discover that 35 to 40 percent of their weight is body fat!

How can I determine my ideal body weight?

In general, weights at the lower end of the range on these charts are recommended for individuals with a low ratio of muscle and bone to fat; those at the upper end are advised for people with more muscular builds (Table 10.2). However, since actual body composition is hard to determine, most charts give a general range.

Table 10.1
Selected Health Consequences of Overweight and Obesity

Premature Death
- Obese individuals have a 50–100% increased risk of death from all causes compared with people of normal weight. Among 25- to 35-year-olds, severe obesity increases the risk of death by a factor of 12.
- At least 300,000 deaths per year may be attributable to obesity.
- The risk of death rises with increasing weight.
- Even moderate excess weight (10–20 pounds for a person of average height) increases risk of death.

Cardiovascular Disease
- High blood pressure is twice as common in obese adults as it is for those who are at healthy weights.
- Incidence of all forms of heart disease is increased among overweight and obese people.
- Obesity is associated with elevated triglycerides and decreased "good" (HDL) cholesterol.

Diabetes
- A weight gain of 11–18 pounds increases a person's risk of developing type 2 diabetes to twice that of individuals who have not gained weight.
- More than 80% of people with diabetes are overweight or obese.

Cancer
- Overweight and obesity are associated with increased risk of endometrial, colon, gallbladder, prostate, kidney, and postmenopausal breast cancer.
- Women gaining more than 20 pounds between age 18 and midlife double their risk of postmenopausal breast cancer compared to women whose weight remains stable.

Additional Health Consequences
- Sleep apnea and asthma are both associated with obesity.
- For every 2-pound increase in weight, the risk of developing arthritis increases by 9–13%.
- Obesity-related complications during pregnancy include increased risk of fetal and maternal death, labor and delivery complications, and increased risk of birth defects.

Source: U.S. Department of Health and Human Services, "The Surgeon General's Call to Action to Prevent and Decrease Overweight and Obesity," 2001, www.surgeongeneral.gov/topics/obesity/calltoaction/fact_consequences.htm; D. Eberwine, "Globesity: The Crisis of Growing Proportions," *Perspectives in Health* 7, no. 3 (2003): 6–11.

Overweight or Obese?

Most of us cringe at the thought of being labeled as one of the "O" words. What is the distinction between the two? **Overweight** refers to increased body weight in relation to height, when compared to a standard such as the height–weight charts in Table 10.2. The excess weight may come from muscle, bone, fat, and/or water. Historically, nutritionists have defined overweight as being 1 to 19 percent above one's ideal weight and obese as being above 19 percent.

Another measurement of overweight and obesity is a mathematical formula known as **body mass index (BMI),** which represents weight levels associated with the lowest overall risk to health (see page 279 to calculate your BMI). Desirable BMI levels may vary with age.[8] About 34 percent of all Americans are classified as being overweight using BMI calculations.

A person may be classified as overweight using these standards even if the weight gain is due to an increase in lean muscle mass. For example, an athlete may be very lean and muscular, with very little body fat, yet she may weigh a lot more than others of the same height who have little muscle tissue. Conversely, a person may proudly proclaim that he weighs the same that he did in high school but have a much greater proportion of body fat, particularly in the hips, buttocks, or thighs, than he did at a younger age. Body weight alone may not be a good indicator of overall fitness.

Another problem with using BMI is that people who have lost muscle mass, such as older adults, people with anorexia, or those who are seriously disabled or bedridden, could be in the "healthy weight" range even though their nutritional reserves are dangerously low. BMI is a useful guideline but by itself is not diagnostic of a person's overall health status.[9]

Obesity is defined as an excessively high amount of body fat (adipose tissue) in relation to lean body mass or a BMI of 30 or more. Over 31 percent of all Americans are obese. It is important to consider both the distribution of fat throughout the body and the size of the adipose tissue deposits. Body fat distribution can be estimated in a variety of ways, as will be discussed shortly. Using traditional standards, people 20 to 40 percent above their ideal weight are labeled as *mildly obese* (90 percent of the obese fall into this category). Those 41 to 99 percent above their ideal weight

Overweight   Increased body weight in relation to height.

Body Mass Index (BMI)   A technique of weight assessment based on the relationship of weight to height.

Obesity   A weight disorder generally defined as an accumulation of fat beyond that considered normal for a person based on age, sex, and body type.

Table 10.2
Healthy Weight Ranges*

Height without Shoes	Weight† without Clothes
4'10"	91–119
4'11"	94–124
5'0"	97–128
5'1"	101–132
5'2"	104–137
5'3"	107–141
5'4"	111–146
5'5"	114–150
5'6"	118–155
5'7"	121–160
5'8"	125–164
5'9"	129–169
5'10"	132–174
5'11"	136–179
6'0"	140–184
6'1"	144–189
6'2"	148–195
6'3"	152–200
6'4"	156–205
6'5"	160–211
6'6"	164–216

* Each data entry applies to both men and women.
† In pounds
Source: Center for Nutrition Policy and Promotion, "Dietary Guidelines for Americans, 2000," 2000, www.usda.gov/cnpp/Pubs/ DG2000.

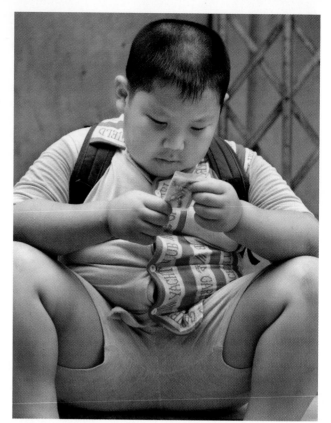

Obesity is increasing especially dramatically among children. Being overweight or obese from an early age can have devastating physical and emotional consequences.

are described as *moderately obese* (about 7 to 8 percent of the obese fit into this category), and 2 to 3 percent of obese people are in the *severely, morbidly,* or *grossly overweight* category, meaning that they are 100 percent or more above their ideal weight. In the last decade, more and more people are at the moderate and severe levels of obesity, meaning increased risks at all ages and stages of their lives.[10]

The difficulty with defining obesity lies in determining what is normal. To date, there are no universally accepted standards for the most "desirable" or "ideal" body weight or *body composition* (the ratio of lean body mass to fat body mass). While sources vary slightly, men's bodies should contain between 11 and 15 percent total body fat and women should be within the range of 18 to 22 percent body fat. At various ages and stages of life, these ranges also vary, but generally, when men exceed 20 percent body fat and women exceed 30 percent body fat, they have slipped into obesity.

Why the difference between men and women? Much of it may be attributed to the normal structure of the female body and to sex hormones. Lean body mass consists of the structural and functional elements in cells, body water, muscle, bones, and other body organs such as the heart, liver, and kidneys. Body fat is composed of two types: essential and storage fat. Essential fat is necessary for normal physiological functioning, such as nerve conduction. Essential fat makes up approximately 3 to 7 percent of total body weight in men and approximately 15 percent of total body weight in women. Storage fat, the part that many of us try to shed, makes up the remainder of our fat reserves. It accounts for only a small percentage of total body weight for very lean people and between 5 and 25 percent of body weight of most American adults. Female bodybuilders, who are among the leanest of female athletes, may have body fat percentages of 8 to 13 percent, nearly all of which is essential fat.

Too Little Fat?

A certain amount of body fat is necessary for insulating the body, cushioning parts of the body and vital organs, and maintaining body functions. In men, this lower limit is approximately 3 to 4 percent. Women generally should not go below 8 percent. Excessively low body fat in females may lead to amenorrhea, a disruption of the normal menstrual cycle. The critical level of body fat necessary to maintain normal menstrual flow is believed to be 8 to 13 percent, but many additional factors can affect the menstrual cycle. Under extreme circumstances, such as starvation diets and certain diseases, the body uses all available fat reserves and begins to break down muscle tissue as a last-ditch effort to obtain nourishment.

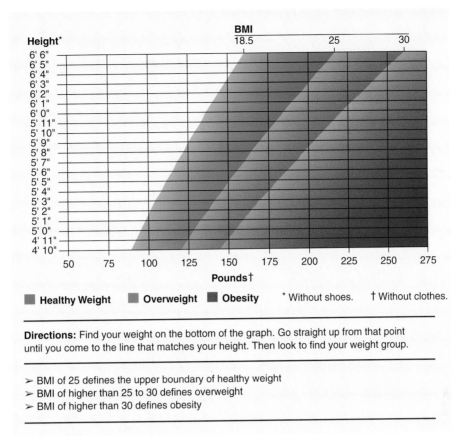

Height*

6' 6"
6' 5"
6' 4"
6' 3"
6' 2"
6' 1"
6' 0"
5' 11"
5' 10"
5' 9"
5' 8"
5' 7"
5' 6"
5' 5"
5' 4"
5' 3"
5' 2"
5' 1"
5' 0"
4' 11"
4' 10"

BMI
18.5   25   30

50   75   100   125   150   175   200   225   250   275

Pounds†

■ **Healthy Weight**   ■ **Overweight**   ■ **Obesity**   * Without shoes.   † Without clothes.

Directions: Find your weight on the bottom of the graph. Go straight up from that point until you come to the line that matches your height. Then look to find your weight group.

➤ BMI of 25 defines the upper boundary of healthy weight
➤ BMI of higher than 25 to 30 defines overweight
➤ BMI of higher than 30 defines obesity

Figure 10.2 ■ Body Mass Index: Are You at a Healthy Weight?

Source: Dietary Guidelines Advisory Committee, USDA Agricultural Research Service, "Dietary Guidelines for Americans," 2000, www.ars.usda.gov/dgac/2kdiet.pdf.

The fact is that too much fat and too little fat are both potentially harmful. The key is to find a healthy level at which you are comfortable with your appearance and your ability to be as active as possible. Many options are available for determining your body fat and weight.

ASSESSING FAT LEVELS

Height–Weight Charts

Today, most weight control authorities believe that looking at where you fall on some arbitrary chart may not be helpful. Height–weight charts may lead some to think they are overweight when they are not, or that they are okay when, in fact, they may be at risk. Other measures exist for calculating body content, and some provide a very precise calculation of body fat. They include body mass index, waist circumference, waist-to-hip ratio, and various measures of body fat.

Body Mass Index

A useful index of the relationship of height and weight, BMI is the measurement of choice for obesity researchers

and health professionals. It is not gender specific. Although it does not directly measure percentage of body fat, it does provide a more accurate measure of overweight and obesity than weight alone.[11]

Follow these steps to determine your BMI using pounds and inches:[12]

1. Multiply your weight in pounds by 704.5.

   For example, Lisa weighs 145 and is 5 feet, 5 inches tall

   $$145 \times 704.5 = 102,152.5$$

2. Divide the result by height in inches.

   $$102,152.5 \div 65 = 1571.6$$

3. Divide that result by height in inches a second time. The result of this step is Lisa's BMI.

   $$(1571.6 \div 65 = 24.1)$$

4. Lisa's BMI is 24.1. Is this a healthy BMI?

Healthy weights are defined as those associated with BMIs of 18.5 to 25, the range of lowest statistical health risk (Figure 10.2).[13] The desirable range for females falls between 21 and 23; for males, it falls between 22 and 24.[14] A BMI greater than 25 indicates overweight and potentially significant health risks. A body mass index of 30 or more is considered obese.[15]

Many experts believe that this number is too high, particularly for younger adults.

Calculating BMI is simple, quick, and inexpensive—but it does have limitations. One problem is that very muscular people may fall into the overweight category when they are actually healthy and fit. In addition, certain population groups, such as Asians, tend to have higher-than-healthy body fat at normal BMI levels, while Polynesians have somewhat lower body fat than other populations at the same BMI.[16]

Waist Circumference and Ratio Measurements

Waist circumference measurement is a useful tool for assessing abdominal fat. Research indicates that a waistline greater than 40 inches (102 cm) in men and 35 inches (88 cm) in women may indicate greater health risk. If a person has a short stature (under 5 feet tall) or has a BMI of 35 or above, waist circumference standards used for the general population might not apply.[17] Measure waist circumference by wrapping a tape measure comfortably around the smallest area below the rib cage and above the belly button.

The *waist-to-hip ratio* measures regional fat distribution. A waist-to-hip ratio greater than 1.0 in men and 0.8 in women indicates increased health risks.[18] Therefore, knowing where your fat is carried may be more important than knowing your total fat content. Men and postmenopausal women tend to store fat in the upper regions of their body, particularly in the abdominal area. Premenopausal women usually store their fat in lower regions of their bodies, particularly the hips, buttocks, and thighs.[19]

Measures of Body Fat

Hydrostatic Weighing Techniques From a clinical perspective, **hydrostatic weighing techniques** offer the most accurate method of measuring body fat. This method measures the amount of water a person displaces when completely submerged. Because fat tissue is less dense than muscle or bone tissue, a relatively accurate indication of actual body fat can be computed by comparing underwater and out-of-water weights.

Pinch and Skinfold Measures The most accurate method of measuring body fat using the skinfold measurement technique is the **skinfold caliper technique.** A specially calibrated instrument called a skinfold caliper is used to measure the fat layer. In making this assessment, a technician pinches a fold of skin on a predetermined body location, such as the triceps areas or waist, with the calipers. Special formulas are employed to arrive at a combined prediction of total body fat.

Bioelectrical Impedance Analysis

Another method, **bioelectrical impedance analysis (BIA),** involves sending a small electrical current through the subject's body. The body's ability to conduct an electrical current reflects the total amount of water in the body. Generally, the more water, the more muscle and lean tissue. The amount of resistance to the current and the person's age, sex, and other physical characteristics are fed into a computer that calculates the total amount of lean and fat tissue.

Total Body Electrical Conductivity One of the newest assessment techniques is **total body electrical conductivity (TOBEC),** which uses an electromagnetic force field to assess relative body fat. Although based on the same principle as impedance, this assessment requires much more elaborate, expensive equipment and therefore is not practical for most people.

Although all of these methods can be useful, they also can be inaccurate and even harmful unless the testers are skillful and well trained. Before undergoing any procedure, make sure you understand the expense, potential for accuracy, risks, and training of the tester.

Try it →NOW_____

Set SMART goals for weight loss. **Give your goals a reality check: Are they Specific, Measurable, Achievable, Relevant, and Time specific? For example, rather than aiming to lose 15 pounds this month (which probably wouldn't be healthy or achievable), set a comfortable goal to lose 5 pounds in a month. Realistic goals will encourage weight loss success by boosting your confidence in your ability to make life-long healthy changes.**

Hydrostatic weighing techniques Method of determining body fat by measuring the amount of water displaced when a person is completely submerged.

Skinfold caliper technique A method of determining body fat whereby folds of skin and fat at various points on the body are grasped between thumb and forefinger and measured with calipers.

Bioelectrical impedance analysis (BIA) A technique of body fat assessment in which electrical currents are passed through fat and lean tissue.

Total body electrical conductivity (TOBEC) Technique using an electromagnetic force field to assess relative body fat.

Globesity: An Epidemic of Growing Proportions

It's not just Americans today who are bigger and less fit than at any time in history. A similar trend is emerging around the world in both developed and developing regions. In countries as diverse as the Czech Republic, Kuwait, and Jamaica, at least half of the population is over-weight and one in five is obese. The highest obesity rate is in Samoa, where two-thirds of all women and half of men are obese. Although rates in Canada and South America are slightly lower than in the United States, residents of the Americas as a whole are among the most over-weight and obese in the world (see details by country in the figure).

While there is growing concern about the epidemic in adults, even more disturbing is the enormous jump in obesity rates among children. Rates of childhood obesity have in-creased 66 percent in the United States and a whopping 240 percent during the same period in Brazil in past decades.

Among the consequences is the parallel rise in type 2 diabetes in the global population; it is nearly five times more prevalent than it was 18 years ago. The dual impact of diabetes and obesity is sure to demand increasing attention to the global health conse-quences and disease burden.

Dietary excesses and sedentary lifestyles are key contributors to the in-creases in obesity. However, accord-ing to Donna Eberwine, editor of the Pan American Health Organization's *Perspectives in Health,* "The growing body of public health literature on the 'globesity' epidemic places the bulk of the blame not on individuals but on globalization and development, with poverty as an exacerbating factor." As entire cultures move away from tradi-tional diets with raw fruits and vegeta-bles and fewer fats to diets heavy in highly processed, high-fat and high-calorie fast food and packaged prod-ucts, the world population is becom-ing supersized along with the products we consume.

Another factor is the increasingly sprawling environment in which peo-ple travel only by car and walking or bicycling is difficult. Lack of health ed-ucation about the risks of obesity also contributes to its increase.

The challenge is daunting. Nations must work together in the decades ahead to educate their populations, promote nutritious diets, and encour-age physical activity.

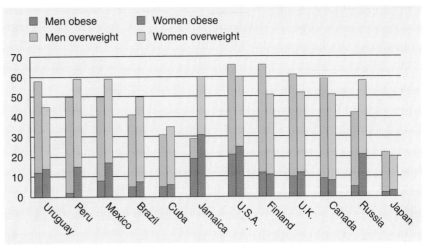

Percentage of Men and Women Who Are Overweight or Obese, by Country

Source: Figure from D. Eberwine, "Globesity: The Crisis of Growing Proportions," *Perspectives in Health* 7, no. 3 (2003):6–11. Reprinted by permission from Pan American Health Organization.

Source: Eberwine, D. "Globesity: The Crisis of Growing Proportions," *Perspectives in Health* 7, no. 3 (2003):6–11.

RISK FACTORS FOR OBESITY

In spite of efforts to keep Americans fit and in good health, obesity is the most common nutritional disorder in the United States, with rates that have increased dramatically among children and adults in recent decades.[20] The prevalence of obesity and overweight is generally higher among minorities, especially minor-ity women.[21]

In a major report, the U.S. Surgeon General stated it quite plainly: "Overweight and obesity result from an energy imbalance. This means eating too many calories and not getting enough exercise."[22] However, many have criticized such a simplistic view. If it were that simple, Americans would merely reevaluate their diets, reduce the amount they eat, and exercise more. In fact, there are probably many factors conspiring to make us fat and keep us fat. Recognizing these factors and making conscious decisions to change lifestyle behav-iors is an important first step in beating the "battle of the bulge." For those who don't currently have a weight problem, knowing how to maintain a healthy weight through a lifetime of temptations and metabolic changes is another important message.

What are some of these factors that influence our collective trend toward weight gain? We know that body weight is a result of genes, metabolism, behavior, environment, culture, and socioeconomic status. Of these, behavior and environment are the easiest to change. Indeed, environmental factors play a large role, especially factors that favor increased energy intake (consuming too much) and decreased energy expenditure (too little physical activity).

Key Environmental Factors

There is a long list of environmental factors that encourage us to consume more, including:

- Bombardment with advertising designed to increase energy intake—ads for high-calorie foods at a low price, marketing super-sized portions (see the Reality Check box).[23] Prepackaged meals, fast food, and soft drinks are all increasingly widespread. High-calorie drinks such as coffee lattes and energy drinks add to daily caloric intake.[24]

- Changes in the number of working women, leading to greater use of restaurant meals, fast foods, and convenience foods. Women now consume, on average, nearly 350 calories per day more than they did in the 1970s.[25]

- Bottle-feeding of infants, which may increase energy intake relative to breast-feeding.[26]

- Misleading food labels that confuse consumers about portion and serving sizes.[27]

Factors contributing to decreased energy expenditure include:

- The increasingly sedentary nature of many jobs.[28]

- Automated equipment and electronic communications, such as cell phones, remote controls, and other labor-saving devices.[29]

- Spending more time in front of the computer and TV and playing video games.[30]

- Fear of playing or being outside based on the threat of violence.

- Decline in physical education requirements in schools.[31]

- Lack of community resources for exercise.

What Do You Think?
In addition to those listed, can you think of other environmental factors that contribute to obesity? ■ What actions could you take to reduce your risk for each of these factors?

Heredity and Genetic Factors

Are some people born to be fat? Several factors appear to influence why one person becomes obese and another remains thin; genes seem to interact with many of these factors.

Body Type and Genes In some animal species, the shape and size of the individual's body are largely determined by its parents' shape and size. Many scientists have explored the role of heredity in determining human body shape. You need only look at your parents and then glance in the mirror to see where you got your own body type. Children whose parents are obese also tend to be overweight. In fact, a family history of obesity has long been thought to increase one's chances of becoming obese by 25 to 30 percent.[32] Some researchers argue that obesity has a strong genetic determinant; they cite the statistic that 80 percent of children who have two obese parents are also obese.[33] Genes play a significant role in how the body balances calories and energy. Also, by influencing the amount of body fat and fat distribution, genes can make a person more susceptible to gaining weight.

Twin Studies Studies of identical twins who were separated at birth and raised in different environments provide the strongest evidence yet that the genes a person inherits are a major factor in determining overweight, leanness, or average weight. Whether raised in family environments with fat or thin family members, twins with obese natural parents tend to be obese in later life.[34] According to another study, sets of identical twins who were separated and raised in different families and who ate widely different diets still grew up to weigh about the same.[35]

Although the exact mechanism remains unknown, it is believed that genes set metabolic rates, which influence how the body handles calories. Other experts believe that this genetic tendency may contribute as much as 25 to 40 percent of the reason for being overweight.[36]

Specific Obesity Genes? In the past decade, more and more research has pointed to the existence of a "fat gene." Rather than inheriting a particular body type that predisposes us to overweight, it may be that our genes predispose us toward certain satiety and feeding behaviors. This "I need to eat" gene may account for up to one-third of our risk for obesity.[37] The most promising candidate is the *GAD2* gene. For some individuals, a variation in this gene increases the production of a chemical that boosts appetite and signals us to eat. Researchers hope that discovery of this gene may one day help those predisposed to obesity take steps to prevent becoming obese.[38]

Are Super-Sized Meals Super-Sizing Americans?

Today, super-sized meals are the norm at many restaurants. Biscuits and gravy, huge steaks, and plate-filling meals are popular fare. Consider the 25-ounce prime rib dinner served at a local steak chain. At nearly 3,000 calories and 150 grams of fat for the meat alone, this meal both slams shut arteries and adds on pounds. Add a baked potato with sour cream and/or butter, a salad loaded with creamy salad dressing, and fresh bread with real butter, and the meal may surpass the 5,000-calorie mark and ring in at close to 300 grams of fat. In other words, it exceeds what most adults should eat in two days!

And this is just the beginning. Soft drinks, once commonly served in 12-ounce sizes, now come in Big Gulps and 1-liter bottles. Cinnamon buns at local chains now come in giant, butter-laden, 700-calorie portions. What is the result? Super-sized portions consumed by super-sized Americans. A quick glance at the fattening of Americans provides growing evidence of a significant health problem. According to Donna Skoda, a dietitian and chair of the Ohio State University Extension Service, "People are eating a ton of extra calories. For the first time in history, more people are overweight in America than are underweight. Ironically, although the U.S. fat intake has dropped in the past 20 years from an average of 40 to 33 percent of calories, the daily calorie intake has risen from 1,852 calories per day to over 2,000 per day. In theory, this translates into a weight gain of 15 pounds a year."

Skoda and others say that the main reason that Americans are gaining weight is that people no longer know what a normal serving size is. In a recent USDA survey, only 1 percent of the respondents could correctly identify the serving sizes recommended in the USDA's dietary guidelines.

The National Heart, Lung, and Blood Institute, part of the National Institutes of Health, has developed a "Portion Distortion" quiz that shows how today's portions compare to those of 20 years

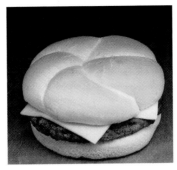

20 years ago

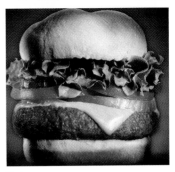

Today

ago. Test yourself online at http://hin.nhlbi.nih.gov/portion to see if you can recognize the differences between today's super-sized meals and those once considered normal. Just one example is the difference between an average cheeseburger 20 years ago (left photo) and the typical cheeseburger of today (right).

According to Carrie Wiatt, a Los Angeles dietitian and author of the recently released book *Portion Savvy,* a telling marker of the big-food trend is that restaurant plates have grown from an average of 9 to 13 inches in the past decade. Studies show that people eat 40 to 50 percent more than usual now that large portions are available.

These statistics alone are alarming; however, they are made worse by a growing trend toward sedentary lifestyles, increased use of technology and gadgetry, and computer-gazing. Americans are taking in more calories and doing less to burn them off. Hence, an epidemic of obesity prevails and is getting worse. Younger and younger kids are eating more and picking up lifetime habits that will be hard to change. To reduce your own risk of super-sizing, follow these simple strategies:

✓ Avoid super-sizing anything. Order the smallest size available when dining out. Focus on taste, not quantity. Get used to eating less and enjoying what you are eating.

✓ Chew your food, and avoid the urge to wash it down with high-calorie drinks. Take time, and let your fullness indicator have a chance to kick in while there is still time to quit.

✓ Serve food on a small or medium plate. Put those big platter-size dinner plates on the top shelf of your cupboard, and leave them there.

✓ Always order dressings, gravies, and sauces on the side. Sprinkle these added calories on carefully, rather than washing your foods down with them. Remember that a tablespoon of gravy could mean an hour on the treadmill to burn off its 200+ calories!

✓ If you order a large muffin or bagel, share it with a friend, or bring only half with you and wrap up the rest. Carry a small zip-lock bag, and use it to take home part of those big portions for another day.

✓ Avoid appetizers in restaurants. They are expensive, in terms of money, calories, and fat content.

✓ Share your dinner with a friend, and order a side salad for each of you. Alternatively, eat only half of your dinner and save the rest for another day.

✓ Measure portions. Before ordering, ask for the size of servings, and always order a size smaller than you really want. When the server tells you it is a "rich dish" or "a lot of food," avoid it.

✓ Avoid buffets and all-you-can-eat establishments. Most of us can eat two to three times what we need—or more.

Source: Some statistics from J. Snow, "Are Super-Sized Meals Super-Sizing Americans?" *Akron Beacon Journal,* May 24, 2000. © 2004 Akron Beacon Journal. All rights reserved. Distributed by Knight Ridder Digital.

Endocrine Influence: The Hungry Hormones

Some researchers are focusing on the hormone *leptin*, which scientists believe signals the brain when you are full and need to stop eating.[39] It is believed that if we can enhance leptin levels in the blood, people may find it easier to control their hunger urges.

A hormone produced in the stomach known as *ghrelin* (GLP-1) may be among the most important players in our collective difficulties in keeping weight off. Researchers at the University of Washington studied a small group of obese people who had lost weight over a six-month period.[40] They noted that ghrelin levels rose before every meal and fell drastically shortly afterward, suggesting that the hormone plays a role in appetite stimulation. Subsequent studies will test the impact of ghrelin-blocking drugs in controlling appetite.

Over the years, many people have attributed obesity to problems with their thyroid gland. They believed that an underactive thyroid impeded their ability to burn calories. However, most authorities agree that less than 2 percent of the obese population have a thyroid problem and can trace their weight problems to a metabolic or hormone imbalance.[41]

Hunger, Appetite, and Satiety

Theories abound concerning the mechanisms that regulate food intake. Some sources indicate that the hypothalamus (the part of the brain that regulates appetite) closely monitors levels of certain nutrients in the blood. When these levels fall, the brain signals us to eat. In the obese person, it is possible that the monitoring system does not work properly and the cues to eat are more frequent and intense than they are in people of normal weight.

Scientists distinguish between **hunger,** an inborn physiological response to nutritional needs, and **appetite,** a learned response to food that is tied to an emotional or psychological craving and is often unrelated to nutritional need. Obese people may be more likely than are thin people to satisfy their appetite and eat for reasons other than nutrition. However, the hypothesis that food tastes better to obese people, thus causing them to eat more, has largely been refuted.

In some instances, the problem with overconsumption may be more related to **satiety** than to appetite or hunger. People generally feel satiated, or full, when they have satisfied their nutritional needs and their stomach signals "no more." For undetermined reasons, obese people may not feel full until much later than thin people do. The leptin and GLP-1 studies seem to support this theory.

Setpoint Theory

Nutritional researchers William Bennett and Joel Gurin developed the **setpoint theory,** which states that a person's body has a setpoint of weight at which it is programmed to be comfortable. If your setpoint is around 160 pounds, you will gain and lose weight fairly easily within a given range of that point. For example, if you gain 5 to 10 pounds on vacation, it will be fairly easy to lose that weight and remain around the 160-pound mark because the body actually tries to maintain this weight. Some people equate this point with the **plateau** that dieters sometimes reach after losing a certain amount of weight. The setpoint theory proposes that after losing a predetermined amount of weight, the body will actually sabotage additional weight loss by slowing down metabolism. In extreme cases, the metabolic rate will decrease to a point at which the body will maintain its weight on as little as 1,000 calories per day.

Can a person change this predetermined setpoint? Proponents of this theory argue that it is possible to raise one's setpoint over time by continually gaining weight and failing to exercise. Conversely, reducing caloric intake and exercising regularly can gradually decrease one's setpoint. Exercise may be the most critical factor in readjusting setpoint, although diet may also be important.

The setpoint theory remains controversial, and many consider it superseded by research into hormonal and other factors. The setpoint theory has also prompted nutritional experts to look more carefully at popular methods of weight loss. If it is correct, an extremely low calorie diet isn't just dangerous; it may also cause the body to protect the dieter from starvation by slowing down metabolism, which makes weight loss even more difficult.

> I exercise and eat right, but I can't seem to lose any more weight. Why?

Hunger An inborn physiological response to nutritional needs.

Appetite A learned response that is tied to an emotional or psychological craving for food; often unrelated to nutritional need.

Satiety The feeling of fullness or satisfaction at the end of a meal.

Setpoint theory A theory of obesity causation that suggests that fat storage is determined by a thermostatic mechanism in the body that acts to maintain a specific amount of body fat.

Plateau That point in a weight loss program at which the dieter finds it difficult to lose more weight.

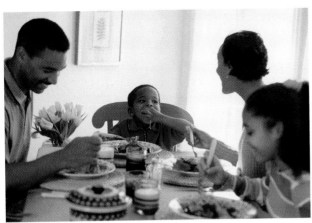

Many factors help determine body type, including heredity and genetic makeup, environmental factors, and learned eating patterns, which are often connected to family habits.

Psychosocial Factors

The relationship of weight problems to deeply rooted emotional insecurities, needs, and wants remains uncertain. Food often is used as a reward for good behavior in childhood. As adults face unemployment, broken relationships, financial uncertainty, fears about health and other problems, the bright spot in the day is often "what's on the table for dinner" or "we're going to that restaurant tonight." Again, the research underlying this theory is controversial. What is certain is that eating tends to be a focal point of people's lives; eating is essentially a social ritual associated with companionship, celebration, and enjoyment. For many people, the social emphasis on the eating experience is a major obstacle to successful weight control. Although some restaurants offer menu items designed to aid dieters, many people have difficulty choosing responsibly when confronted with an entire menu of delicious, fattening foods.

Early Sabotage: Obesity in Youth

Another major factor is the pressure placed on us by the food industry's sophisticated marketing campaigns. There may be salad bars at the local fast-food joints, but customers have to run the gauntlet of starchy, beefy delights and high-fat fries to find them. The food and restaurant industries spend billions each year on ads to entice hungry people to forgo fresh fruit and sliced vegetables for Ring Dings and Happy Meals. Children are among the most vulnerable to these ads.

Children's impulses to eat junk food haven't changed much in recent decades. However, as noted earlier, they are eating larger portions. Social forces mentioned earlier, including the decline of home cooking, increased production of calorie- and fat-laden fast foods, and video technology that encourages kids to surf the Internet rather than ride their bicycles, have converged to increase the number of overweight young Americans. As a direct consequence, over 16 percent of U.S. children and adolescents are now overweight or obese enough to endanger their health.[42] An additional 5 million are on the threshold, and the problem is growing more extreme daily. Obese children suffer both physically and emotionally throughout childhood, and those who stay heavy in adolescence tend to stay fat as adults.[43]

Metabolic Rates and Weight Even at rest, the body consumes a certain amount of energy. The amount of energy your body uses at complete rest is your **basal metabolic rate (BMR).** About 60 to 70 percent of all the calories you consume on a given day go to support your basal metabolism: heartbeat, breathing, maintaining body temperature, and so on. So if you consume 2,000 calories per day, between 1,200 and 1,400 of those calories are burned without your doing any significant physical activity. But unless you exert yourself enough to burn the remaining 600 to 800 calories, you will gain weight.

Your BMR can fluctuate considerably, with several factors influencing whether it slows down or speeds up. In general, the younger you are, the higher your BMR, partly because in young people cells undergo rapid subdivision, which consumes a good deal of energy. BMR is highest during infancy, puberty, and pregnancy, when bodily changes are most rapid.

Body composition also influences BMR. Muscle tissue is highly active—even at rest—compared to fat tissue. In essence, the more lean tissue you have, the greater your BMR, and the more fat tissue you have, the lower your BMR. Men have a higher BMR than women do, at least partly because of their greater proportion of lean tissue. (This is another reason why developing muscular strength and endurance is so important to weight loss and obesity reduction plans.[44])

Age is another factor. After age 30, BMR slows down by about 1 to 2 percent a year. Therefore, people over 30 commonly find that they must work harder to burn off an extra helping of ice cream than they did when in their teens. "Middle-aged spread," a reference to the tendency to put on weight later in life, is partly related to this change. A slower BMR, coupled with less activity, shifting priorities (family and career become more important than fitness), and loss in muscle mass, puts the weight of many middle-aged people in jeopardy.

In addition, the body has self-protective mechanisms that signal BMR to speed up or slow down. For example, when you have a fever, the energy needs of

(Text continues on page 290)

Basal metabolic rate (BMR)   The energy expenditure of the body under resting conditions at normal room temperature.

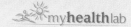

Readiness for Weight Loss

Fill out this assessment online at
www.aw-bc.com/myhealthlab or www.aw-bc.com/donatelle.

How well do your attitudes equip you for a weight-loss program? For each question, circle the answer that best describes your attitude. As you complete each section, tally your score and analyze it according to the scoring guide.

I. Goals, Attitudes, and Readiness

1. Compared to previous attempts, how motivated are you to lose weight this time?

1	2	3	4	5
Not at all motivated	Slightly motivated	Somewhat motivated	Quite motivated	Extremely motivated

2. How certain are you that you will stay committed to a weight loss program for the time it will take to reach your goal?

1	2	3	4	5
Not at all certain	Slightly certain	Somewhat certain	Quite certain	Extremely certain

3. Considering all outside factors at this time in your life—stress at work, family obligations, and so on—to what extent can you tolerate the effort required to stick to a diet?

1	2	3	4	5
Cannot tolerate	Can tolerate somewhat	Uncertain	Can tolerate well	Can tolerate easily

4. Think honestly about how much weight you hope to lose and how quickly you hope to lose it. Figuring a weight loss of one to two pounds per week, how realistic is your expectation?

1	2	3	4	5
Very unrealistic	Somewhat unrealistic	Moderately unrealistic	Somewhat realistic	Very realistic

5. While dieting, do you fantasize about eating a lot of your favorite foods?

1	2	3	4	5
Always	Frequently	Occasionally	Rarely	Never

6. While dieting, do you feel deprived, angry, and/or upset?

1	2	3	4	5
Always	Frequently	Occasionally	Rarely	Never

ANALYZING THIS SECTION

6 to 16: This may not be a good time for you to start a diet. Inadequate motivation and commitment and unrealistic goals could block your progress. Think about what contributes to your unreadiness, and consider changing these factors before undertaking a diet.

17 to 23: You may be close to being ready to begin a program but should think about ways to boost your readiness.

24 to 30: The path is clear: you can decide how to lose weight in a safe, effective way.

II. Hunger and Eating Cues

7. When food comes up in conversation or in something you read, do you want to eat, even if you are not hungry?

1	2	3	4	5
Never	Rarely	Occasionally	Frequently	Always

8. How often do you eat for a reason other than physical hunger?

1	2	3	4	5
Never	Rarely	Occasionally	Frequently	Always

9. Do you have trouble controlling your eating when your favorite foods are around the house?

1	2	3	4	5
Never	Rarely	Occasionally	Frequently	Always

ANALYZING THIS SECTION

3 to 6: You might occasionally eat more than you should, but it does not appear to be due to high responsiveness to environmental cues. Controlling the attitudes that make you eat may be especially helpful.

7 to 9: You may have a moderate tendency to eat just because food is available. Losing weight may be easier for you if you try to resist external cues and eat only when you are physically hungry.

10 to 15: Some or much of your eating may be in response to thinking about food or exposing yourself to temptations to eat. Think of ways to minimize your exposure to temptations so you eat only in response to physical hunger.

III. Controlling Overeating

If the following situations occurred while you were on a diet, would you be likely to eat more or less immediately afterward and for the rest of the day?

10. Although you planned to skip lunch, a friend talks you into going out for a midday meal.

1	2	3	4	5
Would eat much less	Would eat somewhat less	Would make no difference	Would eat somewhat more	Would eat much more

11. You "break" your plan by eating a fattening, "forbidden" food.

1	2	3	4	5
Would eat much less	Would eat somewhat less	Would make no difference	Would eat somewhat more	Would eat much more

12. You have been following your diet faithfully and decide to test yourself by eating something you consider a treat.

1	2	3	4	5
Would eat much less	Would eat somewhat less	Would make no difference	Would eat somewhat more	Would eat much more

ANALYZING THIS SECTION

3 to 7: You recover rapidly from mistakes. However, if you frequently alternate between eating that is out of control and dieting very strictly, you may have a serious eating problem and should get professional help.

8 to 11: You do not seem to let unplanned eating disrupt your program. This is a flexible, balanced approach.

12 to 15: You may be prone to overeat after an event breaks your control or throws you off the track. Your reaction to these problem-causing events can be improved.

IV. Binge Eating and Purging

13. Aside from holiday feasts, have you ever eaten a large amount of food rapidly and felt afterward that this eating incident was excessive and out of control?

2	0
Yes	No

14. If you answered yes to question 13, how often have you engaged in this behavior during the past year?

1	2	3	4	5	6
Less than once a month	About once a month	A few times a month	About once a week	About 3 times a week	Daily

15. Have you purged (used laxatives or diuretics, or induced vomiting) to control your weight?

5	0
Yes	No

16. If you answered yes to question 15, how often have you engaged in this behavior during the past year?

1	2	3	4	5	6
Less than once a month	About once a month	A few times a month	About once a week	About 3 times a week	Daily

(continues)

(continued)

ANALYZING THIS SECTION

0: It appears that binge eating and purging are not problems for you.

2 to 11: Pay attention to these eating patterns. Should they arise more frequently, get professional help.

12 to 19: You show signs of having a potentially serious eating problem. See a counselor experienced in evaluating eating disorders right away.

V. Emotional Eating

17. Do you eat more than you would like to when you have negative feelings such as anxiety, depression, anger, or loneliness?

1	2	3	4	5
Never	Rarely	Occasionally	Frequently	Always

18. Do you have trouble controlling your eating when you have positive feelings—do you celebrate feeling good by eating?

1	2	3	4	5
Never	Rarely	Occasionally	Frequently	Always

19. When you have unpleasant interactions with others in your life or after a difficult day at work, do you eat more than you'd like?

1	2	3	4	5
Never	Rarely	Occasionally	Frequently	Always

ANALYZING THIS SECTION

3 to 8: You do not appear to let your emotions affect your eating.

9 to 11: You sometimes eat in response to emotional highs and lows. Monitor this behavior to learn when and why it occurs, and be prepared to find alternate activities.

12 to 15: Emotional ups and downs can stimulate your eating. Try to deal with the feelings that trigger the eating and find other ways to express them.

VI. Exercise Patterns and Attitudes

20. How often do you exercise?

1	2	3	4	5
Never	Rarely	Occasionally	Somewhat frequently	Frequently

21. How confident are you that you can exercise regularly?

1	2	3	4	5
Not at all confident	Slightly confident	Somewhat confident	Highly confident	Completely confident

22. When you think about exercise, do you develop a positive or negative picture in your mind?

1	2	3	4	5
Completely negative	Somewhat negative	Neutral	Somewhat positive	Completely positive

23. How certain are you that you can work regular exercise into your daily schedule?

1	2	3	4	5
Not at all certain	Slightly certain	Somewhat certain	Quite certain	Extremely certain

ANALYZING THIS SECTION

4 to 10: You're probably not exercising as regularly as you should. Determine whether attitude about exercise or your lifestyle is blocking your way, then change what you must and put on those walking shoes!

11 to 16: You need to feel more positive about exercise so you can do it more often. Think of ways to be more active that are fun and fit your lifestyle.

17 to 20: It looks as if the path is clear for you to be active. Now think of ways to get motivated.

After scoring yourself in each section of this questionnaire, you should be able to better judge your dieting strengths and weaknesses. Remember that the first step in changing eating behavior is to understand the conditions that influence your eating habits.

Source: Reprinted from "The Diet Readiness Test," in Kelly D. Brownell, "When and How to Diet," *Psychology Today,* June 1989, 41–46. Reprinted with permission from *Psychology Today* Magazine, copyright © 1989 (Sussex Publishers, Inc.).

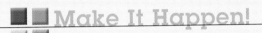

Make It Happen!

Assessment: The Assess Yourself activity identifies six areas of importance in determining your readiness for weight loss. If you should lose weight to improve your health, understanding your attitudes about food and exercise will help you succeed in your plan.

Making a Change: In order to change your behavior, you need to develop a plan. Follow these steps below and complete your Behavior Change Contract to take action.

1. Evaluate your behavior, and identify patterns and specific things you are doing. What can you change now? What can you change in the near future?
2. Select one pattern of behavior that you want to change.
3. Fill out the Behavior Change Contract found at the front of your book. It should include your long-term goal for change, your short-term goals, the rewards you'll give yourself for reaching these goals, potential obstacles along the way, and strategies for overcoming these obstacles. For each goal, list the small steps and specific actions that you will take.
4. Chart your progress in a journal. At the end of a week, consider how successful you were in following your plan. What helped you be successful? What made change more difficult? What will you do differently next week?
5. Revise your plan as needed. Are the short-term goals attainable? Are the rewards satisfying?

Example: Shannon had gained the "freshman 15" and wanted to put together a weight management plan. She assessed her readiness for weight loss and saw that her scores in certain areas highlighted areas that she needed to be aware of to succeed. She had never binged and purged (section IV), she had strong motivation (section I), and she already had an enjoyable, regular exercise program (section VI). However, Shannon also saw that she was not always aware of the eating cues and emotions that caused her to overeat (sections II, III, and V). Although she hadn't realized it, she tended to do most of her snacking while she was studying at night. No matter what else she had eaten during the day, she would end up eating candy and chips from the vending machines. Especially when she was anxious about an upcoming test or bored by her reading, she would eat even though she was already full.

Shannon made a plan that would help her manage her snacking and be part of her weight loss program. She wanted to be aware of what she was eating and how it was contributing to her weight gain. Her first step was to buy some study snacks that were healthier choices than chips and candy, such as grapes and low-fat granola. Her next step was to make a commitment to think about how hungry she was before automatically starting to snack when she was studying. If she was snacking because she was bored or anxious, she would try to restrict her snack to a predetermined amount or to wait until she really was hungry. Shannon tried this plan for two weeks. At the end of two weeks she saw that she had lost 4 pounds. She decided she wanted to address another of her eating habits, which was ordering pizza with her roommates when they watched their favorite TV shows during the week. Even after she had eaten a full dinner, Shannon found herself eating two or three pieces of pizza in front of the TV. Shannon suggested to her roommates that, if they already had eaten dinner, they pop some popcorn to eat instead of the pizza. Not only was this healthier, but it cost less than having a pizza delivered.

your cells increase, which generates heat and speeds up your BMR. In starvation situations, the body protects itself by slowing down BMR to conserve precious energy. Thus, when people repeatedly resort to extreme diets, it is believed that their bodies "reset" their BMRs at lower rates. **Yo-yo diets,** in which people repeatedly gain weight and then starve themselves to lose it, are doomed to fail. When dieters resume eating after their weight loss, their BMR is set lower, making it almost certain that they will regain the pounds they just lost. After repeated cycles of dieting and regaining weight, these people find it increasingly hard to lose weight and increasingly easy to regain it, so they become heavier and heavier.

According to a recent study by Kelly Brownell of Yale University, middle-aged men who maintained a steady weight (even if they were overweight) had a lower risk of heart attack than men whose weight cycled up and down in a yo-yo pattern. Brownell found that small, well-maintained weight losses are more beneficial for reducing cardiovascular risk than large, poorly maintained weight losses.[45]

New research supports the hypothesis that by increasing your muscle mass, you will increase your metabolism and burn more calories each time you exercise (see Chapter 11).

Lifestyle

Of all the factors affecting obesity, perhaps the most critical is the relationship between activity levels and calorie intake. Obesity rates are rising. But how can this be happening? Aren't more people exercising than ever before?

Though the many advertisements for sports equipment and the popularity of athletes may give the impression that Americans love a good workout, the facts are not so positive. Data from the National Health Interview Survey show that 4 in 10 adults in the United States *never* engage in any exercise, sports, or physically active hobbies in their leisure time.[46] Women (43.2 percent) were somewhat more likely than men (36.5 percent) to be sedentary, a finding that was consistent across all age groups. Among both men and women, black and Hispanic adults were more sedentary than white adults.[47] Leisure-time physical activity was also strongly associated with level of education. About 72 percent of adults who never attended high school were sedentary, declining steadily to 45 percent among high school graduates and about 24 percent among adults with graduate-level college degrees.[48]

> **Yo-yo diets** Cycles in which people repeatedly gain weight, then starve themselves to lose weight. This lowers their BMR, which makes regaining weight even more likely.

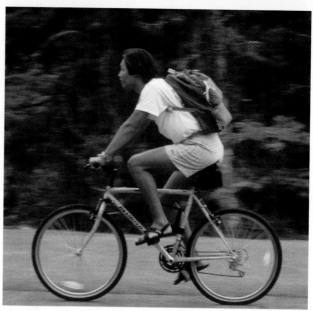

Modern conveniences support a sedentary lifestyle. Small changes to your daily activities can help to increase your activity level and impact your health positively.

Do you know people who seemingly can eat whatever they want without gaining weight? With few exceptions, if you were to follow them around for a typical day and monitor the level and intensity of their activity, you would discover the reason. Even if their schedule does not include jogging or intense exercise, it probably includes a high level of activity. Walking up a flight of stairs rather than taking the elevator, speeding up the pace while mowing the lawn, getting up to change the TV channel rather than using the remote, and doing housework all burn extra calories.

Actually, it may even go beyond that. In studies of calorie burning by individuals placed in a controlled respiratory chamber environment where calories consumed, motion, and overall activity were measured, it was found that some people are better fat burners than others. It is possible that low fat burners may not produce as many of the enzymes needed to convert fat to energy. They may not have as many blood vessels supplying fatty tissue, making it tougher for them to deliver fat-burning oxygen; or, perhaps in subtle ways, these people burn more calories through extra motions. Clearly, any form of activity that burns additional calories helps maintain weight.

Smoking Women who smoke tend to weigh 6 to 10 pounds less than nonsmokers do. After they quit, their weight generally increases to the level found among nonsmokers. Weight gain after smoking cessation may be partly due to nicotine's ability to raise a body's metabolic rate. When smokers stop, they burn fewer calories. Another reason former smokers often gain weight is that they generally eat more to satisfy free-floating cravings.[49]

Gender and Obesity

Throughout our lives, issues of appearance and attractiveness are constantly in the foreground. Only recently have researchers begun to understand just how significant, especially for women, the quest for beauty and the perfect body really is.

Researchers have determined that being severely overweight in adolescence may influence one's social and economic future—particularly for females.[50] Researchers found that obese women complete about half a year less schooling, are 20 percent less likely to get married, and earn thousands less on average per year than their slimmer counterparts. Obese women also have rates of household poverty 10 percent higher than those of women who are not overweight. In contrast, the study found that overweight men are 11 percent less likely to be married than thinner men but suffer few adverse economic consequences.

It may be that women suffer such negative consequences because the social stigma of being overweight is more severe for women than for men. Women are also disadvantaged biologically when it comes to losing weight. Compared to men, they have a lower ratio of lean body mass to fatty mass, in part due to differences in bone size and mass, muscle size, and other variables. Muscle uses more energy than fat does. Because men have more muscle, they burn 10 to 20 percent more calories than women do during rest.[51] (See Chapter 11 for an overview of the role that increased muscle mass has on weight reduction.) After sexual maturity, men have higher metabolic rates, making it easier for them to burn off excess calories. Women also face greater potential for weight fluctuation due to hormonal changes, pregnancy, and other conditions that increase the likelihood of weight gain. Also, as a group, men are more socialized into physical activity from birth. Strenuous work and play are encouraged for men, whereas women's roles have typically been more sedentary and required a lower level of caloric expenditure.

Not only are women more vulnerable to weight gain, but also pressures to maintain and/or lose weight make them more likely to take dramatic measures to lose weight. For example, eating disorders are more prevalent among women, and more women than men take diet pills.

However, males experience these pressures, too. The male image is becoming more associated with the bodybuilder shape and size, and men are becoming more preoccupied with their own physical form. Thus eating disorders, exercise addictions, and other maladaptive responses are on the increase among men as well.

Of increasing interest is an emerging problem seen in both young men and women, known as **social physique anxiety (SPA),** in which the desire to "look good" has a destructive and sometimes disabling effect on one's ability to function effectively in relationships and interactions with others. People suffering from SPA may spend a disproportionate amount of time "fixating" on their bodies, working out, and performing tasks that are ego-centered and self-directed, rather than focusing on interpersonal relationships and general tasks.[52] Incessant worry about their bodies and their appearance permeates their lives. Overweight and obesity are clear risks for these people, and experts speculate that this anxiety may contribute to eating-disorder behaviors.

MANAGING YOUR WEIGHT

At some point in our lives, almost all of us will decide to go on a diet, and many will meet with mixed success. The problem is probably related to the fact that we think about losing weight in terms of dieting rather than in terms of adjusting lifestyle and eating behaviors. It is well documented that hypocaloric (low-calorie) diets produce only temporary losses and may actually lead to disordered binge eating or related problems. While repeated bouts of restrictive dieting may be physiologically harmful, the sense of failure that we get each time we try and fail can also exact far-reaching psychological costs. Drugs and intensive counseling can contribute to positive weight loss, but even then, many people regain weight after treatment.

Social physique anxiety (SPA) A desire to look good that has a destructive effect on a person's ability to function effectively socially.

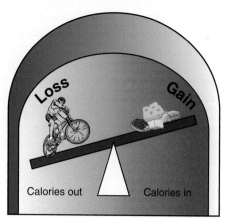

Figure 10.3 ■ The Concept of Energy Balance
How many calories do you need each day? If you consume more calories than you burn, you will gain weight. If you burn more than you consume, you will lose weight, and if both are equal, your weight will not change, according to this concept.

Keeping Weight Control in Perspective

Although experts say that losing weight simply requires burning more calories than are consumed, putting this principle into practice is far from simple (Figure 10.3). According to William W. Hardy, MD, president of the Michigan-based Rochester Center for Obesity, to say weight control is simply a matter of pushing away from the table is ludicrous. Nature is a cheat. Sure, calories in minus calories out equals weight, but people of the same age, sex, height, and weight can have differences of as much as 1,000 calories a day in "resting metabolic rate"—this may explain why one person's gluttony is another's starvation, even if it results in the same read-out on the scale. And, while people of normal weight average 25 to 35 billion fat cells, obese people can inherit a billowing 135 billion. A roll of the genetic dice adds more variety: hundreds of genes can affect weight.[53] Other factors such as depression, stress, culture, and available foods can also play a role.

Weight loss is more difficult for some people and may require supportive friends, relatives, and community resources, plus extraordinary efforts to prime the body for burning extra calories. Being overweight does not mean people are weak-willed or lazy. As scientists unlock the many secrets of genetic messengers that influence body weight and learn more about the role of certain foods in the weight loss equation, dieting may not be the same villain in the future that it is today.

> **Resting metabolic rate (RMR)** The energy expenditure of the body under BMR conditions plus other daily sedentary activities.
>
> **Exercise metabolic rate (EMR)** The energy expenditure that occurs during exercise.

To reach and maintain the weight at which you will be healthy and feel best, you need to develop a program of exercise and healthy eating behaviors that will work for you now and in the long term. You also need to become familiar with important concepts in weight control.

Understanding Calories

A *calorie* is a unit of measure that indicates the amount of energy we obtain from a particular food. One pound of body fat contains approximately 3,500 calories. Each time you consume 3,500 calories more than your body needs to maintain weight, you gain a pound. Conversely, each time your body expends an extra 3,500 calories, you lose a pound. So if you add a can of Coca-Cola or Pepsi (140 calories) to your daily diet and make no other changes in diet or activity, you would gain a pound in 25 days (3,500 calories ÷ 140 calories/day = 25 days). Conversely, if you walk for half an hour each day at a pace of 15 minutes per mile (172 calories burned), you would lose a pound in approximately 20 days (3,500 calories ÷ 172 calories/day = 20.3 days). The two ways to lose weight, then, are to lower calorie intake (through improved eating habits) and to increase exercise (thereby expending more calories).

Adding Exercise

Approximately 90 percent of the daily calorie expenditures of most people occurs as a result of the **resting metabolic rate (RMR).** Slightly higher than the BMR, the RMR includes the BMR plus any additional energy expended through daily sedentary activities such as food digestion, sitting, studying, or standing. Because lean muscle tissue appears to influence metabolic rates, increasing muscle mass may be a factor in burning calories throughout the day (see Chapter 11). The **exercise metabolic rate (EMR)** accounts for the remaining 10 percent of all daily calorie expenditures; it refers to the energy expenditure that occurs during physical exercise. For most of us, these calories come from light daily activities, such as walking, climbing stairs, and mowing the lawn. If we increase the level of physical activity to moderate or heavy, however, our EMR may be 10 to 20 times greater than typical RMRs and can contribute substantially to weight loss.

Increasing BMR, RMR, or EMR levels will help burn calories. An increase in the intensity, frequency, and duration of daily exercise levels can have significant impact on total calorie expenditure.

Physical activity makes a greater contribution to BMR when large muscle groups are used. The energy spent on physical activity is the energy used to move the body's muscles—the muscles of the arms, back, abdomen, legs, and so on—and the extra energy used to

What Triggers Your "Eat" Response?		What Stops Your "Eat" Response?

What Triggers Your "Eat" Response?

- Time of day
- Mood
- Boredom

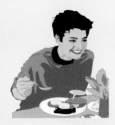

- Nervousness/ anxiety/stress
- Hormonal fluctuations
- Peer/family pressure
- Inattentiveness
- Habit
- Hunger/appetite
- Low self-esteem
- Environment
- Sight and smell of favorite foods

What Stops Your "Eat" Response?

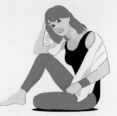

- Acting responsibly in assessing foods
- Practicing stress management
- Breaking the habit
- Remaining active
- Analyzing emotional problems
- Making a conscious effort
- Recognizing true hunger
- Avoiding environment that causes "eat" response
- Selecting alternatives
- Recognizing triggers
- Planning

Figure 10.4 ■ The "Eat" Response
Learn to understand what triggers and stops your "eat" response by keeping a daily log.

speed up heartbeat and respiration rate. The number of calories spent depends on three factors:

1. The amount of muscle mass moved
2. The amount of weight moved
3. The amount of time the activity takes

An activity involving both the arms and legs burns more calories than one involving only the legs. An activity performed by a heavy person burns more calories than one performed by a lighter person. And an activity performed for 40 minutes requires twice as much energy than one performed for only 20 minutes. Thus, obese people walking for 1 mile burn more calories than do slim people walking the same distance. It also may take overweight people longer to walk the mile, which means that they are burning energy for a longer time and therefore expending more overall calories than the thin walkers.

Improving Your Eating Habits

At any given time, many Americans are trying to lose weight. Given the hundreds of different diets and endless expert advice available, why do we find it so difficult?

Determining What Triggers an Eating Behavior

Before you can change a behavior, you must first determine what causes it. Many people have found it helpful to keep a chart of their eating patterns: when they feel like eating, where they are when they decide to eat, the amount of time they spend eating, other activities they engage in during the meal (watching television or reading), whether they eat alone or with others, what and how much they consume, and how they felt before they took their first bite. If you keep a detailed daily log of eating triggers for at least a week, you will discover useful clues about what in your environment or your emotional makeup causes you to

want food (Figure 10.4). Typically, these dietary triggers center on problems in everyday living rather than on real hunger pangs. Many people find that they eat compulsively when stressed. For other people, the same circumstances diminish their appetite, which causes them to lose weight.

Changing Your Triggers

Once you recognize the factors that cause you to overeat, removing the triggers or substituting other activities for them will help you develop more sensible eating patterns. Here are some examples of substitute behaviors.

1. When eating dinner, turn off all distractions, including the television and radio.
2. Instead of gulping your food, chew each bite slowly and savor it.
3. Vary the time of day when you eat. Instead of eating by the clock, do not eat until you are truly hungry.
4. If you find that you generally eat all that you can cram on a plate, use smaller plates.
5. Stop buying high-calorie foods that tempt you to snack, or store them in an inconvenient place.

See the Skills for Behavior Change box on page 294 for more weight management tips.

Try it ►NOW

Healthy substitutions at meal time is the key to weight maintenance success! The next time you make dinner, take a look at the proportions on your plate. Veggies and whole grains should take up the most space; if not, substitute 1 cup of the meat, pasta, or cheese on your plate for 1 cup of legumes, salad greens, or a favorite vegetable. You'll reduce the number of calories in your meal, while eating the same amount of food!

Rather than thinking about the best diet, the key to successful weight management is finding a sustainable way to control food that will work for you. Combine the following strategies with a Behavior Change Contract to develop a weight management plan that is right for you. Remember, you are not going on a diet that you will quit someday. You are making life-long changes that will result in weight loss.

Making a Plan

■ *Think of it as a way of life.* This is a way of improving your body and your health rather than a punishment or a diet.

■ *Assess where you are.* Monitor your eating habits for 2 to 3 days, taking careful note of the good things you are doing and the things that need improvement.

■ *Set realistic goals.* No matter what you do, you may not have a perfect body. Realistically, how do you want to look and feel? Set either a weight or a BMI that you want to achieve. Establish short-term goals on the way to the final goal.

■ *Establish a plan.* What are three dietary changes you can make today? What exercise will you do tomorrow, the next day, and sustain for one week? Once you do one week, plot a course for two weeks. Jot down how you feel after each week's activity.

■ *Be consistent.* Make a number of small changes in what you regularly eat and drink and in your daily activity levels. Make changes that you can stick with and that are comfortable for you (parking farther from a destination and walking, eating cereal and juice for breakfast, walking three days per week, and so on). Set a schedule and try to stick to it, with an alternative time each day in case your plans change. Always have a fallback option for your scheduled exercise.

■ *Look for balance in what you do.* Remember that it's more about balance than about giving things up. If you must have that piece of chocolate cake, enjoy it, but then be sure to do the extra exercise it takes to burn off the calories or for limiting caloric intake the next day. Remember that it's calories taken in and burned over time that makes the difference.

■ *Stay positive.* Focus on the positive steps you are taking and the healthy things you do each week rather than the less healthy things.

■ *Be patient and persistent.* You didn't develop a weight problem overnight. Don't expect instant results. Assess other gains that you make each week: gains in energy level, the fit of your clothes, and how you feel in your body.

■ *Reward successes.* Set short-term goals and reward yourself when you've reached them—new shoes, a new CD, whatever it takes to keep you motivated.

Changing Your Diet

■ *Be adventurous.* Expand your usual meals and snacks to enjoy a wide variety of different options. Focus on the quality of the food rather than the amount you get. Avoid buffets that allow you to replenish your plate several times.

■ *Do not constantly deprive yourself of favorite foods or set unrealistic guidelines.* If you slip and eat something you know you shouldn't, just be more careful the next day. Balance over a week's time is important. Allow slips and reward successes.

■ *Be sensible with your knife and fork.* Enjoy all foods, just don't overdo. When you eat out, eat slowly, cut food into smaller pieces, and think about taking some home for tomorrow's lunch or dinner. Share entrées with a friend, and order salads with dressings on the side.

■ *Eat on a regular schedule.* Do not skip meals or let yourself get too hungry.

■ *Eat breakfast.* This will prevent you from being too hungry and overeating at lunch.

■ *Plan ahead and be prepared for when you might get hungry.* Always have good food available when and where you get hungry.

Changing Your Level of Activity

■ *Be active and slowly increase activity.* If you stick to something, it will gradually take less and less effort to walk that mile, for example. Gradually increase your speed and/or distance (see Chapter 11). Move more, sit less. Remember, every step counts. Purchasing an inexpensive pedometer and recording your daily steps is an excellent way to monitor and improve your level of activity.

■ *Be creative with your physical activity.* Find activities that you really love and stick to them. If you hate to walk in the rain but love to shop, walk in a covered mall and then shop! Try things you haven't tried before. Today, options such as yoga, Pilates, dancing, swimming, skiing, and gardening are available.

■ *Pick an activity that is inexpensive and does not require fancy equipment.* This means you will maintain your fitness program even when you are traveling away from home.

■ *Find an exercise partner to help you stay motivated.* Don't pick your fittest friend. Find someone who is patient, understanding, and supportive. Choose people who need help and commit to helping them. It will also help you get through the difficult days until exercise is part of your lifestyle.

Source: Adapted in part from M. Manore and J. Thompson, "Table 15.3: Techniques to Help an Active Individual Identify and Maintain a Healthy Body Weight Throughout the Life Cycle" in *Sport Nutrition for Health and Performance* (Champaign, IL: Human Kinetics Publishing, 2000), 417.

Selecting a Nutritional Plan

Once you have discovered what factors tend to sabotage your weight-loss efforts, you will be well on your way to healthy weight control. To succeed, however, you must plan for success. The U.S. *Dietary Guidelines for Americans* endorses small weight losses of one-half to 1 pound per week, as well as smaller weight losses of 5 to 10 percent to make a difference toward health.[54]

By setting goals that are unrealistic or too far in the future, you will doom yourself to failure. Do not try to lose 40 pounds in two months. Try, instead, to lose a healthy 1 to 2 pounds during the first week, and stay with this slow and easy regimen. Reward yourself when you lose pounds. If you binge and go off your nutrition plan, get right back on it the next day. Remember that you did not gain 40 pounds in eight weeks, so it is unrealistic to punish your body by trying to lose that amount of weight in such a short time.

Seek assistance from reputable sources in selecting a dietary plan that is nutritious and easy to follow, such as the MyPyramid Plan discussed in Chapter 9. Registered dietitians, some physicians (not all doctors have a strong background in nutrition), health educators and exercise physiologists with nutritional training, and other health professionals can provide reliable information. Beware of people who call themselves nutritionists. There is no such official designation, which leaves the door open for just about anyone to call himself or herself a nutritional expert. Avoid weight-loss programs that promise quick miracle results.

For any weight-loss program, ask about the credentials of the adviser; assess the nutrient value of the prescribed diet; verify that dietary guidelines are consistent with reliable nutrition research; and analyze the suitability of the diet to your tastes, budget, and lifestyle. Any diet that requires radical behavior changes is doomed to failure. The most successful plans allow you to make food choices and do not ask you to sacrifice everything you enjoy. See the New Horizons in Health box on page 296 for information on various popular diets and on low-carbohydrate diets in particular.

Considering Drastic Weight Loss Measures

When nothing seems to work, people often become willing to take significant risks in order to lose weight. Dramatic weight loss may be recommended in cases of extreme health risk. However, even in such situations, drastic dietary, pharmacological, or surgical measures should be considered carefully and discussed with several knowledgeable health professionals.

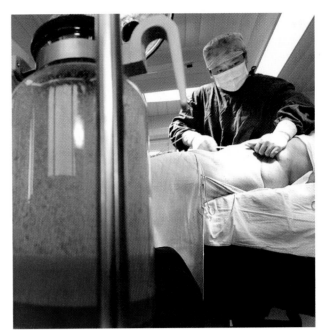

Liposuction is a surgical procedure that removes fat cells from specific areas of the body. It is not a good solution for long-term weight loss.

"Miracle" Diets

Fasting, starvation diets, and other forms of **very low-calorie diets (VLCDs)** have been shown to cause significant health risks. Typically, depriving the body of food for prolonged periods forces it to make adjustments to prevent the shutdown of organs. The body depletes its energy reserves to obtain necessary fuels. One of the first reserves the body turns to in order to maintain its supply of glucose is lean, protein tissue. As this occurs, weight is lost rapidly because protein contains only half as many calories per pound as fat. At the same time, significant water stores are lost. Over time, the body begins to run out of liver tissue, heart muscle, blood, and so on, since these readily available substances are burned to supply energy. Only after depleting the readily available proteins from these sources does the body begin to burn fat reserves. In this process, known as **ketosis,** the body adapts to prolonged fasting or carbohydrate deprivation by converting body fat to ketones, which can be used as fuel for some brain cells. Within about ten days after the typical adult begins a complete fast, the body will have used many of its energy stores, and death may occur.

> **Very low-calorie diets (VLCDs)** Diets with caloric value of 400 to 700 calories per day.
>
> **Ketosis** A condition in which the body adapts to prolonged fasting or carbohydrate deprivation by converting body fat to ketones, which can be used as fuel for some brain activity.

Low carbohydrate diets have attracted millions of Americans with reports of massive, quick weight loss. Bookstores struggle to keep the latest editions of *The Atkins Diet, The South Beach Diet,* and other bestsellers on their shelves. Restaurants have added "low carb" items to their menus, and a multimillion dollar industry of low-carb food products has emerged. The promise? Eliminate nearly all of the bread, pasta, sweets, and high carbohydrate foods from your diet, eat red meat and other high-protein and high-fat foods until you are satisfied, and lose weight.

Many health professionals have spent the past 20 years criticizing low carb diets as dangerous, ineffective, and unhealthy. The American Heart Association and the America Dietetic Association were just two of many professional health groups that issued warnings about the craze. Yet several well-designed clinical trials indicated that low carbohydrate diets were as good as—and in many cases, better than—low-fat diets in helping very overweight people shed pounds.

In these studies, more people stayed with the low carb diet than the low fat one, and, although they ate more fat, they did not experience the harmful changes in blood cholesterol

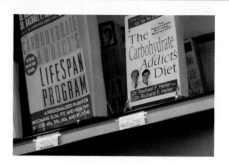

that many expected. In fact, their LDL ("bad") cholesterol and triglycerides were reduced and their HDL ("good") cholesterol increased.

However, these benefits were only short-term, and reports of problems with low carb diets began to surface. A study by the Stanford University Medical Center in conjunction with researchers at Yale University found that although low carbohydrate diets cause weight loss, it's the total caloric reduction and the duration of the reduction that causes the loss, not the reduction in carbohydrate intake per se. The take-home message was that any low calorie diet that a person can stay on long enough will have similar results. Furthermore, people had difficulty in sticking to the rigid dietary requirements. When they lost weight, they gained it back nearly as quickly as they had lost it. People with diabetes had problems because whole grains, beans, and other fiber-rich foods were not allowed. And rather than remembering to cut back on saturated fats, people were gulping down bacon and eggs, eating huge steaks, and feeling good about the guilt-free diet.

A major problem with the Atkins and similar diets is that they assume that virtually any carbohydrate is bad for you. However, they do not account

for the vast difference in nutrient value among carbohydrates and their *glycemic index,* a ranking of foods according to how quickly their sugars are released into the bloodstream. The body converts a food's sugars into glucose, which is released slowly or rapidly into the bloodstream. Insulin is secreted to counter glucose levels and return the body to healthy levels. The amount of insulin a food triggers is referred to as *glycemic load,* which considers both a food's glycemic index and how much carbohydrate the food delivers in one hit in a single serving.

Most fruits, vegetables, beans, and whole grains have low glycemic loads; their sugars enter the bloodstream gradually and trigger only a moderate rise in insulin. High-calorie sugars cause insulin levels to rise, triggering a chain of reactions that ultimately make

In very low-calorie diets, powdered formulas are usually given to patients under medical supervision. These formulas have daily values of 400 to 700 calories plus vitamin and mineral supplements. Although these diets may be beneficial for people who have failed at all conventional weight-loss methods and who face severe health risks due to obesity, they never should be undertaken without strict medical supervision. Problems associated with fasting, VLCDs, and other forms of severe calorie deprivation include blood sugar imbalance, cold intolerance, constipation, decreased BMR, dehydration, diarrhea, emotional problems, fatigue, headaches, heart irregularity, ketosis, kidney infections and failure, loss of lean body tissue, weakness, and eventual weight gain due to the yo-yo effect and other variables. Also consider the nutritional quality of

packaged "low-fat" foods commonly used as part of a low calorie diet. Many of these foods have a high sugar and sodium content to make the food taste better. They might be low-fat but generally are full of salt and empty calories from sugar.

Drug Treatment Experts reason that if obesity is a chronic disease, it should be treated as such, and the treatment for most chronic diseases includes drugs.[55] The challenge is to develop an effective drug that can be used over time without adverse effects or abuse, and no such drug currently exists.

A classic example of a supposedly safe set of drugs that later were found to have dangerous side effects were Pondimen and Redux, known as *fen-phen* (fenfluramine and phentermine), two of the most widely prescribed diet you sluggish, bloated, and feeling hungry, driving you to eat more and continuing the cycle. Ultimately, these high insulin levels can lead to diabetes.

Given this new understanding of carbohydrates, should you do what Atkins suggests and follow a diet that avoids most carbs? No. The bulk of scientific evidence suggests that you should choose foods with low glycemic loads and continue to reduce your total caloric intake and saturated fat intake.

A few examples of the glycemic load of common foods demonstrates the range you may find in your daily diet: a serving of high quality orange juice has nearly three times the glycemic load (13) as an orange; a serving of cornflakes has five times the load (21) as a serving of All Bran (4). Listing for many foods can be found online, particularly in connection with diabetes resources.

However, instead of memorizing glycemic load values for all your favorite foods, try following these general guidelines:

■ *Choose plants.* Pick the fruit rather than its sugar-laden juice counterpart. Eating the skin of apples adds fiber and slows the entry of glucose into the bloodstream. If you must eat potatoes,

eat them with the skin on and cut back on other starches. Instead of potatoes and corn, try sweet potatoes and yams.

■ *Forgo meat in favor of beans.* It isn't necessary to cut all meat-based protein from your diet. However, when you eat meat, opt for the lean cuts and choose poultry over pork or beef. Learn to cook and flavor beans. They are high in protein and other nutrients and have very little effect on blood sugar and insulin.

■ *Go nuts several times a week.* Almonds, hazelnuts, peanuts, pecans, and others are healthy low carbohydrate alternatives to snacking on chips and desserts made from white flour. They are not calorie free, though, so manage your intake based on exercise patterns and calorie needs.

■ *Mix your carbs with other foods.* Eating carbohydrates with other foods such as monounsaturated oils (olive or canola) can slow the rate of carbohydrate absorption. Milk or yogurt with cereal is one example; bananas and cottage cheese in cereal is another.

■ *Make whole-grain breads a staple.* Avoid white bread and look for brown breads with 100 percent whole-wheat or other grains. Consider options such as brown rice and whole-wheat pizza

dough and pasta. These are good choices for slowing your blood sugar rises.

■ *Exercise regularly.* Most people would be shocked if they ate a normal meal, measured their blood sugar, then noted how dramatically their blood sugars go down after a 30-minute walk. It may seem simple, but one of the best ways to keep yourself healthy and still consume the carbs you want is through exercise.

These recommendations hold true no matter what low-fat, low-carb, low-calorie or other plan you choose to follow.

Sources: W. Willet and P. Skerrett, "Going Beyond Atkins," *Newsweek,* January 19, 2004, 46; S. Conner et al., "Should a Low Fat, High-Carb Diet be Recommended for Everyone?" *New England Journal of Medicine* 350 (2004): 1691–1692. F. F. Samaha et al., "A Low-Carbohydrate as Compared with a Low-Fat Diet in Severe Obesity," *New England Journal of Medicine* 348, no. 21 (2003): 2074–2081; G.D. Foster et al., "A Randomized Trial of Low Carbohydrate Diet for Obesity," *New England Journal of Medicine* 348, no. 21 (2003): 2082–2090; D.M. Bravata et al., "Efficacy and Safety of Low-Carbohydrate Diets," *Journal of the American Medical Association* 289, no. 14 (2003): 1837–1850.

drugs in U.S. history.[56] When the drugs were found to damage heart valves and contribute to pulmonary hypertension, a massive recall and lawsuit occurred.

Other diet drugs that you should view with caution include sibutramine, orlistat, herbal weight loss aids, and over-the-counter (OTC) drugs. Sibutramine (Meridia) and orlistat (Xenical) are appetite suppressants but can cause increased blood pressure in some people. Though these drugs have been found to minimize weight regain in those following low-calorie diets, their long-term safety and effectiveness is still unknown.

Surgery When all else fails, a relatively permanent yet risky solution may lie in surgical stapling or gastric bypass surgery (where a portion of the stomach is tied off). This procedure effectively reduces stomach size to

hold only a few tablespoons of food. Patients can't eat enough calories, so they lose weight. Make no mistake about it, this procedure should be reserved only for the morbidly obese who face imminent health risks. Complications are many and include infections, nausea, vomiting, vitamin and mineral deficiencies, and dehydration. (Imagine being really thirsty and only able to drink a few tablespoons of water at a time.) Lifelong medical and sometimes psychological monitoring is needed for those who have this procedure. However, one recent study showed that those who successfully lose weight with this procedure experience clear health benefits and drastic reductions in CVD risk factors, including blood glucose, blood pressure, total cholesterol, high-density lipoprotein cholesterol, and triglycerides.[57]

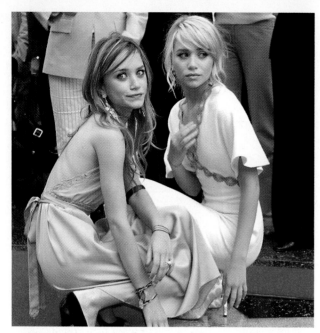
Pressures from society, especially on women, can have a detrimental effect on body image. Mary-Kate Olsen is one celebrity struggling with an eating disorder.

Liposuction is another surgical procedure for spot reducing. Although this technique has garnered much attention, it too is not without risk. Infections, severe scarring, and even death have resulted. Many people who have liposuction regain the fat or require multiple surgeries to repair lumpy, irregular surfaces from which the fat was removed.

TRYING TO GAIN WEIGHT

Although trying to lose weight poses a challenge for many, a smaller group of Americans, for a variety of metabolic, hereditary, psychological, and other reasons, inexplicably start to lose weight or can't seem to gain weight no matter how hard they try. If you are one of these individuals, determining the reasons for your difficulty in gaining weight is a must. For example, among older adults, the senses of taste and smell may decline, which makes food taste differently and be less pleasurable. Visual problems and other disabilities may make meals more difficult to prepare, and dental problems may make it more difficult to eat. People who engage in extreme sports that require extreme nutritional supplementation may be at risk for nutritional deficiencies, which can lead to immune system problems and organ dysfunction, weakness that leads to falls and fractures, slower recovery from diseases, and a host of other problems.

Once you know what is causing a daily caloric deficit, there are steps you can take to gain extra weight.

- *Eat at regularly scheduled times, whether you are hungry or not.*

- *Eat more.* Obviously, you are not taking in enough calories to support whatever is happening in your body. Eat more frequently, spend more time eating, eat the high-calorie foods first if you fill up fast, and always start with the main course. Take time to shop, to cook, to eat slowly. Put extra spreads such as peanut butter, cream cheese, or cheese on your foods. Make your sandwiches with extra-thick slices of bread, and add more filling. Take second helpings whenever possible, and eat high-calorie snacks during the day.

- *Supplement your diet.* Add high-calorie drinks that have a healthy balance of nutrients.

- *Try to eat with people you are comfortable with.* Avoid people who you feel are analyzing what you eat or who make you feel like you should eat less.

- *If you aren't exercising, exercise to increase your appetite.* If you are exercising or exercising to extremes, moderate your activities until weight gain is evident.

- *Avoid diuretics, laxatives, and other medications that cause you to lose body fluids and nutrients.*

- *Relax.* Many people who are underweight operate at high gear most of the time. Slow down, get more rest, and control stress.

THINKING THIN: BODY IMAGE AND MEDIA MESSAGES

Most of us think of the obsession with thinness as a recent phenomenon that began with supermodel Kate Moss in the 1990s. Beyond a doubt, the thin look dominates fashion and the media. However, an obsession with being thin has been a part of our culture for decades. Anorexia nervosa, an eating disorder (see the next section), has been defined as a psychiatric illness since 1873. During the Victorian era, women wore corsets to achieve unrealistically tiny waists. By the 1920s, it was common knowledge that obesity was linked to poor health. The American Tobacco Company coined the phrase "reach for a Lucky instead of a sweet" to promote the idea that cigarettes dulled appetite.

Today more than ever before, underweight models and celebrities exemplify desirability and success, delivering the subtle message that thin is in. Public health warnings that being overweight increases risk for heart disease, certain cancers, and a number of other disorders can send a panic through people when their weight isn't what they think it should be. Some of these distorted views of self-image arise from misinterpreting height–weight charts, making some people strive for the lower readings stipulated for a light-boned person when determining their own normal weight. Increasing

Table 10.3
Does Someone You Are Close to Have an Eating Disorder?

Although every situation is different, there are several things that you can do if you suspect someone is struggling with an eating disorder.

- Learn as much as you can about eating disorders ahead of time.
- Check out resources on your campus and in your local community. Talk to professionals about what approaches and treatments have been most successful. Have a list of referrals ready to give to the person. Be armed with information.
- Set up a time to meet and share your concerns openly, honestly, and in a caring and supportive way. Be a good listener, and don't give advice unless asked.
- Provide examples of why you think there might be a disordered eating problem. Talk about health, relationships, and changes in behaviors.
- Avoid conflicts or battle of the wills with this person. If he or she denies that there is a problem or minimizes it, repeat your concerns in a nonjudgmental way. You want the person to feel comfortable talking to you—not to drive him or her away.

- Never nag, plead, beg, bribe, threaten, or manipulate. Be straightforward, acknowledge it will be hard but that you know he or she can work through this.
- Don't get involved in endless conversations about diet, fatness, or exercise.
- Don't talk about how *thin* they are or focus on weight, diets, or exercise. Remember that the person wants to hear he or she is thin, and if you say it's good he or she is gaining weight, he or she will try to lose it.
- If the person is nervous about seeing a counselor, offer to go along as a support.
- Avoid placing shame, guilt, or accusations. Use "I" words (such as, "I am worried that you won't be able to do such and such if you don't eat,") rather than, "you need to eat or you are going to make yourself really sick."
- Stay calm and realize your own limitations. Be patient and supportive and be there in an emergency if the person asks for your help.

Sources: Adapted from "Anorexia Nervosa and Related Eating Disorders. When you want to help someone you care about," October 2003; National Eating Disorders Association, Communication: What Should I Say?" 2002, www.nationaleatingdisorders.org/p.asp?WebPage-ID=322&Profile-ID=41174.

numbers of adolescents, teens, and adults are so preoccupied with trying to be like the size 4 models that they make themselves ill. Being overweight has become socially unacceptable in many circles, and obese people are increasingly stigmatized in our society.[58] Americans are looking for fast answers: Should we count calories or carbohydrates? Is dietary fat your biggest enemy? Is Pritikin, Atkins, Weight Watchers, or something else your best weight control strategy? Sadly, many people end up answering these questions with disordered eating patterns such as anorexia, bulimia, and binge-eating.

EATING DISORDERS

For an increasing number of people, particularly young women, an obsessive relationship with food develops into **anorexia nervosa,** a persistent, chronic eating disorder characterized by deliberate food restriction and severe, life-threatening weight loss. **Bulimia nervosa,** involves frequent bouts of binge eating followed by purging (self-induced vomiting), laxative abuse, or excessive exercise. **Binge eating disorder (BED)** also involves episodes of binge eating; but, unlike bulimics, binge eaters do not purge after a binge episode. Binge eating episodes are often characterized by eating rapidly, eating large amounts of food even when not feeling hungry, and feeling guilty or depressed after overeating.[59] In the United States, more than 10 million women meet the established criteria for one of these disorders, and their numbers appear to be increasing.[60] Many more suffer from lesser forms of these

conditions—not enough for a true diagnosis but dangerously close to the precipice that will ultimately lead to life-threatening results. Some of the physical complications associated with eating disorders include osteoporosis, heart attack, seizures, anemia, electrolyte imbalances, and tooth erosion. The severity of these conditions varies with the degree and duration of the eating disorder.[61]

Anorexia Nervosa

Anorexia nervosa involves self-starvation motivated by an intense fear of gaining weight along with an extremely distorted body image. When anorexia occurs in childhood, failure to gain weight in a normal growth pattern may be the key indicator; later, anorexia typically results in actual weight loss. Nearly 1 percent of girls in late adolescence meet the full criteria for anorexia; many others suffer from significant symptoms.

Anorexia nervosa Eating disorder characterized by excessive preoccupation with food, self-starvation, and/or extreme exercising to achieve weight loss.

Bulimia nervosa Eating disorder characterized by binge eating followed by inappropriate measures to prevent weight gain.

Binge eating disorder (BED) Eating disorder characterized by recurrent binge eating, without excessive measures to prevent weight gain.

FOOD IS NOT AN ISSUE	CONCERNED WELL	FOOD PREOCCUPIED/ OBSESSED	DISRUPTIVE EATING PATTERNS	EATING DISORDERED
• I am not concerned about what others think regarding what and how much I eat. • I feel no guilt or shame no matter how much I eat or what I eat. • Food is an important part of my life but only occupies a small part of my time. • I trust my body to tell me what and how much to eat.	• I pay attention to what I eat in order to maintain a healthy body. • I may weigh more than what I like, but I enjoy eating and balance my pleasure with eating with my concern for a healthy body. • I am moderate and flexible in goals for eating well. • I try to follow Dietary Guidelines for healthy eating.	• I think about food a lot. • I feel I don't eat well most of the time. • It's hard for me to enjoy eating with others. • I feel ashamed when I eat more than others or more than what I feel I should be eating. • I am afraid of getting fat. • I wish I could change how much I want to eat and what I am hungry for.	• I have tried diet pills, laxatives, vomiting, or extra time exercising in order to lose or maintain my weight. • I have fasted or avoided eating for long periods of time in order to lose or maintain my weight. • I feel strong when I can restrict how much I eat. • Eating more than I wanted to makes me feel out of control.	• I regularly stuff myself and then exercise, vomit, use diet pills or laxatives to get rid of the food or calories. • My friends/family tell me I am too thin. • I am terrified of eating fat. • When I let myself eat, I have a hard time controlling the amount of food I eat. • I am afraid to eat in front of others.

BODY OWNERSHIP	BODY ACCEPTANCE	BODY PREOCCUPIED/ OBSESSED	DISTORTED BODY IMAGE	BODY HATE/ DISASSOCIATION
• Body image is not an issue for me. • My body is beautiful to me. • My feelings about my body are not influenced by society's concept of an ideal body shape. • I know that the significant others in my life will always find me attractive. • I trust my body to find the weight it needs to be so I can move and feel confident of my physical body.	• I base my body image equally on social norms and my own self-concept. • I pay attention to my body because it is important to me, but it only occupies a small part of my day. • I nourish my body so it has the strength and energy to achieve my physical goals. • I am able to assert myself and maintain a healthy body without losing my self-esteem.	• I spend a significant time viewing my body in the mirror. • I spend a significant time comparing my body to others. • I have days when I feel fat. • I am preoccupied with my body. • I accept society's ideal body shape and size as the best body shape and size. • I'd be more attractive if I was thinner, more muscular, etc...	• I spend a significant amount of time exercising and dieting to change my body. • My body shape and size keeps me from dating or finding someone who will treat me the way I want to be treated. • I have considered changing or have changed my body shape and size through surgical means so I can accept myself. • I wish I could change the way I look in the mirror.	• I often feel separated and distant from my body—as if it belongs to someone else. • I hate my body and I often isolate myself from others. • I don't see anything positive or even neutral about my body shape and size. • I don't believe others when they tell me I look OK. • I hate the way I look in the mirror.

Figure 10.5 ■ The Eating Issues and Body Image Continuum

Individuals whose responses fall to the far left side of the continuum have normal eating patterns and are not at risk for an eating disorder. Individuals whose answers fall to the far right of this continuum likely suffer from an eating disorder. Where are your responses on the continuum?

Initially, most people with anorexia lose weight by reducing total food intake, particularly of high-calorie foods, eventually leading to restricted intake of almost all foods. What they do eat, they often purge through vomiting or using laxatives. Although they lose weight, people with anorexia never seem to feel thin enough and constantly identify body parts that are "too fat." Anorexia has the highest death rate (20 percent) of any mental illness.

Bulimia Nervosa

People with bulimia nervosa often binge and then take inappropriate measures, such as secret vomiting, to lose the calories they have just acquired. Up to 3 percent of adolescents and young female adults are bulimic, with male rates being about 10 percent of the female rate. People with bulimia are also obsessed with their bodies, weight gain, and how they appear to others. Unlike those with anorexia, people with bulimia are often hidden from the public eye because their weight may vary only slightly or fall within a normal range. Also, treatment appears to be more effective for bulimia than for anorexia.

One of the more common symptoms of bulimia is tooth erosion, which occurs as a result of the excessive vomiting associated with this disorder. Chronic regurgitation causes hydrochloric acid (stomach acid) to break down the enamel of the teeth. Tooth erosion can also be contributed to the excessive consumption of acidic foods and beverages.[62]

Binge Eating Disorder

Individuals with binge eating disorder binge like their bulimic counterparts but do not take excessive measures to lose the weight that they gain. Often they are clinically obese, and they tend to binge much more often than the typical obese person, who may consume too many calories but spaces his or her eating over a more normal daily eating pattern.

Who's at Risk?

There's no simple explanation for why intelligent, often highly accomplished people spiral downward into the

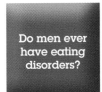

Do men ever have eating disorders?

destructive behaviors associated with eating disorders. Obsessive-compulsive disorder, depression, and anxiety can all play a role, as can a desperate need to win social approval or gain control of their lives through food. Figure 10.5 details the characteristics of those at risk for an eating disorder. Where do you fall on this continuum?

Once believed to be primarily a female issue, eating disorders are on the rise among young men. While it is true that females between ages 12 and 25 make up 85 to 90 percent of people with eating disorders, some 15 percent of people affected are males.[63] Certain athletic competitions appear to put males at much greater risk. Jockeys, bodybuilders, wrestlers, dancers, swimmers, rowers, gymnasts, and runners are at highest risk. At the other end of the continuum are men and women who are so obsessed with bulking up and obtaining "six-pack abs" that they are willing to do just about anything to get "the look."

Treatment for Eating Disorders

Because eating disorders result from many factors spanning many years of development, there are no quick or simple solutions. Table 10.3 details what you can do to help a friend or family member who has eating disorder. Treatment often focuses first on reducing the threat to life; once the patient is stabilized, long-term therapy involves family, friends, and other significant people in the individual's life. Therapy focuses on the psychological, social, environmental, and physiological factors that have led to the problem. Finding a therapist who really understands the multidimensional aspects of the problem is a must. Therapy allows the patient to focus on building new eating behaviors, recognizing threats, building self-confidence, and finding other ways to deal with life's problems. Support groups often help the family and the individual gain understanding and emotional support and learn self-development techniques designed to foster positive reactions and actions. Treatment of underlying depression may also be a focus.

What Do You Think?   Which groups or individuals on your campus appear to be at greatest risk for eating disorders? ■ What social factors might encourage this? ■ Why do you think society tends to overlook eating disorders in males?

Taking Charge

Summary

- Overweight, obesity, and weight-related problems appear to be on the rise in the United States. Obesity is now defined in terms of fat content rather than in terms of weight alone.

- There are many different methods of assessing body fat. Body mass index (BMI) is one of the most commonly accepted measures of weight based on height. Body fat percentages more accurately indicate how fat or lean a person is.

- Many factors contribute to one's risk for obesity, including genetics, setpoint, endocrine influences, psychosocial factors, eating cues, lack of awareness, metabolic changes, lifestyle, and gender. Women often have considerably more difficulty losing weight.

- Exercise, dieting, diet pills, surgery, and other strategies are used to maintain or lose weight. However, sensible eating behavior and adequate exercise offer the best options.

- Eating disorders consist of severe disturbances in eating behaviors, unhealthy efforts to control body weight, and abnormal attitudes about body and shape. Anorexia nervosa, bulimia nervosa, and binge eating disorder are the three main eating disorders. Though prevalent among white women of upper- and middle-class families, eating disorders affect women of all backgrounds and increasing numbers of men.

1. Essential fat makes up approximately _____ percent of total body weight in men and approximately _____ percent of total body weight in women.
   a. 3 to 5; 18
   b. 3 to 7; 15
   c. 5 to 25; 13
   d. 3 to 5; 7

2. The method of determining body fat by measuring the amount of water displaced when a person is completely submerged is called the
   a. skin-fold caliper test.
   b. body mass index.
   c. hydrostatic weighing technique.
   d. bioelectrical impedance analysis.

3. What technique of weight assessment is based on the relationship of weight to height?
   a. body composition index
   b. body mass index
   c. hydrostatic weight
   d. waist-to-hip ratio

4. What percent of all the calories you consume on a given day go to support your basal metabolism?
   a. 10 to 20 percent
   b. 30 to 40 percent
   c. 60 to 70 percent
   d. 80 to 90 percent

5. What theory states that a person's body has a set amount of weight at which it is programmed to be comfortable?
   a. endocrine theory
   b. plateau theory
   c. setpoint theory
   d. adaptive thermogenesis theory

6. Jenny binge eats and then secretly vomits. What eating disorder does she suffer from?
   a. pica
   b. anorexia nervosa
   c. bulimia nervosa
   d. binge eating disorder

7. Tim's desire to look good interferes with his relationship with others. Rather than spending his leisure time with family and friends, he spends a disproportionate amount of time exercising excessively at the gym and worrying about how his body looks. Tim suffers from
   a. social physique anxiety.
   b. appearance anxiety.
   c. obesity anxiety.
   d. anorexia nervosa.

8. What is the death rate for anorexia nervosa?
   a. 1 percent
   b. 5 percent
   c. 10 percent
   d. 20 percent

9. Very low calorie diets (VLCDs) have a caloric value of
   a. 400 to 700 calories per day.
   b. 700 to 1,000 calories per day.
   c. 1,000 to 1,200 calories per day.
   d. 1,200 to 1,400 calories per day.

10. One pound of body fat contains
    a. 1,500 calories.
    b. 3,500 calories.
    c. 5,000 calories.
    d. 7,000 calories.

Answers to these questions can be found on page A-1.

Questions for Discussion and Reflection

1. Discuss the pressures, if any, you feel to improve your personal body image. Do these pressures come from media, family, friends, and other external sources, or from concern for your personal health?

2. What type of measurement would you choose in order to assess your fat levels? Why?

3. List the risk factors for obesity. Evaluate which seem to be most important in determining whether you will be obese in middle age.

4. Create a plan to help someone lose the "freshman 15" over the summer vacation. Assume that the person is male, 180 pounds, and has 15 weeks to lose the excess weight.

5. Differentiate among the three eating disorders. Then give reasons why females might be more prone to anorexia and bulimia than males are.

Accessing Your Health on the Internet

The following websites explore further topics and issues related to personal health. For links to the websites below, visit the Companion Website for *Health: The Basics,* Seventh Edition at www.aw-bc.com/donatelle.

1. *American Dietetic Association.* Includes recommended dietary guidelines and other current information about weight control.

2. *Duke University Diet and Fitness Center.* Includes information about one of the best programs in the country; focuses on helping people live healthier, fuller lives through weight control and lifestyle change.

3. *Helping to End Eating Disorders (HEED).* The website of an organization dedicated to fighting eating disorders and helping individuals through the ordeal. Includes a chatroom for people to exchange thoughts and share support.

4. *Mayo Health Clinic's O@sis.* Summarizes many weight-control issues and concerns.

5. *Shape Up America.* Includes strategies and ideas for getting in shape and staying at your optimal weight.

Further Reading

Brownell, K. and K. Horgen. *Food Fight: The Inside Story of the Food Industry, America's Obesity Crisis, and What We Can Do about It.* New York: McGraw-Hill, 2003.

Director of the Yale Center for Eating and Weight Disorders, Brownell critiques the way that food is marketed and sold to children and places much of the blame for childhood obesity on advertising and unhealthy foods being offered in schools.

Gaesser, G. *Big Fat Lies.* New York: Fawcett Columbine Press, 1997.

Excellent overview of leading theories on fat, obesity, and a host of related problems and issues. Also discusses potential weight-loss strategies that are "keepers" for life.

Piscatella, J. *The Fat-Gram Guide to Restaurant Food,* 3rd ed. New York: Workman Press, 2000.

Excellent guide to fast foods and restaurant fat content.

U.S. Department of Agriculture (USDA). "The Great Nutrition Debate," 2000, www.usda.gov/cnpp.

An online transcript of a day of presentations and panel discussions by leading obesity experts and authors of fad diet books.

References

1. A. Hedley et al., "Prevalence of Overweight and Obesity Among U.S. Children, Adolescents, and Adults," *Journal of the American Medical Association* 291: 2847–2850.

2. Trust for America's Health, 2005, www.healthyamericans.org. (Specific information about how your state ranks is available at www.healthyamericans.org.)

3. Department of Health and Children, National Task Force on Obesity (Dublin, Ireland), "Obesity: The Policy Challenges," 2005, www.dohc.ie/publications.

4. C. Rodrigues, K. Walker-Thurmond, and M. Thun, "Overweight, Obesity, and Cancer Rise," *New England Journal of Medicine* 348 (2003): 1625–1638; S. Konchicah et al., "Obesity and the Rise of Heart Failure," *New England Journal of Medicine* 347 (2002): 305–313.

5. American Diabetes Association, "1 in 3 Americans Born in 2000 Will Develop Diabetes," June 14, 2003, www.diabetes.org/for-media/scientific-sessions/06-14-03-2.jsp.

6. E. A. Finkelstein, I. C. Fiebelkorn, and G. Wang, "National Medical Spending Attributable to Overweight and Obesity: How Much, and Who's Paying?" *Health Affairs*, 2003, http://content.healthaffairs.org/cgi/content/full/hlthaff.w3.219v1/DC1.

7. A. Peeters et al., "Adult Obesity and the Burden of Disability Throughout Life," *Obesity Research* 12 (2004): 1145–1151.

8. U.S. Department of Health and Human Services and U.S. Department of Agriculture, "Dietary Guidelines for Americans," 2005, www.healthierus.gov/dietaryguidelines.

9. R. F. Kushner and D. J. Blatner, "Risk Assessment of the Overweight and Obese Patient," *Journal of the American Dietetic Association* 105: 553–562.

10. Weight Control Information Network, "Statistics Related to Overweight and Obesity," October 2004, www.niddk.nih.gov/statistics.

11. Ibid.

12. American Obesity Association, "AOA Fact Sheets: What Is Obesity?" May 2, 2005, www.obesity.org.

13. Ibid.

14. Ibid.

15. Ibid.

16. D. Eberwine, "Globesity: The Crisis of Growing Proportions," *Perspectives in Health* 7, no. 3 (2003): 9.

17. Ibid.

18. Rush University, "Waist to Hip Ratio Calculator," 2005, www.rush.edu/itools/hip/hipcalc.html.

19. L. Kagan et al., "Chapter 5—Moving Through Menopause," in *Mind Over Menopause,* eds. L. Kagan et al., (New York: Free Press, 2004).

20. S. Kautiainen et al., "Use of Information and Communication Technology and Prevalence of Overweight and Obesity Among Adolescents," *International Journal of Obesity* 29 (2005): 925–933.

21. Ibid.

22. U.S. Department of Health and Human Services, "Surgeon General's Call to Action to Prevent and Decrease Overweight and Obesity" (Rockville MD: U.S. Department of Health and Human Services, Office of the Surgeon General, 2001).

23. A. Drewnowski and N. Darmon, "Food Choices and Diet Costs: An Economic Analysis," *Journal of Nutrition* 135 (2005): 900–904.

24. L. Young and M. Nestle, "Expanding Portion Sizes in the U.S. Marketplace: Implications for Nutrition Counseling," *Journal of the American Dietetic Association* 103 (2003): 231–234.

25. J. D. Wright et al., "Trends in Intake of Energy and Macronutrients—United States 1971–2000," *Morbidity and Mortality Weekly Report* 53, no. 4 (2004): 80–82.

26. M. W. Gillman et al., "Risk of Overweight Among Adolescents Who Were Breastfed as Infants," *Journal of the American Medical Association* 285 (2001): 2461–2467; M. L. Hediger et al., "Association between Infant Breastfeeding and Overweight in Young Children," *Journal of the American Medical Association* 285 (2001): 2453–2460.

27. J. H. Ledikwe et al., "Portion Sizes and the Obesity Epidemic," *Journal of Nutrition* 135:905–909.

28. American Obesity Association, "Obesity: A Global Epidemic," Updated May 2, 2005. www.obesity.org.

29. Ibid.

30. Ibid.

31. Ibid.

32. Mayo Clinic "Special Report: Weight Control," Women's Health-Source (1987): 3.

33. M. Treuth, "Predictors of Body Fat Gain in Non-obese Girls with Familial Predisposition to Obesity," *Journal of Clinical Nutrition* 78, no. 6 (2003): 1051–1052.

34. C. Bouchard et al., "The Response to Long-Term Overfeeding in Identical Twins," *The New England Journal of Medicine* 322 (1990): 1483–1487.

35. Ibid.

36. American Dietetic Society Association, "Position of the American Dietetic Association: Weight Management," *Journal of the American Dietetic Association* 102 (2002): 1145–1155.

37. L. K. Mahan and S. Escott-Stump, *Krause's Food, Nutrition, and Diet Therapy* (Philadelphia: Saunders, 2004).

38. P. Bouth et al., "GAD2 on Chromosome 10p12 Is a Candidate Gene for Human Obesity," *Public Library of Science Biology* 1, no. 3 (2003): e68.

39. S. G. Bouret et al., "Trophic Action of Leptin on Hypothalamic Neurons That Regulate Feeding," *Science* 304 (April 2, 2004) 110–115.

40. D. E. Cummings et al., "Plasma Ghrelin Levels After Diet-Induced Weight Loss or Gastric Bypass Surgery," *New England Journal of Medicine* 346, no. 21 (2002): 1623–1630.

41. Ibid.

42. A. A. Hedley et al., "Overweight and Obesity among US Children, Adolescents, and Adults, 1999–2002," *Journal of the American Medical Association* 291 (2004): 2847–2850.

43. G. B. Forbes, "Childhood and Adolescent Obesity: Causes and Consequences, Prevention and Management," *New England Journal of Medicine* 349 (2003): 619.

44. Centers for Disease Control and Prevention, "Growing Stronger: Strength Training for Older Adults—Why Strength Training," April 2005, www.cdc.gov/nccdphpdnpa/physical/growing_stronger/why.htm.

45. Marchesini et al., "Weight Cycling in Treatment Seeking Obese Persons: Date from the QUOUADIS Study," *International Journal of Obesity* 28: 1456–1462 ; K. Brownell, "Comments on the Latest Study on Yo-Yo Diets by Steven Blair of the Institute for Aerobics Research" (paper originally presented at Oregon State University, Corvallis, OR, 1993; newer report in paper presented by Steven Blair at Oregon State University, Corvallis, OR, Fall, 1998).

46. National Center for Health Statistics, "Prevalence of Sedentary Leisure Time Behavior Among Adults in the United States," February 2005, www.cdc.gov/nchs.

47. Ibid.

48. Ibid.

49. National Institute of Diabetes and Digestive and Kidney Diseases, "You Can Control Your Weight as You Quit Smoking," 2005, www.pueblo.gsa.gov.

50. I. Rashad and M. Grossman, "Economics of Obesity," *The Public Interest* 156 (2004), www.thepublicinterest.com/previous/article3.html.

51. S. Halls, "The BMI Gap Between Men and Women," November 2003, www.halls.md/bmi/gap.htm.

52. N. Diehl, C. Johnson, and R. Rogers, "Social Physique Anxiety and Disordered Eating: What's the Connection?" *Addictive Behaviors* 23 (1998): 1–16.

53. V. Paracchini et al., "Genetics of Leptin and Obesity: A Huge Review," *American Journal of Epidemiology* 162, no. 2: 101–114.

54. J. O. Hill et al., "Weight Maintenance: What's Missing?" *Journal of the American Dietetic Association* 105: S63–S66.

55. Weight Control Information Network, "Prescription Medications for the Treatment of Obesity," http://win.niddk.nih.gov.

56. "Fen-Phen Legal Resources," 2002, www.fen-phen-legal-resources.com.

57. L. Busetto et al., "Short-Term Effects of Weight Loss on the Cardiovascular Risk Factors in Morbidly Obese Patients," *Obesity Research* 12 (2004): 1256–1263.

58. A. Ghosh, "Seminar Explores Obesity Research Stigma," National Institutes of Health, January, 2005, www.nih.gov/nihrecord/01_18_2005/story09.htm.

59. National Institute of Diabetes and Digestive and Kidney Disease, Weight-control Information Network, "Binge Eating Disorder," http://win.niddk.nih.gov/publications/binge.htm.

60. National Eating Disorder Association, "Statistics: Eating Disorders and their Precursors," 2002, www.nationaleatingdisorders.org.

61. The Renfrew Center Foundation for Eating Disorders, "Eating Disorders 101 Guide: A Summary of Issues, Statistics, and Resources," October 2003, www.renfrew.org.

62. M. P. Faine, "Recognition and Management of Eating Disorders in the Dental Office," *The Dental Clinics of North America* 42, no. 9: 395–410.

63. Substance Abuse and Mental Health Services Administration, "SAMHSA's Mental Health Information Center: Eating Disorders," 2004, www.mentalhealth.samhsa.org/publications /allpubs/ KEN98-0047.

I don't want to diet; can I lose weight with exercise alone?

Which factors should I think about as I develop a fitness plan?

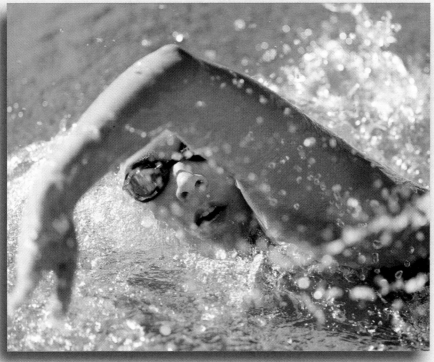

What types of exercises can I do to improve my muscular strength?

How can I prevent an exercise-related injury?

11

Personal Fitness
Improving Health through Exercise

Objectives

- **Describe** the benefits of regular physical activity, including improvements in physical health, mental health, stress management, and life span.
- **Explain** the components of an aerobic exercise program and how to determine the best frequency, intensity, and duration of exercise.

- **Describe** different stretching and strength exercises designed to improve flexibility.
- **Compare** the various types and benefits of resistance exercise programs.
- **Summarize** ways to prevent and treat common fitness injuries.
- **Summarize** the key components of a personal fitness program, and design a program that works for you.

A century ago in the United States, simple survival meant performing physical labor on a daily basis. However, science and technology have transformed our lives. Today most adults in our country lead sedentary lifestyles and perform little physical labor or exercise.[1] The growing percentage of Americans who live sedentary lives has been linked to dramatic increases in the incidence of obesity, diabetes, and other chronic diseases.[2] More than 110 million Americans are overweight or obese, 50 million have high blood pressure, 8 million have type 2 diabetes (which is associated with obesity and physical inactivity), approximately 41 million have "prediabetes," and 1.5 million suffer a heart attack in any given year.[3]

Decades of research show that physical activity has tremendous health-promoting and disease-preventing benefits.[4] Now is an excellent time to develop exercise habits that will improve the quality and duration of your own life.

WHAT IS PHYSICAL FITNESS?

Physical activity is defined as any bodily movement that is produced by the contraction of skeletal muscles and that substantially increases energy expenditure.[5] Physical activities can be done in leisure time, at work, or even for transportation. Walking, swimming, heavy lifting, and housework are all examples of physical activity. Physical activities also may vary by intensity. For example, walking to class may require little effort but walking to class up a hill while carrying a heavy backpack makes the activity more intense.

The term *exercise* is a bit more specific than *physical activity*. Exercise is defined as planned, structured, and repetitive bodily movement done to improve or maintain one or more components of physical fitness such as endurance, flexibility, and strength.[6] **Physical fitness** is the ability to perform moderate-to-vigorous levels of physical activity on a regular basis without

excessive fatigue. Table 11.1 identifies the major health-related components of physical fitness.

The recommendations for physical activity and exercise vary by their goal. Because research shows numerous health benefits from becoming more physically active, the Centers for Disease Control and Prevention (CDC) and American College of Sports Medicine (ACSM) recommend that adults engage in moderate-intensity physical activities for at least 30 minutes on most days of the week.[7] This amount of physical activity will not prepare you for running a marathon, but it can improve your overall health. The ACSM and CDC recommend that if you want to improve your cardiorespiratory fitness, you need to perform vigorous physical activities (e.g., jogging/running, walking hills, circuit weight training, singles tennis) at least 3 days per week for at least 20 minutes at a time.

Some people have physical limitations that make achieving these recommendations difficult, but they can still be active and reap the benefits of regular exercise. For example, a woman with arthritis in the knee and hip joints may find it too painful to jog but can still enjoy water exercise in a swimming pool. A man who uses a wheelchair may be unable to walk but can stay physically fit by playing wheelchair basketball.

What Do You Think? Which of the key aspects of physical fitness do you currently possess?
▧ Which ones would you like to improve or develop?
▧ What types of activities could you do to improve your fitness level?

BENEFITS OF REGULAR PHYSICAL ACTIVITY

Regular physical activity has been shown to improve more than 50 different physiological, metabolic, and psychological aspects of human life.[8]

Improved Cardiorespiratory Fitness

Cardiorespiratory fitness refers to the ability of the circulatory and respiratory systems to supply oxygen to the body during sustained physical activity.[9] Regular exercise makes these systems more efficient by enlarging the heart muscle, enabling more blood to be pumped with each stroke and increasing the number of *capillaries* (smallest blood vessels) in trained skeletal muscles, which supply more blood to working muscles. Exercise improves the respiratory system by increasing the amount of oxygen that is inhaled and distributed to body tissues.[10]

Physical activity   Any bodily movement that is produced by the contraction of skeletal muscles and that substantially increases energy expenditure.

Exercise   Planned, structured, and repetitive bodily movement done to improve or maintain one or more components of physical fitness.

Physical fitness   The ability to perform regular moderate to vigorous physical activity without excessive fatigue.

Cardiorespiratory fitness   The ability of the heart, lungs, and blood vessels to supply oxygen to skeletal muscles during sustained physical activity.

Reduced Risk of Heart Disease Your heart is a muscle made up of highly specialized tissue. Because muscles become stronger and more efficient with use, regular exercise strengthens the heart, which enables it to pump more blood with each beat. This increased efficiency means that the heart requires fewer beats per minute to circulate blood throughout the body. A stronger, more efficient heart is better able to meet the ordinary demands of life.

Prevention of Hypertension *Blood pressure* refers to the force exerted by blood against blood vessel walls, generated by the pumping action of the heart. *Hypertension,* the medical term for abnormally high blood pressure, is a significant risk factor for cardiovascular disease and stroke. Hypertension is particularly prevalent in adult African Americans. Over 38 percent report having high blood pressure, compared with 27 percent of whites and 29 percent of Hispanics.[11] People with consistently elevated blood pressure are more susceptible to heart disease and die at a younger age than people with normal blood pressure.[12] Studies report that moderate exercise can reduce both diastolic and systolic blood pressure by 7 mmHg.[13]

Improved Blood Lipid and Lipoprotein Profile Lipids are fats that circulate in the bloodstream and are stored in various places in the body. Regular exercise is known to reduce the levels of low-density lipoproteins (LDLs, or "bad cholesterol") while increasing the number of high-density lipoproteins (HDLs, or "good cholesterol") in the blood. Higher HDL levels are associated with lower risk for artery disease because they remove some of the bad cholesterol from artery walls and hence prevent clogging. The bottom line: regular exercise lowers the risk of cardiovascular disease. (For more on cholesterol and blood pressure, see Chapter 12).

Reduced Cancer Risk

Regular physical activity appears to lower the risk for some types of cancer. There is strong evidence that physical activity reduces the risk of breast and colon cancer.[14] Experts say that because physical activity makes food move more quickly through your digestive system, there is less time for the body to absorb potential carcinogens and for potential carcinogens to be in contact with the digestive tract. Physical activity also decreases the levels of prostaglandins, substances found in cells of the large intestine that are implicated in cancer.[15]

Improved Bone Mass

A common affliction among older adults is **osteoporosis,** a disease characterized by low bone mass and deterioration of bone tissue, which increase fracture risk.

Table 11.1 **Components of Physical Fitness**	
Cardiorespiratory fitness	Ability to sustain moderate-intensity whole-body activity for extended time periods
Flexibility	Range of motion at a joint or series of joints
Muscular strength and endurance	Maximum force applied with single muscle contraction; ability to perform repeated high-intensity muscle contractions
Body composition	A composite of total body mass fat mass, fat-free mass, and fat distribution

Source: American College of Sports Medicine, "ACSM Position Stand on the Recommended Quantity and Quality of Exercise for Developing and Maintaining Cardiorespiratory and Muscular Fitness and Flexibility in Adults," *Medicine and Science in Sports and Exercise* 30 (1998): 975–991, http://lww.com.

Osteoporosis currently affects 20 to 25 million Americans, 90 percent of them women. About 50 percent of all women eventually develop osteoporosis. Men are not immune; nearly 2 million men have the disease.

Osteoporosis is more common among women than among men for at least three reasons: women live longer, they have lower peak bone mass than men, and they lose bone mass at a faster rate after menopause as their estrogen levels decrease. The incidence of osteoporosis and fractures increases substantially with age in both women and men. Over 300,000 Americans aged 45 years and older are admitted to hospitals each year with osteoporosis-related hip fractures.[16] The estimated national direct expenditures (hospitals and nursing homes) for osteoporotic and associated fractures was $17 billion in 2001 ($47 million each day), and the cost is rising.[17]

Bone, like other human tissues, responds to the demands placed on it. Women (and men) have much to gain by remaining physically active as they age—bone mass levels are significantly higher among active than among sedentary women.[18] New research indicates that by "surprising" bone (by jumping and other sudden activities), young children may improve their bone density.[19] Regular weight-bearing exercise, when combined with a balanced diet containing adequate calcium, will

Osteoporosis A disease characterized by low bone mass and deterioration of bone tissue, which increase risk of fracture.

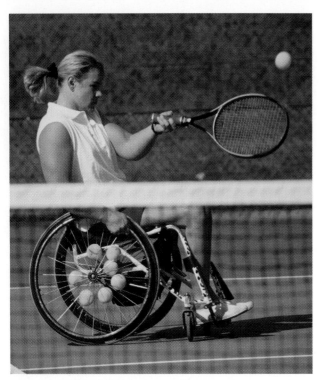
Everyone can attain cardiovascular fitness and muscular endurance.

help keep bones healthy.[20] See Chapter 15 for more information on risk factors for osteoporosis.

Improved Weight Control

Many people start exercising because they want to lose weight. Level of physical activity has a direct effect upon metabolic rate and can raise it for several hours following a vigorous workout. An effective method for losing weight combines regular endurance-type exercises with a moderate decrease in food intake. The ACSM recommends 30 minutes of moderate physical activity daily with an intake between 1,500 to 2,000 calories per day.[21] Cutting daily caloric intake beyond this range ("severe dieting") actually decreases metabolic rate by up to 20 percent and makes weight loss more difficult.

> I don't want to diet; can I lose weight with exercise alone?

The best way to lose weight is a combination of exercise and decreased calorie intake. However, if you want to lose weight only through physical activity, you will have to spend more time exercising than if you reduce your calories at the same time. In addition to helping you lose weight, increasing physical activity also improves your chances at keeping the weight off once you have lost it.[22]

Improved Health and Life Span

Prevention of Diabetes Type 2 diabetes (noninsulin-dependent diabetes) is a complex disorder that affects millions of Americans, many of whom have no idea that they have the disease (see Chapter 14). Risk factors for diabetes include obesity, high blood pressure, and high cholesterol, as well as a family history of the disease.[23] Physicians suggest exercise combined with weight loss and healthy diet to prevent diabetes. In a recent study, people who began a moderate exercise program reduced their risk of getting diabetes by over 50 percent.[24] Exercise also helps manage the disease; walking 30 to 60 minutes a day lowers a diabetic's risk of dying from cardiovascular disease by 40 to 50 percent.[25]

Longer Life Span Several large studies that followed groups of people over time found that those who exercised or were more fit lived longer.[26] In one study, capacity for exercise was a better predictor of whether a man would die in the next few years than were high blood pressure, high cholesterol, or smoking.[27]

Improved Immunity to Disease Regular, consistent exercise promotes a healthy immune system. Research shows that moderate exercise gives the immune system a temporary boost in the production of the cells that attack bacteria.[28] While moderate amounts of exercise can be beneficial, extreme exercise may actually be detrimental. For example, athletes engaging in marathon-type events or very intense physical training have an increased risk of colds and flu.[29]

Just how exercise alters immunity is not well understood. We do know that brisk exercise temporarily increases the number of white blood cells (WBCs), the blood cells responsible for fighting infection. Generally speaking, the less fit the person and the more intense the exercise, the greater the increase in WBCs.[30] Because exercise can reduce illness, many worksites have begun exercise programs for their employees. Reviews of past research shows that employees who regularly exercise take fewer sick-days.[31]

Improved Mental Health and Stress Management

People who engage in regular physical activity also notice psychological benefits. Regular vigorous exercise has been shown to burn off the chemical by-products released by the nervous system during normal response to stress. This reduces stress levels by accelerating the body's return to a balanced state. Regular exercise improves a person's physical appearance by toning and developing muscles and reducing body fat. Feeling good about personal appearance boosts self-esteem. At the same time, as exercisers come to appreciate the improved strength, skills, and flexibility that accompany fitness, they often become less obsessed with physical appearance.[32]

What Do You Think?
Among the many benefits to be derived from physical activity, which two are most important to you? Why? ■ After exercising regularly for several weeks, what benefits do you notice?

IMPROVING CARDIORESPIRATORY FITNESS

There are many options for improving cardiorespiratory fitness. Swimming, cycling, jogging, and in-line skating are just a few options for **aerobic exercise.** The term *aerobic* means "with oxygen" and describes any type of exercise, typically performed at moderate levels of intensity for extended periods of time, that increases your heart rate. A person said to be in good shape has an above-average **aerobic capacity**—a term used to describe the functional status of the cardiorespiratory system (i.e., heart, lungs, blood vessels). Aerobic capacity (commonly written as $VO_{2\ max}$) is defined as the maximum volume of oxygen consumed by the muscles during exercise.

To measure your maximal aerobic capacity, an exercise physiologist or physician typically will have you exercise on a treadmill. You will initially be asked to walk at an easy pace and then, at set time intervals during this **graded exercise test,** will gradually increase the workload (i.e., a combination of running speed and the angle of incline of the treadmill). Generally, the higher your cardiorespiratory endurance level, the more oxygen you can transport to exercising muscles and the longer you can exercise without becoming exhausted. In other words, the higher the $VO_{2\ max}$ value, the higher your level of aerobic fitness.

You can test your own aerobic capacity by using either the 1.5-mile run or the 12-minute run endurance test described in the Assess Yourself box on page 312. However, do not take these tests if you are just starting to exercise.[33] Progress slowly through a walking/jogging program at low intensities before measuring your aerobic capacity with one of these tests. If you have any medical conditions, such as asthma, diabetes, heart disease, or obesity, consult your physician before beginning any exercise program.

Aerobic Fitness Programs

The most beneficial aerobic exercises are total body activities involving all the large muscle groups of your body, for example, swimming, cross-country skiing, and rowing. If you have been sedentary for quite a while, simply initiating a physical activity program may be the hardest task you'll face. The key is to begin at a very low intensity. This will give you confidence to continue and reduce the amount of muscle soreness you may experience.

There are three main components of an aerobic exercise program: frequency, intensity, and duration. The characteristics of these components vary by individual exercise goal and beginning fitness level. You can remember them with the acronym FIT (frequency, intensity, and time/duration).

Determining Exercise Frequency To best improve your cardiovascular endurance, you will need to exercise vigorously at least 3 times a week. If you are a newcomer to exercise, you can still make improvements by doing less intense exercise but doing it more days a week, following the CDC/ACSM recommendations for moderate physical activity at least 5 days a week (Figure 11.1 on page 310).

Determining Exercise Intensity There are several ways to measure exercise intensity. One of the main ways is using your **target heart rate.** To calculate target heart rate, start by subtracting your age from 220 to find your maximum heart rate. Your target heart rate is a certain percentage of this maximum heart rate, often 60 percent. Thus, if you are a 20-year-old female, your 60 percent target heart rate would be

$$(220 - 20) \times 0.60, \text{ or } 120 \text{ beats per minute (bpm)}$$

For moderate-intensity physical activity, you should work out at 50 to 70 percent of your maximum heart

---

Aerobic exercise   Any type of exercise, typically performed at moderate levels of intensity for extended periods of time (typically 20 to 30 minutes or longer), that increases heart rate.

Aerobic capacity   The current functional status of a person's cardiovascular system; measured as $VO_{2\ max}$.

Graded exercise test   A test of aerobic capacity administered by a physician, exercise physiologist, or other trained person; two common forms are the treadmill running test and the stationary bike test.

Target heart rate   Calculated as a percentage of maximum heart rate (220 minus age); heart rate (pulse) is taken during aerobic exercise to check if exercise intensity is at the desired level (e.g., 60 percent of maximum heart rate).

Adults should strive to meet either of the physical activity recommendations:

- Adults should engage in moderate-intensity physical activities for at least 30 minutes on 5 or more days of the week (CDC/ACSM)

- Adults should engage in vigorous-intensity physical activity 3 or more days per week for 20 or more minutes per occasion (*Healthy People 2010*)

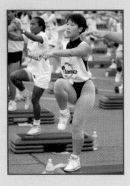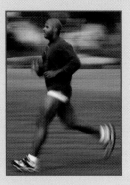

Figure 11.1 ■ Guidelines for Aerobic Activity

Source: National Center for Chronic Disease Prevention and Health Promotion, "Physical Activity Recommendations," 2003, www.cdc.gov.nccdphp/dnpa/physical/recommendations/index.htm.

rate. For more vigorous activities (e.g., running), aim for 70 to 85 percent of your maximum heart rate. People in poor physical condition should set a target heart rate between 40 and 50 percent of maximum and gradually increase the target rate in 5 percent increments.

Once you know your target heart rate, you can take your pulse to determine how close you are to this value during your workout. As you exercise, lightly place your index and middle fingers (don't use your thumb) on your radial artery (inside your wrist, on the thumb side). Using a watch or clock, take your pulse for six seconds and multiply this number by 10 (just add a zero to your count) to get the number of beats per minute. Your pulse should be within a range of 5 beats per minute above or below your target heart rate. If necessary, adjust the pace or intensity of your workout to achieve your target heart rate.

Another way of determining intensity is to use the Borg rating of perceived exertion (RPE) scale (Figure 11.2). Perceived exertion is how hard you feel like you are working. When using this method, you would think about your heart rate, increased breathing rate, sweating, and muscle fatigue. This scale uses a rating from 6 (no exertion at all) to 20 (maximal exertion). This method corresponds to heart rate for most people. Experts agree that RPE ratings of 12 to 14 correspond to moderate intensity activity and 15 to 17 for vigorous activity.

The easiest, but least scientific, method of measuring exercise intensity is the "talk test." If you are exercising moderately, you should be able to carry on a conversation comfortably. If you are too out of breath to carry on a conversation, you are exercising vigorously.

Determining Exercise Duration

Duration refers to the number of minutes of activity performed during any one session. Vigorous activities should be performed for at least 20 minutes at a time and moderate activities for at least 30 minutes at a time.

The lower the intensity of your activity, the longer the duration you'll need to get the same caloric expenditure. For example, a 120-pound woman will burn 180 calories walking for 30 minutes at a 15 min/mile pace, but will burn 330 calories if she jogs for 30 minutes at a 10 min/mile pace. A 180-pound man will expend 210 calories per hour of downhill skiing but 700 calories per hour if he is cross-country skiing.[34] Aim to expend 300 to 500 calories per exercise session, with an eventual weekly calorie expenditure of 1,500 to 2,000 calories. As you progress, add to your exercise load by increasing duration or intensity, but not both at the same time. From week to week, don't increase duration or intensity by more than 10 percent.

A program of repeated sessions of exercise over several months or years—exercise training—changes the way your cardiovascular system meets your body's oxygen requirements at rest and during exercise. Many of the health benefits associated with cardiorespiratory fitness activities (such as lower blood pressure) may take several months of regular exercise to achieve; don't expect improvements overnight.[35] However, any physical activity of low to moderate intensity will benefit your overall health almost from the start (Figure 11.3).

What Do You Think?

Calculate your maximum heart rate. Pick an intensity of exercise that suits your fitness level, for example, 60, 70, or 80 percent of your maximum heart rate. Using a familiar physical activity and monitoring your pulse, experiment by exercising at three different intensities. Do you notice any difference in the way you felt while exercising? Afterward?

IMPROVING MUSCULAR STRENGTH AND ENDURANCE

To get a sense of what resistance training is about, do a resistance exercise. Start by holding your right arm straight down by your side, then turn your hand palm up and bring it up toward your shoulder. That's a resistance exercise: using a muscle, your biceps, to move a resistance, which in this case, is just the weight of your

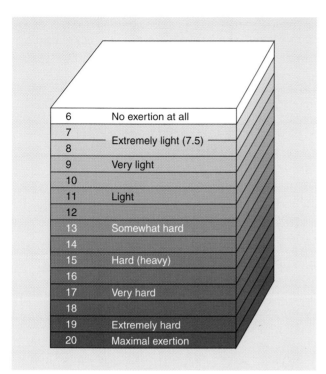

Figure 11.2 ■ Rating of Perceived Exertion (RPE) Scale

Source: G. Borg, *Borg's Perceived Exertion and Pain Scales* (Champaign, IL: Human Kinetics, 1998), 47. Used with permission of Borg Products, USA.

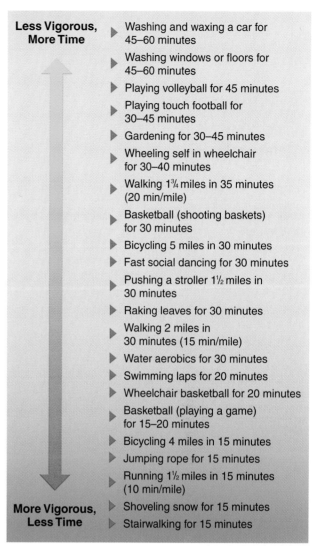

Figure 11.3 ■ Levels of Physical Activity

A moderate amount of physical activity is roughly equivalent to physical activity that uses about 150 calories of energy per day, or 1,000 calories per week. Some activities can be performed at various intensities; the suggested durations correspond to expected intensity effort.

Source: U.S. Department of Health and Human Services, *Physical Activity and Health: A Report of the Surgeon General* (Washington, DC: USDHHS, 1996).

hand—not very much resistance. Resistance training usually involves more weight or tension than this; but, unlike flexibility training, resistance training is usually equipment intense. Free weights (e.g., dumbbells and barbells) various tension-producing machines are usually part of resistance training. It's not just bodybuilding that uses this type of training either. Fitness enthusiasts of all levels and athletes perform resistance training to improve strength and endurance, and resistance exercises are an integral part of rehabilitation programs to help patients recover from muscle and joint injury.

Strength and Endurance

In the field of resistance training, **muscular strength** refers to the amount of force a muscle or group of muscles is capable of exerting. The most common way to assess strength in a resistance exercise program is to measure the **one repetition maximum (1 RM),** which is the maximum amount of weight a person can move one time (but not more) in a particular exercise. For example, 1 RM for the simple exercise done at the beginning of this section is the maximum weight you lift to your shoulder one time. **Muscular endurance** is the ability of muscle to exert force repeatedly without fatiguing. If you can perform the exercise described earlier holding a 5-pound weight in your hand and lifting ten times, you will have greater endurance than

someone who attempts that same exercise but is only able to lift the weight seven times.

Some resistance programs are designed primarily for increasing strength; others are aimed more at

---

Muscular strength   The amount of force that a muscle is capable of exerting.

One repetition maximum (1 RM)   The amount of weight/resistance that can be lifted or moved once, but not twice; a common measure of strength.

Muscular endurance   A muscle's ability to exert force repeatedly without fatiguing.

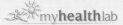

Fill out this assessment online at
www.aw-bc.com/myhealthlab or www.aw-bc.com/donatelle.

Evaluating Your Cardiorespiratory Endurance

After you have exercised regularly for several months, you might want to assess your cardiorespiratory endurance level. Find a local track, typically one quarter mile per lap, to perform your test. You may either *run or walk* for 1.5 miles and measure how long it takes to reach that distance or *run or walk* for 12 minutes and determine the distance you covered in that time. Use the chart below to estimate your cardiorespiratory fitness level based upon your age and sex. Note that women have lower standards for each fitness category because they have higher levels of essential fat than men do.

Age*	1.5-Mile Run/Walk (min:sec)		12-Minute Run/Walk (miles)	
	Women (min:sec)	Men (min:sec)	Women (miles)	Men (miles)
Good				
18–29	<13.24	<11:27	>1.3	>1.5
30–39	<14.03	<12:06	>1.2	>1.4
40–49	<14:29	<12:32	>1:1	>1.4
50+	<15:21	<13:50	>1.0	>1.2
Adequate for most activities				
18–29	13:25–14:55	11:28–12:58	1.1–1.3	1.3–1.5
30–39	14:04–15:21	12:07–13:37	1.1–1.2	1.3–1.45
40–49	14:30–15:47	12:33–14:03	0.99–1.11	1.25–1.4
50+	15:22–16:39	13:25–15:21	0.87–1.0	1.0–1.3
Borderline				
18–29	14:56–15:22	12:59–13:25	0.96–1.2	1.2–1.4
30–39	15.22–15:48	13:38–14:04	0.95–1.05	1.2–1.3
40–49	15:48–16:14	14:04–14:30	0.9–1.0	1.14–1.24
50+	16:40–17:06	14:56–15:48	0.78–0.93	0.87–1.16
Need extra work on cardiovascular fitness				
18–29	>15:22	>13:25	<1.0	<1.3
30–39	>15:448	>14:04	<0.94	<1.18
40–49	>16:14	>14:30	<0.88	<1.14
50+	>17:06	>15:22	<0.84	<1.0

If you are now at the good level, congratulations! Your emphasis should be on maintaining this level for the rest of your life. If you are currently at lower levels, set realistic goals for improvement.

Source: Reprinted by permission from E. T. Howley and B. D. Franks, *Health Fitness Instructor's Handbook,* 3rd ed. (Champaign, IL: Human Kinetics Publishers, 1997), 85.

Make It Happen!

Assessment: Complete the Assess Yourself activity to determine your current cardiorespiratory endurance level. Your results may indicate that you should take steps to improve this component of your physical fitness.

Making a Change: In order to change your behavior, you need to develop a plan. Follow these steps below and complete your Behavior Change Contract to take action.

1. Evaluate your behavior, and identify patterns and specific things you are doing. What can you change now? What can you change in the near future?
2. Select one pattern of behavior that you want to change.
3. Fill out the Behavior Change Contract found at the front of your book. It should include your long-term goal for change, your short-term goals, the rewards you'll give yourself for reaching these goals, potential obstacles along the way, and strategies for overcoming these obstacles. For each goal, list the small steps and specific actions that you will take.
4. Chart your progress in a journal. At the end of a week, consider how successful you were in following your plan. What helped you be successful? What made change more difficult? What will you do differently next week?
5. Revise your plan as needed. Are the short-term goals attainable? Are the rewards satisfying?

Example: Chris decided to measure how long it took him to run 1.5 miles around the school track to determine his level of cardiorespiratory endurance. It took him 13.0 minutes, which, as a 20-year-old, put him into the "borderline" category. Chris had played sports in high school and considered himself in good physical shape. However, he realized he had stopped exercising regularly in his freshman year when he didn't make the baseball team.

Chris decided to start by incorporating more activity into his daily routine. He tended to drive even to places that he could walk or bicycle to as easily. His friends had invited him to join in the pick-up basketball games they played on Saturday afternoons, but he had turned them down in order to play Playstation with his roommate. Chris filled out a Behavior Change Contract with a goal of riding his bicycle the three miles to and from campus three times a week and to play basketball every Saturday. If he did this consistently every week, he would reward himself with a new CD. After a month of this increased activity, Chris was already feeling more fit and was ready to add another aerobic activity. With winter weather coming, he thought he should add an indoor activity and started swimming laps at the school pool. He found swimming boring, so when he realized he was making excuses not to go, Chris switched to using a stair-climbing machine, which he could do while reading *Sports Illustrated* or watching ESPN. He was able to stick to doing this three times a week and made a commitment to go a fourth time whenever he missed his Saturday basketball game.

---

increasing endurance. Winning an Olympic weight-lifting event depends on the amount of weight that is lifted in just a few seconds. Endurance doesn't play a large role. Conversely, a soccer event lasts much longer and requires enormous endurance but less strength than does weight lifting. In football, strength and endurance are both important. Training for endurance includes using lighter weights but repeats an exercise more times than does training for strength. If you were endurance training for performing the hand-to-shoulder exercise described above (called a curl in weight-training circles), you might hold a 5-pound weight in each hand and curl 15 times per exercise segment. In training for strength, 40-pound weights might be used for a five-time curl.

Principles of Strength Development

An effective **resistance exercise program** involves three key principles: tension, overload, and specificity of training.[36]

The Tension Principle The key to developing strength is to create tension within a muscle or group of muscles. Tension is created by resistance provided by weights such as barbells or dumbbells, specially designed machines, or the weight of the body.

The Overload Principle This principle is the most important of our three key principles. Overload doesn't mean forcing a muscle or group of muscles to do too much, which could result in injuries. Rather, overload in resistance training requires muscles to do more than they are used to doing. Everyone begins a resistance training program with an initial level of strength. To become stronger, you must regularly create a degree of tension in your muscles that is greater than

---

Resistance exercise program   A regular program of exercises designed to improve muscular strength and endurance in the major muscle groups.

you are accustomed to. This overload will cause your muscles to adapt to a new level. As your muscles respond to a regular program of overloading by getting larger, they become stronger.

Remember that resistance training exercises cause microscopic damage (tears) to muscle fibers, and the rebuilding process that increases the size and capacity of the muscle takes 24 to 48 hours. Thus, resistance training exercise programs should include at least one day of rest and recovery between workouts before overloading the same muscles again.

The Specificity-of-Training Principle

According to the specificity principle, the effects of resistance exercise training are specific to the muscles being exercised. Only the muscle or muscle group that you exercise responds to the demands placed upon it. For example, if you regularly do curls, the muscles involved—your biceps—will become larger and stronger, but the other muscles in your body won't change. It is important to note that only exercising certain muscle groups may put opposing muscle groups at increased risk for injury. For example, overworking your quadriceps muscles but neglecting your hamstrings can put you at risk for a hamstring muscle pull or strain.

Gender Differences in Weight Training

The results of resistance training in men and women are quite different. Women normally don't develop muscles to the same extent that men do. The main reason for this difference is that men and women have different levels of the hormone testosterone in their blood. Before puberty, testosterone levels are similar for both boys and girls. During adolescence, testosterone levels in boys increase dramatically (about tenfold) while testosterone levels in girls remain unchanged. Muscles will become larger (**hypertrophy**) as a result of resistance training exercise; typically this change is not as dramatic in women as it is in men. To enhance muscle bulk, some bodybuilders (both men and women) take synthetic hormones (anabolic steroids) that mimic the effects of

testosterone. However, using anabolic steroids is a dangerous and illegal practice (see Chapter 7).

Types of Muscle Activity

In the past, the term *contraction* was used to define the tension a muscle produces as it shortens. Since a tension develops as muscles contract, the term *muscle action* is a better descriptor. Skeletal muscle actions fall into three different categories: isometric, concentric, and eccentric.[37] In **isometric muscle action** (Figure 11.4a), force is produced through tension and muscle contraction, not movement. For example, an isometric muscle action would occur in your back, legs, and arms if you try to move a large, immovable object. A **concentric muscle action** (Figure 11.4b), causes joint movement and a production of force while the muscle shortens. An empty-hand curl is a concentric exercise, with joint movement occurring at the elbow. In general, concentric muscle actions produce movement in a direction opposite to the downward pull of gravity.

Eccentric muscle action (Figure 11.4c) describes the ability of a muscle to produce force while returning to its noncontracted state. Typically, eccentric muscle actions occur when movement is in the same direction as the pull of gravity. Once you've brought a weight up during a curl, an eccentric muscle action would be to lower your hand and the weight back to their original position.

Methods of Providing Resistance

There are four commonly used resistance exercise methods: body weight, fixed, variable, and accommodating resistance devices.

What types of exercises can I do to improve my muscular strength?

Body Weight Resistance (Calisthenics)
Strength and endurance training don't have to rely on equipment. You can use your own body weight to develop skeletal muscle fitness. Calisthenics (such as pull-ups or push-ups) use part or all of your body weight to offer resistance during exercise. While less effective than other resistance methods in developing large muscle mass and strength, calisthenics improve general muscular fitness and muscle tone and maintain a level of muscular strength.

Fixed Resistance
Fixed resistance exercises provide a constant amount of resistance throughout the full range of movement. Barbells, dumbbells, and some types of machines provide fixed resistance because their weight, or the amount of resistance, does not change during an

---

Hypertrophy Increased size (girth) above normal levels.

Isometric muscle action Force produced without any resulting joint movement.

Concentric muscle action Force produced while the muscle is shortening.

Eccentric muscle action Force produced while the muscle is returning to its uncontracted state.

---

exercise. Fixed resistance equipment has the potential to strengthen all the major muscle groups in the body.

One advantage of dumbbells and barbells is that they are relatively inexpensive. Fixed resistance exercise machines are commonly available at college recreation/fitness facilities, health clubs, and many resorts and hotels.

Variable Resistance Variable resistance equipment alters the resistance encountered by a muscle during a movement so that the effort by the muscle is more consistent throughout the full range of motion. Variable resistance machines, such as Nautilus and Bowflex, are typically single-station devices; a person stays on the same machine throughout the whole series of exercises. Other types of machines, such as Soloflex, have multiple stations; the person using them moves from one machine to another. While some of these machines are expensive and too big to move easily, others are affordable and more portable. Many forms of variable resistance devices are sold for home use.

Accommodating Resistance Devices
These devices adjust the resistance according to the amount of force generated by the person using the equipment. The exerciser performs at maximal level of effort while the exercise machine controls the speed of the exercise. The machine is set to a particular speed, and muscles being exercised must move at a rate faster than or equal to that speed in order to encounter resistance.

The Benefits of Strength Training

Does strength training offer any benefits beyond simply getting stronger? Regular strength training can reduce the occurrence of lower back pain and joint and muscle injuries. It can also postpone loss of muscle tissue due to aging and a sedentary lifestyle and help prevent osteoporosis.

Strength training enhances muscle definition and tone and improves personal appearance. This, in turn, enhances self-esteem. Strength training even has a hidden benefit: muscle tissue burns calories faster than most other tissues do, even when it is resting—so increasing your muscle mass can help you boost your metabolism and maintain a healthy weight.

What Do You Think?   What types of resistance equipment are currently available to you? ■ Based on what you've read, what actions can you take to increase your muscular strength? Muscular endurance? ■ How would you measure your improvement?

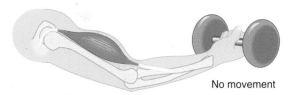

(a) Isometric muscle action
Muscle contracts but does not shorten

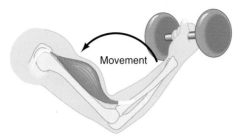

(b) Concentric muscle action

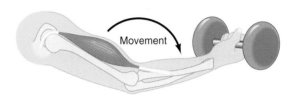

(c) Eccentric muscle action

Figure 11.4 ■ Isometric, Concentric, and Eccentric Muscle Actions

Source: S. Powers and E. Howley, *Exercise Physiology: Theory and Application to Fitness and Performance* (Madison, WI: Brown and Benchmark, 1997).

IMPROVING FLEXIBILITY

Stretching Exercises and Well-Being

Who would guess that improved flexibility can give you a sense of well-being, help you deal with stress better, and stop your joints from hurting as much as they used to? But that's just what people who have improved their flexibility are saying. Stretching exercises are the main way to improve flexibility. Today, they are extremely popular, both because they work and because people can begin them at virtually any age and enjoy them for a lifetime.

Flexibility is a measure of the range of motion (the amount of movement possible) at a particular joint. Improving range of motion through stretching exercises enhances efficiency, extent of movement,

> **Flexibility**   The measure of the range of motion, or the amount of movement possible, at a particular joint.

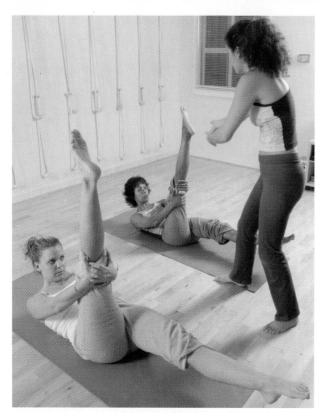
Pilates and other styles of exercise that strengthen core body muscles also enhance flexibility and lower stress levels.

greater flexibility. In stretching exercises a muscle or group of muscles is stretched to a point of slight discomfort, and that position is held for 10 to 30 seconds or more.

Types of Stretching Exercises

In the language of exercise science, all of the commonly practiced stretching exercises fall into two major categories: static and proprioceptive neuromuscular facilitation.[39] **Static stretching** techniques involve the slow, gradual stretching of muscles and their tendons, then holding them at a point. During this holding period—the stretch—participants may feel a mild discomfort and a warm sensation in the muscles that are being stretched. Static stretching exercises involve specialized tension receptors in our muscles. When done properly, static stretching slightly lessens the sensitivity of tension receptors, which allows the muscle to relax and be stretched to greater length.[40] The stretch is followed by a slow return to the starting position. As discussed in the next section, the physical aspect of yoga and tai chi is largely composed of static techniques, as are some of the exercises in Pilates programs.

The second major type of stretching exercise is **proprioceptive neuromuscular facilitation (PNF).** This technique uses various patterns of movement, such as a contraction of a muscle followed by a stretch. While PNF techniques have been shown to be superior to other stretching techniques for improving flexibility, they are, unfortunately, quite complex in their original form. A certified athletic trainer or physical therapist may be required to help in performing PNF exercises correctly; however, several have been simplified to the point that they can be performed with an exercise partner or even alone.

Yoga, Tai Chi, and Pilates

Three major styles of exercise that include stretching have become widely practiced in the United States and other Western countries: yoga, tai chi, and Pilates. All three emphasize a joining of mind and body as a result of intense concentration on breathing and body position.

Yoga One of the most popular fitness and static stretching activities, **yoga** originated in India about 5,000 years ago. Yoga blends the mental and physical aspects of exercise, a union of mind and body that participants find relaxing and satisfying. Done regularly, its combination of mental focus and physical effort improves flexibility, vitality, posture, agility, and coordination.

The practice of yoga focuses attention on controlled breathing as well as purely physical exercise. In addition to its mental dimensions, yoga incorporates a complex array of static stretching exercises expressed as postures (*asanas*). Over 200 postures exist, but only

and posture. Flexibility exercises are effective in reducing the incidence and severity of lower back problems. Improved flexibility also reduces the risk of muscle or tendon injuries that can occur during sports or everyday physical activities. It can also mean less tension and pressure on joints, which results in less joint pain and joint deterioration.[38]

Flexibility is enhanced by the controlled stretching of muscles and muscle attachments that act on a particular joint. Each muscle involved in a stretching exercise is attached to our skeleton by tendons. The goal of stretching is to decrease the resistance of a muscle and its tendons to tension, that is, to reduce resistance to being stretched. Stretching exercises gradually result in

Static stretching Techniques that gradually lengthen a muscle to an elongated position (to the point of discomfort) and hold that position for 10 to 30 seconds.

Proprioceptive neuromuscular facilitation (PNF) Techniques that involve the skillful use of alternating muscle contractions and static stretching in the same muscle.

Yoga A variety of Indian traditions geared toward self discipline and the realization of unity; includes forms of exercise widely practiced in the West today that promote balance, coordination, flexibility, and meditation.

about 50 are commonly practiced. During a session participants move to different asanas and hold them for 30 seconds or more. Yoga not only enhances flexibility, it has the great advantage of being flexible itself. Asanas and combinations of asanas can be changed and adjusted for young and old and to accommodate people with physical limitations or disabilities. Asanas can also be combined to provide even conditioned athletes with challenging sessions.

A typical yoga session will move the spine and joints through their full range of motion. Yoga postures lengthen, strengthen, and balance musculature, leading to increased flexibility, stamina, and strength—and many people report a psychological sense of general well-being too.

There are many styles of yoga. Three of the most popular follow:

- *Iyengar yoga* focuses on precision and alignment in the poses. Standing poses are basic to this style, and poses are often held longer than in other styles.

- *Ashtanga yoga* in its pure form is based on a specific flow of poses with an emphasis on strength and agility that creates internal heat. Power yoga, a style growing in popularity, is a derivative of Ashtanga yoga.

- *Bikram's yoga* (or *hot yoga*) is similar to power yoga but does not incorporate a specific flow of poses. Literally the hottest yoga going, it is performed in temperatures of 100°F, or even a bit higher. Proponents say that the heat increases the body's ability to move and stretch without injury.

Tai chi Tai chi is an ancient Chinese form of exercise that, like yoga, combines stretching, balance, coordination, and meditation. It is designed to increase range of motion and flexibility while reducing muscular tension. Based on Chi Kung, a Taoist philosophy dedicated to spiritual growth and good health, tai chi was developed about 1000 AD by monks to defend themselves against bandits and warlords. It involves a series of positions called *forms* that are performed continuously.

Pilates Compared to yoga and tai chi, **Pilates** is the new kid on the exercise block. It was developed by Joseph Pilates, who came from Germany to New York City in 1926. Shortly after his arrival, he introduced his exercise methodology, which emphasizes flexibility, coordination, strength, and tone. Pilates combines stretching with movement against resistance, which is aided by devices such as tension springs or heavy rubber bands.

Pilates includes a component designed to increase core muscle strength. The method consists of a sequence of carefully performed movements. Some are carried out on specially designed equipment, while others are performed on mats. Each exercise stretches and strengthens the muscles involved and has specific breathing patterns associated with it. A Pilates class focuses on strengthening specific muscle groups by using equipment that provides resistance.

Try it NOW

Stretching exercises aren't just for the gym! Sitting hunched over a pile of books for an extended period of time can be a pain in the neck. Be sure to stretch out every 20 minutes or so by doing shoulder rolls, shrugs, and neck stretches to help work out the kinks. These mini-stretch breaks will ease your muscles and your mind.

BODY COMPOSITION

Body composition is the fourth and final component of a comprehensive fitness program. Body composition describes the relative proportion of lean tissue (muscle, bone, water, organs) and fat tissue in the body. Body composition parameters that can be influenced by regular physical activity include total body mass, fat mass, fat-free mass, and regional fat distribution. Body composition differs significantly for women and men because women have a higher percentage of body fat and a significantly lower percentage of fat-free mass (such as muscle and bone) and bone mineral density.[41] Aerobic activities that improve cardiovascular endurance also help improve body composition because they expend calories, contribute to weight loss, and help with weight loss maintenance.

There are many ways to assess body composition. These range from simple (e.g., height-weight charts) to complex (e.g., underwater weighing) (see Assessing Fat Levels in Chapter 10).

CREATING YOUR OWN FITNESS PROGRAM

Identify Your Fitness Goals

The first step in creating your fitness program is to identify your fitness goals. Do you want to improve your quality of life? Lose weight? Train for an upcoming

---

Tai chi An ancient Chinese form of exercise widely practiced in the West today that promotes balance, coordination, stretching, and meditation.

Pilates Exercise programs that combine stretching with movement against resistance, aided by devices such as tension springs and heavy bands.

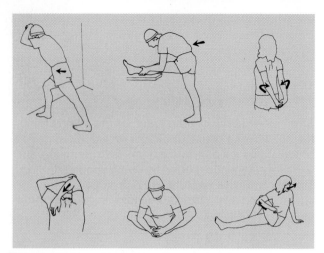

Figure 11.5 ■ Stretching Exercises to Improve Flexibility

Use these stretches as part of your warm-up and cool-down. Hold each stretch for 10 to 30 seconds, and repeat four times for each limb. After only a few weeks of regular stretching, you'll begin to see more flexibility.

Source: Drawings from B. Anderson, *Stretching, 20th Anniversary Revised Edition.* © 2000 Shelter Publications, Box 279, Bolinas, CA 94924.

5K race? Think about a timeline for your goals. Do you want to be able to jog 3 miles before spring break? Hike across campus next semester with a heavy backpack and not be out of breath? Once you develop a specific goal, you can create a plan to help you achieve that goal.

When you become committed to regular physical activity and exercise, you will observe gradual improvements in your functional abilities and note progress toward your goals. Perhaps your most vital goal will be to become committed to fitness for the long haul—to establish a realistic schedule of diverse exercise activities that you can maintain and enjoy throughout your life.

Designing Your Program

Now that you know the fundamentals of fitness, you can design your own personalized fitness program. There are several factors to consider that will boost your chances of successfully achieving your fitness goal. First, choose an activity that is appropriate for you. For example, don't plan on swimming if the pool is difficult to access. Choose activities that you like to do. If you hate to run, don't choose running as your exercise. Be creative in your activity choice; try something new! There are many different classes (e.g., salsa aerobics, boot camp classes) that can keep you motivated—and if you don't like one activity, you can always try another. See the Skills for Behavior Change box on page 323 more tips on getting started on an exercise plan.

> **Which factors should I think about as I develop a fitness plan?**

Your plan should include very specific ways to incorporate physical activity into your lifestyle. When will you exercise? For how long? It is best to write out these goals and put them in your daily planner as you would any other scheduled activity. Lack of time is the number one reason given for not exercising. By looking at your weekly schedule, you can identify segments of time that work for you.

Reevaluate your fitness goal and action plan after 30 days. This time period should give you a good idea of whether or not the program is working for you. Make changes if necessary, and then make a plan to reevaluate after another 30-day period.

Fitness Program Components

The amount and type of exercise required to yield beneficial results vary with the age and physical condition of the exerciser. Men over age 40 and women over age 50 should consult their physicians before beginning any fitness program.

Good fitness programs are designed to improve or maintain cardiorespiratory fitness, flexibility, muscular strength and endurance, and body composition. A comprehensive program could include a warm-up period of easy walking, followed by stretching activities to improve flexibility, then selected strength development exercises, followed by an aerobic activity for 20 minutes or more, and concluding with a cool-down period of gentle flexibility exercises.

Warming Up and Stretching Warming up and stretching prepares your body for exercise and provides a transition from rest to physical activity. A 5-minute warm-up may start with a 5-minute brisk walk to ease your cardiovascular system into the more vigorous activity and to increase blood flow to the exercising muscles. This 5-minute warm up can increase the temperature and elasticity of muscles and connective tissue, making stretching more effective. Add 5 to 10 minutes of stretching to your fitness routine, and you'll be ready to go!

A program of regular stretching exercise doesn't need to take a great deal of time and doesn't require expensive equipment. You can reap the benefits of stretching with just two or three 10-minute sessions per week. Figure 11.5 shows a selection of exercises that will stretch the major muscle groups of your body and can be used as a warm-up for other physical activities and exercise programs, such as jogging and tennis.

Start off slowly with a 5-minute session for the first week, then add a 5-minute session each week until you reach a schedule and comfort level that suit you. A hefty program would consist of five 30-minute sessions each week. Sessions get longer as you slowly increase the time you hold a particular stretch and how many times you repeat each type of stretch.

Strength Training When beginning a resistance exercise program, always consider your age, fitness level, and personal goals. Strength training exercises are done in a set, or a single series of multiple repetitions using the same resistance. For both men and women under the age of 50, the ACSM recommends working major muscle groups with at least one set of eight to ten different exercises 2 to 3 days per week.[42] Weight loads should be at a level to allow up to 8 to 12 repetitions. Beginners should use lighter weights and complete 10 to 15 repetitions. Remember, experts suggest allowing at least one day of rest and recovery between workouts of any specific muscle group. Table 11.2 includes some information on developing a resistance training programe.

Cardiorespiratory Training The greatest proportion of exercise time should be spent developing cardiovascular fitness. Choose an aerobic activity you think you will like. Many people find cross training—alternate-day participation in two or more aerobic activities (i.e., jogging and swimming)—less monotonous and more enjoyable than long-term participation in only one activity. Cross training is also beneficial because it strengthens a variety of muscles, thus helping you avoid overuse injuries to muscles and joints.

Jogging, walking, cycling, rowing, step aerobics, and cross-country skiing are all excellent activities for developing cardiovascular fitness. Most colleges have recreation centers where students can use stair-climbing machines, stationary bicycles, treadmills, rowing machines, and ski-simulators. Table 11.3 on page 320 describes popular workout machines and provides tips for their use.

Cooling Down Just as you ease into a workout with a warm-up, you should slowly transition from activity to rest. At least 5 minutes of your workout should be devoted to a gradual slow-down, decreasing the intensity of your activity. For example, if you jog, walk briskly, then slowly before stretching. Be sure to stretch the major muscle groups to help reduce the amount of soreness from exercise.

Try it ►NOW

Boost daily exercise today with small changes. For example, when you have a choice between elevator and stairs, choose the stairs. Walking up a few flights of stairs a day can be beneficial to your health, especially when you add the weight of a backpack or books. Walking stairs can help strengthen your legs, gets your heart pumping, and contributes to your daily activity level.

Table 11.2
Resistance Training Program Guidelines

- Resistance training should be an integral part of an adult fitness program and be of sufficient intensity to enhance strength and muscular endurance and to maintain fat-free mass.
- Resistance training should be progressive in nature, individualized, and provide a stimulus (overload) to all major muscle groups in the body.
- The exercise sequence should include large before small muscle group exercises, multiple-joint exercises before single-joint exercises, and higher intensity before lower intensity exercises.
- Performing 8 to 10 exercises that train the major muscle groups 2 to 3 days per week is recommended.
- The amount of weight used and number of repetitions vary by individual's target goal, physical capacity, and training status.

Source: W. J. Kraemer et al., "American College of Sports Medicine Position Stand on Progression Models in Resistance Training for Healthy Adults," _Medicine and Science in Sports and Exercise_ 3, no. 2 (2002): 364–380, http://lww.com.

FITNESS INJURIES

Overtraining is the most frequent cause of injuries associated with fitness activities and affects up to 20 percent of all athletes. Enthusiastic but out-of-shape beginners often injure themselves by doing too much too soon. Experienced athletes develop _overtraining syndrome_ by engaging in systematic and progressive increases in training without getting enough rest and recovery time. Eventually, performance begins to decline, and training sessions become increasingly difficult. Adequate rest, good nutrition (including replenishing carbohydrates), and rehydration are important to sustain or improve fitness levels.

Pay attention to your body's warning signs. To avoid injuring a particular muscle group or body part, vary your fitness activities throughout the week to give muscles and joints a rest. Establishing realistic but challenging fitness goals—short-term and long-term—can help you stay motivated without overdoing it. Overtraining injuries occur most often in repetitive activities like skiing, running, bicycling, and step aerobics. However, use common sense, and you're likely to remain injury-free.

Causes of Fitness-Related Injuries

There are two basic types of injuries stemming from fitness-related activities: overuse and traumatic. **Overuse injuries** occur because of cumulative, day-after-day

Overuse injuries Injuries that result from the cumulative effects of day-after-day stresses placed on tendons, muscles, and joints.

Table 11.3

Picking Your Workout Machine

Machine	Advantages	Best Use
Elliptical machine	This machine is designed for nonimpact cardiovascular exercise. Some machines are equipped with handles for arm action that improve the overall workout.	For machines without arm action, pump arms at your sides as you would if you were running. If the machine has arm handles, use resistance by pushing and pulling along with the handles.
Stair climber	This machine is a great lower body workout and most can be adjusted from very easy to very difficult.	Since the degree of workout depends on working against your body weight, stay upright and don't lean on the console. Try not to touch the handrails other than for balance. Keep your steps shallow (no deeper than 6 inches).
Stationary bike	This machine provides an excellent lower body workout. It is generally easy to use and most come with varied resistance programs. Recumbent bikes offer less strain on the back and knees.	Adjust the seat so your leg is almost fully extended when the pedal is at its lowest. Don't grip the handles too tightly.
Treadmill	This machine offers a great lower body workout. It is relatively easy to use.	Most come with an emergency shut-off clip. Be sure to use this for safety. Start gradually and progress to either faster pace or increased incline. Arms should naturally swing at your sides.

stresses placed on tendons, bones, and ligaments during exercise. The forces that occur normally during physical activity are not enough to cause a ligament sprain or muscle strain; but when these forces are applied on a daily basis for weeks or months, they can result in an injury. Common sites of overuse injuries are the leg, knee, shoulder, and elbow joints.

Traumatic injuries occur suddenly and violently, typically by accident. Examples include broken bones, torn ligaments and muscles, contusions, and lacerations. Some traumatic injuries occur quickly and are difficult to avoid—for example, spraining your ankle by landing on another person's foot after jumping up for a rebound in basketball. If your traumatic injury causes a noticeable loss of function and immediate pain or pain that does not go away after 30 minutes, consult a physician.

Prevention

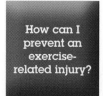

How can I prevent an exercise-related injury?

Exercise clothing is more than a fashion statement—smart choices can help you prevent injuries. For some types of physical activity, you need clothing that allows body heat to dissipate; for example,

light-colored nylon shorts and mesh tank top while running in hot weather. For other types, you need clothing that retains body heat without getting you sweat-soaked; for example, layers of polypropylene and/or wool clothing while cross-country skiing. Today there are high-tech fabrics on the market that can help you stay cool, keep warm, or stay dry. Appropriate quality exercise clothing is a good investment.

Appropriate Footwear When you purchase running shoes, look for several key components. Running is a collision sport: with each stride, the runner's foot collides with the ground with a force three to five times the runner's body weight.[43] The 150-pound runner who takes 1,000 strides per mile applies a cumulative force to his or her body of 450,000 pounds per mile. The force not absorbed by the running shoe is transmitted upward into the foot, leg, thigh, and back. Our bodies are able to absorb forces such as these but may be injured by the cumulative effects of repetitive impacts (e.g., running 40 miles per week). Therefore, the ability of running shoes to absorb shock is critical.

The midsole of a running shoe must absorb impact forces but must also be flexible. To evaluate the flexibility of the midsole, push on both ends of the shoe with your fingers; the shoe should bend easily at the midsole. If you cannot bend the shoe with your index fingers, its midsole is probably too rigid and may irritate your Achilles tendon, among other problems.[44] Other basic characteristics of running shoes include a rigid plastic insert within the heel of the shoe (known as a heel

Traumatic injuries Injuries that are accidental in nature and occur suddenly and violently (e.g., fractured bones, ruptured tendons, and sprained ligaments).

counter) to control the movement of your heel; a cushioned foam pad surrounding the heel of the shoe to prevent Achilles tendon irritation; and a removable thermoplastic innersole that customizes the fit of the shoe by using your body heat to mold it to the shape of your foot (Figure 11.6). Shoes are the runner's most essential piece of equipment, so carefully select appropriate footwear before you start a running program.

Shoe companies also sell cross-training shoes to help combat the high cost of having to buy separate pairs of running shoes, tennis shoes, weight-training shoes, and so on. Although the cross-training shoe can be used for several different fitness activities by the novice or recreational athlete, a distance runner who runs 25 or more miles per week needs a pair of specialty running shoes to prevent injury.

Appropriate Exercise Equipment
Some activities require special protective equipment to reduce chances of injury. Eye injuries can occur in virtually all fitness-related activities, although some activities are more risky than others. As many as 90 percent of the eye injuries resulting from racquetball and squash could be prevented by wearing appropriate eye protection (e.g., goggles with polycarbonate lenses).[45] Nearly 100 million people in the United States ride bikes for pleasure, fitness, or competition. Wearing a helmet while bicycle riding is an important safety precaution. Riding without a bicycle helmet significantly increases the risk of a head injury. Nonhelmeted riders are 14 times more likely to be involved in a fatal crash than helmeted riders; 85 percent of all fatal bicycle accidents are due to head or brain injury, many of which could have been prevented by helmet usage.[46, 47] Look for helmets that meet the standards established by the American National Standards Institute and the Snell Memorial Foundation.

What Do You Think?
Given your activity level, what injury risks are you exposed to on a regular basis? ■ What changes can you make in your equipment and clothing to reduce your risk?

Common Overuse Injuries

Three of the most common overuse injuries are plantar fasciitis, shin splints, and runner's knee.

Plantar Fasciitis
Plantar fasciitis is an inflammation of the plantar fascia, a broad band of dense, inelastic tissue (fascia) that runs from the heel to the toe on the bottom of the foot. Repetitive weight-bearing movements such as walking and running can inflame the plantar fascia. Common symptoms are pain and tenderness under the ball of the foot, at the heel, or at both

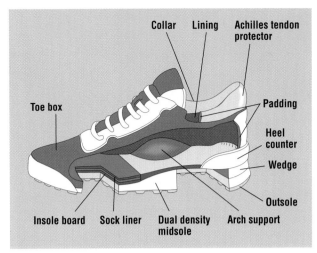

Figure 11.6 ■ Anatomy of a Running Shoe

locations.[48] If not treated properly, plantar fasciitis may progress until weight-bearing exercise is too painful to endure. This injury can often be prevented by regularly stretching the plantar fascia prior to exercise and by wearing athletic shoes with good arch support and shock absorbency. Stretch the plantar fascia by slowly pulling all five toes upward toward your head, holding for 10 to 15 seconds, and repeating this 3 to 5 times on each foot prior to exercise.

Shin Splints
A general term for any pain that occurs below the knee and above the ankle is *shin splints.* This broad description includes more than 20 different medical conditions. Problems range from stress fractures of the tibia (shin bone) to inflammation and irritation in the muscles of the lower leg. Typically, there is pain and swelling along the middle of the shin in the soft tissues, not the bone.

Sedentary people who start a new weight-bearing exercise program are at the greatest risk for shin splints, though well-conditioned aerobic exercisers who rapidly increase their distance or pace may also develop them.[49] To help prevent shin splints, wear athletic shoes with good arch support and shock absorbency. If the pain continues, see your physician. You may need to substitute a nonweight-bearing activity, such as swimming, during your recovery period.

Runner's Knee
Runner's knee describes a series of problems involving the muscles, tendons, and ligaments about the knee. The most common problem identified as runner's knee is abnormal movement of the kneecap, which irritates the cartilage on the back side of the kneecap as well as nearby tendons and ligaments.[50] Women experience this more often than men.[51] Symptoms of runner's knee include pain, swelling, redness, and tenderness around the kneecap.[52] Your physician

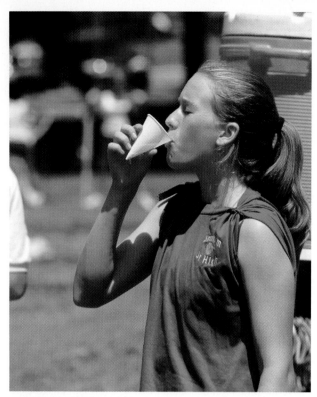
Avoiding dehydration is important when exercising in hot or cold weather.

will probably recommend that you stop running for a few weeks and reduce daily activities that compress the kneecap (e.g., exercise on a stair-climbing machine or doing squats with heavy resistance) until you no longer feel any pain.

Treatment

First aid treatment for virtually all personal fitness injuries involves **RICE: r**est, **i**ce, **c**ompression, and **e**levation. *Rest,* the first component of this treatment, is required to avoid further irritation of the injured body part. *Ice* is applied to relieve pain and constrict the blood vessels to stop any internal or external bleeding.

RICE Acronym for the standard first aid treatment for virtually all traumatic and overuse injuries: rest, ice, compression, and elevation.

Heat cramps Muscle cramps that occur during or following exercise in warm or hot weather.

Heat exhaustion A heat stress illness caused by significant dehydration resulting from exercise in warm or hot conditions; frequent precursor to heat stroke.

Heat stroke A deadly heat stress illness resulting from dehydration and overexertion in warm or hot conditions; can cause body core temperature to rise from normal to 105°F to 110°F in just a few minutes.

Never apply ice cubes, reusable gel ice packs, chemical cold packs, or other forms of cold directly to your skin. Instead, place a layer of wet toweling or elastic bandage between the ice and your skin. Ice should be applied to a new injury for approximately 20 minutes every hour for the first 24 to 72 hours. *Compression* of the injured body part can be accomplished with a 4- or 6-inch-wide elastic bandage; this applies indirect pressure to damaged blood vessels to help stop bleeding. Be careful, though, that the compression wrap does not interfere with normal blood flow. A throbbing, painful hand or foot indicates that the compression wrap should be loosened. *Elevation* of the injured extremity above the level of your heart also helps to control internal or external bleeding by making the blood flow upward to reach the injured area.

Exercising in the Heat

Heat stress, which includes several potentially fatal illnesses resulting from excessive core body temperatures, should be a concern whenever you exercise in warm, humid weather. In these conditions, your body's rate of heat production can exceed its ability to cool itself.

You can help prevent heat stress by following certain precautions. First, proper acclimatization to hot and/or humid climates is essential. The process of heat acclimatization, which increases your body's cooling efficiency, requires about 10 to 14 days of gradually increased activity in the hot environment. Second, avoid dehydration by replacing the fluids you lose during and after exercise. Third, wear clothing appropriate for your activity and the environment. And finally, use common sense—for example, on an 85°F, 80 percent humidity day, postpone your usual lunchtime run until the cool of evening.

The three different heat stress illnesses are progressive in severity: heat cramps, heat exhaustion, and heat stroke. **Heat cramps** (heat-related muscle cramps), the least serious problem, can usually be prevented by warm-ups, adequate fluid replacement, and a diet that includes the electrolytes lost during sweating (sodium and potassium). (For general information on cramps, see the next section.) **Heat exhaustion** is caused by excessive water loss resulting from prolonged exercise or work. Symptoms of heat exhaustion include nausea, headache, fatigue, dizziness and faintness, and, paradoxically, goosebumps and chills. If you are suffering from heat exhaustion, your skin will be cool and moist. Heat exhaustion is actually a mild form of shock in which the blood pools in the arms and legs away from the brain and major organs of the body. **Heat stroke,** often called sunstroke, is a life-threatening emergency with a 20 to 70 percent death rate.[53] Heat stroke occurs during vigorous exercise when the body's heat production significantly exceeds its cooling capacities. Body core temperature can rise from normal (98.6°F) to

The most successful exercise program is one that is realistic and appropriate for your skill level and needs. Be realistic about the amount of time you will need to get into good physical condition and experiment to find an activity that you truly enjoy. Be open to exploring new activities and new exercise equipment.

■ *Start slow.* For the sedentary, first-time exerciser, any type and amount of physical activity will be a step in the right direction. If you are extremely overweight or out of condition, you might only be able to walk for 5 minutes at a time. Don't be discouraged; you're on your way!

■ *Make only one life change at a time.* Success with one major behavioral change will encourage you to make other positive changes.

■ *Set reasonable expectations for yourself and your fitness program.*

Many people become exercise dropouts because their expectations were too high to begin with. Allow sufficient time to reach your fitness goals.

■ *Choose a specific time to exercise and stick with it.* Learning to establish priorities and keeping to a schedule are vital steps toward improved fitness. Experiment by exercising at different times of the day to learn what schedule works best for you.

■ *Exercise with a friend.* It's easier to keep your exercise commitment if you exercise with someone else. Partners can motivate and encourage each other.

■ *Make exercise a positive habit.* Usually, if you are able to practice a desired activity for three weeks, you will be able to incorporate it into your lifestyle.

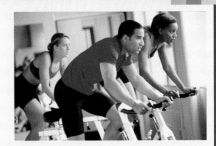

■ *Keep a record of your progress.* Detail your physical activities (duration, intensity), emotions, and personal achievements as you progress.

■ *Reward yourself!* Think about an incentive to use to help you stick to your exercise program.

■ *Take lapses in stride.* Physical deconditioning—a decline in fitness level—occurs at about the same rate as physical conditioning. Renew your commitment to fitness, and then restart your exercise program.

105°F to 110°F within minutes after the body's cooling mechanism shuts down. Rapidly increasing core temperatures can cause brain damage, permanent disability, and death. Common signs of heat stroke are dry, hot, and usually red skin; very high body temperature; and rapid heart rate.

If you experience any of the symptoms mentioned here, stop exercising immediately, move to the shade or a cool spot to rest, and drink large amounts of cool fluids. Be aware that heat stress can also result from prolonged immersion in a sauna or hot tub or by exercising in a plastic or rubber head-to-toe "sauna suit."[54]

Exercising in the Cold

When you exercise in cool weather, **hypothermia**—a potentially fatal condition resulting from abnormally low body core temperature, which occurs when body heat is lost faster than it is produced—may result. Temperatures need not be frigid for hypothermia to occur; it can also result from prolonged, vigorous exercise in 40°F to 50°F temperatures, particularly if there is rain, snow, or a strong wind.

In mild cases of hypothermia, as body core temperature drops from the normal 98.6°F to about 93.2°F,

you will begin to shiver. Shivering increases body temperature by using the heat given off by muscle activity. You may also experience cold hands and feet, poor judgment, apathy, and amnesia.[55] Shivering ceases as body core temperatures drop to between 87°F and 90°F, a sign that the body has lost its ability to generate heat. Death usually occurs at body core temperatures between 75°F and 80°F. To prevent hypothermia, pay attention to weather conditions, dress in layers, avoid dehydration, and exercise with a friend.[56]

Preventing Cramps

Although most of us have experienced the quick, intense pain of muscle cramps, they are poorly understood. According to one theory, when a muscle gets tired, the numerous muscle fibers that comprise the muscle fail to contract in a synchronized rhythm, probably due to overstimulation from the nerves that trigger the muscles to contract.[57]

> **Hypothermia** Potentially fatal condition caused by abnormally low body core temperature.

Although calcium plays a role in muscle contraction and people with a tendency to have cramps are often calcium deficient, exercise physiologists question the validity of the low calcium theory. However, because calcium has many health benefits, experts continue to recommend it for anyone who has a tendency toward cramping.

Lack of sodium is another possible factor. If you exercise a lot and sweat a lot, you will lose sodium through sweat, may develop a sodium imbalance, and experience cramps. This is most likely to occur in endurance sports, particularly if athletes have consumed only plain water (not sodium-containing food or beverages) while exercising.[58]

Drinking enough fluids before, during, and after such activity is important. On a daily basis, drink enough fluid so you have to urinate every two to four hours. Your urine should be pale, and there should be lots of it. In addition, make sure your muscles are warmed up before exercising, and don't strain muscles beyond their limit.

If you get cramps, what should you do? Generally massage, stretching, putting pressure on the painful muscle, and deep breathing are useful remedies.

Taking Charge

Summary

- The physiological benefits of regular physical activity include 1) reduced risk of heart attack, some cancers, hypertension, and diabetes and 2) improved blood profile, skeletal mass, weight control, immunity to disease, mental health and stress management, and physical fitness. Regular physical activity can also increase life span.

- It is recommended that every adult participate in moderate-intensity activities for 30 minutes at least 5 days a week. For improvements in cardiorespiratory fitness, you should work out aerobically for at least 20 minutes, a minimum of 3 days per week. Exercise intensity involves working out at target heart rate. Exercise duration should increase to 30 to 45 minutes; the longer the exercise period, the more calories burned, and the greater the improvement in cardiovascular fitness.

- Key principles for developing muscular strength and endurance are the tension principle, the overload principle, and the specificity-of-training principle. The different types of muscle actions include isometric, concentric, and eccentric. Resistance training programs include body weight resistance (calisthenics), fixed resistance, variable resistance, and accommodating resistance devices.

- Flexibility exercises should involve static stretching exercises performed in sets of four or more repetitions held for 10 to 30 seconds on at least 2 to 3 days a week.

- Planning a fitness program involves setting goals and designing a program to achieve these goals. A comprehensive program would include a warm-up period, stretching activities, strength development exercises, an aerobic activity, and a cool-down period.

- Fitness injuries generally are caused by overuse or trauma; the most common ones are plantar fasciitis, shin splints, and runner's knee. Proper footwear and equipment can help prevent injuries. Exercise in the heat or cold requires special precautions.

Chapter Review

1. The maximum volume of oxygen consumed by the muscles during exercise defines
   a. target heart rate.
   b. muscular strength.
   c. aerobic capacity.
   d. muscular endurance.

2. The main components of an aerobic exercise program include all of the following *except*
   a. intensity.
   b. frequency.
   c. metabolism.
   d. duration.

3. What effect does regular exercise have on lipoproteins?
   a. It reduces the levels of LDLs and HDLs.
   b. It increases the levels of LDLs and HDLs.
   c. It reduces the levels of LDLs and increases the levels of HDLs.
   d. It increases the levels of LDLs and reduces the levels of HDLs.

4. A test of aerobic capacity administered by a physician, exercise physiologist, or other trained person is called a(n)
   a. graded exercise test.
   b. maximum aerobic capacity test.
   c. aerobic endurance test.
   d. cardiac output test.

5. The "talk test" measures
   a. exercise intensity.
   b. exercise duration.
   c. exercise frequency.
   d. metabolism.

6. An effective resistance exercise program involves all of the following three key principles, *except* the
   a. tension principle.
   b. overload principle.
   c. specificity of training principle.
   d. flexibility principle.

7. Yoga, tai chi, and Pilates are three major styles of exercise that focus on
   a. flexibility.
   b. stretching.
   c. endurance.
   d. muscular strength.

8. Theresa wants to lower her ratio of fat weight to her total body weight. She wants to work on her
   a. flexibility.
   b. muscular endurance.
   c. muscular strength.
   d. body composition.

9. Janice has been lifting 95 pounds while doing three sets of 10 leg curls. To become stronger, she began lifting 105 pounds while doing leg curls. What principle of strength development does this represent?
   a. tension principle
   b. overload principle
   c. flexibility principle
   d. specificity-of-training principle

10. Joel enjoys various types of fitness exercises. He alternates his training days with jogging, cycling, and step aerobics. This type of training is called
    a. cardiac fitness training.
    b. static training.
    c. cross training.
    d. multisport training.

Answers to these questions can be found on page A-1.

Questions for Discussion and Reflection

1. How do you define physical fitness? What are the key components of a physical fitness program? What might you need to consider when beginning a fitness program?

2. How would you determine the proper intensity and duration of an exercise program? How often should exercise sessions be scheduled?

3. Why is stretching vital to improving physical flexibility? Why is flexibility important in everyday activities?

4. Identify at least four physiological and psychological benefits of physical fitness. What is the significance of the latest fitness report from the Office of the Surgeon General? How might it help more people realize the benefits of physical fitness?

5. Describe the different types of resistance employed in an exercise program. What are the benefits of each type of resistance?

6. Your roommate has decided to start running first thing in the morning in an effort to lose weight, tone muscles, and improve cardiorespiratory fitness. What advice would you give to make sure your roommate has a good plan and doesn't get injured?

7. What key components would you include in a fitness program for yourself?

Accessing Your Health on the Internet

The following websites explore further topics and issues related to personal health. For links to the websites, below visit the Companion Website for *Health: The Basics,* Seventh Edition at www.aw-bc.com/donatelle.

1. *ACSM Online.* A link with the American College of Sports Medicine and all their resources.

2. *American Council on Exercise.* Information on exercise and disease prevention.

3. *The American Medical Association's Health Insight.* Provides a fitness assessment and guidelines to help you develop your own fitness program.

4. *Just Move.* The American Heart Association's fitness website has the latest information on heart disease and exercise, plus a guide to local, regional, and national fitness events.

5. *National Strength and Conditioning Association.* A resource for personal trainers and others interested in conditioning and fitness.

Further Reading

Fahey, T. D. *Super Fitness for Sports, Conditioning, and Health.* Boston: Allyn & Bacon, 2000.

A brief guide to developing fitness that emphasizes training techniques for improving sports performance.

Powers, S., S. Dodd, and V. Noland *Total Fitness and Wellness,* 4th ed. San Francisco: Benjamin Cummings, 2006.

A complete guide to improving all areas of fitness, including being a smart health consumer, interviews with fitness specialists, and the links between nutrition and fitness.

Schlosberg, S. *The Ultimate Workout Log: An Exercise Diary and Fitness Guide.* Boston: Houghton Mifflin, 1999.

A six-month log that also provides fitness definitions, training tips, and motivational quotes.

References

1. L. Ballu et al., "Surveillance for Certain Behaviors among Selected Local Areas—United States Behavioral Risk Factor Surveillance System," *Morbidity and Mortality Weekly Report* 53, (SS05): 1–100.
2. Centers for Disease Control, "Physical Activity and Health." www.cdc.gov/nccdphp/dnpa/physical/index.htm.
3. National Institutes of Mental Health, "Statistics," 2004, www.nimh.nih.gov/healthinformation/statisticsmenu.cfm; National

Institute of Diabetes and Digestive and Kidney Diseases, "National Diabetes Statistics Fact Sheet: General Information and National Estimates on Diabetes in the United States, 2003," (Bethesda, MD: U.S. Department of Health and Human Services, National Institutes of Health. Rev. ed. Bethesda, MD: U.S. Department of Health and Human Services, National Institutes of Health, 2004); American Heart Association (AHA), *Heart Disease and Stroke Statistics—2005 Update* (Dallas TX: AHA, 2005).

4. C. A. Macera et al., "Prevalence of Physical Activity, Including Lifestyle Activities among Adults—U.S. 2000–2001," *Morbidity and Mortality Weekly Report* 52, no. 32 (2003): 764–769.

5. Centers for Disease Control, "Physical Activity and Health," www.cdc.gov/nccdphp/dnpa/physical/index.htm.

6. Ibid.

7. National Center for Chronic Disease Prevention and Health Promotion, "Nutrition and Physical Activity Recommendations," 2004, www.cdc.gov/nccdphp/dnpa/physical/recommendations/index.htm.

8. Ibid.

9. American College of Sports Medicine, *American College of Sports Medicine Fitness Book,* 3rd ed. (Champaign, IL: Human Kinetics, 2003).

10. A. Colin et al., "Cardiorespiratory Fitness, Physical Activity, and Arterial Stiffness: The Northern Ireland Young Hearts Project," *Hypertension,* 44 (2004): 721–726.

11. American Heart Association, "The Number of Adults in the U.S. with High Blood Pressure Rose in the Last Decade," www .americanheart.org/presenter.jhtml?identifier=3024254.

12. American Heart Association, "Study Shows that Middle Age High Blood Pressure Shortens Life," www.americanheart.org/presenter .jhtml?identifier=3031751.

13. L. S. Pescatello et al., "American College of Sports Medicine Position Stand: Exercise and Hypertension," *Medicine and Science in Sports and Exercise* 36, no. 3 (2004): 533–553.

14. G. A. Colditz et al., "Physical Activity and Risk of Breast Cancer in Premenopausal Women," *British Journal of Cancer* 89, no. 5: 847–851; A. K. Samad et al., "A Meta-Analysis of the Association of Physical Activity with Risk of Colorectal Cancer," *Colorectal Disease* 7, no. 3: 204–213.

15. T. J. Key et al., "Diet, Nutrition, and the Prevention of Cancer," *Public Health Nutrition,* 7(1A) (2005): 187–200.

16. National Osteoporosis Foundation, "Fast Facts," 2004, www.nof.org.

17. National Institutes of Health Osteoporosis and Related Bone Diseases, National Resource Center, "Fast Facts on Osteoporosis," 2004, www.osteo.org/newfile.asp?doc=fast&doctitle=Fast+Facts+ on+Osteoporosis&doctype=HTML+Fact+Sheet.

18. K. J. Stewart et al., "Exercise Effects on Bone Mineral Density: Relationships to Changes in Fitness and Fatness," *American Journal of Preventive Medicine* 28, no. 5 (2005): 453–60.

19. C. Snow and T. Hayes, "Bone Health" (guest lecture in Modern Maladies class, Oregon State University, Corvallis, OR, 2001).

20. B. R. Beck and C. M. Snow, "Bone Health across the Lifespan—Exercising Our Options," *Exercise and Sport Sciences Reviews* 31, no. 3 (2003): 117–122.

21. American College of Sports Medicine, "Exercise Recommendations," *Guidelines for Physical Activity,* www.acsm.org/pdf/Guidelines.pdf.

22. D. Reibe et al., "Long Term Maintenance of Exercise and Healthy Eating Behaviors in Overweight Adults," *Preventive Medicine* 40, no. 6: 769–778.

23. American Diabetes Association, "Diabetes Risk Test," 2004, www.diabetes.org/risk-test.jsp.

24. D. E. Laaksonen et al., "Physical Activity in the Prevention of Type 2 Diabetes: The Finnish Diabetes Prevention Study," *Diabetes,* 54: 158–165.

25. J. Shaw, "The Deadliest Sin," *Harvard Magazine,* March/April 2004.

26. Centers for Disease Control, "Physical Activity and Health."

27. P. Palatini et al., "Exercise Capacity and Mortality," *New England Journal of Medicine* 374, no. 4 (2002): 288.

28. E. Quinn, "Exercise and Immunity," *Sports Medicine,* 2004, http:// sportsmedicine.about.com/cs/exercisephysiology/a/aa100303a.htm.

29. E. Tollier et al., "Intense Training: Mucosal Immunity and Incidence of Respiratory Infections," *European Journal of Applied Physiology* 93, no. 4: 421–428.

30. J. A. Woods, "Physical Activity, Exercise, and Immune Function," *Brain, Behavior, and Immunity* 19, no. 5: 369–370.

31. A. L. Marshall, "Challenges and Opportunities for Promoting Physical Activity in the Workplace," *Journal of Science and Medicine in Sport* 7, no.1 (2004): Suppl. 60–66.

32. L. M. Hays, T. M. Damush, and D.O. Clark, "Relationships between Exercise Self-Definitions and Exercise Participation among Urban Women in Primary Care," *Journal of Cardiovascular Nursing* 20, no. 1 (2005): 9–17.

33. E. T. Howley and D. B. Frinaks, *Health Fitness Instructor's Handbook,* 3rd ed. (Champaign, IL: Human Kinetics, 2003).

34. G. A. Klug and J. Lettunich, *Wellness: Exercise and Physical Fitness* (Guilford, CT: Dushkin Publishing Group, 1992).

35. J. Gavin, *Life Fitness Coaching* (Champaign IL: Human Kinetics, 2005).

36. J. Orvis, *Weight Training Workouts that Work,* 2nd ed. (Crosslake MN: Ideal Publishing, 2004).

37. S. J. Fleck and W. I. Kraemer, *Designing Resistance Training Programs,* 3rd ed. (Champaign, IL: Human Kinetics, 2004).

38. Arthritis Foundation, "Exercise and Arthritis," 2004, www.arthritis .org/conditions/exercise.

39. E. T. Howley and D. B. Frinaks, *Health Fitness Instructor's Handbook,* 3rd ed. (Champaign, IL: Human Kinetics, 2003).

40. Ibid.

41. S. B. Heymsfield et al., *Human Body Composition,* 2nd ed. (Champaign, IL: Human Kinetics, 2005).

42. M. L. Pollock and W. J. Evans, "Resistance Training for Health and Disease: Introduction," *Medicine and Science in Sports and Exercise* 31 (1999): 10–11.

43. W. C. Whiting and R. F. Zernicke, *Biomechanics of Musculoskeletal Injury* (Champaign, IL: Human Kinetics, 1998).

44. American Academy of Podiatric Sports Medicine, "Selecting an Athletic Shoe," 2005, www.aapsm.org/fit_shoes.htm.

45. J. C. Erie, "Eye Injuries: Prevention, Evaluation, and Treatment," *The Physician and Sports Medicine* 19 (11): 108–122.

46. Bicycle Helmet Safety Institute, "A Compendium of Statistics," 2004, www.bhsi.org/stats.htm.

47. Ibid.

48. D. Ritchie, "Plantar Fasciitis: Treatment Pearls," American Academy of Podiatric Sports Medicine, www.aapsm.org/plantar_fasciitis.html.

49. American College of Sports Medicine, *American College of Sports Medicine Fitness Book.*

50. Ibid.

51. American College of Sports Medicine, "Female Athlete Issues for the Team Physician: A Consensus Statement," *Medicine & Science in Sports & Exercise* 35, no.10 (2003):1785–1793.

52. American Academy of Orthopaedic Surgeons, "Runner's knee," 2003, http://orthoinfo.aaos.org/fact/thr_report.cfm?Thread_ID =417&topcategory=Knee.

53. N.M. Lugo-Amador , T. Rothenhaus, and P. Mover, "Heat-Related Illness," *Emergency Medical Clinics of North America* 22, no. 2 (2004): 315–327.

54. International Fitness Association, *Aerobics and Fitness Institute Certification Coursebook* (Orlando, FL: International Fitness Association, 2004), http://ifafitness.com/book1.

55. Mayo Clinic Medical Services, "Hypothermia," www.mayoclinic.com.

56. M. Nimmo, "Exercising in the Cold," *Journal of Sports Sciences* 22, no. 10 (2004): 898–915.

57. American Academy of Orthopaedic Surgeons, "Muscles Cramps," 2001, http://orthoinfo.aaos.org/fact/thr_report.cfm?Thread_ID =270&topcategory=Sports.

58. Medicine Consumer Health, "Heat Cramps," 2005, www.emedic-inehealth.com/articles/6186-2.asp; N. Clark, "Muscle Cramps: Do They Cramp Your Style?" Newsletter of the American College of Sports Medicine, (Summer 2001): 7.

What's the difference between good and bad cholesterol?

Does cardiovascular disease run in families?

What's the best way to eat for a healthy heart?

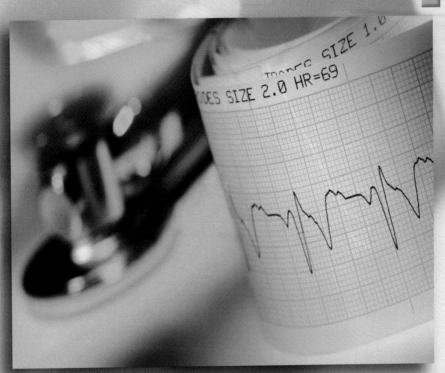

Does red wine really prevent heart disease?

12 Cardiovascular Disease
Reducing Your Risk

Objectives

- **Discuss** the incidence, prevalence, and outcomes of cardiovascular disease in the United States, including its impact on society.
- **Describe** the anatomy and physiology of the heart and circulatory system and the importance of healthy heart function.
- **Review** major types of cardiovascular disease, factors that contribute to their development, and diagnostic and treatment options.

- **Discuss** controllable risk factors for cardiovascular disease, including smoking, cholesterol, diet and obesity, exercise, hypertension, diabetes mellitus, and stress. Examine your own risk profile, and determine which risk factors you can and cannot control.
- **Discuss** the issues surrounding cardiovascular disease risk and disease burden in women.

Despite the many medical advances we enjoy, diseases of the heart and cardiovascular system continue to be a significant health threat in the United States (Figure 12.1). In fact, cardiovascular disease (CVD) remains the leading single cause of death in the global population.[1]

AN EPIDEMIOLOGICAL OVERVIEW

In 2002, **cardiovascular disease (CVD),** the broad term used to describe diseases of the heart and blood vessels, accounted for approximately 38 percent of all deaths in the United States. CVD continues to claim more lives each year than the next five leading causes of death combined (cancer, chronic lower respiratory diseases, accidents, diabetes, and influenza/pneumonia).[2] CVD has been the number one killer in the United States for all ages since 1900 in every year but one—1918, when another killer, a particularly virulent strain of influenza (flu), struck with blinding force. For the population as a whole, CVD remains the greatest killer; but in 2005 researchers reported that among Americans under 85 years of age, cancer surpassed CVD as the leading cause of death (see Chapter 13). To realize the prevalence of CVD, consider these facts:[3]

- More than 2,600 Americans die of CVD each day; that's more than 1.4 million CVD-related deaths each year.

- Many of these fatalities are **sudden cardiac deaths,** meaning that these Americans die from sudden, abrupt loss of heart function (cardiac arrest), either instantly or shortly after symptoms occur.

- If all forms of major CVD were eliminated, life expectancy would rise by almost seven years. If all forms of cancer were eliminated, the gain would be three years.

- The probability at birth of eventually dying of CVD is 47 percent; of dying from cancer, 22 percent; from accidents, 3 percent; from diabetes, 2 percent; and from HIV, 0.7 percent.

- In terms of total deaths, in every year since 1984, CVD has claimed the lives of more women than men.

Today, nearly 70 million Americans live with one of the major categories of CVD. Many people with CVD do not know they have a serious problem.[4] Nearly 13 million of them have a history of heart attack,

---

Cardiovascular disease (CVD) Term encompassing a variety of diseases of the heart and blood vessels.

Sudden cardiac death Death that occurs as a result of sudden, abrupt loss of heart function.

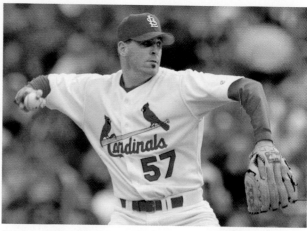

Cardiovascular disease can affect even the youngest and most fit people. Daryl Kile, a 33-year-old professional baseball player, died suddenly from atherosclerosis. It was discovered after his death that two of the main arteries in his heart were 80 to 90 percent blocked. His heart was also enlarged, weighing 20 percent more than normal.

angina pectoris (chest pain), or both.[5] In spite of major improvements in medication, surgery, and other health care procedures, the prognosis for many of these individuals is not good. In fact, within six years of a recognized heart attack, 18 percent of men and 35 percent of women will have another heart attack, 7 percent of men and 6 percent of women will experience sudden death, and about 22 percent of men and 46 percent of women will be disabled with heart failure.[6]

Although it is impossible to place a monetary value on human life, the economic burden of cardiovascular disease on our society is staggering—estimated at more than $393 billion in 2005.[7] This figure includes the cost of physician and nursing services, hospital and nursing home services, medications, and lost productivity resulting from disability. As Americans live longer with chronic diseases, costs will continue to increase, resulting in a tremendous burden on the health care system. The many Americans who think that CVD can be cured with a bypass or other surgical procedure, after which life simply returns to normal, are wrong. The effects of CVD can be far reaching and take a toll on quality of life. Even the best treatments exact a heavy toll on families, individuals, and society.

The best line of defense against CVD is to prevent it from developing in the first place. How can you cut your risk? Take steps now to change certain behaviors. Controlling high blood pressure and reducing intake of saturated fats and cholesterol are two examples of things you can do to lower your chances of heart attack. By maintaining your weight, exercising, decreasing your intake of sodium, not smoking, and changing your lifestyle to reduce stress, you can lower your blood pressure. You can also monitor the levels of fat and cholesterol in your blood and adjust your diet to prevent

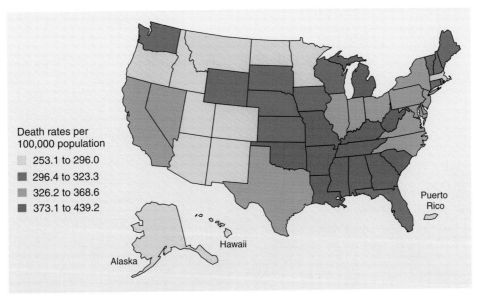

Figure 12.1 ■ Total Cardiovascular Disease, Age-Adjusted Death Rates by State, 2001

Source: American Heart Association, *Heart Disease and Stroke Statistics—2005 Update* (Dallas, TX: American Heart Association, 2005). © 2005 American Heart Association. Reproduced by permission. www.americanheart.org

Death rates per 100,000 population
- 253.1 to 296.0
- 296.4 to 323.3
- 326.2 to 368.6
- 373.1 to 439.2

arteries from becoming blocked. Having combinations of risk factors seems to increase overall risk by a factor greater than those of the combined risks. Happily, the converse is also true: reducing several risk factors can have a dramatic effect. Answer the questions in the Assess Yourself box on page 332 to determine your overall coronary risk. Understanding how your cardiovascular system works will help you understand your risk and how to reduce it.

What Do You Think? Consider what happens when people who suffer a heart attack survive. What unique challenges do they face? ■ What might it be like to live in fear that your heart might give out or a problem could crop up at any time? ■ What support services are available for coping with the unique anxieties faced by CVD survivors and their families?

UNDERSTANDING THE CARDIOVASCULAR SYSTEM

The **cardiovascular system** is the network of elastic tubes through which blood flows as it carries oxygen and nutrients to all parts of the body. It includes the *heart, arteries, arterioles* (small arteries), and *capillaries* (minute blood vessels). It also includes *venules* (small veins) and *veins,* the blood vessels though which blood

flows as it returns to the heart and lungs, carrying carbon dioxide and other waste products.

The Heart: A Mighty Machine

The heart is a muscular, four-chambered pump, roughly the size of your fist. It is a highly efficient, extremely flexible organ that manages to contract 100,000 times each day and pumps the equivalent of 2,000 gallons of blood to all areas of the body. In a 70-year lifetime, an average human heart beats 2.5 billion times. This number is significantly higher for hearts that must work to keep people moving who are out of shape and overweight.

Under normal circumstances, the human body contains approximately 6 quarts of blood. This blood transports nutrients, oxygen, waste products, hormones, and enzymes throughout the body. Blood also aids in regulating body temperature, cellular water levels, and acidity levels of body components, and in bodily defense against toxins and harmful microorganisms. An adequate blood supply is essential to health and well-being.

The heart has four chambers that work together to recirculate blood constantly throughout the body

> **Cardiovascular system**   A complex system consisting of the heart and blood vessels. It transports nutrients, oxygen, hormones, and enzymes throughout the body and regulates temperature, the water levels of cells, and the acidity levels of body components.

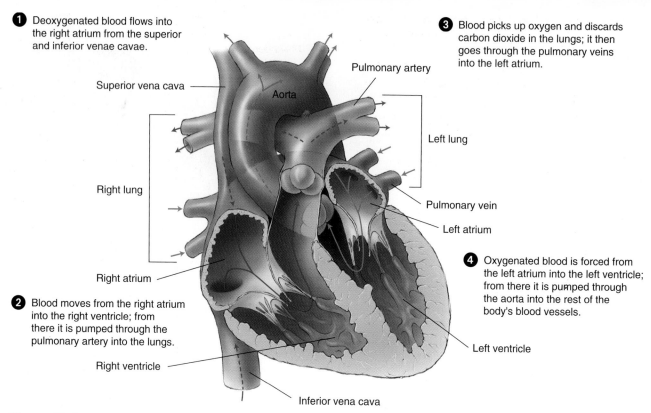

① Deoxygenated blood flows into the right atrium from the superior and inferior venae cavae.

③ Blood picks up oxygen and discards carbon dioxide in the lungs; it then goes through the pulmonary veins into the left atrium.

Superior vena cava

Pulmonary artery

Aorta

Left lung

Right lung

Pulmonary vein

Left atrium

Right atrium

④ Oxygenated blood is forced from the left atrium into the left ventricle; from there it is pumped through the aorta into the rest of the body's blood vessels.

② Blood moves from the right atrium into the right ventricle; from there it is pumped through the pulmonary artery into the lungs.

Left ventricle

Right ventricle

Inferior vena cava

Figure 12.2 ■ Anatomy of the Heart

(Figure 12.2). The two upper chambers of the heart, called **atria,** are large collecting chambers that receive blood from the rest of the body. The two lower chambers, known as **ventricles,** pump the blood out again. Small valves regulate the steady, rhythmic flow of blood between chambers and prevent inappropriate backwash. The *tricuspid valve* (located between the right atrium and the right ventricle), the *pulmonary valve* (between the right ventricle and the pulmonary artery), the *mitral (bicuspid) valve* (between the left atrium and left ventricle), and the *aortic valve* (between the left ventricle and the aorta) permit blood to flow in only one direction.

Atria The two upper chambers of the heart that receive blood.

Ventricles The two lower chambers of the heart that pump blood through the blood vessels.

Arteries Vessels that carry blood away from the heart to other regions of the body.

Arterioles Branches of the arteries.

Capillaries Minute blood vessels that connect the arterioles and venules; their thin walls permit exchange of oxygen, carbon dioxide, nutrients, and waste products with body cells.

Heart Function Heart activity depends on a complex interaction of biochemical, physical, and neurological signals. Here are the basic steps involved in heart function.

1. Deoxygenated blood enters the right atrium after having been circulated through the body.

2. From the right atrium, blood moves to the right ventricle and is pumped through the pulmonary artery to the lungs, where it receives oxygen.

3. Oxygenated blood from the lungs then returns to the left atrium of the heart.

4. Blood from the left atrium moves into the left ventricle.

5. The left ventricle pumps blood through the aorta to all body parts.

Different types of blood vessels are required for different parts of this process. **Arteries** carry blood away from the heart; all arteries carry oxygenated blood *except* for pulmonary arteries, which carry deoxygenated blood to the lungs, where the blood picks up oxygen and gives off carbon dioxide. As they branch off from the heart, the arteries divide into smaller blood vessels called **arterioles,** and then into even smaller blood vessels called **capillaries.** Capillaries have thin walls that permit the exchange of oxygen, carbon dioxide, nutrients, and waste products with body cells.

Carbon dioxide and other waste products are transported to the lungs and kidneys through **veins** and **venules** (small veins).

For the heart to function properly, the four chambers must beat in an organized manner. Your heartbeat is governed by an electrical impulse that directs the heart muscle to move when the impulse moves across it, which results in a sequential contraction of the four chambers. This signal starts in a small bundle of highly specialized cells, the **sinoatrial node (SA node)**, located in the right atrium. The SA node serves as a natural pacemaker for the heart. People with a damaged SA node must often have a mechanical pacemaker implanted to ensure the smooth passage of blood through the sequential phases of the heartbeat.

The average adult heart at rest beats 70 to 80 times per minute, although a well-conditioned heart may beat only 50 to 60 times per minute to achieve the same results. When overly stressed, a heart may beat more than 200 times per minute, particularly in an individual who is overweight or out of shape. A healthy heart functions more efficiently and is less likely to suffer damage from overwork.

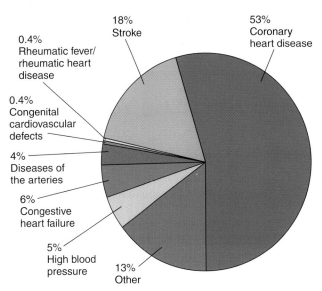

Figure 12.3 ■ Percentage Breakdown of Deaths from Cardiovascular Disease in the United States, 2002

Source: American Heart Association, *Heart Disease and Stroke Statistics— 2005 Update* (Dallas, TX: American Heart Association, 2005). © 2005 American Heart Association. Reproduced by permission. www.americanheart.org

TYPES OF CARDIOVASCULAR DISEASE

There are several different types of cardiovascular disease (Figure 12.3):

- Atherosclerosis (fatty plaque buildup in the arteries)
- Coronary heart disease (CHD)
- Chest pain (angina pectoris)
- Irregular heartbeat (arrhythmia)
- Congestive heart failure (CHF)
- Congenital and rheumatic heart disease
- Stroke (cerebrovascular accident)

Prevention and treatment of these diseases range from changes in diet and lifestyle to medications and surgery.

Atherosclerosis

Arteriosclerosis, thickening and hardening of arteries, is a condition that underlies many cardiovascular health problems and is believed to be the biggest contributor to disease burden globally.[8] **Atherosclerosis** is actually a type of arteriosclerosis and is characterized by deposits of fatty substances, cholesterol, cellular waste products, calcium, and fibrin (a clotting material in the blood) in the inner lining of an artery. Eventually, the artery becomes clogged or narrows, restricting blood flow. Often, atherosclerosis is called *coronary artery disease (CAD)* because of the resultant damage done to coronary arteries. **Hyperlipidemia** (an abnormally high blood

lipid level) is a key factor in this process, and the resulting buildup is referred to as **plaque**.[9] Plaque buildup begins early in life; even in early childhood, blood vessel walls begin to show evidence of fatty deposits.

Genetics, high blood pressure surges, elevated cholesterol and triglyceride levels in the blood (i.e., hyperlipidemia), and cigarette smoking are the main suspects in causing this injury to artery walls.[10] As a result of national campaigns aimed at reducing dietary fats, millions of people cut down on animal fat and dairy products. However, despite massive lifestyle changes and

Veins   Vessels that carry blood back to the heart from other regions of the body.

Venules   Small veins that empty the capillaries into the larger veins.

Sinoatrial node (SA node)   Cluster of electrical-generating cells that act as a natural pacemaker for the heart.

Arteriosclerosis   A general term for thickening and hardening of the arteries.

Atherosclerosis   Condition characterized by deposits of fatty substances, cholesterol, cellular waste products, calcium, and fibrin in the inner lining of an artery.

Hyperlipidemia   Elevated levels of lipids in the blood.

Plaque   Buildup of deposits of cholesterol, lipids, and cellular debris in the arteries.

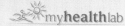

Fill out this assessment online at
www.aw-bc.com/myhealthlab or www.aw-bc.com/donatelle.

Understanding Your CVD Risk

Each of us has a unique level of risk for various diseases. Some of these risks are things you can take action to change; others are risks that you need to consider as you plan a lifelong strategy for overall risk reduction. Complete each of the following questions and total your points in each section. If you score between 1 and 5 in any section, consider your risk. The higher the number, the greater your risk. If you answered "don't know" for any question, talk to your parents or other family members as soon as possible to find out if you have any unknown risks.

Part I: Assess Your Family Risk for CVD

1. Do any of your primary relatives (mother, father, grandparents, siblings) have a history of heart disease or stroke? ❑ Yes (1 point) ❑ No (0 points) ❑ Don't Know

2. Do any of your primary relatives (mother, father, grandparents, siblings) have diabetes? ❑ Yes (1 point) ❑ No (0 points) ❑ Don't Know

3. Do any of your primary relatives (mother, father, grandparents, siblings) have high blood pressure? ❑ Yes (1 point) ❑ No (0 points) ❑ Don't Know

4. Do any of your primary relatives (mother, father, grandparents, siblings) have a history of high cholesterol? ❑ Yes (1 point) ❑ No (0 points) ❑ Don't Know

5. Would you say that your family consumed a high fat diet (lots of red meat, dairy, butter/margarine) during your time spent at home? ❑ Yes (1 point) ❑ No (0 points) ❑ Don't Know

Total Points _____

Part II: Assess Your Lifestyle Risk for CVD

1. Is your total cholesterol level higher than it should be? ❑ Yes (1 point) ❑ No (0 points) ❑ Don't Know
2. Do you have high blood pressure? ❑ Yes (1 point) ❑ No (0 points) ❑ Don't Know
3. Have you been diagnosed as prediabetic or diabetic? ❑ Yes (1 point) ❑ No (0 points) ❑ Don't Know
4. Do you smoke? ❑ Yes (1 point) ❑ No (0 points) ❑ Don't Know
5. Would you describe your life as being highly stressful? ❑ Yes (1 point) ❑ No (0 points) ❑ Don't Know

Total Points _____

Part III: Assess Your Additional Risks for CVD

1. How would you best describe your current weight?
   a. Lower than what it should be for my height and weight (0 points)
   b. About what it should be for my height and weight (0 points)
   c. Higher than it should be for my height and weight (1 point)
2. How would you describe the level of exercise that you get each day?
   a. Less than what I should be exercising each day (1 point)
   b. About what I should be exercising each day (0 points)
   c. More than what I should be exercising each day (0 points)
3. How would you describe your dietary behaviors?
   a. Eating only the recommended number of calories/day (0 points)
   b. Eating *less* than the recommended number of calories each day (0 points)
   c. Eating *more* than the recommended number of calories each day (1 point)

4. Which of the following best describes your typical dietary behavior?
   a. I eat from the major food groups, trying hard to get the recommended fruits and vegetables (0 points)
   b. I eat too much red meat and consume much saturated fat from meats and dairy products each day (1 point)
   c. Whenever possible, I try to substitute olive oil or canola oil for other forms of dietary fat. (0 points)
5. Which of the following best describes you?
   a. I watch my sodium intake and try to reduce stress in my life (0 points)
   b. I have a history of *Chlamydia* infection (1 point)
   c. I try to eat 5 to 10 milligrams of soluble fiber each day and to substitute a soy product for an animal product in my diet at least once each week. (0 points)

Total Points _____

Make It Happen!

Assessment: The Assess Yourself activity evaluates your risk of heart disease and the status of your LDL cholesterol. Based on your results and the advice of your physician, you may need to reduce your cholesterol level and risk of CVD.

Making a Change: In order to change your behavior, you need to develop a plan. Follow these steps below and complete your Behavior Change Contract to take action.

1. Evaluate your behavior, and identify patterns and specific things you are doing. What can you change now? What can you change in the near future?
2. Select one pattern of behavior that you want to change.
3. Fill out the Behavior Change Contract found at the front of your book. It should include your long-term goal for change, your short-term goals, the rewards you'll give yourself for reaching these goals, potential obstacles along the way, and strategies for overcoming these obstacles. For each goal, list the small steps and specific actions that you will take.
4. Chart your progress in a journal. At the end of a week, consider how successful you were in following your plan. What helped you be successful? What made change more difficult? What will you do differently next week?
5. Revise your plan as needed. Are the short-term goals attainable? Are the rewards satisfying?

Example: Nathan knew that his father had a history of heart disease, so he knew it was important to monitor his own risk. Using the results from his most recent checkup, he completed the self-assessment. Although his initial score for ten-year risk of heart attack (in step one of the assessment) was less than 10 percent, the combination of two major coronary risk factors (high systolic blood pressure and family history of CVD) with an LDL level of 140 showed in step 2 of the assessment that he needed to start making some lifestyle changes. At 6 feet in height, he weighed 220 pounds, which he discovered is close to obese according to the Body Mass Index calculations. He decided to manage his weight through exercise and improved eating habits. He also expected a modified diet would help lower his cholesterol levels.

Nathan's first step was to keep track of everything he normally ate for a week. When he analyzed his food journal, he saw that he rarely ate breakfast, which made him more likely to grab a doughnut later in the morning and a big lunch. He bought some whole wheat, high-fiber cereal and skim milk and started getting up 15 minutes earlier so he had time to eat his healthy breakfast. For the days when he didn't feel like eating cold cereal, he bought some five-minute oatmeal that also had healthy fiber and nutrients and had been shown to lower LDL levels. Nathan found that he was not as tempted by the doughnuts and other unhealthy snacks during the day, and that he didn't overeat as much at lunch. He even had more energy during the day. As he started to lose weight, he felt more able to begin a moderate exercise program. All of these changes—losing weight, eating more fiber and less fat, and adding some exercise to his life—made Nathan confident that his next checkup with his doctor would show a lower LDL level and, perhaps, lower blood pressure. When Nathan is in a healthier range on these measures, he plans to buy himself a new DVD player.

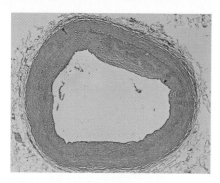

(a)

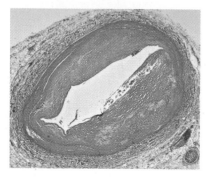

(b)

(a) Cross section of a normal coronary artery. **(b)** A coronary artery narrowed by plaque.

the use of cholesterol-lowering drugs, CVDs continue to be the leading cause of death in the United States, Europe, and most of Asia.[11]

Inflammatory Risks Today, scientists are beginning to look for other factors in the formation of atherosclerotic lesions. Many experts believe that atherosclerosis is an *inflammatory* disease and that inflamed vessels are more prone to plaque formation. What causes this inflammation in artery walls? While researchers aren't sure, there is evidence that a pathogen may be at the root of it. The most likely culprits are *Chlamydia pneumoniae* (a sexually transmitted infection), *Helicobacter pylori* (which causes ulcers), *herpes simplex virus* (a virus the majority of Americans have been exposed to by the age of 5), and *cytomegalovirus* (another herpes virus transmitted through body fluids and infecting most Americans before the age of 40). Clearly, if findings about these viruses holds up, there will be yet another good reason to avoid unprotected sex.

During an inflammatory reaction, *C-reactive proteins (CRPs)* tend to be present at high levels. If levels are high, action could be taken to prevent progression to heart attack or other coronary event. Today, many scientists believe that these elevated CRP levels are markers for CVD risk, even though a causative link between the two has yet to be established. In the near future, the high sensitive assay test (hs-CRP), which looks for CRPs, might be given as routinely as cholesterol screening tests for heart disease.[12] Other possible causes of inflammation and high levels of CRP include elevated low-density lipoproteins, free radicals caused by cigarette smoking, high blood pressure, diabetes mellitus, and the amino acid homocysteine (see the New Horizons in Health box).

The good news is that the same lifestyle changes that help to lower cholesterol can also reduce CRP levels. Regular exercise, weight reduction and control, smoking cessation, and moderation of alcohol intake are steps individuals can take to reduce CRP and cholesterol levels. We will talk more about risk factors you can control later in this chapter.

Metabolic Syndrome

Metabolic syndrome is a group of obesity-related health risk factors that dramatically increase the risk of heart disease and diabetes. Also known as syndrome X or MetS, metabolic syndrome is believed to increase the risk for atherosclerotic cardiovascular disease by as much as threefold.[13] Affecting over 26 percent of adults or 50 million people, this disease has gained increasing attention in the last two to three years worldwide.[14]

How does one develop MetS? Weight gain, particularly in the abdominal area, and insulin resistance are two of the main characteristics of metabolic syndrome. Insulin resistance is not clearly understood, but it means cells don't work properly in handling blood glucose levels. High blood pressure is also a common characteristic of metabolic syndrome. The combination of excess weight, high blood sugar, and high blood pressure can be life-threatening. Today, scientists indicate that when there are three or more of the following, the diagnosis is metabolic syndrome:

- Abdominal obesity (waist measurement of more than 40 inches in men or 35 in women)
- Elevated blood fat (triglycerides greater than 150)
- Low levels of "good" cholesterol (high density lipoprotein, or HDL); less than 40 in men and less than 50 in women
- Elevated blood pressure (greater than 130/85)
- Elevated fasting glucose (greater than 100 mg/dL, a sign of insulin resistance)

For those who have an increased risk for insulin resistance, criteria for diagnosis may be a bit lower.[15]

Metabolic syndrome   A group of obesity-related health risk factors that increase the risk for heart disease and diabetes.

Is it time to forget the cholesterol and fat in your diet altogether and focus on other risks? No. However, researchers are investigating new factors that may contribute to CVD risk as much as that juicy steak or high-fat ice cream.

Like C-reactive protein (CRP), researchers have discovered another substance that may signal increased risk for CVD. Recent studies indicate that *homocysteine,* an amino acid normally present in the blood, may be related to higher risk of coronary heart disease, stroke, and peripheral vascular disease when present at high levels. In fact, it is hypothesized that ho-

mocysteine may work in much the same way as CRP, inflaming the inner lining of arteries and promoting fat deposits on the damaged walls and development of blood clots.

Folic acid and other B vitamins (such as B_6 and B_{12}) help break down homocysteine in the body; many scientists are currently assessing the precise role of high homocysteine levels in increased CVD risk and the role folic acid and B vitamins might play in reducing CVD risk. Because conclusive evidence of risk reduction from folic acid is not available, authorities such as the American Heart Association do not recommend taking folic acid sup-

plements to lower homocysteine levels and prevent CVD. For now, a healthy, balanced diet that includes at least five servings of fruits and vegetables a day is the best preventive action. Citrus fruit, tomatoes, vegetables, and grain products that are fortified with folic acid are good sources of the recommended 400 micrograms.

Sources: American Heart Association, "Homocysteine, Folic Acid, and Cardiovascular Disease," 2004, www.americanheart.org; J. K. Victanen et al., "Homocysteine as a Risk Factor for CVD Mortality in Men with Other CVD Risk Factors: The Kuopio Ischemic Heart Risk Factor (KIHD) Study," *Journal of Internal Medicine* 257, no. 3 (2005): 209–317.

Coronary Heart Disease

Of all the major cardiovascular diseases, coronary heart disease (CHD) is the greatest killer. In fact, this year well over 1,200,000 people will suffer a heart attack, and over 40 percent of them will die.[16] A **myocardial infarction (MI),** or **heart attack,** involves an area of the heart that suffers permanent damage because its normal blood supply has been blocked. This condition is often brought on by a **coronary thrombosis,** or blood clot in a coronary artery, or through an atherosclerotic narrowing that blocks an artery. When blood does not flow readily, there is a corresponding decrease in oxygen flow. If the blockage is extremely minor, an otherwise healthy heart will adapt over time by using small unused or underused blood vessels to reroute needed blood through other areas. This system, known as **collateral circulation,** is a form of self-preservation that allows an affected heart muscle to cope with the damage.

When heart blockage is more severe, however, the body is unable to adapt on its own, and outside lifesaving support is critical. The hour following a heart attack is the most crucial period—over 40 percent of heart attack victims die within this time. These sudden deaths are caused by cardiac arrest that usually results from *ventricular fibrillation,* or irregular, inefficient heartbeats. See the Skills for Behavior Change box on page 336 to learn what to do in case of a heart attack.

What Do You Think?

What risk factors might typical college-age students have for plaque formation? ■ What information should new CVD prevention guidelines include if the new theories discussed in this section prove true?

Angina Pectoris

Atherosclerosis and other circulatory impairments often reduce the heart's blood and oxygen supply, a condition known as **ischemia.** People with ischemia often suffer

---

Myocardial infarction (MI) Heart attack.

Heart attack A blockage of normal blood supply to an area in the heart.

Coronary thrombosis A blood clot occurring in a coronary artery.

Collateral circulation Adaptation of the heart to partial damage accomplished by rerouting needed blood through unused or underused blood vessels while the damaged heart muscle heals.

Ischemia Reduced oxygen supply to a body part or organ.

What to Do in the Event of a Heart Attack

Because heart attacks are so frightening, we would prefer not to think about them. However, knowing how to act in an emergency could save your life or that of somebody else.

Know the Warning Signs of a Heart Attack

- Uncomfortable pressure, fullness, squeezing, or pain in the center of the chest that lasts two minutes or longer
- Jaw pain and/or shortness of breath
- Pain spreading to the shoulders, neck, or arms
- Dizziness, fatigue, fainting, sweating, and/or nausea

Not all these warning signs occur in every heart attack. For instance, women's heart attacks tend to show up as shortness of breath, fatigue, and jaw pain, stretched out over hours rather than minutes. If some of these symptoms do appear, however, don't wait. Get help immediately!

Know What to Do in an Emergency

- Find out which hospitals in your area have 24-hour emergency cardiac care.
- Determine (in advance) the hospital or medical facility that's nearest your home and office, and tell your family and friends to call this facility in an emergency.
- Keep a list of emergency rescue service numbers next to your telephone and in your pocket, wallet, or purse.
- If you have chest or jaw discomfort that lasts more than two minutes, call the emergency rescue service. Do not drive yourself to the hospital.

Be a Heart Saver

- If you're with someone who is showing signs of a heart attack and the warning signs last for two minutes or longer, act immediately.
- Expect a denial. It's normal for a person with chest discomfort to deny the possibility of anything as serious as a heart attack. Don't take no for an answer, however. Insist on taking prompt action.
- Call the emergency rescue service or get to the nearest hospital emergency room that offers 24-hour emergency cardiac care.
- Give CPR (cardiopulmonary resuscitation, or mouth-to-mouth breathing and chest compression) if it's necessary and if you're properly trained to do it.

Source: American Heart Association, *Heart and Stroke Facts* (Dallas: Author, 2004). www.americanheart.org

---

from varying degrees of **angina pectoris**, or chest pain. In fact, an estimated 2.6 million men and 4.2 million women suffer mild to crushing forms of chest pain each day.[17] Many people experience short episodes of angina whenever they exert themselves physically. Symptoms may range from slight indigestion to a feeling that the heart is being crushed. Generally, the more serious the oxygen deprivation, the more severe the pain. Although angina pectoris is not a heart attack, it does indicate underlying heart disease.

Currently, there are several methods of treating angina. In mild cases, rest is critical. The most common treatments for more severe cases involve using drugs that affect either the supply of blood to the heart muscle or the heart's demand for oxygen. Pain and discomfort are often relieved with *nitroglycerin,* a drug used to relax (dilate) veins, thereby reducing the amount of blood returning to the heart and thus lessening its workload. Patients whose angina is caused by spasms of the coronary arteries are often given drugs called *calcium channel blockers,* drugs that prevent calcium atoms from passing through coronary arteries and causing heart contractions. They also appear to reduce blood pressure and slow heart rate. *Beta blockers,* the other major type of drugs used to treat angina, control potential overactivity of the heart muscle.

Arrhythmias

Over 4 million Americans experience some type of **arrhythmia**, an irregularity in heart rhythm; about 480,400 result in death.[18] A person who complains of a racing heart in the absence of exercise or anxiety may be experiencing *tachycardia,* the medical term for abnormally fast heartbeat. On the other end of the continuum is *bradycardia,* or abnormally slow heartbeat. When a heart goes into **fibrillation**, it beats in a

Angina pectoris   Chest pain occurring as a result of reduced oxygen flow to the heart.

Arrhythmia   An irregularity in heartbeat.

Fibrillation   A sporadic, quivering pattern of heartbeat that results in extreme inefficiency in moving blood through the cardiovascular system.

sporadic, quivering pattern that results in extreme inefficiency in moving blood through the cardiovascular system. If untreated, fibrillation may be fatal.

Not all arrhythmias are life threatening. In many instances, excessive caffeine or nicotine consumption can trigger an arrhythmia episode. However, severe cases may require drug therapy or external electrical stimulus to prevent serious complications.

Congestive Heart Failure

When the heart muscle is damaged or overworked and lacks the strength to keep blood circulating normally through the body, its chambers are often taxed to the limit. **Congestive heart failure (CHF)** affects over 5 million Americans and dramatically increases risk of premature death.[19] The heart muscle may be injured by a number of health conditions, including rheumatic fever, pneumonia, heart attack, or other cardiovascular problems. In some cases, the damage is due to radiation or chemotherapy treatments for cancer. These weakened muscles respond poorly, impairing blood flow out of the heart through the arteries. The return flow of blood through the veins begins to back up, causing congestion in body tissues. This pooling of blood enlarges the heart, makes it less efficient, and decreases the amount of blood that can be circulated. Fluid begins to accumulate in other body areas, such as the vessels in the legs, ankles, or lungs, where it can leak into surrounding tissues and cause swelling or difficulty in breathing.

Today, CHF is the single most frequent cause of hospitalization in the United States.[20] If untreated, congestive heart failure can be fatal. However, most cases respond well to treatment that includes *diuretics* (such as water pills) to relieve fluid accumulation; drugs, such as *digitalis,* that increase the pumping action of the heart; and drugs called *vasodilators* that expand blood vessels and decrease resistance, allowing blood to flow more easily and making the heart's work easier.

Congenital and Rheumatic Heart Disease

Approximately 1 out of every 125 children is born with some form of **congenital heart disease** (disease present at birth). These forms may be relatively minor, such as slight *murmurs* (low-pitched sounds caused by turbulent blood flow through the heart) that result from valve irregularities, which some children outgrow. Other congenital problems involve serious complications in heart function that can be corrected only with surgery. Their underlying causes are unknown but may be related to hereditary factors; maternal diseases, such as rubella, that occur during fetal development; or chemical intake (particularly alcohol) by the mother during pregnancy. Because of advances in pediatric cardiology, the prognosis for children with congenital heart defects is better than ever.

Rheumatic heart disease can cause similar heart problems in children. It is attributed to rheumatic fever, an inflammatory disease that may affect many connective tissues of the body, especially those of the heart, joints, brain, or skin, and is caused by an unresolved *streptococcal infection* of the throat (strep throat). In a small number of cases, this infection can lead to an immune response in which antibodies attack the heart as well as the bacteria. Many of the 82,000 annual operations on heart valves in the United States are related to rheumatic heart disease.[21]

Stroke

Like heart muscle, brain cells must have a continuous adequate supply of oxygen in order to survive. A **stroke** (also called a *cerebrovascular accident*) occurs when the blood supply to the brain is interrupted. Strokes may be caused by a **thrombus** (a clot in a blood vessel), an **embolus** (a clot that is floating in the bloodstream), or an **aneurysm** (a weakening in a blood vessel that causes it to bulge and in severe cases burst, or *hemorrhage*). Figure 12.4 on page 338 illustrates these blood vessel disorders. When any of these events occur, oxygen deprivation kills brain cells, which do not have the capacity to heal or regenerate. Some strokes are mild and cause only temporary dizziness or slight weakness or numbness. More serious interruptions in blood flow may cause speech impairments, memory problems, and loss of motor control.

Other strokes affect parts of the brain that regulate heart and lung function and kill within minutes. Stroke killed 275,000 Americans in 2002 and accounted for 1 in 15 of our total deaths, surpassed only by CHD and cancer. Each year, about 700,000 people experience a

---

Congestive heart failure (CHF) An abnormal cardiovascular condition that reflects impaired cardiac pumping and blood flow; pooling blood leads to congestion in body tissues.

Congenital heart disease Heart disease that is present at birth.

Rheumatic heart disease A heart disease caused by untreated streptococcal infection of the throat.

Stroke A condition occurring when the brain is damaged by disrupted blood supply.

Thrombus Clot in a blood vessel.

Embolus Clot that is forced through the circulatory system.

Aneurysm A weakened blood vessel that may bulge under pressure and, in severe cases, burst.

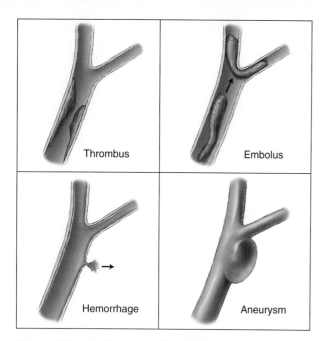

Figure 12.4 ■ Common Blood Vessel Disorders

new or recurrent stroke, which averages out to one person suffering a stroke every 45 seconds, and one person dying as a result every 3 minutes.[22]

About one in ten major strokes is preceded days, weeks, or months earlier by **transient ischemic attacks (TIAs)**, brief interruptions of the blood supply to the brain that cause only temporary impairment. Symptoms of TIAs include dizziness, particularly at first rising in the morning, weakness, temporary paralysis or numbness in the face or other regions, temporary memory loss, blurred vision, nausea, headache, slurred speech, or other unusual physiological reactions. TIAs are often indications of an impending major stroke.

Warning signs of stroke include:

■ Sudden weakness or numbness of the face, arm, or leg on one side of the body

■ Sudden dimness or loss of vision, particularly in only one eye

■ Loss of speech, or trouble talking or understanding speech

■ Sudden, severe headaches with no known cause

■ Unexplained dizziness, unsteadiness, or sudden falls, especially with any of the previously listed symptoms

If you experience any of these symptoms, or if you are with someone who does, be sure to seek medical help

Transient ischemic attack (TIA)   Brief interruption of the blood supply to the brain that causes only temporary impairment; often an indicator of impending major stroke.

immediately. The earlier treatment starts, the more effective it will be.

One of the greatest medical successes in recent years has been the decline in the fatality rates from strokes, a rate that has dropped by one-third in the United States since the 1980s and continues to fall. Improved diagnostic procedures, better surgical options, clot-busting drugs injected soon after a stroke has occurred, and acute care centers specializing in stroke treatment and rehabilitation have all been factors. Increased awareness of risk factors for stroke, especially high blood pressure, knowledge of warning signals, and an emphasis on prevention also have contributed. It is estimated that more than half of all remaining strokes could be avoided if more people followed the recommended preventive standards.

Unfortunately, those who survive a stroke do not always make a full recovery. Some 50 to 70 percent of stroke survivors regain functional independence, while 15 to 30 percent are permanently disabled and require assistance. Today stroke is a leading cause of serious long-term disability and contributes a significant amount to Medicaid and Medicare expenses for older Americans.[23]

REDUCING YOUR RISK FOR CARDIOVASCULAR DISEASES

Factors that increase the risk for cardiovascular problems fall into two categories: those we can control and those we cannot. Fortunately, we can take steps to minimize many risk factors.

Risks You Can Control

Avoid Tobacco   In 1964, the Surgeon General of the United States asserted that smoking was the greatest risk factor for heart disease. Today, more than one in five deaths from CVD are directly related to smoking. The risk for cardiovascular disease is 70 percent greater for smokers than for nonsmokers. Smokers who have a heart attack are more likely to die suddenly (within one hour) than are nonsmokers. Evidence also indicates that chronic exposure to environmental tobacco smoke (ETS, or secondhand smoke) increases the risk of heart disease by as much as 30 percent.[24]

How does smoking damage the heart? There are two plausible explanations. One is that nicotine increases heart rate, heart output, blood pressure, and oxygen use by heart muscles. Because the carbon monoxide in cigarette smoke displaces oxygen in heart tissue, the heart is forced to work harder to obtain sufficient oxygen. The other explanation states that chemicals in smoke damage the lining of the coronary arteries and cause inflammation, allowing cholesterol and plaque to accumulate more easily. This additional buildup constricts the vessels, increasing blood pressure and forcing the heart to work harder.

When people stop smoking, regardless of how long or how much they've smoked, their risk of heart disease declines rapidly. Three years after quitting, the risk of death from heart disease and stroke for people who smoked a pack a day or less is almost the same as for people who never smoked. Although the exact reasons are unknown, new findings from the Lung Health Study indicate that women have greater lung function improvements than their male counterparts after sustained smoking cessation.[25]

Cut Back on Saturated Fats and Cholesterol

The National Heart, Lung, and Blood Institute's *Third Report on Detection, Evaluation, and Treatment of Cholesterol National Guidelines* show that cholesterol levels are out of control in the United States. Nearly 36 million people in the United States—one-fifth of all adults—require medications to avoid cardiovascular problems.[26]

Why all the fuss about fats and cholesterol? Diets high in saturated fat are known to raise cholesterol levels, send the body's blood-clotting system into high gear, and make the blood more viscous in just a few hours, increasing the risk of heart attack or stroke. Switching to a low-fat diet lowers the risk of clotting.

What's the difference between good and bad cholesterol?

A fatty diet also increases the amount of cholesterol in the blood, contributing to atherosclerosis. See Table 12.1 for cholesterol level recommendations. People with multiple risk factors for CVD are advised to follow even more stringent guidelines.[27]

However, it isn't just the total cholesterol level that you should be concerned about. Cholesterol comes in two main varieties: **low-density lipoprotein (LDL)** and **high-density lipoprotein (HDL)**. Low-density lipoprotein, often referred to as "bad" cholesterol, is believed to build up on artery walls. In contrast, high-density lipoprotein, or "good" cholesterol, appears to remove cholesterol from artery walls, thus serving as a protector. In theory, if LDL levels get too high or HDL levels too low—largely because of too much saturated fat in the diet, lack of exercise, high stress levels, or genetic predisposition—cholesterol will accumulate inside arteries and lead to cardiovascular problems. A lipoprotein component of HDL, Lp(a), plays an important role in plaque accumulation and increased risk for stroke and coronary events, particularly in males. The higher the Lp(a) level, the higher the risk.[28]

The goal is to manage the ratio of HDL to total cholesterol by lowering LDL levels, raising HDL, or both. Regular exercise and a healthy diet low in

Table 12.1
Classification of LDL, Total, and HDL Cholesterol (mg/dL) and Recommended Levels for Adults

LDL Cholesterol

< 100	Optimal
100–129	Near optimal/above optimal
130–159	Borderline high
160–189	High
≥ 190	Very high

Total Cholesterol

<200	Desirable
200–239	Borderline high
≥ 240	High

HDL Cholesterol

<40	Low/increased risk
≥ 60	High/decreased risk

Triglycerides

<150	Normal
150–199	Borderline high
≥ 200	High

Source: National Heart, Lung, and Blood Institute, *Detection, Evaluation, and Treatment of High Blood Cholesterol in Adults* (NIH Publication No. 02-5215), 2002, www.nhlbi.nih.gov/guidelines/cholesterol/atp3_rpt.htm.

saturated fat continue to be the best methods for maintaining healthy ratios. However, if dietary efforts and exercise do not reduce total cholesterol or LDL, several medications are available that may help.

Triglycerides, another type of fat in the blood, also appear to promote atherosclerosis. As people get older, heavier, or both, their triglycerides and cholesterol levels tend to rise. A causal link between high triglyceride levels and CVD has yet to be established. It may be that high triglyceride levels do not directly cause atherosclerosis but, rather, are among the abnormalities that speed its development.

Current guidelines suggest that you should reduce consumption of saturated fat (which comes mostly from animal products) to less than 7 percent of your total

Low-density lipoproteins (LDLs) Compounds that facilitate the transport of cholesterol in the blood to the body's cells; "bad" cholesterol.

High-density lipoproteins (HDLs) Compounds that facilitate the transport of cholesterol in the blood to the liver for metabolism and elimination from the body; "good" cholesterol.

Triglycerides The most common form of fat in the body; excess calories are converted into and stored as body fat.

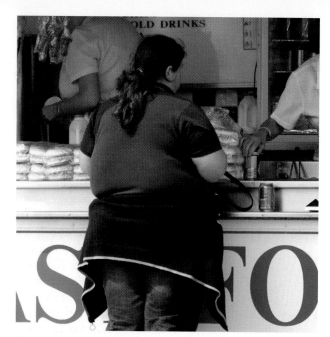

Excessive body weight increases the risk of developing CVD. Weight management should be a primary goal for CVD prevention.

daily caloric intake and minimize your consumption of *trans* fat (see Chapter 9), which is found in partially hydrogenated products such as most margarines, many fast foods, and many packaged foods. By cutting your intake of saturated fats and *trans* fats, experts from the National Heart, Lung, and Blood Institute (NHLBI) believe that you can reduce your LDL levels by as much as 10 percent.[29] In addition, NHLBI experts indicate that you should consume fewer than 200 milligrams per day of cholesterol (found mainly in eggs and meat), which may reduce LDL by as much as 5 percent.[30]

While it is wise to cut back on saturated fat, be aware that some fat is necessary to overall health. Try to eat foods with olive oil, canola oil, and other mononounsaturated fats instead of consuming low-fat or no-fat products. (For a complete discussion of this topic, see Chapter 9.) Of course, all fat intake should be in moderation.

Monitor Your Cholesterol Levels To get an accurate assessment of your total cholesterol and LDL and HDL levels, consider a *lipoprotein analysis*. This analysis should be done by a reputable health provider and requires that you not eat or drink anything for 12 hours prior to the test.

In general, LDL is more closely associated with cardiovascular risk than is total cholesterol. However, most authorities agree that looking only at LDL ignores the positive effects of HDL. Perhaps the best method of evaluating risk is to examine the ratio of HDL to total cholesterol, or the percentage of HDL in total cholesterol. If the HDL level is lower than 35, the risk increases dramatically.

Change Lifestyle to Reduce Your Risk

Of the more than 100 million Americans who need to worry about their cholesterol levels, almost half, particularly those at the low-to-moderate risk levels, should be able to reach their LDL and HDL goals through lifestyle changes alone. People who are at higher risk or those for whom lifestyle modifications are not effective may need to take cholesterol-lowering drugs while they continue modifying their lifestyle. Among the most commonly prescribed drugs are statins (Lipitor, Baycol, and Pravachol are examples), which are very effective in reducing LDL levels. Be sure to speak with your doctor about possible side effects before beginning a drug therapy program. Folic acids and niacin drugs are often prescribed for people with low HDL and high triglyceride levels.

Maintain a Healthy Weight No question about it—body weight plays a role in CVD. Researchers are not sure whether high-fat, high-sugar, high-calorie diets are a direct risk for CVD or whether they invite risk by causing obesity, which strains the heart, forcing it to push blood through the many miles of capillaries that supply each pound of fat. A heart that has to continuously move blood through an overabundance of vessels may become damaged.

Overweight people are more likely to develop heart disease and stroke even if they have no other risk factors. If you're heavy, losing even 5 to 10 pounds can make a significant difference. This is especially true if you're an "apple" (thicker around your upper body and waist) rather than a "pear" (thicker around your hips and thighs). (See Chapter 10 for more tips on weight management.)

Modify Other Dietary Habits The NHLBI guidelines recommend the following dietary changes to reduce CVD risk:

> What's the best way to eat for a healthy heart?

- Consume 5 to 10 milligrams per day of *soluble fiber* from sources such as psyllium seeds, oat bran, fruits, vegetables, and legumes (see Chapter 9). Even this small dietary modification may result in a 5 percent drop in LDL levels.

- Consume about 2 grams per day of *plant sterols* or sterol derivatives from substances such as Benecol or Take Control margarine. These are the first widely available sources of sterols, but more will be on the market soon. This has the potential to reduce LDL by another 5 percent.

- Although less widely supported by rigorous research findings, many experts believe that consuming at least 25 grams of *soy protein* from various soy foods, instead of dairy sources, could reduce LDL by 5 percent.

Exercise Regularly Inactivity is a clear risk factor for CVD. The good news is that you do not have to be an exercise fanatic to reduce your risk. Even modest levels of low-intensity physical activity—walking, gardening, housework, dancing—are beneficial if done regularly and over the long term (see Chapter 11). Exercise can increase HDL, lower triglycerides, and reduce coronary risks in several ways. Exercise could reduce LDL levels by as much as 35 percent—similar to taking any of the statin drugs typically prescribed. Despite recommendations, and the clear benefits of regular exercise, only 31.3 percent of American adults aged 18 and older engage in any regular physical activity.[31]

Control Diabetes The recent NHLBI guidelines underscore the unique CVD risks for people with diabetes. Diabetics who have taken insulin for a number of years have a greater chance of developing CVD. In fact, CVD is the leading cause of death among diabetic patients. Because overweight people have a higher risk for diabetes, distinguishing between the effects of the two conditions is difficult. Diabetics also tend to have elevated blood fat levels, increased atherosclerosis, and a tendency toward deterioration of small blood vessels, particularly in the eyes and extremities. However, through a prescribed regimen of diet, exercise, and medication, diabetics can control much of their increased risk for CVD (see Chapter 14).

Control Your Blood Pressure Hypertension refers to sustained high blood pressure. If it cannot be attributed to any specific cause, it is known as **essential hypertension.** Approximately 90 percent of all cases of hypertension fit this category. **Secondary hypertension** refers to hypertension caused by specific factors, such as kidney disease, obesity, or tumors of the adrenal glands. In general, the higher your blood pressure, the greater your risk for CVD.

Hypertension is known as the "silent killer" because it usually has no symptoms. Its prevalence has increased by over 30 percent in the last 10 years; over one-third of all adults have blood pressure problems and may be on medication, working to reduce risk factors, or unaware that they have a problem.[32]

Blood pressure is measured in two parts and is expressed as a fraction—for example, 110/80, or "110 over 80." Both values are measured in *millimeters of mercury* (mm Hg). The first number refers to **systolic pressure,** or the pressure being applied to the walls of the arteries when the heart contracts, pumping blood to the rest of the body. The second value is **diastolic pressure,** or the pressure applied to the walls of the arteries during the heart's relaxation phase. During this phase, blood is reentering the chambers of the heart, preparing for the next heartbeat.

Normal blood pressure varies depending on weight, age, physical condition, and for different groups of people, such as women and minorities. Systolic blood pressure tends to increase with age, while diastolic blood pressure increases until age 55 and then declines. As a rule, men have a greater risk for high blood pressure than women until age 55, when their risks become about equal. After age 75, women are more likely to have high blood pressure than men.[33]

For the average person, 110/80 is a healthy blood pressure level. High blood pressure (HBP) is usually diagnosed when systolic pressure is 140 or above. Diastolic pressure does not have to be high to indicate high blood pressure. When only systolic pressure is high, the condition is known as *isolated systolic hypertension (ISH),* the most common form of high blood pressure in older Americans.[34] If your blood pressure exceeds 140/90, you need to take steps to lower it. See Table 12.2 on page 342 for a summary of blood pressure values and what they mean.

Treatment of hypertension can involve dietary changes (reducing salt and calorie intake), weight loss (when appropriate), the use of diuretics and other medications (only when prescribed by a physician), regular exercise, and the practice of relaxation techniques and effective coping and communication skills.

Try it ▸NOW_____

Eat heart healthy foods! **Omega-3 fatty acids occur naturally in a variety of foods, and this nutrient has proven benefits to heart health. Start adding foods like walnuts (in your salad), salmon and tuna, and soy products such as tofu or soy milk to your snacks and meals several times a week. Add these foods to your diet now to reduce your risk of CHD later in life.**

Manage Stress Some scientists have noted a relationship between CVD risk and a person's stress level, behavior habits, and socioeconomic status.

Hypertension Sustained elevated blood pressure.

Essential hypertension Hypertension that cannot be attributed to any specific cause.

Secondary hypertension Hypertension caused by specific factors, such as kidney disease, obesity, or tumors of the adrenal glands.

Systolic pressure The upper number in the fraction that measures blood pressure; it indicates pressure on the walls of the arteries when the heart contracts.

Diastolic pressure The lower number in the fraction that measures blood pressure; it indicates pressure on the walls of the arteries during the relaxation phase of heart activity.

Table 12.2
Blood Pressure Classifications

Classification	Systolic Reading (mm Hg)		Diastolic Reading (mm Hg)
Normal	<120	and	<80
Prehypertension	120–139	or	80–89
Hypertension			
Stage 1	140–159	or	90–99
Stage 2	≥ 160	or	≥ 100

Note: If systolic and diastolic readings fall into different categories, treatment is determined by the highest category. Readings are based on the average of two or more properly measured, seated readings on each of two or more health care provider visits.
Source: National Heart, Lung, and Blood Institute, *The Seventh Report of the Joint National Committee on Prevention, Detection, Evaluation, and Treatment of High Blood Pressure* (NIH Publication No. 03-5233) (Bethesda, MD: National Institutes of Health, May 2003).

These factors may influence established risk factors. For example, people under stress may start smoking or smoke more than they otherwise would. In one study, researcher-physician Robert S. Eliot demonstrated that approximately one out of five people has an extreme cardiovascular reaction to stressful stimulation (see Chapter 3). These people are called *hot reactors*. Although their blood pressure may be normal when they are not under stress—for example, in a doctor's office—it increases dramatically in response to even small amounts of everyday tension. *Cold reactors* are those who are able to experience stress without showing harmful cardiovascular responses. Cold reactors may internalize stress, but their self-talk and perceptions about the stressful events lead them to a nonresponse state in which their cardiovascular system remains virtually unaffected.[35]

Since Eliot's early work, research in this area has been inconclusive, although more recent studies suggest that personality does indeed play an important role in effective coping. See Chapter 3 for tips on managing your stress, whether you are a hot or cold reactor.

Risks You Cannot Control

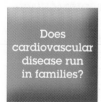

Does cardiovascular disease run in families?

There are, unfortunately, some risk factors for CVD that we cannot prevent or control. The most important are these:

- *Heredity.* A family history of heart disease appears to increase the risk significantly. Whether the increase is due to genetics or environment is unresolved.

- *Age.* Seventy-five percent of all heart attacks occur in people over age 65. The risk for CVD increases with age for both sexes.

- *Gender.* Men are at greater risk for CVD until about age 60. Women under 35 have a fairly low risk unless they have high blood pressure, kidney problems, or diabetes. Using oral contraceptives and smoking also increase the risk. Hormonal factors appear to reduce risk for women, although after menopause or after estrogen levels are otherwise reduced (e.g., because of hysterectomy), women's LDL levels tend to go up, which increases their chances for CVD. (For more on the gender factor, see the next section.)

- *Race.* African Americans have a 45 percent greater risk for hypertension and thus a greater risk for CVD than whites. In addition, African Americans are less likely to survive a heart attack.

The Health in a Diverse World box describes the impact of race, gender, and age on CVD risk.

Try it ▶NOW

Modify risk factors now to prevent heart disease later! Right now, find out if you are prone for CVD, and take steps to modify your risk. Does heart disease, high blood pressure, or high cholesterol run in your family? If so, discuss steps you can take to reduce your risk and monitor your heart health with your health care provider. Though you can't control your genetic susceptibility, you can make other positive lifestyle changes to reduce your risk now.

WOMEN AND CARDIOVASCULAR DISEASE

Although men tend to have more heart attacks and to suffer them earlier in life than do women, some interesting trends in survivability have emerged. In 2002, CVD claimed the lives of 433,825 men and a surprising 493,623 women.[36] Why do more men have heart attacks but more women die of them? Why do some studies say that women have about the same mortality rate after an MI and others indicate that there are vast differences, supported by actual numbers? Although we understand the mechanisms that cause heart disease in men and women (or at least we think we do!), their experiences in the health care system, their reactions to life-threatening diseases, and a host of other technological and environmental factors may play a role in these statistics.

Cardiovascular disease is not an equal opportunity disease. In fact, when it comes to risk of attack and eventual mortality, there are huge disparities based on gender, race, and age. Consider the following.

■ African American and Mexican American women have a higher risk of CVD than do white women of comparable socioeconomic status (SES). The striking differences by both ethnicity and SES underscore the critical need to improve screening, early detection, and treatment of CVD-related conditions for African American and Mexican American women, as well as for women of lower SES in all ethnic groups.

■ Among American Indians/Alaskan Natives aged 18 and older, 63.7 percent of men and 61.4 percent of women have one or more CVD risk factors (hypertension, current cigarette smoking, high blood cholesterol, obesity, or diabetes). If data on physical activity had been included in this analysis, the prevalence of risk factors would have been much higher.

■ In 2002, the prevalence of CVD was 34.3 percent for white males and 41.5 percent for African American males at all ages and stages of life. The rate for Mexican Americans was 29.2 percent.

■ In 2002, the prevalence of CVD was 32.4 percent for white females, 44.7 percent for African American females, and 29.3 percent for Mexican American females.

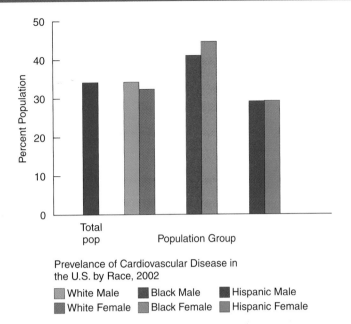

Prevelance of Cardiovascular Disease in the U.S. by Race, 2002

■ White Male ■ Black Male ■ Hispanic Male
■ White Female ■ Black Female ■ Hispanic Female

Prevalence of Cardiovascular Disease in the United States by Race, 2002.

Source: American Heart Association, *Heart Disease and Stroke Statistics—2005 Update* (Dallas: American Heart Association, 2005). © 2005 American Heart Association. Reproduced by permission. www.americanheart.org.

■ African Americans are 60 percent more likely to suffer a stroke than are whites, and two and one half times more likely to die from a stroke.

■ A family history of diabetes, gout, high blood pressure, or high cholesterol increases one's risk of heart disease. African Americans are more likely to have these familial risk factors, which increases their overall chances for CVD.

■ Cholesterol levels higher than 200 milligrams per deciliter (mg/dL) in those aged 20 and over are found in:

- 53 percent of non-Hispanic white females
- 47 percent of non-Hispanic African American females
- 43 percent of Mexican Americans
- 28 percent of American Indian/Alaskan Natives
- 27 percent of Asian/Pacific Islanders

Source: American Heart Association, *Heart Disease and Stroke Statistics—2003 Update* (Dallas, TX: American Heart Association, 2003).

Risk Factors for Heart Disease in Women

Premenopausal women are unlikely candidates for heart attacks unless they suffer from diabetes, high blood pressure, kidney disease, or a genetic predisposition to high cholesterol levels. Family history, use of birth control pills, and smoking also increase the risk.

The Role of Estrogen Once a woman's estrogen production drops with menopause, her chance of developing CVD rises rapidly. A 60-year-old woman has the same heart attack risk as a 50-year-old man. By her late seventies, a woman has the same heart attack risk as a man her age. To date, much of this changing risk has been attributed to the aging process, but the role of estrogen and other hormones remains unclear. Early

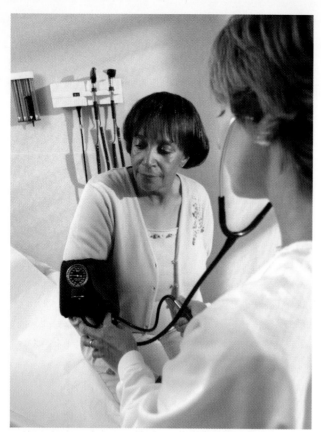

Women at risk for heart disease need to have their blood pressure and other CVD risk factors carefully monitored.

studies of various **hormone replacement therapies (HRTs)** indicated that HRT might reduce the risk of CVD. However, newer findings throw a huge wrench in what was previously believed to be the health-enhancing powers of HRT. A 2002 study in the *Journal of the American Medical Association* confirmed that HRT will not reduce the risk of cardiovascular disease in women.[37]

Cholesterol It's true that women age 25 and over tend to have lower cholesterol levels than men of the same age; but when they reach 45, things change. Most men's cholesterol levels become more stable, while both LDL and total cholesterol levels in women start to rise. The gap widens further beyond age 55.[38]

Before age 45, women's total blood cholesterol levels average below 220 mg/dL. By the time she is 45 to 55, the average woman's blood cholesterol rises to

---

Hormone replacement therapies (HRTs)
Therapies that replace estrogen and progestin in post-menopausal women.

---

between 223 and 246 mg/dL. Studies of men have shown that for every 1 percent drop in cholesterol, there is a 2 percent decrease in CVD risk.[39] If this holds true for women, prevention efforts focusing on dietary intervention and exercise may significantly help post-menopausal women.

Neglect of Heart Disease Symptoms in Women During the past decade, research has suggested three main reasons why signs of heart disease in women may get overlooked: (1) physicians may be gender-biased in their delivery of health care, tending to concentrate on women's reproductive organs rather than on the whole body; (2) physicians tend to view male heart disease as a more severe problem because men have traditionally had a higher incidence of the disease; (3) women decline major procedures more often than men do. Other explanations for diagnostic and therapeutic difficulties encountered by women with heart disease include:[40]

- Delay in diagnosing a possible heart attack due to the complexity of interpreting chest pain and because symptoms of heart attack often differ for women and men.

- Typically less aggressive treatment of female heart attack victims

- Their older age, on average, and greater frequency of other health problems

- Women's coronary arteries are often smaller than men's, making surgical or diagnostic procedures more difficult technically

- Their increased incidence of postinfarction angina and heart failure

---

What Do You Think? How do men and women differ in their experiences related to CVD? ■ Why do you think women's risks largely were ignored until fairly recently? ■ What actions do you think individuals can take to help improve the situation for both men and women? ■ What actions can communities and medical practitioners take?

NEW WEAPONS AGAINST HEART DISEASE

The victim of a heart attack today has many options that were not available a generation ago. Medications can strengthen heartbeat, control arrhythmias, remove fluids in case of congestive heart failure, and relieve pain. New surgical procedures are saving many lives.

Techniques for Diagnosing Heart Disease

Several techniques are used to diagnose heart disease, including electrocardiogram, angiography, and positron emission tomography scans. An **electrocardiogram (ECG)** is a record of the electrical activity of the heart. Patients may undergo a stress test, such as walking or running on a treadmill while their hearts are monitored. A more accurate method of testing for heart disease is **angiography** (often referred to as *cardiac catheterization*), in which a needle-thin tube called a *catheter* is threaded through heart arteries, a dye is injected, and an X ray is taken to discover which areas are blocked. A more recent and even more effective method of measuring heart activity is **positron emission tomography (PET scan)**, which produces three-dimensional images of the heart as blood flows through it. During a PET scan, a patient receives an intravenous injection of a radioactive tracer and is then monitored at rest and during exercise. As the tracer decays, it emits positrons that are picked up by the scanner and transformed by a computer into color images of the heart. Newer *single-photon emission computed tomography (SPECT)* scans provide an even better view. Other tests include:

- *Radionuclide imaging* (includes tests such as thallium test, multinucleated gated angiography [MUGA] scan, and acute infarct scintigraphy). In these procedures, substances called radionuclides are injected into the bloodstream. Computer-generated pictures can then show them in the heart. These tests can show how well the heart muscle is supplied with blood, how well the heart's chambers are functioning, and which part of the heart has been damaged by a heart attack.

- *Magnetic resonance imaging (MRI).* This test uses powerful magnets to look inside the body. Computer-generated pictures can show the heart muscle and help physicians identify damage from a heart attack, diagnose congenital heart defects, and evaluate disease of larger blood vessels such as the aorta.

- *Ultrafast computed tomography (CT).* This is an especially fast form of X ray of the heart designed to evaluate bypass grafts, diagnose ventricular function, and measure calcium deposits.

- *Digital subtraction angiography (DSA).* This modified form of computer-aided imaging records pictures of the heart and its blood vessels.

Angioplasty versus Bypass Surgery

Coronary bypass surgery has helped many patients who suffered coronary blockages or heart attacks. In coronary bypass surgery, a blood vessel is taken from

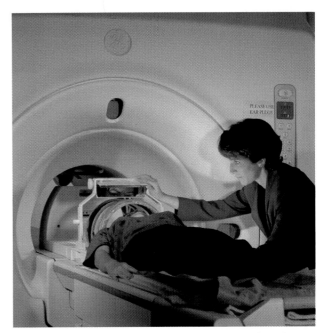

Magnetic resonance imaging is one of several methods to detect heart damage, abnormalities, or defects.

another site in the patient's body (usually the *saphenous vein* in the leg or the *internal mammary artery*) and implanted to "bypass" blocked arteries and transport blood. Bypass patients typically spend four to seven days in the hospital to recuperate. The average cost of the procedure itself is well over $50,000, and the additional intensive care treatments and follow-ups often result in total medical bills of $125,000. Death rates are generally much lower at medical centers where surgical teams and intensive care teams see large numbers of patients.[41]

Another procedure, **angioplasty** (sometimes called *balloon angioplasty*), carries fewer risks and may be

---

Electrocardiogram (ECG)   A record of the electrical activity of the heart.

Angiography   A technique for examining blockages in heart arteries.

Positron emission tomography scan (PET scan)   Method for measuring heart activity by injecting a patient with a radioactive tracer that is scanned electronically to produce a three-dimensional image of the heart and arteries.

Coronary bypass surgery   A surgical technique whereby a blood vessel is implanted to bypass a clogged coronary artery.

Angioplasty   A technique in which a catheter with a balloon at the tip is inserted into a clogged artery; the balloon is inflated to flatten fatty deposits against artery walls, which allows blood to flow more freely. A stent is typically inserted to keep the artery open.

more effective than bypass surgery in selected cases. As in angiography, a thin catheter is threaded through blocked heart arteries. The catheter has a balloon at the tip, which is inflated to flatten fatty deposits against the artery walls, allowing blood to flow more freely. A *stent* (a mesh-like tube) is then inserted into the artery to keep it from collapsing. Angioplasty patients are generally awake but sedated during the procedure and spend only one or two days in the hospital after treatment. Most people can return to work within five days. In about 30 percent of patients, the treated arteries become clogged again within six months. Some patients may undergo the procedure as many as three times within a five-year period. Some surgeons argue that given this high rate of recurrence, bypass may be a more effective treatment.

Today, newer forms of laser angioplasty and atherectomy, a procedure that removes plaque, are being done in several clinics. These procedures are often followed by procedures in which the affected area has a stent inserted.

Research suggests that in many instances, drug treatments may be just as effective in prolonging life as invasive surgical techniques, but it is critical that doctors prescribe an aggressive drug treatment program and that patients comply with it. Among the most effective are beta blockers and calcium channel blockers to reduce high blood pressure and treat other symptoms. Cholesterol-lowering drugs are also effective.

Aspirin for Heart Disease: Can It Help?

Research indicates that low doses of aspirin (80 milligrams daily or every other day) are beneficial to heart patients because of its blood-thinning properties. Higher levels do not provide significantly more protection. Aspirin has even been advised as a preventive strategy for people with no current heart disease symptoms. However, major problems associated with chronic aspirin use are gastrointestinal intolerance and a tendency for some people to have difficulty with blood clotting, and these factors may outweigh aspirin's benefits in some cases. People taking aspirin face additional risks from emergency surgery or accidental bleeding. Although the findings concerning aspirin and heart disease are still inconclusive, the research seems promising.[42] Aspirin should only be taken as a preventative measure if your physician recommends it. See the New Horizons in Health box for more on promising new research to control CVD risk.

Thrombolysis   Injection of an agent to dissolve clots and restore some blood flow, thereby reducing the amount of tissue that dies from ischemia.

Thrombolysis

Whenever a heart attack occurs, prompt action is vital. When a coronary artery is blocked, the heart muscle doesn't die immediately, but time determines how much damage occurs. If a victim reaches an emergency room and is diagnosed fast enough, a form of reperfusion therapy called **thrombolysis** can be performed. Thrombolysis involves injecting an agent such as TPA (tissue plasminogen activator) to dissolve the clot and restore some blood flow, thereby reducing the amount of tissue that dies from ischemia.[43] These drugs must be administered within one to three hours after a heart attack for best results.

What Do You Think?   With all the new diagnostic procedures, treatments, and differing philosophies about prevention and intervention techniques, how can health consumers ensure that they will get the best treatment? ■ Where can they go for information? ■ Why might patients need a health advocate who can help them get through the system?

Cardiac Rehabilitation

Every year, nearly 1 million people survive heart attacks. Over 7 million more have unstable angina, and about 650,000 undergo bypass surgery or angioplasty. Heart failure is the most common discharge diagnosis for hospitalized Medicare patients and the fourth most common diagnosis among all patients hospitalized in the United States. Most of these patients are eligible for cardiac rehabilitation (including exercise training and health education classes on good nutrition and CVD risk management), needing only a doctor's prescription for these services. However, many Americans do not have access to these programs. Even larger numbers are finding it difficult to afford them in light of skyrocketing costs for prescription drugs. While some patients must choose between home health care and cardiac rehabilitation, others stay away from such programs because of cost, transportation, or other factors. Perhaps the biggest deterrent is fear of having another attack due to exercise. The benefits of cardiac rehabilitation (including increased stamina and strength and faster recovery), however, far outweigh the risks when these programs are run by certified health professionals.

Personal Advocacy and Heart-Smart Behaviors

People who suspect they have cardiovascular disease are often overwhelmed and frightened. Where should they go for diagnosis? What are the best treatments?

Just when we thought that indulging in certain dietary delights should be avoided, there is growing evidence that the antioxidant compound known as flavonoids, found in fruits, teas, red wine, and cocoa, may protect us from risks for heart disease, stroke, and even diabetes. Sound too good to be true? Exciting new research is indicating that the flavonoids in red wine in particular, may act as an anti-inflammatory and protect us from CVD. Though the evidence supporting these claims is promising, research into these compounds and exactly how they protect against CVD is still in its infancy, and scientists warn that it is too early to come to a solid conclusion.

Does red wine really prevent heart disease?

Consider results from these studies:

■ At a 2005 conference held in Switzerland on the health benefits of cocoa, researchers revealed that cocoa flavonol molecules may reduce the risk of blood clotting and improve blood flow in the brain.

■ Results from over 51 epidemiological studies suggest that risk of CHD may decrease by as much as 20 percent when 0 to 2 alcoholic drinks per day are consumed.

■ In a study of 329 heart disease patients, the intake of a small amount of wine or tea daily corresponded to a 24 percent decrease in CHD risk.

■ Results from the Health Professionals Follow-Up Study, a study in which 38,077 male health professionals who were free of cardiovascular disease were observed for 12 years, suggested that drinking 1 to 2 drinks per day, 3 to 4 days per week decreased the risk of having a heart attack by as much as 32 percent. In the same study, it was found that light alcohol consumption can reduce the risk of stroke by 20 percent.

In spite of the promising nature of these studies, most experts warn that nondrinkers should not begin drinking to improve overall health. While the benefits of light alcohol consumption are suggested, they still do not outweigh the overall risk of alcohol consumption (see Chapter 8 for more on the risks of alcohol consumption). Likewise, balanced nutrition should not be abandoned for a daily chocolate bar. However, what this research does indicate is that perhaps some day scientists will discover how to isolate the beneficial compounds found in these foods and offer them to people in the form of preventive medications for those at risk for CVD.

Sources: C. Keen, "Specific Compound Identified Behind Aspirin-Like Effect" (presentation, Cocoa Flavonols Meeting, Lucerne, Switzerland, July 25–27, 2002); P. Lagiou et al., "Intake of Specific Flavonoid Classes and Coronary Heart Disease— A Case-Control Study in Greece," *European Journal of Clinical Nutrition* 58, no. 12(4):1643–1648; P. Szmitko and V. Subodh, "Red Wine and Your Heart," *Circulation* 111 (2004). e10-e11.

Answering these questions becomes even more difficult if they are upset, scared, or tend to listen unquestioningly to doctors' orders. If you or a loved one must face a CVD crisis, it is important to act with knowledge, strength, and assertiveness. The following suggestions will help you deal with hospitals and health care providers in the wake of a cardiac event or any major health problem:

1. *Know your rights as a patient.* Ask about the risks and costs of various diagnostic tests. Some procedures, particularly angiography, may pose significant risks for people who are older, have a history of minor strokes, or have had chemotherapy or other treatments that can have damaged their blood vessels. Ask for test results and an explanation of any abnormalities.

2. *Find out about informed consent procedures, living wills, durable power of attorney, organ donation, and other legal issues before you become sick.* Having someone shove a clipboard in your face and ask you if life support can be terminated in case of a problem is one of the great horrors of many people's hospital experiences. Be prepared.

3. *Ask about alternative procedures.* If possible, seek a second opinion at a different health care facility (in other words, get at least two opinions from doctors who are not in the same group and who cannot read each other's diagnoses). New research indicates that doctors may not use drug treatments as aggressively as they could and that medications may be as effective as major bypass or open heart surgeries. Ask, ask, and ask again.

4. *Remain with your loved one as a personal advocate.* If your loved one is unable to ask questions, ask the questions yourself. Inquire about new medications, tests, and other potentially risky procedures that may be undertaken during the course of treatment or recovery. If you feel your loved one is being removed from intensive care or other closely monitored areas prematurely, ask if the hospital is taking this action to comply with DRGs (established limits of treatment for certain conditions in **d**iagnosis-**r**elated **g**roups) and if this action is warranted. Most hospitals have waiting areas or special rooms so family members can stay close to a patient. Exercise your right to this option.

5. *Monitor the actions of health care providers.* To control costs, some hospitals are hiring nursing aides and other personnel who may lack the training that registered nurses have in handling patients with CVD. Ask about the patient-to-nurse ratio, and make sure that people monitoring you or your loved ones have appropriate credentials.

6. *Be considerate of your care provider.* One of the most stressful jobs any person can be entrusted with is care of a critically ill person. Although questions are appropriate and your emotions are running high, be as tactful and considerate as possible. Nurses often carry a disproportionate responsibility for the care of patients during critical times and are often forced to carry a higher than optimal patient load. Try to remain out of their way, ask questions as necessary, and report any irregularities in care to the supervisor.

7. *Be patient with the patient.* The pain, suffering, and fears associated with a cardiac event often cause otherwise nice people to act in not-so-nice ways. Be patient and helpful, and allow time for the person to rest. Talk with the patient about his or her feelings, concerns, and fears. Do not ignore these concerns to ease your own anxieties.

We still have much to learn about CVD and its causes, treatments, and risk factors. Staying informed is an important part of staying healthy. Good dietary habits, regular exercise, stress management, prompt attention to suspicious symptoms, and other healthy behaviors will greatly enhance your chances of remaining CVD-free. Other factors that influence risk include how much emphasis our health care systems place on access to health care for all underserved populations, education about risk, and other community-based interventions. Action on both community and individual levels can help address the challenge of CVD.

▪ Taking Charge

Summary

- Cardiovascular disease (CVD) incidence and prevalence rates have changed considerably in the past 50 years. Certain segments of the population have disproportionate levels of risk.

- The cardiovascular system consists of the heart and circulatory system and is a carefully regulated, integrated network of vessels that supply the body with the nutrients and oxygen necessary to perform daily functions.

- There are many types of CVD, including atherosclerosis, heart attack, angina pectoris, arrhythmias, congestive heart failure, congenital and rheumatic heart disease, and stroke. These combine to make CVD the leading cause of death in the United States today.

- Many risk factors for CVD can be controlled, such as cigarette smoking, high blood cholesterol and triglyceride levels, hypertension, lack of exercise, high-fat diet, obesity, diabetes, and emotional stress. Some risk factors, such as age, gender, and heredity, cannot be controlled. Many of these factors have a compounded effect when combined. Dietary changes, exercise, weight reduction, and attention to lifestyle risks can greatly reduce susceptibility to CVD.

- Women face a unique challenge in controlling their risk for CVD, particularly after menopause, when estrogen levels are no longer sufficient to be protective.

- New methods developed for treating heart blockages include coronary bypass surgery and angioplasty.

Drugs such as beta blockers and calcium channel blockers can reduce high blood pressure and treat other symptoms. Research has provided important clues on how to best prevent or reduce risk of CVD today. Recognizing your own risks and acting now to reduce risk are important elements of lifelong cardiovascular health.

Chapter Review

1. Vessels that carry blood away from the heart to other regions of the body are called the
   a. atrium.
   b. veins.
   c. capillaries.
   d. arteries.

2. What type of blood vessels have thin walls that permit the exchange of oxygen, carbon dioxide, nutrients, and waste products with body cells?
   a. arteries
   b. arterioles
   c. capillaries
   d. veins

3. Severe chest pain occurring as a result of reduced oxygen flow to the heart is called
   a. angina pectoris.
   b. arrhythmias.
   c. myocardial infarction.
   d. congestive heart failure.

4. The heart is a _____ -chambered pump.
   a. two
   b. three
   c. four
   d. five

5. Chest pain is also called
   a. arrhythmia.
   b. angina pectoris.
   c. atherosclerosis.
   d. cerebrovascular accident.

6. What serves as a natural pacemaker for the heart?
   a. arterioles
   b. arteriosclerosis
   c. collateral circulation
   d. the sinoatrial node

7. What disease is caused by an unresolved strepto-coccal infection of the throat?
   a. atherosclerosis
   b. congestive heart failure
   c. rheumatic heart disease
   d. congenital heart disease

8. A thrombus, an embolus, or an aneurysm can cause
   a. strokes.
   b. atherosclerosis.
   c. coronary heart disease.
   d. congestive heart failure.

9. Which of the following methods involves injecting a person with a radioactive tracer that is scanned electronically to produce a three-dimensional image of the heart and arteries?
   a. angiography
   b. electrocardiogram
   c. magnetic resonance imaging
   d. positron emission tomography

10. Nitroglycerin, calcium channel blockers, and beta blockers are used to treat
    a. angina pectoris.
    b. coronary heart disease.
    c. atherosclerosis.
    d. strokes.

Answers to these questions can be found on page A-1.

Questions for Discussion and Reflection

1. Trace the path of a drop of blood from the time it enters the vena cava until it reaches your little finger. Be sure to include the types of blood vessels involved.

2. List the different types of CVD. Compare and contrast their symptoms, risk factors, prevention, and treatment.

3. What are the major indicators that CVD poses a particularly significant risk to people of your age?

To the elderly? To people from selected minority groups?

4. Discuss the role that exercise, stress management, dietary changes, medical checkups, sodium reduction, and other factors can play in reducing risk for CVD. What role may chronic infections play in CVD risk?

5. Discuss why age is such an important factor in women's risk for CVD. What can be done to decrease women's risk in later life?

6. Describe some of the diagnostic and treatment alternatives for CVD. If you had a heart attack today, which treatment would you prefer? Explain why.

Accessing Your Health on the Internet

The following websites explore further topics and issues related to personal health. For links to the websites, below visit the Companion Website for *Health: The Basics,* Seventh Edition at www.aw-bc.com/donatelle.

1. *American Heart Association.* Home page for the leading private organization dedicated to heart health. This site provides information, statistics, and resources regarding cardiovascular care, including an opportunity to test your own risk for CVD.

2. *Johns Hopkins Cardiac Rehabilitation Homepage.* Information about prevention of heart disease and rehabilitation from CVD from one of the best cardiac care centers in the United States. Includes information about programs to help individuals stop smoking, lose weight, lower blood pressure and blood cholesterol, and reduce emotional stress.

3. *National Heart, Lung, and Blood Institute.* A valuable resource for information on all aspects of cardiovascular health and wellness.

4. *U.S. National Library of Medicine: Health Services/ Technology Assessment Text.* Provides access to numerous databases of health care documents outlining procedures for clinicians and patients. Choose the database for the Agency for Health Care Policy and Research (AHCPR) to review various guidelines regarding all forms of cardiac care.

Further Reading

American Heart Association. *Heart Disease and Stroke Statistics—2005.* Dallas, TX: American Heart Association.

An annual overview providing facts and figures concerning CVD in the United States. Supplement provides key statistics about current trends and future directions in treatment and prevention.

Gersh, Bernard and Michael Wood, eds. *The Mayo Clinic Heart Book.* New York: William Morrow, 2000.

Pashkow, Frederic and Charlotte Libov. *The Women's Heart Book.* New York: Hyperion, 2001.

Both The Mayo Clinic Heart Book and The Women's Heart Book provide overviews of heart disease in America, including risk factors, trends, and options for patients.

McCrum, Robert. *My Year Off: Recovering after a Stroke.* New York: Broadway Books, 1999.

The chronicle of a young man's recovery from a severe stroke.

References

1. World Health Organization, *The World Health Report,* 2004, www.who.int/whr/2004/en.
2. American Heart Association, *Heart Disease and Stroke Statistics— 2005.* (Dallas: Author, 2005), www.americanheart.org.
3. Ibid.
4. Ibid.
5. Ibid.
6. Ibid.
7. Ibid.
8. Ibid.
9. American Heart Association, *Heart Disease and Stroke Statistics— 2005.*
10. Ibid.
11. World Health Organization, *The World Health Report;* American Heart Association, *Heart Disease and Stroke Facts.*
12. L. Best et al., "C-Reactive Proteins as a Predictor of Cardiovascular Risk in a Population with High Prevalence of Diabetes," *Circulation* 112, no. 9 (2005): 1289–1295; C. Boos and G. Lip, "Elevated High Sensitive C-Reactive Protein, Large Arterial Stiffness and Atherosclerosis: A Relationship between Inflammation and Hypertension, *Journal of Human Hypertension* 19, no. 7 (2005): 511–513.
13. S. Mora et al., "Enhanced Risk Assessment in Asymptomatic Individuals with Exercise Testing and Framingham Risk Scores," *Circulation* 112, no. 11 (2005): 1566–1572.
14. G. Hu et al., "Prevalence of the Metabolic Syndrome and Its Relation to All-cause and Cardiovascular Mortality in Non-Diabetic European Men and Women," *Archives of Internal Medicine* 164, no. 10:1066–1076; L. Girman et al., "An Exploratory Analysis of Criteria for the Metabolic Syndrome and ITS Prediction of Cardiovascular Outcomes: The Hoorn Study," *American Journal of Epidemiology* 162, no. 5 (2005): 438–447; J. Ford et al., "Risks for All-Cause Mortality, Cardiovascular Disease, and Diabetes Associated with the Metabolic Syndrome: A Summary of Evidence," *Diabetes Care* 28, no. 7 (2005): 1769–1778; J. Bertrais et al., "Sedentary Behaviors, Physical Activity, and Metabolic Syndrome in Middle-aged French Subjects," *Obesity Research* 13, no. 6 (2005): 936–944.
15. American Heart Association, *Heart Disease and Stroke Statistics— 2005.*
16. Ibid.
17. Ibid.
18. Ibid.
19. Ibid.
20. Ibid.
21. Ibid.
22. Ibid.
23. Ibid.
24. Ibid.
25. N. R. Anthonisen et al for the Lung Health Study Research Group, "The Effects of a Smoking Cessation Intervention on 14.5 Year Mortality: A Randomized Controlled Trial," *Annals of Internal Medicine* 142 (2005): 223–239.
26. National Heart, Lung, and Blood Institute, "Third Report of the National Cholesterol Education Program (NCEP) Expert Panel on Detection, Evaluation and Treatment of High Blood Cholesterol in Adults (Adult Treatment Panel III)," May 2001, www.nhlbi.nih. gov/guidelines/cholesterol/index.htm.
27. Ibid.
28. S. M. Marovina et al., "NHLBI Workshop on Lipoprotein(a) and CVD: Recent Advances and Future Directions," 2004, www.nhlbi.nih.gov; A. Ariyo, C. Thach, and R. Tracy, "Lp(a) Lipoprotein, Vascular Disease, and Mortality in the Elderly," *New England Journal of Medicine* 349, no. 22 (2003): 2108–2115.
29. National Heart, Lung, and Blood Institute, "Third Report of the NCEP."
30. Ibid.
31. Center for Disease Control and Prevention, National Center for Health Statistics, "Vital and Health Statistics," series 10 (219), February 2004.
32. L. E. Fields et al, "The Burden of Adult Hypertension in the United States 1999 to 2000: A Rising Tide," *Hypertension* 44 (2004): 1–7.
33. Ibid.
34. Ibid.
35. R. Eliot, "Changing Behavior: A New Comprehensive and Quantitative Approach" (keynote address, Annual Meeting of the American College of Cardiology on Stress and the Heart, Jackson Hole, WY, July 3, 1987).
36. American Heart Association, "Women and Cardiovascular Diseases — Statistics Updated 2005," www.americanheart.org/presenter.jhtml?identifier=3000941.
37. D. Grady et al., "Cardiovascular Disease Outcomes During 6.8 Years of Hormone Therapy: Heart and Estrogen/Progestin Replacement Study Follow-up (HERS II)", *Journal of the American Medical Association* 288, no. 1:11–128.
38. Ibid.
39. Ibid.
40. National Heart, Lung, and Blood Institute, *Heart Memo: The Cardiovascular Health of Women* (Bethesda, MD: Author, 1995), 5.
41. American Heart Association, *Heart Disease and Stroke Facts.*
42. J. E. Willard, R. A. Lange, and D. L. Hillis, "The Use of Aspirin in Ischemic Heart Disease," *New England Journal of Medicine* 327 (1992): 175–179.
43. Agency for Healthcare Policy and Research, *Cardiac Rehabilitation: Exercise, Training, Education, Counseling, and Behavioral Interventions* (Publication #96-0672) (Rockville, MD: Author, 1996).

Does being overweight cause cancer?

Is a tanning booth safer than the sun?

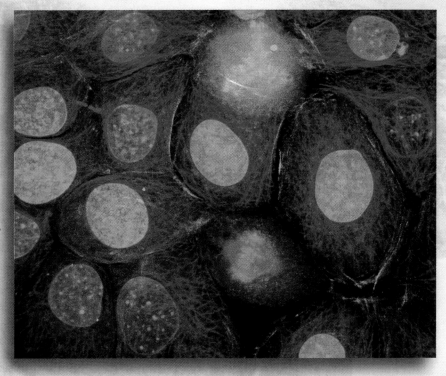

If I am already a smoker, will quitting now reduce my risk of lung cancer?

What are some ways cancer is detected?

13

Cancer
Reducing Your Risk

Objectives

- **Define** cancer, and understand its causes and how it develops.
- **Describe** the different types of cancer and the risks they pose to people at different ages and stages of life.
- **Explain** the importance of self-exams, medical exams, and recognizing symptoms related to different types

of cancer. Explain the importance of early detection.
- **Discuss** cancer diagnosis and treatment, including radiation therapy, chemotherapy, immunotherapy, and other common methods of detection and treatment.

In February 2005 a startling chronic disease statistic was revealed: cancer has become the leading cause of death for Americans under the age of 85, overtaking heart disease for the first time ever.[1] According to American Cancer Society data, 476,009 Americans under 85 died of cancer, compared to 450,637 who died of heart disease deaths. Why was this news surprising to public health experts? Cancer-related mortality rates have declined over the last decade and five-year survival rates (the relative survival rates in persons who are living cancer-free five years after diagnosis) for all cancers diagnosed between 1995 and 2000 were 64 percent, up dramatically from the 50 percent survivals in the 1970s.[2] However, while cancer-related deaths have declined over the last decade, they have not declined as quickly as deaths related to heart disease. New drug regimens, surgical techniques, and other anti–heart disease measures have been largely responsible for declines in heart disease (see Chapter 12). Although noteworthy improvements have been made in many cancer survival rates, certain cancers such as pancreatic and liver, remain particularly resistant to treatment.

Despite recent data, there is still hope in the battle against cancer. Our arsenal of weapons against cancer grows daily, and new research into causes and possible methods of prevention and treatment provides new hope for survivors. Early detection and vast improvements in technology have dramatically improved prognosis for many cancer patients. We also know that there are many actions we can take individually and as a society to prevent cancer. Knowing the facts about cancer, recognizing your own risk, and taking action to reduce your risk are important steps in the battle.

Cancer   A large group of diseases characterized by the uncontrolled growth and spread of abnormal cells.

Neoplasm   A new growth of tissue that serves no physiological function and results from uncontrolled, abnormal cellular development.

Tumor   A neoplasmic mass that grows more rapidly than surrounding tissue.

Malignant   Very dangerous or harmful; refers to a cancerous tumor.

Benign   Harmless; refers to a noncancerous tumor.

Biopsy   Microscopic examination of tissue to determine if a cancer is present.

Metastasis   Process by which cancer spreads from one area to another in the body.

Mutant cells   Cells that differ in form, quality, or function from normal cells.

AN OVERVIEW OF CANCER

What Is Cancer?

Cancer is the name given to a large group of diseases characterized by the uncontrolled growth and spread of abnormal cells.[3] Think of a healthy cell as a small computer programmed to operate in a particular fashion. Under normal conditions, healthy cells are protected by a powerful overseer, the immune system, as they perform their daily functions of growing, replicating, and repairing body organs. When something interrupts normal cell programming, however, uncontrolled growth and abnormal cellular development result in a new growth of tissue serving no physiological function—a **neoplasm.** This neoplasmic mass often forms a clumping of cells known as a **tumor.**

Not all tumors are **malignant** (cancerous); in fact, most are **benign** (noncancerous). Benign tumors are generally harmless unless they grow in such a fashion that they obstruct or crowd out normal tissues. A benign tumor of the brain, for instance, is life threatening if it grows enough to restrict blood flow and cause a stroke. The only way to determine whether a given tumor or mass is malignant is through **biopsy,** or microscopic examination of cell development.

Benign and malignant tumors differ in several key ways. Benign tumors generally consist of ordinary-looking cells enclosed in a fibrous shell or capsule that prevents their spreading to other body areas. Malignant tumors are usually not enclosed in a protective capsule and can therefore spread to other organs. This process, known as **metastasis,** makes some forms of cancer particularly aggressive in their ability to overcome the body's defenses. By the time they are diagnosed, malignant tumors have frequently metastasized throughout the body, which makes treatment extremely difficult. Unlike benign tumors, which merely expand to take over a given space, malignant cells invade surrounding tissue and emit clawlike protrusions that disturb the RNA and DNA within normal cells. Disrupting these substances, which control cellular metabolism and reproduction, produces **mutant cells** that differ in form, quality, and function from normal cells. Assess your own cancer risk by completing the Assess Yourself box on page 354.

Who Gets Cancer?

The American Cancer Society estimates that in 2005, more than 1,372,910 new cancer cases will be diagnosed, and about 570,280 Americans will die of cancer. Today, cancer accounts for nearly 1 of every 4 deaths, and untold pain and suffering for patients and their loved ones. Of these cancers, one-third are believed to be related to poor nutrition, physical inactivity and obesity, which means that they could have been prevented. Heredity, behavioral factors such as cigarette smoking,

Table 13.1

Table 13.1
Probability of Developing Invasive Cancers Over Selected Age Intervals, by Sex, United States, 1999–2001[*]

		Birth to 39 (%)	40 to 59 (%)	60 to 79 (%)
All sites[†]	Male	1.41	8.52	34.63
	Female	1.97	9.10	22.51
Breast	Female	0.48	4.18	7.49
Colon and rectum	Male	0.07	0.90	3.96
	Female	0.06	0.69	3.04
Lung and bronchus	Male	0.03	1.06	5.75
	Female	0.03	0.81	3.91
Melanoma of skin	Male	0.13	0.51	1.08
	Female	0.21	0.40	0.53
Prostate	Male	0.01	2.58	14.76

[*]For those free of cancer at beginning of age interval. Based on cancer cases diagnosed during 1999–2001.
[†]All sites exclude basal and squamous cell skin cancers and in situ carcinomas except urinary bladder.
Source: DEVCAN: Probability of Developing or Dying of Cancer Software, Version 5.2. Statistical Research and Applications Branch, National Cancer Institute, 2004, http://srab.cancer.gov/devcan; American Cancer Society, Surveillance Research, 2005.

certain dietary patterns, certain infectious agents, environmental exposures, stress, and a host of other factors combine to contribute to cancer development. How great is your risk? Table 13.1 helps put this into perspective. Age and gender have a great deal to do with who gets cancer and who does not. For example, women under age 39 have a relatively low rate of breast cancer (1 in 207). However, women aged 60 and older face a dramatic increase in risk of breast cancer, at 1 in 13.[4]

Disparities in Cancer Rates

There are many demographic and socioeconomic factors associated with health-related disparities, including income, race/ethnicity, culture, geography (urban vs. rural), age, sex, sexual orientation, and literacy.[5] The Institute of Medicine (IOM) has published a comprehensive review of racial and ethnic disparities in health care.[6]

Poverty is widely believed to be the most important factor affecting health and longevity. People from lower socioeconomic levels tend to smoke more and are greater targets for predatory tobacco marketing, are more likely to be obese and sedentary, have less access to healthy fruits and vegetables, are often under- or uninsured and therefore lack access to health care, may not be able to afford medications or health care, and have difficulty communicating with their health care providers.[7] Cultural factors, including ability to speak English, beliefs about the benefits and risks of treatment, beliefs about illness, and other factors may also affect the ability to access quality health care.

How serious are the disparities? Consider the following:[8]

- Of all racial or ethnic groups in the United States, African Americans have the highest death rates from all cancer sites combined and from malignancies of the lung and bronchus, colon and rectum, female breast, prostate, and uterine cervix. Death rates for African American males are 1.4 times higher than whites, and for females, they are 1.2 times higher.

- African Americans, American Indians, Alaska Natives, and Asian American and Pacific Island women have a lower five-year survival than non-Hispanic whites.

- A person living in an affluent census tract has a five-year survival rate that is 10 percent higher than a person living in a tract below the poverty level; 24 percent of African Americans live below the poverty line, compared to 8 percent of non-Hispanic whites.

- Thirty-two percent of Hispanics and 20 percent of African Americans have no medical insurance.

- Men from poorer census counties have a 22 percent higher death rate from prostate cancer than their affluent county comparison groups.

To reduce these disparities, the American Cancer Society plans to increase advocacy, research, and education. The goal is to help those who are subject to disparities navigate and utilize the health care system in the hope of improving outcome for cancer patients and reducing risk.

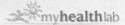

Fill out this assessment online at
www.aw-bc.com/myhealthlab or www.aw-bc.com/donatelle.

Cancer: Understanding Your Personal Risk

Although you may be predisposed to some types of cancer due to genetic, biological, and/or environmental causes, there are many more that may be prevented through lifestyle changes and risk reduction strategies. If you carefully assess your risks, you can then make behavior changes that may make you less susceptible to various cancers. The following questions will give you an indication of your susceptibility. Of course, no single instrument can serve as a complete risk assessment or diagnostic guide. These questions merely serve as the basis for personal introspection and thoughtful planning about ways to reduce your risk.

Read each question and circle the number in parentheses next to your response. Be honest and accurate in order to get the most complete understanding of your cancer risks. Individual scores for specific questions should not be interpreted as a precise measure of relative risk, but the totals in each section give a general indication of your risk.

	Yes	No
Section 1: Breast Cancer		
1. Do you check your breasts at least monthly using breast self-examination (BSE) procedures?	1	2
2. Do you look at your breasts in the mirror regularly, checking for any irregular indentations/lumps, discharge from the nipples, or other noticeable changes	1	2
3. Has your mother, sister, or daughter been diagnosed with breast cancer?	1	2
4. Have you ever been pregnant?	1	2
5. Have you had a history of lumps or cysts in your breasts or underarm?	1	2

Total Points _____

	Yes	No
Section 2: Skin Cancer		
1. Do you spend a lot of time in the sun, either at work or at play?	1	2
2. Do you use sunscreens with an SPF rating of 15 or more when you are in the sun?	1	2
3. Do you use tanning beds or sun booths regularly to maintain a tan?	1	2
4. Do you examine your skin once a month, checking any moles or other irregularities, particularly in hard-to-see areas such as your back, genitals, neck, and under your hair?	1	2
5. Do you purchase and wear sunglasses that adequately filter out harmful sun rays?	1	2

Total Points _____

Section 3: Cancers of the Reproductive System

	Yes	No
MEN		
1. Do you examine your penis regularly for unusual bumps or growths?	1	2
2. Do you perform regular testicular self-examination?	1	2
3. Do you have a family history of prostate or testicular cancer?	1	2
4. Do you practice safer sex and wear condoms with every sexual encounter?	1	2
5. Do you avoid exposure to harmful environmental hazards such as mercury, coal tars, benzene, chromate, and vinyl chloride?	1	2

Total Points _____

	Yes	No
WOMEN		
1. Do you have a regularly scheduled Pap test?	1	2
2. Have you been infected with the human papillomavirus, Epstein-Barr virus, or other viruses believed to increase cancer risk?	1	2
3. Has your mother, sister, or daughter been diagnosed with breast, cervical, endometrial, or ovarian cancer (particularly at a young age)?	1	2
4. Do you practice safer sex and use condoms with every sexual encounter?	1	2
5. Are you obese, taking estrogen, and/or consuming a diet that is very high in saturated fats?	1	2

Total Points _____

	Yes	No

Section 4: Cancers in General

	Yes	No
1. Do you smoke cigarettes on most days of the week?	1	2
2. Do you consume a diet that is rich in fruits and vegetables?	1	2
3. Are you obese and/or do you lead a primarily sedentary lifestyle?	1	2
4. Do you live in an area with high air pollution levels and/or work in a job where you are exposed to several chemicals on a regular basis?	1	2
5. Are you careful about the amount of animal fat in your diet, substituting olive oil or canola oil for animal fat whenever possible?	1	2
6. Do you limit your overall consumption of alcohol?	1	2
7. Do you eat foods rich in lycopenes (such as tomatoes) and antioxidants?	1	2
8. Are you "body aware" and alert for changes in your body?	1	2
9. Do you have a family history of ulcers or of colorectal, stomach cancer, or other digestive system cancers?	1	2
10. Do you avoid unnecessary exposure to radiation, cell phone emissions, and microwave emissions?	1	2

Total Points _____

ANALYZING YOUR SCORES

Take a careful look at each question for which you received a "2" score. Are there any areas in which you received mostly "2s"? Did you receive total points of 6 or higher in Sections 1 through 3? Did you receive total points of 11 or higher in Section 4? If so, you have at least one identifiable risk. The higher the score, the more risks you may have.

However, rather than focusing just on your score, focus on which items you might change. Review the suggestions throughout this chapter and list actions that you could take right now that might help you reduce your risk for these cancers.

Make It Happen!

Assessment: The Assess Yourself activity above identifies certain behaviors that can contribute to increased cancer risks. If you have identified particular behaviors that may be putting you at risk, consider steps you can take to change these behaviors and improve your future health.

Making a Change: In order to change your behavior, you need to develop a plan. Follow these steps below and complete your Behavior Change Contract to take action.

1. Evaluate your behavior, and identify patterns and specific things you are doing. What can you change now? What can you change in the near future?
2. Select one pattern of behavior that you want to change.
3. Fill out the Behavior Change Contract found at the front of your book. It should include your long-term goal for change, your short-term goals, the rewards you'll give yourself for reaching these goals, potential obstacles along the way, and strategies for overcoming these obstacles. For each goal, list the small steps and specific actions that you will take.
4. Chart your progress in a journal. At the end of a week, consider how successful you were in following your plan. What helped you be successful? What made change more difficult? What will you do differently next week?

5. Revise your plan as needed. Are the short-term goals attainable? Are the rewards satisfying?

Example: Keisha's assessment showed that, while she was taking precautions to reduce her cancer risk in most areas, she was not doing what she should about her breast cancer risk. Her score in this area was 8, because she did not regularly examine her breasts, her mother had been diagnosed with breast cancer two years ago, and she had never been pregnant. Keisha decided she needed to learn how to examine her breasts and to make a plan to ensure she did it every month. After studying this textbook's illustrations, she made an appointment with her gynecologist. While she was there, she asked the doctor to confirm that she was doing the examination correctly.

Next, Keisha decided that she would spend the first ten minutes of her morning once a month to do the exam and that she would give herself a reward for each month that she examined herself on schedule. On her way to campus after doing the exam, she would treat herself to a latte and a scone. After she stuck with her schedule for six months in a row, she would buy herself a new outfit. She also resolved to talk to her younger sister, who was also at risk, about the importance of the exam.

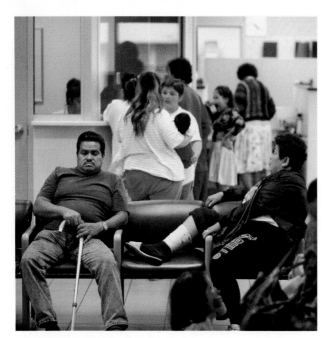

Ethnic and racial minorities often have no health insurance and have difficulty obtaining the type of regular medical care and prevention education that plays a role in reducing the overall risk of cancer.

WHAT CAUSES CANCER?

After decades of research, most cancer epidemiologists believe that cancers are preventable, at least in theory, and many could be avoided by suitable choices in lifestyle and environment.[9] Many specific causes of cancer are well documented, the most important of which are smoking, obesity, and a few organic viruses. However, wide global variations in common cancers, such as those of the breast, prostate, colon, and rectum, remain unexplained (Figure 13.1.)

Most research supports the idea that cancer is caused by both *external* (chemicals, radiation, viruses, and lifestyle) and *internal* (hormones, immune conditions, and inherited mutations) factors. Causal factors may act together or in sequence to promote cancer development. We do not know why some people have malignant cells in their body and never develop cancer while others may take ten years or more to develop the disease.

Carcinogens   Cancer-causing agents.

Oncogenes   Suspected cancer-causing genes present on chromosomes.

Protooncogenes   Genes that can become oncogenes under certain conditions.

Cellular Change/Mutation Theories

One theory of cancer development proposes that cancer results from spontaneous errors that occur during cell reproduction. Perhaps cells that are overworked or aged are more likely to break down, causing genetic errors that result in mutant cells.

Another theory suggests that cancer is caused by some external agent or agents that enter a normal cell and initiate the cancerous process. Numerous environmental factors, such as radiation, chemicals, hormonal drugs, immunosuppressant drugs (drugs that suppress the normal activity of the immune system), and other toxins, are considered possible **carcinogens** (cancer-causing agents); perhaps the most common carcinogen is the tar in cigarettes. The greater the dose or exposure to environmental hazards, the greater the risk of disease. People who are forced to work, live, and pass through areas that have high levels of environmental toxins may be at greater risk for several types of cancers.[10]

A third theory came out of research on certain viruses that are believed to cause tumors in animals. Scientists discovered **oncogenes,** suspected cancer-causing genes that are present on chromosomes. Although oncogenes are typically dormant, scientists hypothesized that certain conditions such as age, stress, and exposure to carcinogens, viruses, and radiation may activate them. Once activated, they grow and reproduce in an out-of-control manner.

Scientists are uncertain whether only people who develop cancer have oncogenes or whether we all have **protooncogenes,** genes that can become oncogenes under certain conditions. Many physicians who specialize in the treatment of malignancies believe that the oncogene theory may lead to a greater understanding of how individual cells function and bring us closer to developing effective treatments.

Many factors are believed to contribute to cancer, and combining risk factors can dramatically increase a person's risk of the disease.

Risks for Cancer: Lifestyle

Anyone can develop cancer; however, most cases affect adults beginning in middle age. In fact, nearly 80 percent of cancers are diagnosed at ages 55 and over.

Cancer researchers refer to one's *cancer risk* when they assess risk factors. *Lifetime risk* refers to the probability that an individual, over the course of a lifetime, will develop cancer or die from it. In the United States, men have a lifetime risk of about one in two; women have a lower risk of one in three.[11]

Relative risk is a measure of the strength of the relationship between risk factors and a particular cancer. Basically, relative risk compares your risk if you engage in certain known risk behaviors with that of someone who does not engage in such behaviors. For example, if you are a male and smoke, you have a 20-fold relative risk of developing lung cancer compared to a non-smoker: your chances of getting lung cancer are about 20 times greater.[12]

Over the years, researchers have found that people who engage in certain behaviors show a higher incidence of cancer. In particular, diet, sedentary lifestyle (and resultant obesity), consumption of alcohol or cigarettes, stress, and other lifestyle factors seem to play a role. Likewise, colon and rectal cancer occur more frequently among persons with a high-fat, low-fiber diet; in those who don't eat enough fruits and vegetables; and in those who are inactive. (See Chapter 9 for more information on healthy nutrition.)

Keep in mind that a high relative risk does not guarantee cause and effect. It merely indicates the likelihood of a particular risk factor being related to a particular outcome.

Smoking and Cancer Risk

Of all the potential risk factors for cancer, smoking is among the greatest; it is the leading cause of preventable death in the world today. In the United States, tobacco is responsible for nearly one in five deaths annually. Nearly one-half of all Americans who smoke will die from a tobacco-related illness.[13] Trying to quit? See Chapter 8 for more information on smoking cessation strategies.

Recent declines in smoking have likely had a direct effect on the overall decrease in lung cancer rates; however, lung cancer remains the leading cause of cancer death in men and women.[14] (See Chapter 8 for more on global trends in tobacco use.)

Researchers once believed that cigarettes caused only cancers of the lung, pancreas, bladder, and kidney, and (synergistically with alcohol) the larynx, mouth, pharynx, and esophagus. However, recent evidence indicates that several other types of cancer are also related to tobacco. Most notably, cancers of the stomach, liver, and cervix seem to be directly related to long-term smoking.

Obesity and Cancer Risk

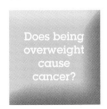

It is difficult to sort through the accumulated evidence about the role of nutrients, obesity, sedentary lifestyle, and related variables. Nevertheless, research points to a potential cancer link. Cancer is more common among people who are overweight, and risk increases as obesity increases. A recent study of over 900,000 U.S. adults indicates a significant relationship between a high body mass index and death rates for cancers such as esophagus, colon, rectum, liver, kidney, and pancreas. Women with a high BMI have a higher mortality rate from breast, uterine, cervical and ovarian cancers; men with a high BMI have higher death rates from

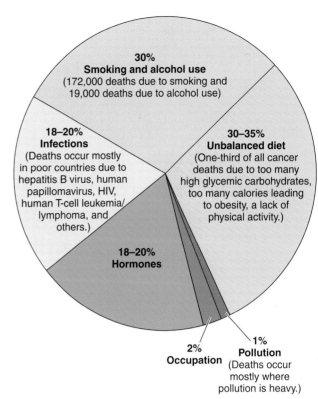

Figure 13.1 ■ **Factors Believed to Contribute to Global Causes of Cancer**

Sources: S. Heacht et al., Public Session/Panel Discussion (Linus Pauling Institute International Conference on Diet and Optimum Health, Portland, OR, May 2001); American Cancer Society, *Cancer Facts and Figures 2005* (Atlanta: American Cancer Society, 2005).

prostate and stomach cancers. In this study, 34 percent of all cancer deaths were attributable to overweight and obesity.[15] A number of other studies also support the link between cancer and obesity:[16]

■ The relative risk of breast cancer in postmenopausal women is 50 percent higher for obese women.

■ The relative risk of colon cancer in men is 40 percent higher for obese men.

■ The relative risks of gallbladder and endometrial cancer are five times higher in obese individuals compared to individuals of "healthy" weight.

Biological Factors

Early theorists believed that we inherit a genetic predisposition toward certain forms of cancer. Cancers of the breast, stomach, colon, prostate, uterus, ovaries, and lungs appear to run in families. For example, a woman runs a much higher risk of breast cancer if her mother, sisters, or daughters (primary relatives) have had the disease, particularly if they had it at a young age. Hodgkin's disease and certain leukemias show similar familial patterns. Can we attribute these patterns to genetic susceptibility? To date, the research in this area is inconclusive. It is possible that we can inherit a

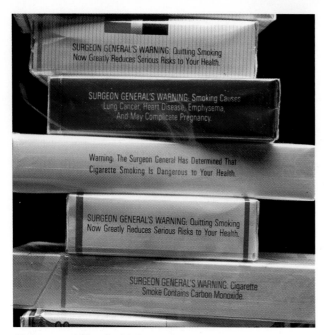
Of the several lifestyle risk factors for cancer, tobacco use is perhaps the most significant and the most preventable.

tendency toward a cancer-prone, weak immune system or, conversely, that we can inherit a cancer-fighting potential. But the complex interaction of hereditary predisposition, lifestyle, and environment on the development of cancer makes it a challenge to determine a single cause.

Gender also affects the likelihood of developing certain forms of cancer. For example, breast cancer occurs primarily among females, although men do occasionally get breast cancer. However, while gender plays a role in certain cases of cancer, other variables such as lifestyle are probably more significant.

Reproductive and Hormonal Risks for Cancer The effects of reproductive factors on breast and cervical cancer have been well-documented. Pregnancy and estrogen supplementation in the form of oral contraceptives or hormone replacement therapy increase a woman's chances of breast cancer. Late menarche, early menopause, early first childbirth, and high parity (having many children) have been shown to reduce a woman's risk of breast cancer. A higher risk of endometrial cancer is also associated with hormone replacement therapy.[17]

Breast cancer is much more common in most Western countries than in developing countries. This is partly—and perhaps largely—accounted for by dietary effects (consuming a diet high in calories and fat), combined with later first childbirth, lower parity (having fewer children), shorter breastfeeding, and higher obesity rates.[18]

Environmental Cancer Risks Environmental factors such as smoking, diet, and infectious diseases, as well as chemicals and radiation, cause an estimated three-quarters of all cancer deaths in the United States. As indicated earlier, tobacco, obesity and physical activity are major sources of risk when compared to trace levels of pollution in food, drinking water, contact exposures, and air. However, the degree of risk from pollutants depends on the concentration, intensity, and duration of exposure. If you live and work in close proximity to carcinogens or handle them through work activity, you face an increased risk. Working with herbicides and pesticides, certain metals, and several chemicals (benzene, asbestos, vinyl chloride, arsenic, and aflatoxin) have been shown to cause cancer in humans. Others, such as DDT (the insecticide), formaldehyde, polychlorinated biphenyls (PCBs), and polycyclic aromatic hydrocarbons are highly suspect carcinogens.[19]

Radiation: Ionizing and Nonionizing
Ionizing radiation (IR)—radiation from X rays, radon, cosmic rays, and ultraviolet (UV) radiation (primarily ultraviolet B, or UVB, radiation)—is the only form of radiation proven to cause human cancer (see the section on skin cancer). Evidence that high-dose IR causes cancer comes from studies of atomic bomb survivors, patients receiving radiotherapy, and certain occupational groups (for example, uranium miners). Virtually any part of the body can be affected by IR, but bone marrow and the thyroid are particularly susceptible. Radon exposures in homes can increase lung cancer risk, especially in cigarette smokers. To reduce the risk of harmful effects, diagnostic medical and dental X rays are set at the lowest dose levels possible. Nonionizing radiation–producing items such as cell phones, microwaves, electric blankets, and other products have been a topic of great concern in recent years, but research has not proven excess risk to date.[20]

Social and Psychological Factors Many researchers claim that social and psychological factors play a major role in determining whether a person gets cancer. Stress has been implicated in increased susceptibility to several types of cancers. By reducing stress levels in your daily life, you may, in fact, lower your risk for cancer. A number of therapists have even established preventive treatment centers where the primary focus is on being happy and thinking positive thoughts. However, to date, no controlled studies have proven that laughter or positive thoughts can reduce cancer risks.

Although medical personnel are skeptical of overly simplistic solutions, we cannot rule out the possibility that negative emotional states contribute to illness. People who are under chronic, severe stress or who suffer from depression or other persistent emotional problems show higher rates of cancer than their healthy counterparts. Sleep disturbances, diet, or a combination of factors may weaken the body's immune system, increasing susceptibility to cancer. Although psychological factors may play a part in cancer development, exposure to

Table 13.2

Preventing Cancer through Diet and Lifestyle

Type of Cancer	Factors that Decrease Risk	Factors that Increase Risk
Breast	Engage in physical activity for at least 4 hours per week; consume lots of fruits and vegetables	Obesity and weight gain; alcohol consumption; hormone replacement therapy
Colorectal	Engage in regular, moderate physical activity; consume lots of fruits and vegetables	High intake of red meat; smoking; alcohol consumption; obesity
Lung	Consume at least 5 servings of fruits and vegetables daily	Tobacco use; some occupations
Oral/Throat	Consume at least 5 servings of fruits and vegetables daily; engage in regular, moderate physical activity	Tobacco use; obesity; alcohol consumption; salted foods
Prostate	Consume at least 5 servings of fruits and vegetables daily	High intake of red meat and high-fat dairy products
Stomach	Consume at least 5 servings of fruits and vegetables daily; refrigerate food	Salted foods; *Helicobacter pylori* bacteria

Here are some additional tips issued by a panel of cancer researchers:
- Avoid being underweight or overweight, and limit weight gain during adulthood to less than 11 pounds.
- If you don't get much exercise at work, take a 1-hour brisk walk or similar exercise daily, and exercise vigorously for at least 1 hour a week.
- Eat 8 or more servings a day of cereals and grains (such as rice, corn, breads, and pasta), legumes (such as peas), roots (such as beets, radishes, and carrots), tubers (such as potatoes), and plantains (including bananas).
- Limit consumption of refined sugar.
- Limit alcoholic drinks to less than 2 a day for men and 1 for women.
- Limit intake of red meat to less than 3 ounces a day, if eaten at all.
- Limit consumption of salted foods and use of cooking and table salt. Use herbs and spices to season foods.

Sources: World Cancer Research Fund, American Institute for Cancer Research, "Food, Nutrition and the Prevention of Cancer," www.wecf-uk.org; American Cancer Society, "The Complete Guide: Nutrition and Physical Activity," www.cancer.org.

substances such as tobacco and alcohol is far more important. Cancers of the mouth and throat pose significant risks for smokers.[21]

Chemicals in Foods

Among the food additives suspected of causing cancer is *sodium nitrate*, a chemical used to preserve and give color to red meat. Research indicates that the actual carcinogen is not sodium nitrate but *nitrosamines*, substances formed when the body digests the chemical. Sodium nitrate has not been banned, primarily because it kills the bacterium *Clostridium botulinum*, which causes botulism, a highly virulent foodborne disease. It should also be noted that the bacteria found in the human intestinal tract may contain more nitrates than a person could ever take in from eating cured meats or other nitrate-containing food products. Nonetheless, concern about the carcinogenic properties of nitrates has led to the introduction of meats that are nitrate-free or contain reduced nitrate levels.

There is also concern about the possible harm caused by pesticide and herbicide residues. Although some of these chemicals cause cancer at high doses in experimental animals, the very low concentrations found in some foods are well within established government safety levels. Continued research regarding pesticide and herbicide use is essential, and the continuous monitoring of agricultural practices is necessary to ensure a safe food supply. Scientists and consumer groups stress the importance of a balance between chemical use and the production of quality food products. Prevention efforts should focus on policies to protect consumers, develop low-chemical pesticides and herbicides, and reduce environmental pollution. See Table 13.2 for more information on preventing cancer through diet and lifestyle.

Infectious Diseases and Cancer

According to recent estimates, 17 percent of new cancers worldwide will be attributable to infection in 2005.[22] Infections are thought to influence cancer development in several ways, most commonly through chronic inflammation, suppression of the immune system, and/or chronic stimulation.

HBV, HCV, and Liver Cancer Viruses such as hepatitis B (HBV) and C (HCV) are believed to stimulate cancer cells in the liver because they are chronic diseases that cause inflammation of liver tissue. This may prime the liver for cancer or make it more hospitable for cancer development. Global increases in HBV and HCV rates and concurrent increases in liver cancer rates seem to provide evidence of such an association.

HPV and Cervical Cancer Nearly 100 percent of women with cervical cancer have evidence of human papillomavirus (HPV) infection, believed to be a major cause of cervical cancer. Fortunately, only a small percentage of HPV cases progress to cervical cancer.[23]

Medical Factors

Some medical treatments increase the risk of cancer. One famous example is the prescription drug *diethylstilbestrol (DES),* widely used from 1940 to 1960 to control problems with bleeding during pregnancy and reduce the risk of miscarriage. Not until the 1970s did the dangers of this drug became apparent. Although DES caused few side effects in the millions of women who took it, their daughters were found to have an increased risk for cancer of the reproductive organs. Another example is the use of estrogen in treating menopausal symptoms, which has been the basis for numerous conflicting reports on cancer risk over the years. Ironically, another medical factor is chemotherapy, which while being used to treat one cancer may increase the patient's risk of other forms of cancer.

What Do You Think?

How do we determine whether a given factor is a risk factor for a disease? ■ Although a direct causal relationship between lung cancer and smoking has not been proved, the evidence supporting such a relationship is strong. Must a clearly established causal link exist before consumers are warned about risk? ■ How does the consumer know what to believe?

TYPES OF CANCERS

As mentioned earlier, the term *cancer* refers not to a single disease but to hundreds of different diseases. They are grouped into four broad categories based on the type of tissue from which the cancer arises.

Oncologists Physicians who specialize in the treatment of malignancies.

Classifications of Cancer

- *Carcinomas.* Epithelial tissues (tissues covering body surfaces and lining most body cavities) are the most common sites for cancers. Carcinomas of the breast, lung, intestines, skin, and mouth are examples. These cancers affect the outer layer of the skin and mouth as well as the mucous membranes. They metastasize through the circulatory or lymphatic system initially and form solid tumors.

- *Sarcomas.* Sarcomas occur in the mesodermal, or middle, layers of tissue—for example, in bones, muscles, and general connective tissue. They metastasize primarily via the blood in the early stages of disease. These cancers are less common but generally more virulent than carcinomas. They also form solid tumors.

- *Lymphomas.* Lymphomas develop in the lymphatic system—the infection-fighting regions of the body—and metastasize through the lymphatic system. Hodgkin's disease is an example. Lymphomas also form solid tumors.

- *Leukemias.* Cancer of the blood-forming parts of the body, particularly the bone marrow and spleen, is called leukemia. A nonsolid tumor, leukemia is characterized by an abnormal increase in the number of white blood cells.

Trained **oncologists,** doctors who specialize in cancer treatment, determine the seriousness and general prognosis of a particular cancer. Once laboratory results and clinical observations have been made, cancers are rated by level and stage of development. Those diagnosed as "carcinoma in situ" are localized and often curable. Cancers with higher level, or stage, ratings have spread farther and are less likely to be cured. Figure 13.2 shows the most common cancer sites and the number of annual deaths from each type.

Lung Cancer

Lung cancer killed an estimated 163,510 people in 2005, and it continues to be the leading cancer killer for men and women.[24] Since 1987, more women have died each year from lung cancer than from breast cancer, which for over 40 years had been the major cancer killer in women. As smoking rates have declined over the past 30 years, we have seen significant declines in male lung cancer. These rates have not dropped among women but have recently plateaued.

Symptoms of lung cancer include persistent cough, blood-streaked sputum, chest pain, and recurrent attacks of pneumonia or bronchitis. Treatment depends on the type and stage of the cancer. Surgery, radiation therapy, and chemotherapy are all options. If the cancer is localized, surgery is usually the treatment of choice. If it has spread, surgery is combined with radiation and chemotherapy. Unfortunately, despite advances in

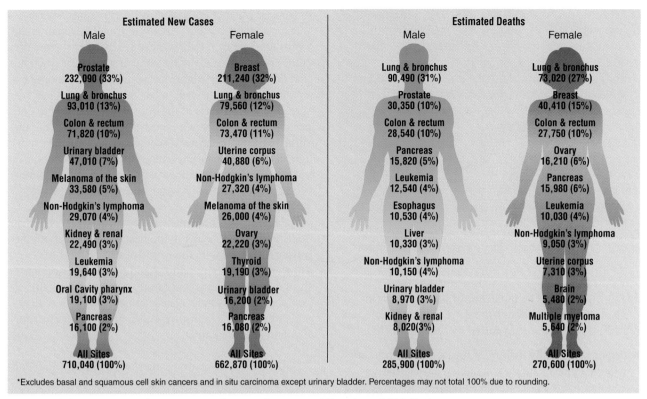

Estimated New Cases

Male	Female
Prostate 232,090 (33%)	Breast 211,240 (32%)
Lung & bronchus 93,010 (13%)	Lung & bronchus 79,560 (12%)
Colon & rectum 71,820 (10%)	Colon & rectum 73,470 (11%)
Urinary bladder 47,010 (7%)	Uterine corpus 40,880 (6%)
Melanoma of the skin 33,580 (5%)	Non-Hodgkin's lymphoma 27,320 (4%)
Non-Hodgkin's lymphoma 29,070 (4%)	Melanoma of the skin 26,000 (4%)
Kidney & renal 22,490 (3%)	Ovary 22,220 (3%)
Leukemia 19,640 (3%)	Thyroid 19,190 (3%)
Oral Cavity pharynx 19,100 (3%)	Urinary bladder 16,200 (2%)
Pancreas 16,100 (2%)	Pancreas 16,080 (2%)
All Sites 710,040 (100%)	All Sites 662,870 (100%)

Estimated Deaths

Male	Female
Lung & bronchus 90,490 (31%)	Lung & bronchus 73,020 (27%)
Prostate 30,350 (10%)	Breast 40,410 (15%)
Colon & rectum 28,540 (10%)	Colon & rectum 27,750 (10%)
Pancreas 15,820 (5%)	Ovary 16,210 (6%)
Leukemia 12,540 (4%)	Pancreas 15,980 (6%)
Esophagus 10,530 (4%)	Leukemia 10,030 (4%)
Liver 10,330 (3%)	Non-Hodgkin's lymphoma 9,050 (3%)
Non-Hodgkin's lymphoma 10,150 (4%)	Uterine corpus 7,310 (3%)
Urinary bladder 8,970 (3%)	Brain 5,480 (2%)
Kidney & renal 8,020 (3%)	Multiple myeloma 5,640 (2%)
All Sites 285,900 (100%)	All Sites 270,600 (100%)

*Excludes basal and squamous cell skin cancers and in situ carcinoma except urinary bladder. Percentages may not total 100% due to rounding.

Figure 13.2 ■ Leading Sites of New Cancer Cases and Deaths—2005 Estimates

Source: Reprinted by permission of the American Cancer Society, *Cancer Facts and Figures 2005* (Atlanta: American Cancer Society, 2005).

medical technology, survival rates for lung cancer have improved only slightly over the past decade. Just 13 percent of lung cancer patients live five or more years after diagnosis. These rates improve to 47 percent with early detection, but only 15 percent of lung cancers are discovered in their early stages.[25]

Prevention Smokers, especially those who have smoked for over 20 years, and people who have been exposed to industrial substances such as arsenic and asbestos or to radiation are at the highest risk for lung cancer. Quitting smoking, and not starting if you don't, are the best measures you can take to prevent lung cancer. Those who quit do reduce their risk of developing cancer and other diseases associated with smoking and will live longer than those who do smoke, regardless of age.[26]

> If I am already a smoker, will quitting now reduce my risk of lung cancer?

Breast Cancer

In 2005, approximately 211,240 women in the United States were diagnosed with invasive breast cancer for the first time. In addition, 58,490 new cases of in situ breast cancer, typically ductal carcinoma in situ (DCIS), a more localized cancer, were diagnosed. The increase in detection of DCIS is a direct result of earlier detection through mammography. In the same year, about

1,690 new cases of breast cancer were diagnosed in men. About 40,410 women (and 460 men) died, making breast cancer the second leading cause of cancer death for women. According to the most recent data, mortality rates went down dramatically from 1990 to 2000, with the largest decrease in women under the age of 50. This decline may be due to earlier diagnosis and better treatment, as numerous studies have shown that early detection increases survival and treatment options.[27]

The earliest signs of breast cancer are usually observable on mammograms, often before lumps can be felt. However, mammograms are not foolproof: regular breast self-examination and careful attention to subtle body changes are important. If a mammogram detects a suspicious mass, a biopsy is performed to provide a more definitive assessment. Once breast cancer has grown to where it can be palpated, symptoms may include persistent breast changes, such as a lump in the breast or surrounding lymph nodes, thickening, dimpling, skin irritation, distortion, retraction or scaliness of the nipple, nipple discharge, or tenderness. Breast pain is commonly due to noncancerous conditions, such as fibrocystic breasts, and is not usually a first symptom. However, any time pain or tenderness persists in the breast or underarm area, it is a good idea to seek medical attention. Women who have ignored this symptom have been shocked to find out later that it was, for them, a sign of cancer.

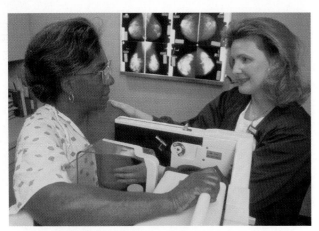

Early detection through mammography and other techniques greatly increases a woman's chance of surviving breast cancer.

Risk Factors The incidence of breast cancer increases with age. Although there are many possible risk factors, those that are supported by research include:[28]

- Personal or family history of breast cancer (primary relatives such as mother, daughter, sister); the younger the relative was when diagnosed, the greater the family risk
- Biopsy-confirmed atypical hyperplasia (excessive increase in the number of cells or tissue growth)
- Long menstrual history (menstrual periods that started early and ended late in life)
- Obesity after menopause
- Recent use of oral contraceptives or postmenopausal estrogens or progestin
- Never having children or having a first child after age 30
- Consuming two or more drinks of alcohol per day
- Higher education and socioeconomic status

Risk factors that need more rigorous research before being firmly established as risks include:[29]

- Consuming a diet high in saturated fats
- Exposure to pesticides and other chemicals
- Weight gain, particularly after menopause
- Physical inactivity
- Genetic predisposition through *BRCA1* and *BRCA2* genes (Genes appear to account for approximately 5 percent of all cases of breast cancer. When counseling is available, screening for these genes is recommended for women with a family history of breast cancer.)

Although risk factors are useful indicators, they do not always predict individual susceptibility. However, because of increased awareness, better diagnostic techniques, and improved treatments, breast cancer patients have a better chance of surviving today. The five-year survival rate for people with localized breast cancer (which includes all people living five years after diagnosis, whether the patient is in remission, disease-free, or under treatment) has risen from 72 percent in the 1940s to 98 percent today. These statistics vary dramatically, however, based on the stage of the cancer when it is first detected. If the cancer has spread to surrounding tissue, the five-year survival rate is 80 percent; if it has spread to distant parts of the body, these rates fall to 26 percent; and if the breast cancer has not spread at all, the survival rate approaches 100 percent. Survival after a diagnosis of breast cancer continues to decline beyond five years. Seventy-seven percent of women diagnosed with breast cancer survive 10 years, and 59 percent survive 15 years.[30]

Patients who become actively involved in treatment decision making, seek out the best oncologists with the most experience with their type of cancer, become knowledgeable about options and treatments, and have the support of friends and family often fare best. Of course, this takes time, access to health care providers, and attention to health-promoting lifestyles before, during, and after treatment.

Prevention A study of the role of exercise in reducing the risk for breast cancer generated much excitement in the scientific community. The study, involving 1,090 women who were 40 or younger (545 with breast cancer and 545 without), analyzed subjects' exercise patterns since they began menstruating. The risk of those who averaged four hours of exercise a week since menstruation was 58 percent lower than that of women who did no exercise at all. Subjects did not have to be avid exercisers to reduce their risk. Researchers speculate that exercise may protect women by altering the production of the ovarian hormones estrogen and progesterone during menstrual cycles.

International differences in breast cancer incidence correlate with variations in diet, especially fat intake, although a causal role for these dietary factors has not been firmly established. A high BMI or sudden weight gain has also been implicated. Exciting new research in susceptibility genes for breast cancer offers new hope for early detection.

Regular self-examination (Figure 13.3) and mammograms are the best ways to detect breast cancer early. The American Cancer Society offers guidelines for how often women should get mammograms and checkups (Table 13.3 on page 364). All women, regardless of age, should be in the habit of breast self-examination every month.

Treatment Today, people with breast cancer (like people with nearly any type of cancer) have many treatment options to choose from. It is important to thoroughly check out a physician's track record and his or her philosophy on the best treatment. Is the physician's recommendation consistent with that of major cancer centers in the country? Check out the doctor's credentials and the experiences of other patients, and do the same for the surgeon who will perform your biopsy and other surgical

How to Examine Your Breasts

The best time for a woman to examine her breasts is when the breasts are not tender or swollen. Women who are pregnant, breast-feeding, or have breast implants can also choose to examine their breasts regularly.

1. Lie down and place your right arm behind your head. The exam is done while lying down, not standing up, because when lying down the breast tissue spreads evenly over the chest wall and it is as thin as possible, making it much easier to feel all the breast tissue.

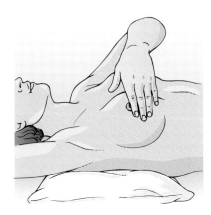

2. Use the finger pads of the three middle fingers on your left hand to feel for lumps in the right breast. Use overlapping dime-sized circular motions of the finger pads to feel the breast tissue.

3. Use three different levels of pressure to feel all the breast tissue. Light pressure is needed to feel the tissue closest to the skin; medium pressure to feel a little deeper; and firm pressure to feel the tissue closest to the chest and ribs. A firm ridge in the lower curve of each breast is normal. If you're not sure how hard to press, talk with your doctor or nurse. Use each pressure level to feel the breast tissue before moving on to the next spot.

4. Move around the breast in an up and down pattern starting at an imaginary line drawn straight down your side from the underarm and moving across the breast to the middle of the chest bone. Be sure to check the entire breast area going down until you feel only ribs and up to the neck or collar bone (clavicle).

   There is some evidence to suggest that the up and down pattern (sometimes called the vertical pattern) is the most effective pattern for covering the entire breast without missing any breast tissue.

5. Repeat the exam on your left breast, using the finger pads of the right hand.

6. While standing in front of a mirror with your hands pressing firmly down on your hips, look at your breasts for any changes of size, shape, contour, or dimpling. (The pressing down on the hips position contracts the chest wall muscles and enhances any breast changes.)

7. Examine each underarm while sitting up or standing and with your arm only slightly raised so you can easily feel in this area. (Raising your arm straight up tightens the tissue in this area and makes it difficult to examine.)

Figure 13.3 ▪ Breast Self-Examination

Follow these instructions for breast self-examination (BSE), the ten-minute habit that could save your life. Note that the American Cancer Society recommends the use of mammography and clinical breast exam in addition to self-examination.

Source: American Cancer Society, "Breast Awareness and Self-Examination," 2004, www.cancer.org/docroot/CRI/content/ CRI_2_4_3X_Can_breast_cancer_be_found_early_5.asp?siterea=.

techniques. If possible, seek a facility that has a significant number of breast cancer patients, does many surgeries, is regarded as a "teaching facility" for new oncologists, has the "latest and greatest" in terms of technology, and is highly regarded by past patients. Nurses are also an important part of hospital care, so be sure to check on their level of knowledge, experience, and nurse-to-patient ratio. Often, cancer support groups can provide invaluable information and advice. Treatments range from a lumpectomy to radical mastectomy to various combinations of radiation or chemotherapy. Among nonsurgical options, promising results have been noted among women using *selective estrogen-receptor modulators (SERMs)* such as tamoxifen and raloxifen, particularly among women whose cancers appear to grow in response to estrogen.[31] Remember that it is always a good idea to seek more than one opinion before making a decision.

Colon and Rectum Cancers

Colorectal cancers (cancers of the colon and rectum) continue to be the third most common cancer in both men and women, with over 145,240 cases diagnosed in 2005.[32] Although colon cancer rates have increased steadily in recent decades, many people are unaware of their risk. In its early stages, colorectal cancer has no symptoms. Bleeding from the rectum, blood in the stool, and changes in bowel habits are the major warning signals.

Anyone can get colorectal cancer, but people who are over age 50, who are obese, who have a family history of colon and rectal cancer, a personal or family history of polyps (benign growths) in the colon or rectum, or inflammatory bowel problems such as colitis run an increased risk. Other possible risk factors include diets high in fat or low in fiber, smoking, sedentary lifestyle, high alcohol consumption, and low intake of fruits and vegetables. Indeed, approximately 90 percent of all colorectal cancers are preventable. Recent studies have suggested that estrogen replacement therapy and nonsteroidal anti-inflammatories such as aspirin may reduce colorectal risk.[33]

Because colorectal cancer tends to spread slowly, the prognosis is quite good if it is caught early. Early screening can detect and remove precancerous polyps

Table 13.3

Recommendations for the Early Detection of Cancer in Asymptomatic People

Site	Recommendation
Cancer-Related Checkup	For individuals undergoing periodic health examinations, a cancer-related checkup should include health counseling and, depending on a person's age, might include examination for cancers of the thyroid, oral cavity, skin, lymph nodes, testes, and ovaries, as well as for some nonmalignant diseases.
Breast	Women 40 and older should have an annual mammogram and an annual clinical breast exam (CBE) performed by a health care professional and should perform monthly breast self-examination (BSE). Ideally, the CBE should occur before the scheduled mammogram.
	Women ages 20–39 should have a CBE performed by a health care professional every 3 years and should perform monthly breast self-examination.
Colon and Rectum	Beginning at age 50, men and women should follow one of the examination schedules below: ■ A fecal occult blood test (FOBT) every year, or ■ A flexible sigmoidoscopy (FSIG) every five years, or ■ Annual fecal occult blood test and flexible sigmoidoscopy every 5 years.* ■ A double-contrast barium enema every 5 to 10 years. ■ A colonoscopy every 10 years.
Prostate	The American Cancer Society recommends that both the prostate-specific antigen (PSA) blood test and the digital rectal examination be offered annually, beginning at age 50, to men who have a life expectancy of at least 10 more years.
	Men at high risk (African American men and men with a strong family history of one or more primary relatives diagnosed with prostate cancer at an early age) should begin testing at age 45.
	Information should be provided to patients about what is known and what is uncertain about the benefits and limitations of early detection and treatment of prostate cancer, so that they can make an informed decision.
Uterus	**Cervix:** Screening should begin approximately 3 years after a woman begins having vaginal intercourse, but no later than 21 years of age. Screening should be done every year with Pap tests or every 2 years using liquid-based tests. At or after age 30, women who have had 3 normal tests in a row may get screened every 2–3 years, unless they have certain risk factors, such as HIV infection or a weak immune system.
	Endometrium: The American Cancer Society recommends that all women should be informed about the risks and symptoms of endometrial cancer, and strongly encouraged to report any unexpected bleeding or spotting to their physicians. Annual screening for endometrial cancer with endometrial biopsy beginning at age 35 should be offered to women with or at risk for hereditary nonpolyposis colon cancer (HNPCC).

*Combined testing is preferred over either annual FOBT or FSIG every 5 years alone. People who are at moderate or high risk for colorectal cancer should talk with a doctor about a different testing schedule.
Source: American Cancer Society, *Cancer Facts and Figures 2005* (Atlanta: American Cancer Society, 2005). Reprinted with permission.

and diagnose disease at more treatable stages. However, in spite of major educational campaigns, only 21 percent of all Americans over age 50 have had the most basic screening test—the fecal occult blood test—in the last five years, and 33 percent have had a colonoscopy during that same time period. Colonoscopy or barium enemas are recommended screening tests for at-risk populations and everybody over age 50.

Treatment often consists of radiation or surgery. Chemotherapy, although not used extensively in the past, is today a possibility. A permanent *colostomy,* the creation of an abdominal opening to eliminate body wastes, is seldom required for people with colon cancer and even less frequently for those with rectum cancer.

African Americans appear to have the highest risk of colorectal cancer, followed by whites, Asians/Pacific Islanders, American Indians/Alaska Natives, and Hispanics.[34]

Prevention and Screening Regular exercise, a diet with lots of fruits and plant-origin foods, a healthy weight, and moderation in alcohol consumption appear to be among the most promising prevention strategies. New research also suggests that aspirin-like drugs, postmenopausal hormones, folic acid, calcium supplements, selenium, and vitamin E may also contribute to prevention; however, more research must be conducted to conclusively determine if and how these substances reduce risk.[35]

Prostate Cancer

The prostate is a muscular, walnut-sized gland that surrounds part of the urethra, the tube that transports urine and sperm out of the body. Cancer of the prostate is the most common cancer in American males today (excluding skin cancer) and the second leading cause of cancer death in men, after lung cancer. In 2005, about 232,090 new cases of prostate cancer were diagnosed nationwide. About 1 man in 6 will be diagnosed with prostate cancer during his lifetime, but only 1 man in 33 will die of it.[36] Put into perspective, prostate cancer accounts for about 10 percent of cancer-related deaths in men each year.

Symptoms Most symptoms of prostate cancer mimic signs of infection or an enlarged prostate. Symptoms include weak or interrupted urine flow; difficulty starting or stopping urination; feeling the urge to urinate frequently; pain upon urination; blood in the urine; or pain in the lower back, pelvis, or thighs. Many men have no symptoms in the early stages, which is why testing and early diagnosis are so important. Most prostate cancers grow slowly and are believed to take years to develop. New research that is particularly relevant to college-age men has found that prostate cancer may begin with a condition called *prostatic intraephithelial neoplasia (PIN)*. In this condition, there are changes in the microscopic appearance of prostate gland cells, ranging from a bit different than normal to abnormal; PIN may appear in men in their twenties, and by the time men reach age 50, nearly 50 percent of them have these changes.[37]

Risk Factors Several factors appear to increase the risk of prostate cancer, including:[38]

- *Age.* More than 70 percent of cancers are diagnosed in men over the age of 65. Usually the disease has progressed to the point of displaying symptoms in these older men, or they receive a screening test.

- *Race.* African American men are 60 percent more likely to develop prostate cancer than white men and are much more likely to be diagnosed at an advanced stage. Prostate cancer is less common among Asian men and occurs at about the same rates among Hispanic men as it does among white men.

- *Nationality.* Prostate cancer is most common in North America and northwestern Europe and less common in Asia, Africa, Central America, and South America. The reasons for these differences are not well understood but may be due to the fact that men in these countries are less likely to receive PSA testing (see the following section).

- *Family history.* Having a father or brother with prostate cancer more than doubles a man's risk of getting prostate cancer.

- *Diet.* Men in countries where they consume high-fat diets may have a greater risk of prostate cancer than men in countries with lower fat diets of rice, soybean products, and vegetables. Lycopenes (found in tomatoes, pink grapefruit, and watermelon), vitamin D, vitamin E, and the mineral selenium are being studied for their possible role in reducing prostate risk.

- *Physical activity and overweight/obesity.* Some studies have suggested that regular physical activity and maintaining a healthy weight may reduce the risk of developing or dying from prostate cancer; however, this link is not clear.

Prevention and Treatment Some risk factors for prostate cancer, such as age and race, are beyond your control. However, there are other steps you could take that appear promising. Eating more fruits and vegetables and taking 50 milligrams (400 IU, or international units) of vitamin E and adequate amounts of selenium may reduce risk, while consuming high levels of vitamin A may increase your risk. The best advice is to follow the MyPyramid dietary recommendations discussed in Chapter 9. Otherwise, keeping your weight levels healthy, getting regular amounts of exercise and sleep, and reducing stress levels keeps your immune system functioning effectively and may help you resist some forms of cancer.

Another important strategy is to get diagnostic tests on the schedule recommended by the American Cancer Society and the National Cancer Institute (see Table 13.3). The American Cancer Society recommends that men aged 50 and over have an annual **prostate-specific antigen (PSA)** test, a blood test that can detect a specific antigen found in those with prostate cancer.

Fortunately, even with so many generalized symptoms, 83 percent of all prostate cancers are detected while they are still in the local or regional stages and tend to progress slowly. The five-year survival rate in these early stages is 100 percent. Because most men develop the disease in their late sixties and early seventies, it is likely that they will die of other causes first. For this reason, some health care groups question the cost effectiveness and necessity of prostate surgeries and other costly procedures that may have little real effect on life expectancy. Over the past 20 years, the survival rate for all stages combined has increased from 67 percent to 96 percent, largely due to earlier diagnosis and improved treatment.

> **Prostate-specific antigen (PSA)** An antigen found in the blood of prostate cancer patients.

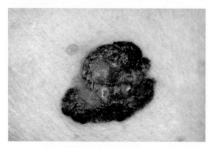 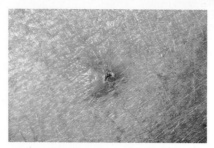 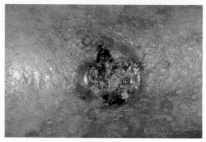

Prevention of skin cancer includes keeping a careful watch for any new pigmented growths and for changes to any moles. Melanoma symptoms, as shown in the left photo, include scalloped edges, asymmetrical shapes, discoloration, and an increase in size. Basal cell carcinoma and squamous cell carcinoma (middle and right photos) should be brought to your physician's attention but are not as deadly as melanoma.

Skin Cancer: Sun Worshipers Beware

If you are one of the millions of people who try to get a "healthy tan" each year, think again. As the primary cause of more than 1 million cases of skin cancer in the United States this year, many of which will disfigure or permanently change the person's appearance, the sun may just be the skin's public enemy number one.[39] Skin cancer is one of the most common forms of cancer in the United States today, affecting over 1 million people in 2005.[40] Last year 10,590 people died of skin cancer. Of those, 7,770 died of melanoma and 2,820 of other forms of skin cancer.

Malignant melanoma, the deadliest form of skin cancer, is beginning to occur at a much higher rate in women under age 40. In fact, while relatively few people die from the highly treatable *basal* or *squamous cell skin cancers,* the highly virulent malignant melanoma has become the most frequent cancer in women aged 25 to 29 and runs second only to breast cancer in women aged 30 to 34. If you think skin cancer is something that only older people get, think again![41]

What happens when you expose yourself to the ultraviolet radiation in sunlight? Biologically, the skin responds to photodamage by increasing its thickness and the number of pigment cells (melanocytes), which produce the "tan" look. However, photodamage also impairs the skin's immune system, priming it for cancer.[42] Photodamage also causes wrinkling by impairing the elastic substances (collagens) that keep skin soft and pliable.

Although sun exposure risks have been widely reported, over 60 percent of Americans aged 25 years and under report that they are "working on a tan" at some point during the year. These numbers spike dramatically just prior to spring break as tanning booths fill with students and others trying to get "starter tans" before heading out to tropical climates for spring vacations. Fewer than one in three sunbathers bothers to wear sunscreen.

Tanning booths and other artificial tans are *not* a safe alternative (see the Reality Check box).

The risk of skin cancer is greatest for people who:

- Have traits such as fair skin; blonde, red, or light brown hair; blue, green, or gray eyes
- Always burn before tanning, or don't tan easily, but spend lots of time outdoors
- Burn easily and peel readily
- Have previously been treated for skin cancer or have a family history of skin cancer (If you have a family history of melanoma, see your physician for regular skin exams.)
- Live in or take regular vacations to high altitudes (UV exposure increases with altitude)
- Work indoors all week and try to play tanning "catch-up" on weekends
- Use no or low-SPF sunscreens

Many people do not know what to look for when examining themselves for skin cancer. Basal and squamous cell carcinomas can be a recurrent annoyance, showing up most commonly on the face, ears, neck, arms, hands, and legs as warty bumps, colored spots, or scaly patches. Bleeding, itchiness, pain, or oozing are other symptoms that warrant attention. Changes such as a new spot or a change in size, shape, or color should be examined by a physician.

In striking contrast is the insidious melanoma, an invasive killer that quickly spreads to regional organs and throughout the body, accounting for over 75 percent of all skin cancer deaths. Risks increase dramatically among whites after age 20.[43] Often, melanoma starts as a normal-looking mole but quickly develops abnormal characteristics. A simple *ABCD* rule outlines the warning signs of melanoma:

- *Asymmetry.* One half of the mole does not match the other half.
- *Border irregularity.* The edges are uneven, notched, or scalloped.
- *Color.* Pigmentation is not uniform. Melanoma may vary in color from tan to deeper brown, reddish black, black, or deep bluish black.

Malignant melanoma A virulent cancer of the melanocytes (pigment-producing cells) of the skin.

Reality Check

Artificial Tans: Sacrificing Health for Beauty?

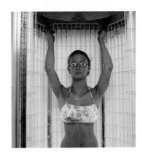

Men and women of all ages, shapes, and sizes are searching for an easy way to get that glamorous tan before or instead of spending time in the sun. Are any of the sun substitutes a safe alternative?

Tanning Booths and Beds

On an average day, more than 1.3 million Americans visit a tanning salon including many teenagers and young adults. Researchers using data from the *National Longitudinal Study of Adolescent Health* report that more than 25 percent of white female adolescents and 11 percent of males used tanning booths at least three times in the last year. Adolescents who tanned easily were more likely to visit tanning booths, while women who reported higher levels of physical activity were less likely to use them.

Most tanning salon patrons incorrectly believe that tanning booths are safer than sitting in the sun. However,

Is a tanning booth safer than the sun?

the truth is that there is no such thing as a safe tan from *any* source! Essentially, a tan is the skin's response to an injury; and every time you tan, you accumulate injury and increase your risk for disfiguring forms of skin cancer, premature aging, eye problems, unsightly skin spots, wrinkles and leathery skin, and possible death from melanoma. To make matters worse, the industry is difficult to monitor and regulate because of the many salons that are springing up across the country. Dermatologists cite additional factors that make tanning in a

salon as bad or worse than getting a tan the old fashioned way of sitting in the sun:

✓ Tanning facilities sometimes fail to enforce regulations, such as insuring that customers wear eye protection and that overexposure does not occur.

✓ Some tanning facilities do not calibrate the ultraviolet (UV) output of their tanning bulbs or ensure sufficient rotation of newer and older bulbs, which can lead to more or less exposure than you paid for. Tanning facility patrons often try for a total body tan. The buttocks and genitalia are particularly sensitive to UV radiation and are prone to develop skin cancer.

✓ Another concern is hygiene. Don't assume that those little colored water sprayers used to "clean" the inside of the beds are sufficient to kill organisms. Any time you come in contact with body secretions from others, you run the risk of an infectious disease.

Spray-On Tans

Some companies offer a sunless option that involves spraying customers in a tanning booth with the color additive dihydroxyacetone (DHA), which interacts with the dead surface cells in the outermost layer of the skin to darken skin color. Dihydroxyacetone has been approved by the FDA for use in coloring the skin since 1977 and has typically been used in lotions and creams. Its use is restricted to external application, which means that it shouldn't be sprayed in or on the mouth, eyes, or nose because the risks, if any, are unknown. If you choose to use DHA spray at home or in tanning booths, be sure to cover these areas. Remember that the spray

is a dye and does not increase your protection from the damaging rays of the sun.

Tanning Pills

Although there are no tanning pills approved by the FDA, some companies market pills that contain the color additive canthaxanthin. When large amounts of canthaxanthin are ingested, the substance can turn the skin a range of colors, from orange to brown. However, canthaxanthin is only approved for use as a color additive in foods and oral medications—and only in small amounts. Tanning pills have been associated with health problems, including an eye disorder called canthaxanthin retinopathy, which is the formation of yellow deposits on the eye's retina. Canthaxanthin has also been reported to cause liver injury and a severe itching condition called urticaria, according to the American Academy of Dermatology.

Sources: C. A. Demko et al., "Teenagers in the UV Tanning Booth?" *Archives of Pediatric and Adolescent Medicine* 157, no. 9 (2003): 854–860; University of Alabama at Birmingham, "Dear Doctor column: Tanning Beds," 2002, www.health.uab.edu; University of Alabama at Birmingham, "Dear Doctor column: Tanning (Sunless)," 2004, www.health.uab.edu; U.S. Food and Drug Administration, "Protect the Skin You're In!" *The FDA and You* 3 (2004), www.fda.gov/cdrh/fdaandyou/issue 03.html.

■ *Diameter.* Greater than 6 millimeters (about the size of a pea).

If you notice any of these symptoms, consult a physician promptly.

Treatment of skin cancer depends on its seriousness. Surgery is performed in 90 percent of all cases.

Radiation therapy, *electrodesiccation* (tissue destruction by heat), and *cryosurgery* (tissue destruction by freezing) are also common forms of treatment. For melanoma, treatment may involve surgical removal of the regional lymph nodes, radiation, or chemotherapy.

How to Examine Your Testicles

The best time to perform a testicular self-examination is after a warm shower or bath, when the testicles descend and the scrotal skin is relaxed.

1. Use a mirror to examine the scrotum for any visible swelling.

2. Using both hands, place the index and middle fingers of each hand on the underside of the testicle and the thumbs on top. Gently roll the testicle between the thumbs and fingers.

3. Identify the epididymis, the structure behind the testicle that carries sperm, so that you don't confuse it for a lump.

Lump

Figure 13.4 ■ Testicular Self-Examination

Testicular Cancer

Testicular cancer is one of the most common types of solid tumors found in young adult males, affecting nearly 7,500 young men per year. Those between the ages of 15 and 35 are at greatest risk; there has been a steady increase in tumor frequency over the past several years in this age group.[44] Although the cause of testicular cancer is unknown, several risk factors have been identified. Males with undescended testicles appear to be at greatest risk, and some studies indicate a genetic influence.

In general, testicular tumors first appear as an enlargement or thickening in testicular tissue. Because this enlargement is often painless, it is extremely important to practice regular testicular self-examination (Figure 13.4).

One of the most remarkable testicular cancer stories is the survival of Tour de France champion Lance Armstrong. Struck by an invasive form of testicular cancer that had spread to several parts of his body, including his brain, Armstrong's indomitable spirit set a wonderful example of hope for thousands of young men afflicted with the disease. He survived through a combination of superior medical care, exercise, and dietary and lifestyle changes, as well as a spiritual journey.

Ovarian Cancer

Ovarian cancer is the fifth leading cause of cancer death for women, diagnosed in almost 22,220 women in 2004 and killing over 16,210. Ovarian cancer causes more deaths than any other cancer of the reproductive system because its insidious, often silent, course means women tend not to discover it until the cancer is at an advanced stage. The most common symptom is enlargement of the abdomen (or a feeling of bloating) in women over age 40. Abnormal vaginal bleeding or discharge is rarely a symptom until the disease is advanced. Other symptoms include vague digestive disturbances (stomach discomfort, gas, pressure, distention), fatigue, pain during intercourse, unexplained weight loss, unexplained changes in bowel or bladder habits, urinary frequency, and incontinence.[45]

Risk Factors Studies show that the following factors may increase chances of developing the disease:[46]

- *Family history and genetic predisposition.* Primary relatives (mother, daughter, sister) of a woman who has had ovarian cancer are at increased risk. The likelihood is especially high if two or more primary relatives have had it. A family history of breast or colon cancer is also associated with increased risk. Gene mutation and a genetic syndrome called hereditary nonpolyposis colon cancer have also been linked to increased risk.

- *Age.* Chances of developing ovarian cancer increase with age. Most cases occur in women over age 50, with the highest risk in women over 60.

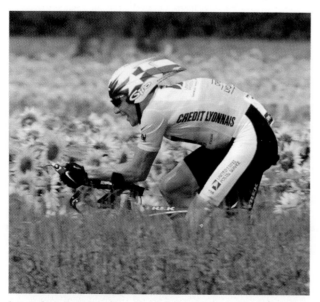

Lance Armstrong's battle with testicular cancer brought attention to a disease that strikes men who may consider themselves "too young" to be at risk for cancer.

- *Childbearing.* Women who have never been pregnant are more likely to develop ovarian cancer than those who have had a child; and the more children a woman has had, the less risk she faces. This may be related to exposure to the hormone estrogen. Women who use oral contraceptives that contain estrogen are also at lower risk.

- *Cancer history.* Women who have had breast or colon cancer have a greater chance of developing ovarian cancer than women who have not had either cancer.

- *Fertility drugs.* Drugs that cause a woman to ovulate may slightly increase her chance of developing ovarian cancer. Researchers are studying this possible association.

- *Hormone replacement therapy (HRT).* Some evidence suggests that women who use HRT after menopause may have a slightly increased risk. This research is controversial, and more studies are needed.

Prevention An early Yale University study indicated that diet may play a role in ovarian cancer.[47] When comparing 450 Canadian women with newly diagnosed ovarian cancer with 564 demographically similar, healthy women, the researchers found that the women without ovarian cancer had a diet lower in saturated fat. The study also found that each full-term pregnancy lowered risk by about 20 percent and each year of oral contraceptive use lowered it by 5 to 10 percent. So, should you go out and get pregnant or start taking birth control pills to reduce risk? No. However, these results, particularly when combined with cardiovascular risks and other health information, provide yet another reason to eat plenty of vegetables and cut down on your fat intake. General prevention strategies focusing on diet, exercise, sleep, stress management, and weight control are good ideas for this and any of the cancers discussed in this chapter, as substantiated by recent research studying the role of lifestyle in breast and ovarian cancer.[48]

To protect yourself, annual thorough pelvic examinations are important. Women over the age of 40 should have a cancer-related checkup every year. Transvaginal ultrasound and a tumor marker, CA125, may assist in diagnosis but are not recommended for routine screening.[49] If you have any symptoms of ovarian cancer and they persist, see your doctor promptly.

Try it →NOW

Perform self-exams for early detection. **The survival rate of breast and testicular cancer patients greatly increases with early detection. Make a commitment to perform a breast or testicular self-exam monthly (see pages 363 and 368 for instructions). Knowing your body and detecting abnormalities is one way you can take an active role in cancer prevention.**

Cervical and Endometrial (Uterine) Cancer

In 2005, an estimated 10,370 new cases of cervical cancer and 40,880 cases of endometrial cancer were diagnosed in the United States. Most uterine cancers develop in the body of the uterus, usually in the endometrium (lining of the uterus). The rest develop in the cervix, located at the base of the uterus. The overall incidence of early-stage uterine cancer—that is, cervical cancer—has increased slightly in recent years in women under age 50. In contrast, invasive, later-stage forms of the disease appear to be decreasing. This may be due to more regular screenings using the **Pap (Papanicolaou) test,** a procedure in which cells taken from the cervical region are examined for abnormal cellular activity. Although Pap tests are very effective for detecting early-stage cervical cancer, they are less effective for detecting cancers of the uterine lining and not effective at all for detecting cancers of the uterine tubes or ovaries.

Risk factors for cervical cancer include early age at first intercourse, multiple sex partners, cigarette smoking, and certain sexually transmitted infections, including human papillomavirus (the cause of genital warts) and herpesvirus. For endometrial cancer, risk factors include age, endometrial hyperplasia, estrogen replacement therapy, being overweight, diabetes and high blood pressure, a history of other cancers, race (white women are at higher risk), and treatment with tamoxifen for breast cancer. (Doctors emphasize that the benefits of tamoxifen far outweigh its possible risks, and close monitoring for endometrial cancer is an important part of tamoxifen treatment.) Other factors include having few or no children and entering menopause late in life.

Early warning signs of uterine cancer include bleeding outside the normal menstrual period or after menopause or persistent unusual vaginal discharge. These symptoms should be checked by a physician immediately.[50]

Cancer of the Pancreas

The incidence of cancer of the pancreas, known as a "silent" disease, has increased substantially during the last 25 years to 32,180 cases in 2005. Chronic inflammation of the pancreas, obesity, physical inactivity, diabetes, cirrhosis, and a high-fat diet may contribute to its development. Smokers have double the risk of nonsmokers.[51]

> **Pap test** A procedure in which cells taken from the cervical region are examined for abnormal cellular activity.

Unfortunately, pancreatic cancer is one of the worst cancers to get. Only 4 percent of patients live more than five years after diagnosis, usually because the disease is well advanced by the time there are any symptoms.

Leukemia

Leukemia is a cancer of the blood-forming tissues that leads to proliferation of millions of immature white blood cells. These abnormal cells crowd out normal white blood cells (which fight infection), platelets (which control hemorrhaging), and red blood cells (which carry oxygen to body cells). As a result, symptoms such as fatigue, paleness, weight loss, easy bruising, repeated infections, nosebleeds, and other forms of hemorrhaging occur. In children, these symptoms can appear suddenly.

Leukemia can be acute or chronic and can strike both sexes and all age groups. Although many people think of it as a childhood disease, leukemia struck over ten times more adults than children in 2005. Chronic leukemia can develop over several months and have few symptoms. The five-year survival rate varies by type of leukemia; for patients with chronic lymphocytic leukemia, one of the most common types, it has risen to 73 percent.[52]

Try it ▸NOW_____

Take steps to prevent cancer. **There are many actions you can take right away to improve your lifestyle and prevent your risk of developing cancer. Take advantage of the salad bar in your dining hall, and load up on greens or request veggies like steamed broccoli or sautéed spinach. Don't forget the sunscreen—make applying a sunscreen with SPF 15 (at least) part of your daily routine, and stay in the shade from noon to 2 PM (the sun's strongest time period).**

FACING CANCER

Based on current rates, about 83 million Americans—or one in three of us now living—will eventually develop cancer. Many factors have contributed to the rise in cancer

Magnetic resonance imaging (MRI)   A device that uses magnetic fields, radio waves, and computers to generate an image of internal tissues of the body for diagnostic purposes without the use of radiation.

Computed tomography (CT scan)   A machine that uses radiation to view internal organs not normally visible on X rays.

mortality, but the increased incidence of lung cancer, a largely preventable disease, is probably the most important. Despite these gloomy predictions, recent advancements in diagnosis and treatment have reduced much of the fear and mystery that once surrounded cancer.

Detecting Cancer

What are some ways cancer is detected?

The earlier cancer is diagnosed, the better the prospect for survival. Several high-tech tools have been developed to detect cancer. They include the following:

■ New high-technology diagnostic imaging techniques have replaced exploratory surgery for some cancer patients. In **magnetic resonance imaging (MRI),** a huge electromagnet detects hidden tumors by mapping the vibrations of the various atoms in the body on a computer screen. The **computed tomography scan (CT scan)** uses X rays to examine parts of the body. In both of these painless, noninvasive procedures, cross-sectioned pictures can reveal a tumor's shape and location more accurately than using conventional X rays.

■ *Prostatic ultrasound* (a rectal probe using ultrasonic waves to produce an image of the prostate) is being investigated as a means to increase the early detection of prostate cancer. Prostatic ultrasound has been combined with the PSA blood test.

Such medical techniques, along with regular self-examinations and checkups, play an important role in the early detection and secondary prevention of cancer.

Most of the sites that pose the highest risk for cancer have screening tests available for early detection. Other common forms of cancer have readily identifiable symptoms. The key seems to be whether people have the financial resources (insurance) to seek medical diagnosis and early treatment.

The best way to detect cancer early is to stay actively involved in your own health care. Table 13.4 lists seven warning signals of cancer. If you notice any of these signals and they don't appear to be related to anything else, see a doctor immediately. For example, difficulty swallowing may be due to a cold or flu. But if you are otherwise symptomless and the difficulty continues, consult your physician. Make sure you receive all appropriate diagnostic tests.

Also, make a realistic assessment of your own risk factors, and avoid the ones that you can control. Do you have a family history of cancer? If so, what types? Make sure you know which symptoms to watch for and follow the recommendations for self-exams and medical checkups in Table 13.3. Avoid known carcinogens—such as tobacco—and other environmental hazards. Eat a nutritious diet. Heeding the suggestions for primary prevention can significantly decrease your risk.

New Hope in Cancer Treatments

Although cancer treatments have changed dramatically over the past 20 years, surgery, in which the tumor and surrounding tissue are removed, is still common. Today's surgeons tend to remove less surrounding tissue than previously and to combine surgery with either **radiotherapy** (the use of radiation) or **chemotherapy** (the use of drugs) to kill cancerous cells.

Radiation works by destroying malignant cells or stopping cell growth. It is most effective in treating localized cancer masses. When cancer has spread throughout the body, it is necessary to use some form of chemotherapy. Unfortunately, chemotherapy attacks both healthy cells and the cancerous ones. Ongoing research will result in new drugs that are less toxic to normal cells and more potent against tumor cells.

Whether used alone or in combination, radiotherapy and chemotherapy have side effects, including extreme nausea, nutritional deficiencies, hair loss, and general fatigue. Long-term damage to the cardiovascular system and other body systems can be significant. It is important to discuss these matters with doctors when making treatment plans.

Today, researchers are targeting cancer as a genetic disease that is brought on by some form of mutation, either inherited or acquired. Promising treatments focus on stopping the cycle of these mutant cells, targeting toxins through monoclonal antibodies, and rousing the immune system to be more effective.

Participation in clinical trials has provided a new source of hope for many individuals undergoing cancer treatment. Clinical trials are people-based studies of new drugs or procedures. Because of the many unknown variables, deciding whether or not to participate in a clinical trial can be a very difficult decision. Despite the risks, which should be carefully considered, thousands have benefited from treatments that would otherwise be unavailable to them.

Talking with Your Doctor about Cancer

Any time cancer is suspected, people react with anxiety, fear, and anger. Emotional distress is sometimes so intense that they are unable to make critical health care decisions. If you find it difficult to know what to ask your doctor during a routine exam, imagine how hard it would be to discuss life-or-death options for yourself or a loved one. Before you arrive at the doctor's office, prepare a list of important questions to discuss. Remember, your health care provider should be your partner and help you make the best decisions for you.

If the diagnosis is cancer, here are some questions to ask:

Table 13.4
Cancer's Seven Warning Signals

1. Changes in bowel or bladder habits
2. A sore that does not heal
3. Unusual bleeding or discharge
4. Thickening or lump in breast or elsewhere
5. Persistent indigestion or difficulty in swallowing
6. Obvious change in a wart or mole
7. Nagging cough or hoarseness

If you have a warning signal, see your doctor.

- What kind of cancer do I have? What stage is it in? Based on my age and cancer stage, what prognosis do I have?
- What are my treatment choices? Which do you recommend? Why?
- What are the benefits of each kind of treatment? What are the risks and possible side effects?
- Would a clinical trial be appropriate for me?

If surgery is recommended, ask:

- What kind of operation will it be, and how long will it take? What form of anesthesia will be used? How many similar procedures has this surgeon done in the past month? What is his or her success rate?
- How will I feel after surgery? If I have pain, how will you help me?
- Where will the scars be? What will they look like? Will they cause disability?
- Will I have any activity limitations after surgery? What kind of physical therapy, if any, will I need? When will I get back to normal activities?

If radiation is recommended, you may want to know:

- Why do you think this treatment is better than my other options?
- How long will I need to have treatments, and what will the side effects be in the short and long term? What body organs or systems may be damaged?
- What can I do to take care of myself during therapy? Are there services available to help me?
- What is the long-term prognosis for people of my age with my type of cancer who are using this treatment?

Questions to ask about chemotherapy include:

- Why do you think this treatment is better than other options?

Radiotherapy   Use of radiation to kill cancerous cells.

Chemotherapy   Use of drugs to kill cancerous cells.

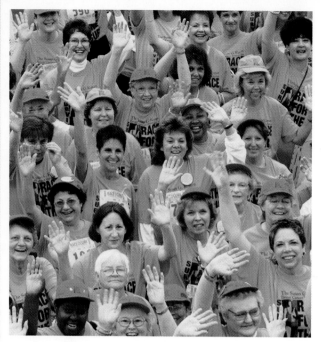

Cancer survivors can live long and health lives. Some, such as these breast cancer survivors and their supporters, participate in walkathons and other activities to raise money for cancer research and treatment and to raise public awareness about prevention.

- Which drug combinations pose the fewest risks and most benefits?

- What will be the short- and long-term side effects?

Before beginning any form of cancer therapy, it is imperative to be a vigilant and vocal consumer. Read and seek information from cancer support groups. Check the skills of your surgeon, your radiation therapist, and your doctor in terms of clinical experience and interpersonal interactions.

Cancer Survivors: Life after Cancer

Heightened public awareness and an improved prognosis have made the cancer experience less threatening and isolating than it once was. While you may have once heard stories of recovering cancer patients experiencing job discrimination or being unable to obtain health or life insurance, these cases are decreasing. Several states have even enacted legislation to prevent insurance companies from canceling policies or instituting other forms of discrimination. Since health insurance can be obtained through large employers and large companies spread the insurance risk among many employees, insurance companies often accept new employees without underwriting.

In fact, assistance for the cancer patient is more readily available than ever before. Cancer support groups, information workshops, and low-cost medical consultation are just a few of the forms of assistance now offered in many communities. Government funding for cancer research has increased substantially over the past decade. The battle for funds continues. Increasing efforts in cancer research, improvements in diagnostic equipment, and advances in treatment provide hope for the future.

Taking Charge

Summary

- Cancer is a group of diseases characterized by uncontrolled growth and spread of abnormal cells. These cells may create tumors. Benign (noncancerous) tumors grow in size but do not spread; malignant (cancerous) tumors spread to other parts of the body.

- Several causes of cancer have been identified. Lifestyle factors include smoking and obesity. Biological factors include inherited genes and gender. Occupational and environmental hazards are carcinogens present in people's home or work environments. Chemicals in foods that may act as carcinogens include preservatives and pesticides. Infectious diseases that may lead to cancer include herpes, mononucleosis, and human papillomavirus (which causes genital warts). Medical factors include certain drug therapies given for other conditions that may elevate the chance of cancer. Combined risk refers to a combination of the above factors, which tends to compound the risk for cancer.

- There are many different types of cancer, each of which poses different risks, depending on a number of factors. Common cancers include lung, breast, colon and rectal, prostate, skin, testicular, ovarian, uterine, and pancreatic cancers, as well as leukemia.

- Early diagnosis improves survival rate. Self-exams for breast, testicular, and skin cancer and knowledge of the seven warning signals of cancer aid early diagnosis.

- New types of cancer treatments include combinations of radiotherapy, chemotherapy, and immunotherapy.

Chapter Review

1. Suspected cancer-causing genes that are present on chromosomes are called
   a. epigenes.
   b. oncogenes.
   c. primogenes.
   d. metastogenes.

2. What is the lifetime risk for developing cancer in the United States?
   a. Men have a lifetime risk of 1 in 2; women have a lifetime risk of 1 in 3.
   b. Women have a lifetime risk of 1 in 2; men have a lifetime risk of 1 in 3.
   c. Men and women have a lifetime risk of 1 in 4.
   d. Men and women have a lifetime risk of 1 in 8.

3. The most common sites for cancers are
   a. bone marrow.
   b. lymphatic system.
   c. epithelial tissues.
   d. mesodermal tissues.

4. Barbara is a physician who specializes in the treatment of malignancies. Barbara is an
   a. internist.
   b. oncologist.
   c. endocrinologist.
   d. epidemiologist.

5. The fecal occult blood test is the most basic screening test used for
   a. lung cancer.
   b. prostate cancer.
   c. cervical cancer.
   d. colorectal cancer.

6. Late menarche, early menopause, early first childbirth, and high parity have been shown to reduce a woman's risk of
   a. breast cancer.
   b. ovarian cancer.
   c. uterine cancer.
   d. endometrial cancer.

7. Environmental factors such as smoking, diet, and infectious diseases, as well as chemicals, cause _____ of all cancer deaths in the United States.
   a. one-fourth
   b. one-half
   c. two-thirds
   d. three-fourths

8. A study of the role of exercise in reducing the risk for breast cancer found that the risk of those who averaged four hours of exercise a week since menstruation was _____ than that of women who did no exercise at all.
   a. 58 percent higher
   b. 80 percent higher
   c. 58 percent lower
   d. 80 percent lower

9. Hodgkin's disease is a type of
   a. sarcoma.
   b. carcinoma.
   c. lymphoma.
   d. leukemia.

10. In general, ordinary-looking cells enclosed in a fibrous shell or capsule that prevents their spreading to other body areas are called
   a. mutant cells.
   b. malignant tumors.
   c. benign tumors.
   d. metastatic tumors.

Answers to these questions can be found on page A-1.

Questions for Discussion and Reflection

1. What is cancer? How does it spread? What is the difference between a benign and a malignant tumor?

2. List the likely causes of cancer. Do any of them put you at greater risk? What can you do to reduce your risk? What risk factors do you share with family members? With friends?

3. What are the symptoms of lung, breast, prostate, and testicular cancer? What can you do to reduce your risk of developing these cancers or increase your chances of surviving them?

4. What are the differences between carcinomas, sarcomas, lymphomas, and leukemia? Which is the most common? Least common?

5. Why are breast and testicular self-exams important for women and men? What could be the consequences of not doing these exams regularly?

6. Discuss the seven warning signals of cancer. What could signal that you have cancer instead of a minor illness? How soon should you seek treatment for any of the warning signs?

Accessing Your Health on the Internet

The following websites explore further topics and issues related to personal health. For links to the websites below, visit the Companion Website for *Health: The Basics,* Seventh Edition at www.aw-bc.com/donatelle.

1. *American Cancer Society.* Home page for the leading private organization dedicated to cancer prevention. This site provides information, statistics, and resources regarding cancer.

2. *International Cancer Information Center.* Sponsored by the National Cancer Institute, this site is designed to be a comprehensive information resource on cancer for patients and health professionals.

3. *National Cancer Institute.* Check here for information on clinical trials and the Physician Data Query (PDQ), a comprehensive database of cancer treatment information.

4. *National Women's Health Information Center (NWHIC).* Provides a wealth of information about cancer in women. Cosponsored by the National Cancer Institute.

5. *Oncolink.* Sponsored by the University of Pennsylvania Cancer Center, this site seeks to educate cancer patients and their families by offering information on support services, cancer causes, screening, prevention, and common questions.

Further Reading

Journal of the National Cancer Institute. Bethesda, MD (published monthly).

> *Focuses on current risk factors, prevention, and treatment research in the area of cancer.*

American Cancer Society. *Cancer Facts and Figures.* Atlanta: Author (published annually).

> *A summary of major facts relating to cancer. Provides information on incidence, prevalence, symptomology, prevention, and treatment. Available through local divisions of the American Cancer Society.*

American Cancer Society. *A Breast Cancer Journey: Your Personal Guidebook,* 2nd ed. Atlanta: American Cancer Society, 2004.

> *Contains up-to-date information on treatments, medicines, reconstructive surgery, and complementary and alternative options. Also includes information for caregivers, family, and friends.*

Armstrong, L. *It's Not about the Bike: My Journey Back to Life.* New York: Penguin, 2000.

> *Armstrong's incredible description of his triumph over testicular cancer and his Tour de France victories. A book full of inspiration for young men with this disease, their families, and anyone facing cancer.*

Nutrition and Cancer Journal, Lawrence Erlbaum Associates. Mahwah, NJ (published monthly).

> *Focuses on etiological aspects of various dietary factors and research on risks for cancer development. Also includes current research on dietary factors and prevention.*

References

1. A. Jemal et al., "Cancer Statistics," *CA: A Cancer Journal for Clinicians* 55 (2005): 10–30.
2. American Cancer Society, *Cancer Facts and Figures 2005* (Atlanta: Author, 2005).
3. Ibid.
4. Ibid.
5. Ibid.
6. B. D. Smedley, A. Y. Stith, and A. R. Nelson, eds., *Unequal Treatment: Confronting Racial and Ethnic Disparities in Health Care* (Washington, DC: National Academies Press, 2003).
7. H. P. Freeman, "Commentary on the Meaning of Race in Science and Society," *Cancer Epidemiology Biomarkers and Prevention* 12, no. 3 (2003): 232S–236S.
8. American Cancer Society, *Cancer Facts and Figures 2005.*
9. J. Peto, "Cancer Epidemiology in the Last Century and Next Decade," *Nature* 411 (2001): 390–395.
10. American Cancer Society, *Cancer Facts and Figures 2005.*
11. Ibid.
12. Ibid
13. A. H. Mokdad et al., "Actual Causes of Death in the United States," *Journal of the American Medical Association* 291, no. 10 (2000): 1238–1245.
14. American Cancer Society, *Cancer Facts and Figures 2005.*
15. E. Calle et al., "Overweight, Obesity and Mortality from Cancer in a Prospectively Studied Cohort of U.S. Adults," *New England Journal of Medicine* 348, no. 77: 1625–1638; L. Cooney and C. Gufer, "Hyperglycemia, Obesity, and Cancern Risk on the Horizon," *Journal of the American Medical Association,* 293: 235–236.
16. Ibid.
17. International Agency for Research on Cancer (IARC), "Hormonal Contraception and Post-Menopausal Hormonal Therapy," (IARC Monographs on the Evaluation of Carcinogenic Risks to Humans) (Lyon, France: IARC, 1999), 72.
18. J. Peto, "Cancer Epidemiology in the Last Century."
19. American Cancer Society, *Cancer Facts and Figures 2005.*
20. A. Swerdlow, *British Journal of Cancer,* (2005):
21. American Cancer Society, *Cancer Facts and Figures 2005.*
22. Ibid.; P. Pisani, *Estimates of Number of Cancer Cases throughout the World Attributable to Infectious Diseases* (Lyon, France: International Agency for Research on Cancer, 2004).
23. B. W. Stewart and P. Kleihues, eds., "Cancers of the Female Reproductive Tract," *World Cancer Report* (Lyon, France: IARC Press, 2003), 215–222.
24. American Cancer Society, *Cancer Facts and Figures 2005.*
25. Ibid.
26. Ibid.
27. Ibid.
28. Ibid.
29. Ibid.
30. Ibid.
31. Ibid.
32. Ibid.
33. Ibid.
34. American Cancer Society, *Cancer Facts and Figures 2005.*
35. Ibid.
36. Ibid.
37. Ibid.
38. American Cancer Society, *Cancer Facts and Figures 2005.*
39. University of Wisconsin Health Service, "Sunburn: Prevention Treatment," 2002, www.uhs.wisc.edu/ex/selfcare/resource/sunburn.php.
40. American Cancer Society, *Cancer Facts and Figures 2005.*
41. Ibid.
42. Ibid.
43. Ibid.
44. Ibid.
45. Ibid.
46. Ibid.
47. A. Harvey et al., "Dietary Fat Intake and Risk of Epithelial Ovarian Cancer," *Journal of the National Cancer Institute* 86 (1994): 21.
48. G. C. Zografos, M. Panou, and N. Panou, "Common Risk Factors of Breast and Ovarian Cancer: Recent Review," *International Journal of Gynecological Cancer* 14, no. 5 (2004): 721–740; C. T. Berkelman, "Risk Factors and Risk Reduction of Breast and Ovarian Cancer," *Current Opinion in Obstetrics and Gynecology* 15, no. 1 (2003): 63–68.
49. Ibid.
50. American Cancer Society, *Cancer Facts and Figures 2005.*
51. Ibid.
52. Ibid.

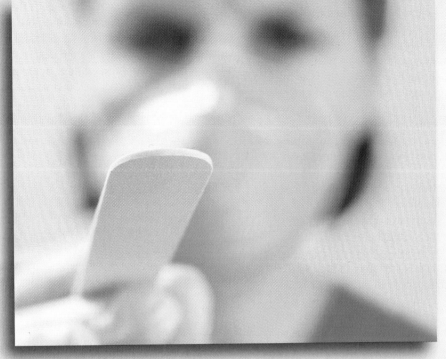

Will vitamin C cure my cold?

Can I get a sexually transmitted infection from "outercourse"?

How does my body fight a disease?

What can I do to reduce my risk for diabetes?

14 Infectious and Noninfectious Conditions
Risks and Responsibilities

Objectives

- *Explain* how your immune system works to protect you and what you can do to boost its effectiveness.
- *Describe* the most common pathogens infecting humans today and the major emerging and resurgent diseases affecting humans.
- *Discuss* the various sexually transmitted infections, their means of transmission, and actions that can be taken to prevent their spread.
- *Discuss* human immunodeficiency virus (HIV) and acquired immunodeficiency syndrome (AIDS), trends in infection and treatment, and the impact on special populations.
- *Discuss* noninfectious diseases, including diabetes, asthma, and lower back pain.

Every moment of every day, you are in contact with microscopic organisms that have the ability to cause illness or even death. These disease-causing agents, known as **pathogens,** are found in air and food and on nearly every object or person with whom you come in contact. Although new varieties of pathogens arise all the time, scientific evidence indicates that many have existed for as long as there has been life on the planet. Fossil evidence shows that infections, cancer, heart disease, and a host of other ailments afflicted the earliest humans. At times, infectious diseases wiped out whole groups of people through epidemics such as the Black Death, or bubonic plague, which killed up to one-third of the population of Europe in the 1300s. A pandemic, or global epidemic, of influenza killed more than 20 million people in 1918, while strains of tuberculosis and cholera continue to cause premature death throughout the world.

In spite of our best efforts to eradicate them, these diseases continue to be a menace. The news isn't all bad; even though we are bombarded by potential pathogenic threats, our immune systems are remarkably adept at protecting us. *Endogenous microorganisms* are those that live in peaceful coexistence with their human hosts most of the time. For people in good health and whose immune systems are functioning properly, endogenous organisms are usually harmless; but, in sick people or those with weakened immune systems, these normally harmless pathogenic organisms can cause serious health problems.

Exogenous microorganisms are organisms that do not normally inhabit the body. When they do, however, they are apt to produce an infection and/or illness. The more easily these pathogens can gain a foothold in the body and sustain themselves, the more **virulent,** or aggressive, they may be in causing disease. However, if your immune system is strong, you will often be able to fight off even the most virulent attacker. Several factors influence your susceptibility to disease.

Pathogen A disease-causing agent.

Virulent Strong enough to overcome host resistance and cause disease.

Multifactorial disease Disease caused by interactions of several factors.

Sickle cell disease Genetic disease commonly found among African Americans; results in organ damage and premature death.

Immunological competence Ability of the immune system to defend the body from pathogens.

Botulism A form of food-poisoning caused by toxins produced by a resistant food borne bacteriam that is extremely virulent.

ASSESSING YOUR DISEASE RISKS

Most diseases are **multifactorial diseases**—that is, they are caused by the interaction of several factors from inside and outside the person. For a disease to occur, the *host* must be *susceptible*, which means that the immune system must be in a weakened condition; an *agent* (or *vector*) capable of transmitting a disease must be present; and the *environment* must be hospitable to the pathogen in terms of temperature, light, moisture, and other requirements. Other risk factors also apparently increase or decrease susceptibility. Figure 14.1 summarizes the body's defenses against invasion.

Risk Factors You Can't Control

Unfortunately, some risk factors are beyond our control. Here are some of the most common.

Heredity Perhaps the single greatest factor influencing longevity is the longevity of a person's parents. Being born into a family in which heart disease, cancer, or other illnesses are prevalent seems to increase risk. Still other diseases are caused by direct chromosomal inheritance. For example, **sickle cell disease,** an inherited blood disease that primarily affects African Americans, is often transmitted to the fetus if both parents carry the sickle cell trait. It is often unclear whether hereditary diseases occur as a result of inherited chromosomal traits or inherited insufficiencies in the immune system.

Aging After age 40 we become more vulnerable to most of the chronic diseases. Moreover, as we age, our immune systems respond less efficiently to invading organisms, thus increasing risk for infection and illness. The same flu that produces an afternoon of nausea and diarrhea in a younger person may cause days of illness or even death in an older person. The very young are also at risk for many diseases, particularly if they are not vaccinated against them.

Environmental Conditions Unsanitary conditions and the presence of drugs, chemicals, and hazardous pollutants and wastes in food and water probably have a great effect on our immune systems. It is well documented that poor environmental conditions can weaken **immunological competence**—the body's ability to defend itself against pathogens.

Organism Resistance Some organisms, such as the foodborne organism that causes **botulism** (a severe type of food poisoning), are particularly virulent, and

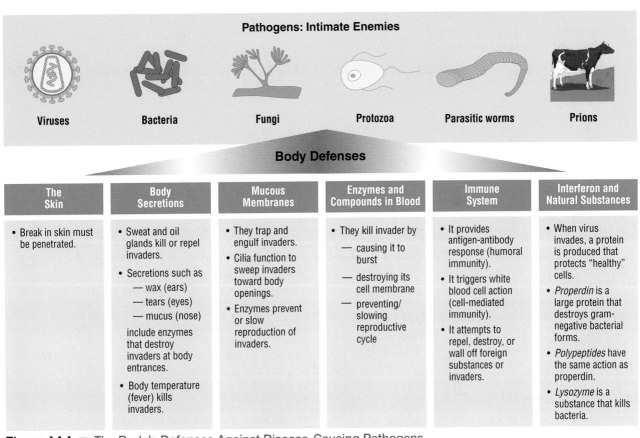

Figure 14.1 ■ The Body's Defenses Against Disease-Causing Pathogens

even tiny amounts may make the most hardy of us ill. Other organisms have mutated and are resistant to the body's defenses as well as to conventional treatments designed to protect against them. Still other, newer pathogens pose unique challenges that our bodily defenses are ill adapted to fight.

Risk Factors You Can Control

The good news is that we all have some degree of personal control over many risk factors for disease. Too much stress, inadequate nutrition, a low physical fitness level, lack of sleep, misuse or abuse of legal and illegal substances, poor personal hygiene, high-risk behaviors, and other variables significantly increase the risk for a number of diseases. Various chapters of this text discuss these variables. Several factors influence our individual susceptibility to various diseases. Factors we can control at least partly through lifestyle decisions and behaviors include vigor of immune response; preexisting level of immunity; nutritional status; preexisting diseases; habits such as smoking, drinking, drugs; and psychological factors such as stress, depression, and anxiety.[1]

TYPES OF PATHOGENS AND ROUTES OF TRANSMISSION

Pathogens enter the body in several ways. They may be transmitted by *direct contact* between infected persons, such as during sexual relations, kissing, or touching, or by *indirect contact*, such as by touching an object the infected person has had contact with. Table 14.1 on page 378 lists the common routes of transmission.

The hands are probably the greatest source of infectious disease transmission. You may also **autoinoculate** yourself, or transmit a pathogen from one part of your body to another. For example, you may touch a sore on your lip that is teeming with viral herpes, then transmit the virus to your eye when you scratch your itchy eyelid.

Your best friend may be the source of *animal-borne pathogens*. Dogs, cats, livestock, and wild animals can spread numerous diseases through their bites or feces or by carrying infected insects into living areas and transmitting diseases either directly or indirectly. Although

Autoinoculation Transmission of a pathogen from one part of the body to another.

Table 14.1
Routes of Disease Transmission

Mode of Transmission	Aspects of Transmission
Contact	Either *direct* (e.g., skin or sexual contact) or *indirect* (e.g., infected blood or body fluid)
Food- or waterborne	Eating or coming in contact with contaminated food or water or products passed through them
Airborne	Inhalation; droplet spread as through sneezing, coughing, or talking
Vectorborne	Vector-transmitted via secretions, biting, egg-laying, as done by mosquitoes, ticks, snails, avians, etc; depends on how infectious the organism is
Perinatal	Similar to contact infection; happens in the uterus or as the baby passes through the birth canal

interspecies transmission of diseases (diseases passed from humans to animals and vice versa) is rare, it does occur.

We can categorize pathogens into six major types: bacteria, viruses, fungi, protozoa, parasitic worms, and prions.

Bacteria

Bacteria are single-celled organisms that are plantlike in nature but lack chlorophyll (the pigment that gives plants their green coloring). There are three major types

Interspecies transmission Transmission of disease from humans to animals or from animals to humans.

Bacteria Single-celled organisms that may cause disease.

Toxins Poisonous substances produced by certain microorganisms that cause various diseases.

Staphylococci Round, gram-positive bacteria, usually found in clusters.

Epidermis The outermost layer of the skin.

Toxic shock syndrome (TSS) A potentially life threatening bacterial infection that is most common in menstruating women who use tampons.

Streptococcus Round bacteria, usually found in chain formation.

Meningitis An infection of the meninges, the membranes that surround the brain and spinal cord.

of bacteria: cocci, bacilli, and spirilla. Bacteria can be viewed under a standard light microscope.

Although there are several thousand species of bacteria, only approximately 100 cause diseases in humans. In many cases, it is not the bacteria themselves that cause disease but rather the poisonous substances, called **toxins,** that they produce. The following are the most common bacterial infections.

Staphylococcal Infections **Staphylococci** are normally present on our skin at all times and usually cause few problems; but, when there is a cut or break in the **epidermis,** or outer layer of the skin, staphylococci may enter and cause a localized infection. If you have ever suffered from acne, boils, styes (infections of the eyelids), or infected wounds, you have probably had a "staph" infection. Although most such infections are readily defeated by your immune system, resistant forms of staph bacteria are on the rise. These bacteria must be treated with heavy doses of antibiotics and pose serious risks to those infected.

At least one staph-caused disorder, **toxic shock syndrome (TSS),** is potentially fatal. Though most common in menstruating women, men can be susceptible too. To reduce the likelihood of toxic shock syndrome, take the following precautions: (1) avoid superabsorbent tampons except during the heaviest menstrual flow; (2) change tampons at least every four hours; (3) use napkins at night instead of tampons; and (4) make sure cuts and wounds remain clean and seek medical attention if there are signs of skin infection such as redness, swelling, or abnormal drainage near the wound.[2]

Streptococcal Infections At least five types of the **streptococcus** microorganism are known to cause bacterial infections. Group A streptococci cause the most common diseases, such as streptococcal pharyngitis (strep throat) and scarlet fever. Group B streptococci can cause illness in newborn babies, pregnant women, the elderly, and adults with other illnesses such as diabetes or liver disease.[3]

Meningitis **Meningitis** is an infection of the *meninges,* the membranes that surround the brain and spinal cord. Meningitis can cause acute inflammation of the brain. Some forms of bacterial meningitis are contagious and can be spread through contact with saliva, nasal discharge, feces, or respiratory and throat secretions. Pneumococcal meningitis is the most common form of meningitis and is the most dangerous form of bacterial meningitis. Approximately 6,000 cases of pneumococcal meningitis are reported in the United States each year.

College students living in dormitories have a higher risk of contracting meningococcal meningitis, a virulent form of meningitis that has risen dramatically on college campuses in recent years. The signs of meningitis are sudden fever, severe headache, and a stiff neck, particularly, and having difficulty touching your chin to your chest. Pneumococcal meningitis symptoms may include nausea and vomiting, confusion and disorientation, drowsiness, and poor appetite. Persons who are suspected of having meningitis should receive immediate, aggressive medical treatment. The infection can progress quickly, and early treatment is critical to the outcome.

Pneumonia In the early twentieth century, **pneumonia** was a leading cause of death in the United States. This lung disease is characterized by chronic cough, chest pain, chills, high fever, fluid accumulation, and eventual respiratory failure. One of the most common forms of pneumonia is caused by bacterial infection and responds readily to antibiotic treatment in the early stages. Other forms are caused by viruses, chemicals, or other substances in the lungs and are more difficult to treat. Although medical advances have reduced the overall incidence of pneumonia, it continues to be a major threat in the United States and throughout the world. Vulnerable populations include the poor, the elderly, and those already suffering from other illnesses.[4]

Tuberculosis A major killer in the United States in the early twentieth century, **tuberculosis (TB)** was largely controlled in America by 1950 due to improved sanitation, isolation of infected persons, and treatment with drugs such as *rifampin* or *isoniazid*. Though many health professionals assumed that TB had been conquered, that appears not to be the case. During the past 20 years, several factors have led to an epidemic rise in the disease: deteriorating social conditions, including overcrowding and poor sanitation; failure to isolate active cases of TB; a weakening of public health infrastructure, which has led to less funding for screening; and migration of TB to the United States through international travel. In 2003, there were over 14,874 active cases of TB in the United States.[5] The U.S. statistics pale by comparison to the staggering tuberculosis burden in the global population. The World Health Organization (WHO) estimates that in the first two decades of the twenty-first century, 1 billion people will acquire a new tuberculosis infection, 200 million will develop active disease, and 35 million will die.[6]

Tuberculosis is caused by bacterial infiltration of the respiratory system that results in a chronic inflammatory reaction in the lungs. Airborne transmission via the respiratory tract is the primary and most efficient mode of transmitting TB. Symptoms include persistent coughing, weight loss, fever, and spitting up blood. If you or someone you know has these symptoms, check with a doctor. Infected people can be contagious without actually showing any symptoms themselves and can transmit the disease while talking, coughing, sneezing, or singing.

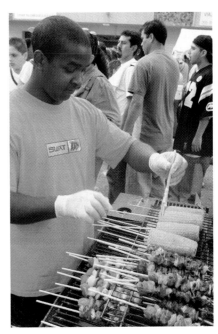

Food workers should always wear latex or plastic gloves to prevent foodborne illness.

Fortunately, TB is fairly difficult to catch, and prolonged exposure, rather than single exposure, is the typical mode of infection. Only about 20 to 30 percent of those exposed to an active case will become infected.[7] Treatments are effective for most nonresistant cases. Treatment includes rest, careful infection-control procedures, and drugs to combat the infection.

Viruses

Viruses are the smallest pathogens, approximately 1/500th the size of bacteria. Because of their tiny size, they are visible only under an electron microscope and were not identified until the twentieth century.[8] More than 150 viruses are known to cause disease in humans, although their role in various cancers and chronic diseases is still unclear.

Essentially, a virus consists of a protein structure that contains either *ribonucleic acid (RNA)* or *deoxyribonucleic acid (DNA)*. Incapable of carrying out the normal cell functions of respiration and metabolism, a virus cannot reproduce on its own and can exist only in a parasitic relationship with the cell it invades.

> **Pneumonia** Disease of the lungs characterized by chronic cough, chest pain, chills, high fever, and fluid accumulation; may be caused by bacteria, viruses, chemicals, or other substances.
>
> **Tuberculosis (TB)** A disease caused by bacterial infiltration of the respiratory system.
>
> **Viruses** Minute parasitic microbes that live inside another cell.

Viral diseases can be difficult to treat because many viruses can withstand heat, formaldehyde, and large doses of radiation with little effect on their structure. Some viruses have **incubation periods** (the length of time required to develop fully and cause symptoms in their hosts) that last for years, which delays diagnosis. Drug treatment for viral infections is also limited. Drugs powerful enough to kill viruses generally kill the host cells too, although some medications block stages in viral reproduction without damaging host cells. When exposed to certain viruses, the body produces a protein substance known as **interferon.** Interferon does not destroy the invading microorganisms but sets up a protective mechanism to aid healthy cells in their struggle against the invaders. Although interferon research is promising, it should be noted that not all viruses stimulate interferon production.

The Common Cold
Colds are responsible for more days lost from work and more uncomfortable days spent at work than any other ailment. Caused by any number of viruses (some experts claim there may be over 100 different viruses responsible), colds are **endemic** (always present to some degree) throughout the world. Current research indicates that otherwise healthy people carry cold viruses in their noses and throats most of the time. These viruses are held in check until the host's resistance is lowered. In the true sense of the word, it is possible to "catch" a cold—from the airborne droplets of another person's sneeze or from skin-to-skin or mucous membrane contact—although the hands are the greatest avenue for transmitting colds and other viruses.

Will vitamin C cure my cold?

Although numerous ideas exist concerning how to cure the common cold, including taking megadoses of vitamin C, little hard evidence supports any of them. The best rule of thumb is to keep your resistance level high with sound nutrition, adequate rest, stress reduction, and regular exercise. Avoid people with newly developed colds (colds appear to be

most contagious during the first 24 hours of onset). If you contract a cold, bed rest, plenty of fluids, and aspirin or over-the-counter preparations to relieve symptoms are tried-and-true remedies for adults. Children should not be given aspirin because this could lead to *Reye's syndrome,* a potentially fatal disease.

Influenza
In otherwise healthy people, **influenza,** or flu, is usually not life-threatening. However, in combination with disorders such as respiratory or heart disease or among people over age 65 or under age 5, the flu can be very serious. How do you know if you have a cold, or a case of the flu? See Figure 14.2.

To date, three major varieties of flu virus have been discovered, with many different strains existing within each variety. The A form of the virus is generally the most virulent, followed by the B and C varieties. For more on the emerging strain of avian flu, see the New Horizons in Health box on page 382. If you contract one form of influenza you may develop immunity to it, but you will not necessarily be immune to other forms of the disease. Little can be done to treat flu patients once the infection has become established.

Some vaccines have proven effective against certain strains of flu virus, but they are totally ineffective against others. In spite of minor risks, people over age 65, pregnant women, people with heart or lung disease, and those with certain other illnesses should be vaccinated. Because flu shots take two to three weeks to become effective, you should get these shots in the fall before the flu season begins. An inhaled vaccine called FluMist is available for healthy, nonpregnant adults up to age 49. Because the vaccine contains a weakened version of the live virus, people who receive the vaccine may pose a risk to anyone with a weakened immune system who is around them. More investigation into the risks are needed.[9]

Infectious Mononucleosis
Initial symptoms of **mononucleosis,** or "mono," include sore throat, fever, headache, nausea, chills, and pervasive weakness/fatigue. As the disease progresses, lymph nodes may enlarge and jaundice, spleen enlargement, aching joints, and body rashes may occur.

Caused by the *Epstein-Barr virus,* mono is readily detected through a *monospot test,* a blood test that measures the percentage of specific forms of white blood cells. Because many viruses are caused by transmission of body fluids, many people once believed that young people contracted mono through kissing (hence its nickname, "the kissing disease"). Although a possible cause, mono is not believed to be highly contagious and does not appear to be easily spread through normal, everyday personal contact.

Treatment of mono is often a lengthy process that involves bed rest, balanced nutrition, and medications. Gradually, the body develops immunity to the disease, and the person returns to normal activity.

Incubation period   The time between exposure to a disease and the appearance of symptoms.

Interferon   A protein substance produced by the body that aids the immune system by protecting healthy cells.

Endemic   Describing a disease that is always present to some degree.

Influenza   A common viral disease of the respiratory tract.

Mononucleosis   A virus characterized by fatigue, sore throat, chills, fever, enlarged lymph nodes and spleen. Not highly contagious; is treated with bed rest, good nutrition.

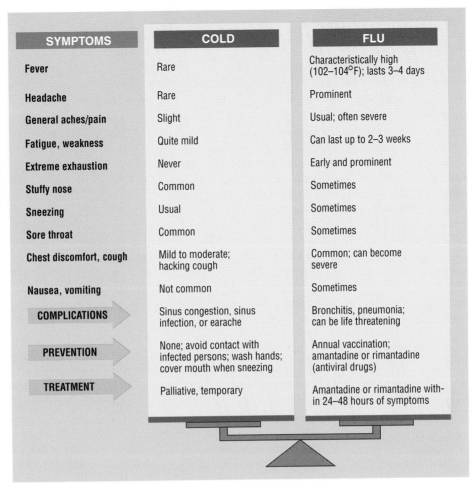

SYMPTOMS	COLD	FLU
Fever	Rare	Characteristically high (102–104°F); lasts 3–4 days
Headache	Rare	Prominent
General aches/pain	Slight	Usual; often severe
Fatigue, weakness	Quite mild	Can last up to 2–3 weeks
Extreme exhaustion	Never	Early and prominent
Stuffy nose	Common	Sometimes
Sneezing	Usual	Sometimes
Sore throat	Common	Sometimes
Chest discomfort, cough	Mild to moderate; hacking cough	Common; can become severe
Nausea, vomiting	Not common	Sometimes
COMPLICATIONS	Sinus congestion, sinus infection, or earache	Bronchitis, pneumonia; can be life threatening
PREVENTION	None; avoid contact with infected persons; wash hands; cover mouth when sneezing	Annual vaccination; amantadine or rimantadine (antiviral drugs)
TREATMENT	Palliative, temporary	Amantadine or rimantadine within 24–48 hours of symptoms

Figure 14.2 ■ Is It a Cold or the Flu?

Source: Adapted from the National Institute of Allergy and Infectious Diseases, "Is It a Cold or the Flu?" 2000. www.niald.nin.gov

Measles **Measles** is a viral disorder that often affects young children. Symptoms, appearing about ten days after exposure, include an itchy rash and a high fever. **Rubella (German measles)** is a milder viral infection that is believed to be transmitted by inhalation, after which it multiplies in the upper respiratory tract and passes into the bloodstream. It causes a rash, especially on the upper extremities. It is not generally a serious health threat and usually runs its course in three to four days. The major exceptions to this rule are newborns and pregnant women. Rubella can damage a fetus, particularly during the first trimester, by creating a condition known as congenital rubella in which the infant may be born blind, deaf, cognitively impaired, or with heart defects. Immunization has reduced the incidence of both measles and rubella. Infections in children not immunized against measles can lead to fever-induced problems such as rheumatic heart disease, kidney damage, and neurological disorders.

Hepatitis One of the most highly publicized viral diseases is **hepatitis,** a virally caused inflammation of the liver. Hepatitis symptoms include fever, headache, nausea, loss of appetite, skin rashes, pain in the upper right abdomen, dark yellow (with brownish tinge) urine, and jaundice (yellowing of the whites of the eyes and the skin). In some regions of the United States and among certain segments of the population, hepatitis has reached epidemic proportions. Internationally, viral hepatitis is a major contributor to liver disease and accounts for high morbidity and mortality. Currently, there are seven known forms, with hepatitis A, B, and C having the highest rate of incidence.

■ *Hepatitis A (HAV)*. HAV is contracted from eating food or drinking water contaminated with human excrement. Infected food handlers, people who ingest

Measles A viral disease that produces symptoms including an itchy rash and a high fever.

Rubella (German measles) A milder form of measles that causes a rash and mild fever in children and may cause damage to a fetus or a newborn baby.

Hepatitis A virally caused disease in which the liver becomes inflamed, which produces symptoms such as fever, headache, and jaundice.

As the flu season of 2005–2006 approached, headlines warning of a massive flu pandemic and images of chickens and other birds going to slaughter across Asia and Europe began to emerge. The media flurry was sparked by concern in the international community over a strain of avian (bird) influenza called H5N1. This newly emerging virulent flu strain began to emerge in bird populations throughout Asia, including domestic birds like chickens and ducks, as early as 1997. Why all of the concern now? Scientists have noted that recently bird flu has appeared in regions of the world previously unaffected. As of this book's publication, bird flu, which is highly contagious and fatal, has spread to parts of Eastern Europe and Russia, further fueling speculation of not *if*, but *when* the H5N1 strain will be readily passed from human to human.

The Threat to Human Health

Many scientists suggest that this virus is virulent enough to surpass the lethality of the Influenza epidemics of 1918 and 1919 which swept the global community, causing millions of deaths. In a 2005 World Health Organization (WHO) meeting devoted to the H5N1 bird flu strain, public health officials warned that a global bird flu pandemic could easily kill millions of people and cost the global economy more than $800 billion.

Why does bird flu pose such a severe threat to humans? The H5N1 strain is so new and unique that human beings have no natural immunity to it. With the common flu virus, our immune system is able to recognize the antigens, and develop antibodies to fight back. H5N1 is considered a threat because it is so different from other flu antigens. Although the virus has yet to mutate into a form highly infectious to humans, outbreaks in rural areas of the world (where people often live in close proximity to poultry and other animals) have occurred. As of January, 2006, bird flu has caused 78 deaths worldwide.

Preventing a Pandemic

WHO officials warn that the world is not prepared to fight a flu pandemic. The current spread of H5N1 throughout global bird populations has seemed to spark international governments into action, however. Countries around the globe are working to develop strategic action plans and early warning systems, prevent the spread of disease, and create vaccines. However, developing countries are of great concern, because the same resources are not available to them. African nations and rural areas of Asia could be devastated by a pandemic.

Research studies are under way to develop a vaccine, but no vaccine is currently ready for production, and when it is ready, producing enough vaccine for an epidemic will present another challenge. Despite this, there

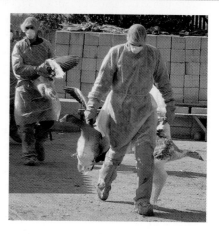

are some promising treatments, and tips for prevention.

■ Antiviral medication, such as Tamiflu, can reduce the severity and duration of illness. Countries worldwide and the WHO are stockpiling of these medications and developing plans for rapid distribution, should an outbreak occur.

■ To date, researchers do not believe the virus can be transmitted via cooked poultry, but caution should be used when eating poultry or eggs in countries experiencing outbreaks. Foods should be properly cooked and handled during food preparation. Exposure could occur during preparation of raw poultry for cooking.

■ Wash your hands (see the Try it Now on page 386 for tips on proper hand-washing). This is one of the best defenses against infection. If you cannot wash your hands with soap and water, consider using an alcohol-based hand sanitizer.

---

seafood from contaminated water, and those who use contaminated needles are also at risk. Fortunately, individuals infected with hepatitis A do not become chronic carriers, and vaccines for HAV are available.[10]

■ *Hepatitis B (HBV).* This disease is spread primarily via body fluids being shared through unprotected sex but also is contracted via sharing needles when injecting drugs, needlesticks on the job, or, in the case of a newborn baby, from an infected mother. Although 30 percent of those who are infected have no symptoms, symptoms can include jaundice, fatigue, abdominal pain, loss of appetite, nausea and vomiting, and joint pain. HBV can lead to chronic liver disease or liver cancer. It is one of the fastest growing sexually transmitted infections in the United States, with over 300,000 new cases per year. It is possible to become a chronic HBV carrier and infect others;

more than 1.2 million people are chronic carriers.[11] Fortunately, a vaccine for HBV is now available, making it one of the only vaccine-preventable sexually transmitted infections.

- *Hepatitis C (HCV).* HCV infections are on an epidemic rise in many regions of the world, as resistant forms are emerging. Some cases can be traced to blood transfusions or organ transplants. Over 85 percent of those infected develop chronic infections, and if the infection is left untreated, the person may develop cirrhosis of the liver, liver cancer, or liver failure. Liver failure due to chronic hepatitis C is the leading cause of liver transplants in the United States.[12] Although there is no vaccine for HCV, one is currently being tested and may be available shortly.[13]

In the United States, hepatitis continues to be a major threat in spite of a safe blood supply and massive efforts at education about hand washing (for HAV) and safer sex (primarily for HBV). Treatment of all forms of viral hepatitis is somewhat limited.

Other Pathogens

Fungi Hundreds of species of **fungi,** multicellular or unicellular primitive plants, inhabit our environment. Many fungi are useful, providing such foodstuffs as edible mushrooms and some cheeses. But some species of fungi can produce infections. *Candidiasis* (a vaginal yeast infection), athlete's foot, ringworm, and jock itch are examples of fungal diseases. Keeping the affected area clean and dry plus treatment with appropriate medications will generally bring prompt relief.

Protozoa **Protozoa** are microscopic, single-celled organisms that are generally associated with tropical diseases such as African sleeping sickness and malaria. Although these pathogens are prevalent in nonindustrialized countries, they are largely controlled in the United States. The most common protozoal disease in the United States is *trichomoniasis*, which we will discuss later in this chapter's section on sexually transmitted infections. A common waterborne protozoan disease in many regions of the country is *giardiasis*. People who drink or are exposed to the *Giardia* pathogen may suffer intestinal pain and discomfort weeks after infection. Protection of water supplies is the key to prevention.

Parasitic Worms **Parasitic worms** are the largest of the pathogens. Ranging in size from the small pinworms typically found in children to the relatively large tapeworms found in all warm-blooded animals, most parasitic worms are more a nuisance than a threat. Of special note today are the worm infestations associated with eating raw fish in Japanese sushi restaurants. Cooking fish and other foods to temperatures sufficient to kill the worms and their eggs can prevent this.

Prions A **prion,** or unconventional virus, is a self-replicating, protein-based agent that can infect humans and other animals. Believed to be the underlying cause of spongiform diseases such as "mad cow disease," this agent systematically destroys brain cells. We will say more about prion-based diseases later in this chapter.

YOUR BODY'S DEFENSES: KEEPING YOU WELL

Although all the pathogens just described pose a threat if they take hold in your body, the chances that they will do so are actually quite small. First, they must overcome a number of effective barriers, many of which were established in your body before you were born. Table 14.2 on the next page lists actions you can take to keep your body's defenses healthy.

Physical and Chemical Defenses

Perhaps our single most critical early defense system is the skin. Layered to provide an intricate web of barriers, the skin allows few pathogens to enter. **Enzymes,** complex proteins manufactured by the body that appear in body secretions such as sweat provide additional protection, destroying microorganisms on skin surfaces by producing inhospitable pH levels. Normal body pH is 7.0, but enzymatic or biochemical changes may cause the body chemistry to become more acidic (pH of less than 7.0) or more alkaline (pH of more than 7.0). In either case, microorganisms that flourish at a selected pH will be weakened or destroyed as these changes occur. Only when cracks or breaks occur in the skin can pathogens gain easy access to the body.

The linings of the body provide yet another protection. Mucous membranes in the respiratory tract and other linings of the body trap and engulf invading organisms. *Cilia,* hairlike projections in the lungs and respiratory tract, sweep invaders toward body openings,

---

Fungi A group of plants that lack chlorophyll and do not produce flowers or seeds; several microscopic varieties are pathogenic.

Protozoa Microscopic, single-celled organisms.

Parasitic worms The largest of the pathogens, most of which are more a nuisance than a threat.

Prions A self-replicating protein-based agent that systematically destroys brain cells.

Enzymes Organic substances that cause bodily changes and destruction of microorganisms.

Table 14.2

Keeping Defenses Healthy

■ Limit exposure to germs	Limit contact with those who are getting colds or have symptoms. Wash your hands and avoid touching hands to eyes and mouth. Avoid antibacterial soaps, which contribute to germ resistance.
■ Exercise regularly	Exercising raises core body temperature, which kills many invaders.
■ Get enough sleep	Refresh your body regularly. Take time out and time off. Experience your spiritual side.
■ Eat healthy foods	Follow established guidelines, consuming adequate amounts of water, protein, carbohydrates, fats, vitamins, and minerals. Moderation in using supplements is recommended.
■ Don't overuse antibiotics	"Use it and lose it" is a phrase that aptly describes what has happened as antibiotics are used over and over again and bacteria adapt to become more resistant to them. Many antibiotics are used inappropriately because patients demand them.
■ Manage stress	Use strategies such as exercise and relaxation techniques to lower stress levels in your life.

Source: Adapted from T. Mitchell, "Make Your Immnue System Invincible," *USA Weekend,* January 7–9, 2000. Reprinted by permission of T. L. Mitchell, USA Weekend Health Editor.

where they are expelled. Tears, nasal secretions, ear wax, and other secretions found at body entrances contain enzymes designed to destroy or neutralize pathogens. Finally, any organism that manages to breach these initial lines of defense faces a formidable specialized network of defenses thrown up by the immune system.

The Immune System: Your Body Fights Back

How does my body fight a disease?

Immunity is a condition of being able to resist a particular disease by counteracting the substance that produces the disease. Any substance capable of triggering an immune response is called an **antigen.** An antigen can be a virus, a bacterium, a fungus, a parasite, or a tissue or cell from another individual. When invaded by an antigen, the body responds by forming substances called **antibodies** that are matched to that specific antigen

Antigen Substance capable of triggering an immune response.

Antibodies Substances produced by the body that are individually matched to specific antigens.

much as a key is matched to a lock. Antibodies belong to a mass of large molecules known as *immunoglobulins,* a group of nine chemically distinct protein substances, each of which plays a role in neutralizing, setting up for destruction, or actually destroying antigens.

Once an antigen breaches the body's initial defenses, the body begins a process of antigen analysis. It considers the size and shape of the invader, verifies that the antigen is not part of the body itself, and then produces a specific antibody to destroy or weaken the antigen. This process, which is much more complex than described here, is part of a system called *humoral immune responses*. Humoral immunity is the body's major defense against many bacteria and bacterial toxins.

Cell-mediated immunity is characterized by the formation of a population of lymphocytes that can attack and destroy the foreign invader. These lymphocytes constitute the body's main defense against viruses, fungi, parasites, and some bacteria. Key players in this immune response are specialized groups of white blood cells known as *macrophages* (a type of phagocytic, or cell-eating, cell) and *lymphocytes,* other white blood cells found in the blood, lymph nodes, bone marrow, and certain glands.

Two forms of lymphocytes in particular, the *B lymphocytes* (B cells) and *T lymphocytes* (T cells), are involved in the immune response. There are different types of B cells, which are manufactured and mature in the soft tissue of the hollow shafts of the long bones. T cells, in contrast, are manufactured in long bones and mature in the thymus, a multilobed organ that lies behind the breastbone.

T cells assist the immune system in several ways. *Regulatory T cells* help direct the activities of the immune system and assist other cells, particularly B cells, to produce antibodies. Dubbed "helper T cells," these cells are essential for activating B cells, other T cells, and macrophages. Another form of T cell, known as the *killer T cells* or *cytotoxic T cells,* directly attacks infected or malignant cells. Killer T cells enable the body to rid itself of cells that have been infected by viruses or transformed by cancer; they are also responsible for the rejection of tissue and organ grafts. The third type of T cells, *suppressor T cells,* turns off or suppresses the activity of B cells, killer T cells, and macrophages. Suppressor T cells circulate in the bloodstream and lymphatic system, neutralizing or destroying antigens, enhancing the effects of the immune response, and helping to return the activated immune system to normal levels.

After a successful attack on a pathogen, some of the attacker T and B cells are preserved as *memory T and B cells,* enabling the body to quickly recognize and respond to subsequent attacks by the same kind of organism at a later time. Thus macrophages, T and B cells, and antibodies are the key factors in mounting an immune response.

Once people have survived certain infectious diseases, they become immune to those diseases, meaning that in all probability they will not develop them again. Upon subsequent attack by the disease-causing microorganisms, their memory T and B cells are quickly activated to come to their defense.

Autoimmune Diseases

Although white blood cells and the antigen–antibody response generally work in our favor by neutralizing or destroying harmful antigens, the body sometimes makes a mistake and targets its own tissue as the enemy, builds up antibodies against that tissue, and attempts to destroy it. This is known as *autoimmune disease* (*auto* means "self"). Common autoimmune disorders are rheumatoid arthritis, systemic lupus erythematosus (SLE), and myasthenia gravis.

In some cases, the antigen–antibody response completely fails to function. The result is a form of *immunodeficiency syndrome.* Perhaps the most dramatic case of this syndrome was the "bubble boy," a youngster who died in 1984 after living his short life inside a sealed-off environment designed to protect him from all antigens. A much more common immune system disorder is *acquired immunodeficiency syndrome (AIDS),* which we will discuss later in this chapter (page 395).

Fever

If an infection is localized, pus formation, redness, swelling, and irritation often occur. These symptoms indicate that the invading organisms are being fought systematically. Another indication is the development of a fever, or a rise in body temperature above the average norm of 98.6°F. Fever is frequently caused by toxins secreted by pathogens that interfere with the control of body temperature. Although extremely elevated temperatures are harmful to the body, a mild fever is believed to act as a form of protection: raising body temperature by one or two degrees provides an environment that destroys some disease-causing organisms. A fever also stimulates the body to produce more white blood cells, which destroy more invaders.

Pain

Although we do not usually think of pain as a defense mechanism, it is a response to injury and plays a valuable role in the body's response to invasion. Pain may be *direct,* caused by the stimulation of nerve endings in an affected area, or *referred,* meaning it is present in one place although the source is elsewhere. An example of **referred pain** is the pain in the arm or jaw often experienced by someone having a heart attack. Most pain responses are accompanied by inflammation. Pain tends to be the earliest sign that an injury has occurred and often causes the person to slow down or stop the activity that was aggravating the injury, thereby protecting against further damage. Because it is often one of the first warnings of disease, persistent pain should not be overlooked or masked with short-term pain relievers.

Vaccines: Bolstering Your Immunity

Recall that once people have been exposed to a specific pathogen, subsequent attacks will activate their memory T and B cells, thus giving them immunity. This is the principle on which **vaccination** is based.

A vaccine consists of killed or attenuated (weakened) versions of a disease-causing microorganism or an antigen that is similar to but less dangerous than the disease antigen. It is administered to stimulate the person's immune system to produce antibodies against future attacks—without actually causing the disease.

Referred pain Pain that is present at one point but whose source is elsewhere.

Vaccination Inoculation with killed or weakened pathogens or similar, less dangerous antigens in order to prevent or lessen the effects of some disease.

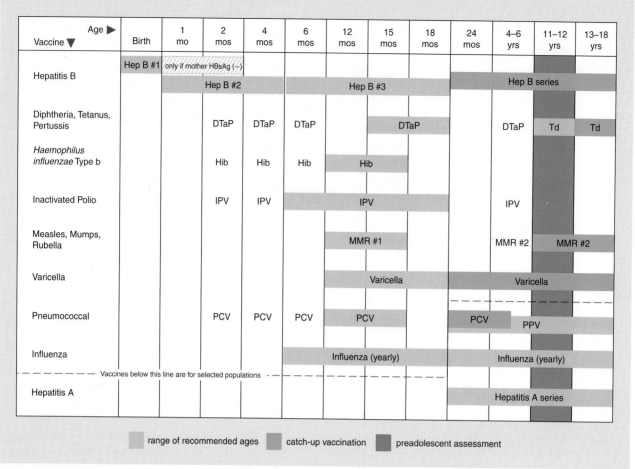

Age ► Vaccine ▼	Birth	1 mo	2 mos	4 mos	6 mos	12 mos	15 mos	18 mos	24 mos	4–6 yrs	11–12 yrs	13–18 yrs
Hepatitis B	Hep B #1	only if mother HBsAg (–)										
		Hep B #2			Hep B #3				Hep B series			
Diphtheria, Tetanus, Pertussis		DTaP	DTaP	DTaP		DTaP			DTaP	Td	Td	
Haemophilus influenzae Type b		Hib	Hib	Hib	Hib							
Inactivated Polio		IPV	IPV		IPV				IPV			
Measles, Mumps, Rubella					MMR #1				MMR #2	MMR #2		
Varicella					Varicella			Varicella				
Pneumococcal		PCV	PCV	PCV	PCV			PCV	PPV			
Influenza				Influenza (yearly)					Influenza (yearly)			
— — — Vaccines below this line are for selected populations — — —												
Hepatitis A									Hepatitis A series			

▢ range of recommended ages ▢ catch-up vaccination ▢ preadolescent assessment

Figure 14.3 ▢ Recommended Childhood and Adolescent Immunization Schedule, 2003

Source: Centers for Disease Control and Prevention, "Recommended Childhood and Adolescent Immunization Schedule, July–December 2004," www.cdc.gov/nip/recs/child~schedule.htm.

Vaccines typically are given orally or by injection, and this form of immunity is termed artificially **acquired active immunity,** in contrast to **naturally acquired active immunity** (which is obtained by exposure to antigens in the normal course of daily life) or *naturally acquired passive immunity* (as occurs when a mother passes to her fetus via their shared blood supply or to an infant via breast milk).

Depending on the virulence of the organism, vaccines containing live, attenuated, or dead organisms are given for a variety of diseases. In some instances, if a person is already weakened by other health problems, vaccination may provoke an actual mild case of the disease. Figure 14.3 shows the recommended schedule for childhood vaccinations.

Acquired active immunity   Immunity developed during life in response to disease, vaccination, or exposure.

Natural active immunity   Immunity passed to a fetus by its mother.

Try it ►NOW_____

Wash your hands to prevent infection. A quick rinse under cold water won't cut it. Wet your hands with warm water and lather up with soap, scrubbing for about 20 seconds—try counting to 20 or saying the alphabet. Rinse well and dry your hands. Start following this basic procedure today whenever you use the bathroom, eat or prepare food, blow your nose, cough, or sneeze.

EMERGING AND RESURGENT DISEASES

Although our immune systems are remarkably adept at responding to challenges, microbes appear to be gaining ground. Within the past decade, rates for infectious diseases have rapidly increased, particularly for reemerging diseases such as tuberculosis. This can be attributed to a combination of overpopulation, inadequate health care systems, increasing poverty, extreme environmental degradation, and drug resistance.[14] As international travel increases (over 1 million people per day cross international boundaries), with germs transported from remote regions to huge urban centers within hours, the likelihood of infection by microbes previously unknown on U.S. soil increases.

Tiny Microbes: Lethal Threats

Today's arsenal of antibiotics appears to be increasingly ineffective. Penicillin-resistant strains of diseases are on the rise as bacteria become able to outlast and outsmart even the best of our antibiotic weapons, and viruses are constantly mutating, making them potentially more lethal.[15] Old scourges are back, and new ones are emerging.

"Mad Cow Disease" The American cattle industry is under new scrutiny, with the first confirmed case of *bovine spongiform encephalopathy* (BSE, or "mad cow disease") being detected in late 2003. Evidence indicates that there is a relationship between ongoing outbreaks in Europe of BSE and a disease in humans known as *new variant Creutzfeldt-Jakob disease (nvCJD)*.[16] Both disorders are invariably fatal brain diseases with unusually long incubation periods (the time between exposure and the appearance of symptoms) measured in years, and both are caused by unconventional transmittable agents known as *prions*.

BSE is thought to have been transmitted when cows were fed slaughterhouse leftovers from sheep and other cows as a protein source. Failure to treat this protein by-product sufficiently to kill the BSE organism allowed it to infect the cows, and the disease is believed to be transmitted to humans through the meat. The resultant variant of BSE in humans, nvCJD, is characterized by progressively worsening neurological damage and death.

As scientists continue to investigate the presence of BSE in U.S. cattle, several possible cases have been identified. To date, there have been no known human infections from U.S. beef. More rigorous testing of cattle is currently being implemented.

Severe Acute Respiratory Syndrome (SARS) SARS is a viral respiratory illness that first emerged in Asia in February 2003 and eventually infected over 8,000 people worldwide, with 774 deaths. Caused by a coronavirus, SARS is thought to be spread by close personal contact with those infected, though research on other methods of transmission is ongoing. Symptoms of SARS include a high fever, body aches, headache, diarrhea, and a cough. Eventually, this cough can progress to a pneumonia-like upper respiratory illness.[17]

West Nile Virus This virus is spread by the bite of an infected mosquito. Until 1999, few Americans had heard of *West Nile Virus (WNV)*; today, only a few states remain disease-free, and during 2005, there were over 1,800 cases of WNV reported, and 52 deaths nationwide.

Most people who become infected with West Nile Virus will have either mild symptoms or none at all. Rarely, West Nile Virus infection can result in severe and sometimes fatal illness. Symptoms include fever, headache, and body aches, often with skin rash and swollen lymph glands, and a form of encephalitis (inflammation of the brain). There is no vaccine or specific treatment for WNV, but avoiding mosquito bites is the best way to prevent WNV. Strategies to prevent mosquito bites include using a bug repellent with DEET (diethyl tolumide) and wearing long-sleeved clothing and long pants when outdoors; staying indoors during dawn, dusk and other peak mosquito feeding times; and removing any standing water sources around the home.

Ebola Hemorrhagic Fever (Ebola HF)
Another emerging disease, Ebola HF is a severe, often fatal disease in humans and nonhuman primates (monkeys, gorillas, and chimpanzees). Researchers believe the Ebola virus is zoonotic (animal-borne) and normally occurs in animal hosts that are native to the African continent.[18] The virus is spread via direct contact with blood and/or secretions and may be aerosol disseminated (airborne). With an incubation period of 2 to 21 days, the course of the disease is quick and characterized by fever, headache, joint and muscle aches, sore throat, and weakness, followed by diarrhea, vomiting, and stomach pain.[19] Fortunately, Ebola is not as prevalent worldwide as many other diseases.

Escherichia coli O157:H7 *E. coli* O157:H7, as it is commonly referred to, is one of over 170 types of *E. coli* bacteria that can infect humans. While most *E. coli* organisms are harmless and live in the intestines of healthy animals and humans, *E. coli* O157:H7 produces a lethal toxin and can cause severe illness or death.

E. coli O157:H7 can live in the intestines of healthy cattle and then contaminate food products at slaughterhouses. Eating ground beef that is rare or undercooked, drinking unpasteurized milk and juice, or swimming in sewage-contaminated water or public pools can cause infection via ingestion of feces that contain *E. coli*. Several children were infected at a fair in Oregon when they petted infected farm animals and did not wash their hands.

A symptom of infection is nonbloody diarrhea, usually 2 to 8 days after exposure; however, asymptomatic cases have been noted. Children, older adults, and people whose immune systems have been weakened by other diseases are particularly vulnerable to serious side effects such as kidney failure.

While *E. coli* organisms continue to pose threats to public health, strengthened regulations on the cooking of meat and regulation of chlorine levels in pools have helped. Recent findings indicate that eliminating grains from the diet of cattle in the days prior to slaughter may reduce the growth of *E. coli* in their stomachs.

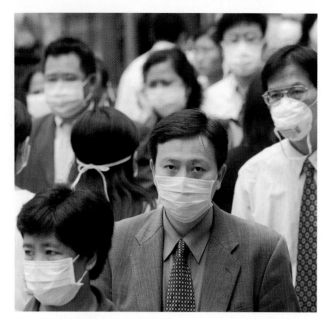

Emerging diseases such as SARS can cause communities to take widespread precautions to prevent transmission.

Cholera An infectious disease transmitted through fecal contamination of food or water, cholera has been rare in the United States for most of this century. Recent epidemics in the Western Hemisphere—over 900,000 cases—however, have started to affect the United States. One theory of how cholera is introduced into distant regions of the world is that ships from endemic areas release contaminated bilge water into port towns, contaminating local shellfish.[20] Efforts to control cholera may be increasingly difficult as international travel and trade increase.

Hantavirus Transmitted via rodent urine and feces, this virus was responsible for many deaths in the southwestern United States in 1994 before experts were able to identify the culprit. Victims were believed to have come into contact with this organism through breathing the virus-laden dust in rodent-infested homes. Within hours, victims showed serious symptoms as their lungs filled with fluid; they subsequently experienced respiratory collapse and died. Today, cases of hantavirus have been noted in more than 20 states, and vaccines are being developed to counteract it.

Bioterrorism: The New Global Threat

The idea of using infectious microorganisms as weapons is not new. In fact, during the seventeenth century wars, the English traded blankets impregnated with scabs from smallpox patients with the American Indians in hopes of causing disease.[21] The threat of delivering a lethal load of anthrax or other deadly microorganisms in the warheads of missiles or by a single person is a topic of much discussion among today's world leaders, particularly after the cases of anthrax delivered by mail following the September 11, 2001, terrorist attacks. For more information on what you can do to protect yourself from bioterrorism, see Chapter 4.

SEXUALLY TRANSMITTED INFECTIONS

Sexually transmitted infections (STIs) have been with us since our earliest recorded days on Earth. Today, there are more than 20 known types of STIs. Once referred to as "venereal diseases" and then "sexually transmitted diseases," the current terminology is more reflective of the number and types of these communicable diseases. More virulent strains and more antibiotic-resistant forms spell trouble in the days ahead.

Sexually transmitted infections affect men and women of all backgrounds and socioeconomic levels. The most recent report issued by the Centers for Disease Control and Prevention (CDC) indicates that there are 19 million annual new occurrences of STIs each year.[22] Exact numbers are not available for each STI, and a significant number of cases go unreported each year. However, syphilis is among those showing the greatest increase, while gonorrhea seems to have hit a historic low.[23]

Early symptoms of an STI are often mild and unrecognizable (Figure 14.4). Left untreated, some of these infections can have grave consequences, such as sterility, blindness, central nervous system destruction, disfigurement, and even death. Infants born to mothers carrying the organisms for these infections are at risk for a variety of health problems.

As with many communicable diseases, much of the pain, suffering, and anguish associated with STIs can be eliminated through education, responsible action, simple preventive strategies, and prompt treatment. Although STIs can happen to anyone, they won't if you take appropriate precautions when you decide to engage in a sexual relationship.

Possible Causes: What's Your Risk

Several reasons have been proposed to explain the present high rates of STIs. The first relates to the moral and social stigma associated with these infections. Shame and embarrassment often keep infected people from seeking treatment. Unfortunately, they usually continue to be

Sexually transmitted infections (STIs) Infectious diseases transmitted via some form of intimate, usually sexual, contact.

sexually active, thereby infecting unsuspecting partners. People who are uncomfortable discussing sexual issues may also be less likely to use and ask their partners to use condoms to protect against STIs and pregnancy.

Another reason proposed for the STI epidemic is our culture's casual attitude about sex. Bombarded by media hype that glamorizes easy sex, many people take sexual partners without considering the consequences. Generally, the more sexual partners a person has, the greater the risk for contracting an STI. Evaluate your own attitude about STIs by completing the Assess Yourself box on page 390.

Ignorance—about the infections, their symptoms, and the fact that someone can be asymptomatic (symptom-free) but still infected—is also a factor. A person who is infected but asymptomatic can unknowingly spread an STI to an unsuspecting partner, who may, in turn, ignore or misinterpret any symptoms. By the time either partner seeks medical help, he or she may have infected several others.

How STIs Are Transmitted

STIs are generally spread through some form of intimate sexual contact. Sexual intercourse, oral–genital contact, hand–genital contact, and anal intercourse are the most common modes of transmission. More rarely, pathogens for STIs are transmitted from mouth to mouth or through contact with fluids from body sores. Although each STI is a different infection caused by a different pathogen, all STI pathogens prefer dark, moist places, especially the mucous membranes lining the reproductive organs. Most of them are susceptible to light, excess heat, cold, and dryness, and many die quickly on exposure to air. Although most STIs are passed on by sexual contact, other kinds of close contact, such as sleeping on sheets used by someone who has pubic lice, may also infect you. Like other communicable infections, STIs have both pathogen-specific incubation periods and periods of time during which transmission is most likely, called *periods of communicability*.

> Can I get a sexually transmitted infection from "outercourse"?

Chlamydia

Chlamydia, a disease that often presents no symptoms, tops the list of the most commonly reported infections in the United States. Chlamydia infects about 2.8 million people annually in the United States, the majority of them women.[24] Public health officials believe that the actual number of cases is probably higher because these figures represent only those cases reported. College students account for over 10 percent of infections, and these numbers seem to be increasing yearly.

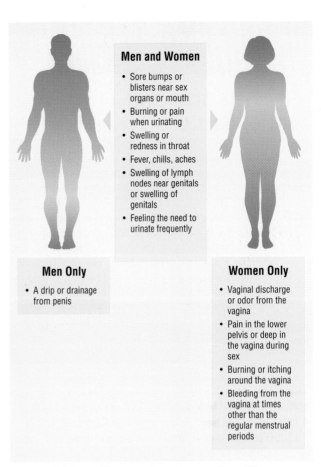

Figure 14.4 ■ Signs or Symptoms of an STI

In males, early symptoms may include painful and difficult urination, frequent urination, and a watery, puslike discharge from the penis. Symptoms in females may include a yellowish discharge, spotting between periods, and occasional spotting after intercourse. However, many chlamydia victims display no symptoms and therefore do not seek help until the disease has done secondary damage. Females are especially likely to be asymptomatic; over 70 percent do not realize they have the disease until secondary damage occurs.

The secondary damage resulting from chlamydia is serious in both genders. Men can suffer injury to the prostate gland, seminal vesicles, and bulbourethral glands as well as arthritis-like symptoms and damage to the blood vessels and heart. In women, chlamydia-related inflammation can injure the cervix or uterine tubes, causing sterility, and damage the inner pelvic structure, leading to pelvic inflammatory disease. If an infected woman becomes pregnant, she has a high risk for miscarriage and stillbirth. Chlamydia may also be

(Text continues on page 392)

> **Chlamydia**   Bacterially caused STI of the urogenital tract; most common STI in the United States.

STI Attitude and Belief Scale

myhealthlab

Fill out this assessment online at
www.aw-bc.com/myhealthlab or www.aw-bc.com/donatelle.

The following quiz will help you evaluate whether your beliefs and attitudes about STIs lead you to behaviors that increase your risk of infection. Indicate that you believe the following items are true or false by circling the T or the F. Then consult the answer key that follows.

1. You can usually tell whether someone is infected with an STI, especially HIV infection.   T   F
2. Chances are that if you haven't caught an STI by now, you probably have a natural immunity and won't get infected in the future.   T   F
3. A person who is successfully treated for an STI needn't worry about getting it again.   T   F
4. So long as you keep yourself fit and healthy, you needn't worry about STIs.   T   F
5. The best way for sexually active people to protect themselves from STIs is to practice safer sex.   T   F
6. The only way to catch an STI is to have sex with someone who has one.   T   F
7. Talking about STIs with a partner is so embarrassing that it's better not to raise the subject and instead hope the other person will.   T   F
8. STIs are mostly a problem for people who have numerous sex partners.   T   F
9. You don't need to worry about contracting an STI so long as you wash yourself thoroughly with soap and hot water immediately after sex.   T   F
10. You don't need to worry about AIDS if no one you know has ever come down with it.   T   F
11. When it comes to STIs, it's all in the cards. Either you're lucky or you're not.   T   F
12. The time to worry about STIs is when you come down with one.   T   F
13. As long as you avoid risky sexual practices, such as anal intercourse, you're pretty safe from STIs.   T   F
14. The time to talk about safer sex is before any sexual contact occurs.   T   F
15. A person needn't be concerned about an STI if the symptoms clear up on their own in a few weeks.   T   F

SCORING KEY

1. *False.* While some STIs have telltale signs, such as the appearance of sores or blisters on the genitals or disagreeable genital odors, others do not. Several STIs, such as chlamydia, gonorrhea (especially in women), internal genital warts, and even HIV infection in its early stages, cause few if any obvious signs or symptoms. You often cannot tell whether your partner is infected with an STI. Many of the nicest-looking and well-groomed people carry STIs, often unknowingly. The only way to know whether a person is infected with HIV is by means of an HIV-antibody test.

2. *False.* If you practice unprotected sex and have not contracted an STI to this point, count your blessings. The thing about good luck is that it eventually runs out.

3. *False.* Sorry. Successful treatment does not render immunity against reinfection. You still need to take precautions to avoid reinfection, even if you have had an STI in the past and were successfully treated. If you answered true to this item, you're not alone. About one in five college students polled in a recent survey of more than 5,500 college students across Canada believed that a person who gets an STI cannot get it again.

4. *False.* Even people in prime physical condition can be felled by the tiniest of microbes that cause STIs. Physical fitness is no protection against these microscopic invaders.

5. *True.* If you are sexually active, practicing safer sex is the best protection against contracting an STI.

6. *False.* STIs can also be transmitted through nonsexual means, such as by sharing contaminated needles or, in some cases, through contact with disease-causing organisms on towels and bedsheets or even toilet seats.

7. *False.* Because of the social stigma attached to STIs, it's understandable that you may feel embarrassed about raising the subject with your partner. But don't let embarrassment prevent you from taking steps to protect your own and your partner's welfare.

8. *False.* While it stands to reason that people who are sexually active with numerous partners stand a greater chance that one of their sexual partners will carry an STI, all it takes is one infected partner to pass along an STI to you, even if he or she is the only partner you've had or even if the two of you had sex only once. STIs are a potential problem for anyone who is sexually active.

9. *False.* While washing your genitals immediately after sex may have some limited protective value, it is no substitute for practicing safer sex.

10. *False.* You can never know whether you may be the first among your friends and acquaintances to become infected. Moreover, symptoms of HIV infection may not appear for years after initial infection with the virus, so you may have sexual contacts with people who are infected but don't know it and who are capable of

passing along the virus to you. You in turn may then pass it along to others, whether or not you are aware of any symptoms.

11. *False.* Nonsense. While luck may play a part in determining whether you have sexual contact with an infected partner, you can significantly reduce your risk of contracting an STI.

12. *False.* The time to start thinking about STIs (thinking helps, but worrying only makes you more anxious than you need be) is now, not after you have contracted an infection. Some STIs, like herpes and AIDS, cannot be cured. The only real protection you have against them is prevention.

13. *False.* Any sexual contact between the genitals, or between the genitals and the anus, or between the mouth and genitals, is risky if one of the partners is infected with an STI.

14. *True.* Unfortunately, too many couples wait until they have commenced sexual relations to have "a talk." By then it may already be too late to prevent the transmission of an STI. The time to talk is before any intimate sexual contact occurs.

15. *False.* Several STIs, notably syphilis, HIV infection, and herpes, may produce initial symptoms that clear up in

a few weeks. But while the early symptoms may subside, the infection is still at work within the body and requires medical attention. Also, as noted previously, the infected person is capable of passing along the infection to others, regardless of whether noticeable symptoms were ever present.

INTERPRETING YOUR SCORE

First, add up the number of items you got right. The higher your score, the lower your risk. The lower your score, the greater your risk. A score of 13 correct or better may indicate that your attitudes toward STIs would probably decrease your risk of contracting them. Yet even one wrong response on this test may increase your risk of contracting an STI. You should also recognize that attitudes have little effect on behavior unless they are carried into action. Knowledge alone isn't sufficient to protect yourself from STIs. You need to ask yourself how you are going to put knowledge into action by changing your behavior to reduce your chances of contracting an STI.

Source: From Jeffrey S. Nevid with Fern Gotfried, *Choices: Sex in the Age of STDs,* 10-13. (c) Copyright 1995 by Allyn & Bacon. Reprinted by permission.

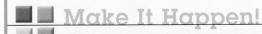

Make It Happen!

Assessment: The Assess Yourself activity gave you the chance to consider your beliefs and attitudes about STIs, and possible risks you may be facing. Now that you have considered these results, you can begin to change behaviors that may be putting you at risk.

Making a Change: In order to change your behavior, you need to develop a plan. Follow these steps below and complete your Behavior Change Contract to take action.

1. Evaluate your behavior, and identify patterns and specific things you are doing. What can you change now? What can you change in the near future?
2. Select one pattern of behavior that you want to change.
3. Fill out the Behavior Change Contract found at the front of your book. It should include your long-term goal for change, your short-term goals, the rewards you'll give yourself for reaching these goals, potential obstacles along the way, and strategies for overcoming these obstacles. For each goal, list the small steps and specific actions that you will take.
4. Chart your progress in a journal. At the end of a week, consider how successful you were in following your plan. What helped you be successful? What made change more difficult? What will you do differently next week?
5. Revise your plan as needed. Are the short-term goals attainable? Are the rewards satisfying?

Example: Carlos had never thought that he was at risk for an STI. He only dated one woman at a time, and he had

never had an STI himself. After he reviewed his answers to the self-assessment, however, he saw that there were several ways in which he was putting himself at risk.

He had thought that he would be able to tell whether someone was infected with an STI but question 1's answer described how, especially among women, there are few if any obvious signs or symptoms of some STIs. Carlos also believed that he was not at risk because he dated only one woman at a time, but the answer to question 8 pointed out that a person can pass on an STI that he or she contracted from a previous sex partner. Carlos decided it was time to take responsibility for his sexual activity. He had been on three dates with Sherry and felt things were progressing toward a more intimate stage; he wanted to be sure that they discussed STIs before they put themselves at risk.

Carlos was nervous when he thought about talking to Sherry, so he wrote out a few ideas of ways to bring up the subject. This made him more confident that he would be able to talk honestly with Sherry. He also made sure that he had a supply of condoms, so there wouldn't be any reason not to practice safer sex. During their next date, Carlos asked Sherry if they could have a serious conversation about the next step. When he told her that he wanted to talk about STIs, she told him that she was relieved that he had brought up the subject. She knew that she was healthy and hadn't been sure how to find out his status. Carlos was relieved that Sherry was as concerned about the issue as he was, and they were both glad that embarrassment had not prevented them from having this conversation.

responsible for one type of **conjunctivitis,** an eye infection that affects not only adults but also infants, who can contract the disease from an infected mother during delivery. Untreated conjunctivitis can cause blindness.

If detected early, chlamydia is easily treatable with antibiotics. Unfortunately, chlamydia tests are not a routine part of many health clinics' testing procedures. Usually a person must specifically request a chlamydia check.

Pelvic Inflammatory Disease

Pelvic inflammatory disease (PID) is a term used to describe a number of infections of the uterus, uterine tubes, and ovaries. Although PID often results from an untreated sexually transmitted infection, especially chlamydia or gonorrhea, it is not actually an STI.

Symptoms of PID vary but generally include lower abdominal pain, fever, unusual vaginal discharge, painful intercourse, painful urination, and irregular menstrual bleeding.[25] Risk factors include young age at first sexual intercourse, multiple sex partners, high frequency of sexual intercourse, and change of sexual partners within the past 30 days. Regular gynecological examinations and early treatment for STI symptoms reduce risk.

Gonorrhea

Gonorrhea is one of the most common STIs in the United States, surpassed only by chlamydia in number of cases. The CDC estimates that there are over 700,000 cases per year, plus numbers that go unreported.[26] Caused by the bacterial pathogen *Neisseria gonorrhoeae,* gonorrhea primarily infects the linings of the urethra, genital tract, pharynx, and rectum. It may spread to the eyes or other body regions via the hands or body fluids, typically during vaginal, oral, or anal sex. Most cases are males between the ages of 20 and 24, with sexually active females between the ages of 15 and 19 also at high risk.[27] In males, a typical symptom is a white, milky discharge from the penis accompanied by painful, burning urination two to nine days after contact. This is usually enough to send most men to the physician for treatment. However, about 20 percent of all males with gonorrhea are asymptomatic.

In females, the situation is just the opposite: only 20 percent experience any discharge, and few develop a burning sensation upon urinating until much later in the course of the infection (if ever). The organism can remain in the woman's vagina, cervix, uterus, or uterine tubes for long periods with no apparent symptoms other than an occasional slight fever. Thus a woman can be unaware that she has been infected and that she is infecting her sexual partners.

If the infection is detected early, antibiotic treatment is generally effective. If the infection goes undetected in a woman, it can spread to the uterine tubes and ovaries, causing sterility, or at the very least, severe inflammation and PID. The bacteria can also spread up the reproductive tract, or more rarely, through the blood and infect the joints, heart valves, or brain. If an infected woman becomes pregnant, the infection can cause conjunctivitis in her infant. To prevent this, physicians routinely administer silver nitrate or penicillin preparations to the eyes of newborn babies.

In a man, untreated gonorrhea may spread to the prostate, testicles, urinary tract, kidney, and bladder. Blockage of the vasa deferentia due to scar tissue may cause sterility. In some cases, the penis develops a painful curvature during erection.

Syphilis

Syphilis is also caused by a bacterial organism, *Treponema pallidum.* Because the organism is extremely delicate and dies readily upon exposure to air, dryness, or cold, it is generally transferred through direct sexual contact. Typically, this means contact between sexual organs during intercourse, but in rare instances, the organism enters the body through a break in the skin, through deep kissing in which body fluids are exchanged, or through some other transmission of body fluids.

Syphilis is called the "great imitator" because its symptoms resemble those of several other infections. Left untreated, syphilis generally progresses through several distinct stages. It should be noted, however, that some people experience no symptoms at all.

Primary Syphilis The first stage of syphilis, particularly for males, is often characterized by the development of a **chancre** (pronounced "shank-er"), a sore located most frequently at the site of initial infection. Although painless, the dime-sized chancre is oozing with bacteria, ready to infect an unsuspecting partner. Usually it appears three to four weeks after contact.

In males, the site of the chancre tends to be the penis or scrotum because this is where the organism first enters the body. But, if the infection was contracted

---

Conjunctivitis Serious inflammation of the eye caused by any number of pathogens or irritants; can be caused by STIs such as chlamydia.

Pelvic inflammatory disease (PID) Term used to describe various infections of the female reproductive tract.

Gonorrhea Second most common STD in the United States; if untreated, may cause sterility.

Syphilis One of the most widespread STDs; characterized by distinct phases and potentially serious results.

Chancre Sore often found at the site of syphilis infection.

through oral sex, the sore can appear in the mouth, throat, or other "first contact" area. In females, the site of infection is often internal, on the vaginal wall or high on the cervix. Because the chancre is not readily apparent, the likelihood of detection is not great. In both males and females, the chancre will completely disappear in three to six weeks.

Secondary Syphilis A month to a year after the chancre disappears, secondary symptoms may appear, including a rash or white patches on the skin or on the mucous membranes of the mouth, throat, or genitals. Hair loss may occur, lymph nodes may enlarge, and the victim may develop a slight fever or headache. In rare cases, sores develop around the mouth or genitals. As during the active chancre phase, these sores contain infectious bacteria, and contact with them can spread the infection. Because symptoms vary so much and appear so much later than the sexual contact that caused them, the victim seldom connects the two. The infection thus often goes undetected even at this second stage. Symptoms typically disappear, leaving the person thinking that all is well.

Latent Syphilis After the secondary stage, the syphilis bacteria begin to invade body organs. The infection now is rarely transmitted to others, except during pregnancy, when it can be passed to the fetus. The child will then be born with *congenital syphilis*, which can cause death or severe birth defects such as blindness, deafness, or disfigurement. One way that some states protect against congenital syphilis is by requiring prospective marriage partners to be tested for syphilis prior to obtaining a marriage license.

Late Syphilis Years after syphilis has entered the body, its effects become all too evident. Late-stage syphilis indications include heart and central nervous system damage, blindness, deafness, paralysis, premature senility, and, ultimately, dementia.

Treatment for Syphilis Because the organism is bacterial, it is treated with antibiotics. The major obstacles to treatment are misdiagnosis of this "imitator" infection and lack of access to health care.

Herpes

Herpes is a general term for a family of infections characterized by sores or eruptions on the skin. Herpes infections range from mildly uncomfortable to extremely serious. There are many different herpesviruses, but it is *herpes simplex viruses (HSV)* that affect the reproductive tract.

There are two types of HSV. Historically, the herpes simplex type 2 virus (HSV-2) was considered the primary culprit in **genital herpes,** and herpes simplex type

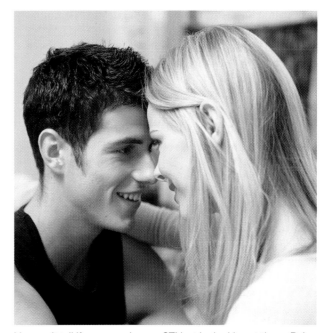

You can't tell if someone has an STI just by looking at them. Being open and honest with your partners (and expecting the same from them) about sexual history and STI testing is an important part of prevention.

1 (HSV-1) was thought to affect the area of the lips and other body areas.[28] We now know that both HSV-1 and HSV-2 can infect any area of the body, producing sores in and around the vaginal area, on the penis, around the anal opening, and on the buttocks or thighs. For example, you may have an HSV-1 infection on your lip and transmit the organism to your partner's genitals during oral sex. Practically speaking, the resulting symptoms would be virtually the same as if you had transmitted HSV-2. Occasionally, sores appear on other parts of the body. The virus remains in certain nerve cells for life and can flare up, or cause symptoms, when the body's ability to maintain itself is weakened.

The precursor phase of the infection is characterized by a burning sensation and redness at the site of infection. During this time prescription medicines such as acyclovir and over-the-counter medications such as Abreva will often keep the disease from spreading. However, this phase of the disease is quickly followed by the second phase, in which a blister filled with a clear fluid containing the virus forms. Over a period of days, the unsightly blister will crust over, dry up, and disappear, and the virus will travel to the base of an affected nerve supplying the area and become dormant. Only when the victim becomes overly stressed, when diet and sleep are inadequate, when the immune system is overworked, or when excessive exposure to sunlight or other stressors occurs will the virus become

Genital herpes STI caused by the herpes simplex virus.

reactivated (at the same site every time) and begin the blistering cycle all over again.

These sores shed viruses that can be highly infectious. If you pick at this blister or otherwise touch the site and spread this fluid with fingers, lipstick, lip balm, or other products, you can autoinoculate other body parts. Particularly dangerous is the possibility of spreading the infection to your eyes; a herpes lesion on the eye can cause blindness. It is important to note that a herpes site can shed the virus even when no overt sore is present, particularly during the interval between early symptoms and blistering. People may get genital herpes by having sexual contact with others who don't know they are infected or who are having outbreaks of herpes without any sores. A person with genital herpes can also infect a sexual partner during oral sex. The virus is spread only rarely, if at all, by touching objects such as a toilet seat or hot tub seat.[29]

Genital herpes is especially serious in pregnant women because the baby can be infected as it passes through the vagina during birth. Many physicians recommend cesarean deliveries for infected women. Additionally, women with a history of genital herpes appear to have a greater risk of developing cervical cancer.

Although there is no cure for herpes at present, certain drugs can reduce symptoms. Although lip balms and cold-sore medications may provide temporary anesthetic relief, remember that rubbing anything on a herpes blister can spread herpes-laden fluids to other body parts.

Preventing Herpes You can take precautions to reduce your risk of herpes:

- Avoid any form of kissing if you notice a sore or blister on your partner's mouth. Although there is no set time period for safe kissing, the longer you refrain from deep kissing after a herpes sore has been present, the better. (Sores typically take two to four weeks to heal, depending on the health of the immune system.[30])

- Be extremely cautious if you have casual sexual affairs. Not every partner will feel obligated to tell you that he or she has a problem. It's up to you to protect yourself. If you have herpes, be responsible in your sexual contacts with others.

- Wash your hands immediately with soap and water after any form of sexual contact.

Pubic lice (crabs) Parasites that can inhabit various body areas, especially the genitals.

Genital warts Warts that appear in the genital area or the anus; caused by the human papillomaviruses.

Human papillomavirus (HPV) A small group of viruses that cause genital warts.

- If you have questionable sores or lesions, seek medical help at once. Do not be afraid to name your contacts.

- Reduce your risk of herpes outbreaks by avoiding excessive stress, sunlight, or whatever else appears to trigger an episode.

- Do not share lip balms or lipstick.

Pubic Lice

Pubic lice, often called "crabs," are small parasites that are usually transmitted during sexual contact. More annoying than dangerous, they move easily from partner to partner during sex. They have an affinity for pubic hair and attach themselves to the base of these hairs, where they deposit their eggs (nits). One to two weeks later, these nits develop into adults that lay eggs and migrate to other body parts, thus perpetuating the cycle.

Treatment includes washing clothing, furniture, and linens that may harbor the eggs. It usually takes two to three weeks to kill all larval forms. Although sexual contact is the most common mode of transmission, you can "catch" pubic lice from lying on sheets that an infected person has slept on.

Genital Warts (Human Papillomavirus)

Genital warts (also known as venereal warts or condylomas) are caused by a group of viruses known as **human papillomaviruses (HPVs).** A person becomes infected when HPV penetrates the skin and mucous membranes of the genitals or anus through sexual contact. This is among the most common forms of STI, infecting over 5.5 million Americans each year, and appears to be relatively easy to catch. The typical incubation period is six to eight weeks after contact. Many people have no symptoms, particularly if the warts are located inside the reproductive tract, while others may notice itchy bumps on the genitals. Genital warts are of two different types: (1) *full-blown genital warts* that are noticeable as tiny bumps or growths, and (2) the much more prevalent *flat warts* that are not usually visible to the naked eye.

Risks and Treatments of Genital Warts
Many genital warts eventually disappear on their own. Others grow and generate unsightly flaps of irregular flesh on the external genitalia. If they grow large enough to obstruct urinary flow or become irritated by clothing or sexual intercourse, they can cause significant problems.

The greatest threat from genital warts lies in the apparent relationship between them and a tendency for *dysplasia,* or changes in cells that may lead to a precancerous condition. Exactly how HPV infection leads to cervical cancer is uncertain—but, within five years after infection, 30 percent of all HPV cases will progress to the precancerous stage. Of those cases that become precancerous and are left untreated, 70 percent will eventually result in actual cancer. (See Chapter 13 for more on cervical cancer.)

Genital warts can be treated with topical medications or removed by being frozen with liquid nitrogen. Large warts may require surgical removal.

Candidiasis (Moniliasis)

Unlike many STIs, which are caused by pathogens that come from outside the body, **candidiasis** (the yeastlike fungus caused by the *Candida albicans* organism) normally inhabits the vaginal tract in most women. Only under certain conditions, in which the normal chemical balance of the vagina is disturbed, will these organisms multiply and cause problems.

Symptoms of candidiasis include severe itching and burning of the vagina and vulva, swelling of the vulva, and a white, cheesy vaginal discharge. These symptoms are collectively called **vaginitis,** or inflammation of the vagina. When this microbe infects the mouth, whitish patches form, and the condition is referred to as *thrush*. This infection also occurs in males and is easily transmitted between sexual partners.

Antifungal drugs applied on the surface or by suppository usually cure it in just a few days. For approximately one out of ten women, however, nothing seems to work, and the infection returns again and again. Symptoms can be aggravated by contact of the vagina with soaps, douches, perfumed toilet paper, chlorinated water, and spermicides. Tight-fitting jeans and pantyhose can provide the combination of moisture and irritant the organism thrives on.

Trichomoniasis

Unlike many STIs, **trichomoniasis** is caused by a protozoan. Although as many as half of the men and women in the United States may carry this organism, most remain free of symptoms until their bodily defenses are weakened. Symptoms include a foamy, yellowish, unpleasant-smelling discharge accompanied by a burning sensation, itching, and painful urination. Although usually transmitted by sexual contact, the "trich" organism can also be spread by toilet seats, wet towels, or other items that have discharged fluids on them. You can also contract trichomoniasis by sitting naked on the locker room bench at your local gym. Treatment includes oral metronidazole, usually given to both sexual partners to avoid the possible "ping-pong" effect of repeated cross-infection so typical of STIs.

General Urinary Tract Infections

Although *general urinary tract infections (UTIs)* can be caused by various factors, some forms are sexually transmitted. Anytime invading organisms enter the genital area, they can travel up the urethra and enter the bladder. Similarly, organisms normally living in the rectum, urethra, or bladder may travel to the sexual organs and eventually be transmitted to another person.

Women, with their shorter urethras, are more likely than men to contract UTIs. Handwashing with soap and water prior to sexual intimacy, foreplay, and so on, is recommended. Treatment depends on the nature and type of pathogen.

HIV/AIDS

Acquired immunodeficiency syndrome (AIDS) is a significant global health threat. Since 1981, when AIDS was first recognized, over 60 million people in the world have become infected with **human immunodeficiency virus (HIV),** the virus that causes AIDS. Today, over 42 million people are estimated to be living with HIV or AIDS.[31] In the United States, as of 2002, over 859,000 men, women, and children with AIDS have been reported to the CDC, and at least 501,669 have died.[32] The CDC estimates that at least 40,000 new infections occur each year in the United States.

A Shifting Epidemic

Initially, people with HIV were diagnosed as having AIDS only when they developed blood infections, the cancer known as Kaposi's sarcoma, or any of 21 other indicator diseases, most of which were common in male AIDS patients. The CDC has expanded the indicator list to include pulmonary tuberculosis, recurrent pneumonia, and invasive cervical cancer. Perhaps the most significant indicator today is a drop in the level of the body's

---

Candidiasis   Yeastlike fungal disease often transmitted sexually.

Vaginitis   Set of symptoms characterized by vaginal itching, swelling, and burning.

Trichomoniasis   Protozoan infection characterized by foamy, yellowish discharge and unpleasant odor.

Acquired immunodeficiency syndrome (AIDS) Extremely virulent sexually transmitted disease that renders the immune system inoperative.

Human immunodeficiency virus (HIV)   The slow-acting virus that causes AIDS.

master immune cells, called CD4s, to 200 per cubic millimeter (one-fifth the level in a healthy person).

AIDS cases have been reported state by state throughout the United States since the early 1980s. Today, the CDC recommends that all states report HIV infections as well as AIDS. Because of medical advances in treatment and increasing numbers of HIV-infected persons who do not progress to AIDS, it is believed that AIDS incidence statistics may not provide a true picture of the epidemic, the long-term costs of treating HIV-infected individuals, and other key information. HIV incidence data also provide a better picture of infection trends. Currently, most states mandate that those who test positive for the HIV antibody be reported. Although there is significant pressure to mandate reporting in all states, there is controversy over implementing such a mandate. Many believe that if we require reporting of HIV-positive tests, many people will refuse to be tested even if they suspect they are infected.

Women and AIDS

HIV is an equal-opportunity pathogen that can attack anyone who engages in high-risk behaviors. This is true regardless of race, gender, sexual orientation, or socioeconomic status. However, some groups seem to be at greater risk. Today women account for an increasing proportion of this epidemic. In 2002, 32 percent of reported HIV infections and 26 percent of AIDS cases were among women, with African American and Hispanic women making up a staggering 81 percent of new cases.[33]

Compounding the problems of women with HIV are serious deficiencies in our health and social service systems, including inadequate treatment for female addicts and lack of access to child care, health care, and social services for families headed by single women.

Special Concerns for Women with HIV/AIDS
Women are 4 to 10 times more likely than men to contract HIV through unprotected sexual intercourse with an infected partner. Unlike the penis, female anatomy can facilitate entry of HIV. The vaginal area is more likely to incur microtears, and a woman is exposed to more semen than is the male to vaginal fluids, during sexual intercourse. Women who have STIs are more likely to be asymptomatic and therefore unaware they have a disease; STIs increase the risk of HIV transmission.

Socioeconomic factors also contribute to a woman's likelihood to contract HIV. Women have been underrepresented in clinical trials for HIV treatment and prevention and may be less likely to seek medical treatment because of caregiving burdens, transportation problems, and lack of money.

In some cultures, women are subordinate to men, especially in developing nations. This reduces women's decision-making power and ability to negotiate safer sex. These women are also more likely to be involved in nonconsensual sex or sex without condoms.

What Do You Think?
Why do you think HIV/AIDS is increasing among women and minority groups in America? ■ Why are some women particularly vulnerable? ■ What actions can we take as a nation to reduce the spread of HIV/AIDS among women and among minority groups? ■ Should Americans be concerned about the global HIV/AIDS epidemic? Why or why not?

How HIV Is Transmitted

HIV typically enters one person's body when another person's infected body fluids (semen, vaginal secretions, blood, etc.) gain entry through a breach in body defenses. Mucous membranes of the genital organs and the anus provide the easiest route of entry. If there is a break in the mucous membranes (as can occur during sexual intercourse, particularly anal intercourse), the virus enters and begins to multiply. After initial infection, HIV multiplies rapidly, invading the bloodstream and cerebrospinal fluid. It progressively destroys helper T cells, weakening the body's resistance to disease. The virus also changes the genetic structure of the cells it attacks. In response to this invasion, the body quickly begins to produce antibodies.

Despite some myths, HIV is not highly contagious. Studies of people living in households with an AIDS patient have turned up no documented cases of HIV infection due to casual contact.[34] Other investigations provide overwhelming evidence that insect bites do not transmit HIV.

Engaging in High-Risk Behaviors
AIDS is not a disease of gay people or minority groups. If you engage in high-risk behaviors, you increase your risk for the disease. If you do not practice these behaviors, your risk is minimal. It is as simple as that.

Unfortunately, the message has not gotten through to many Americans. They assume that because they are heterosexual, do not inject illegal drugs, and do not have sex with sex workers, they are not at risk. They couldn't be more wrong. Anyone who engages in unprotected sex is at risk, especially sex with a partner who has engaged in other high-risk behaviors. Sex with multiple partners is the greatest threat. You can't determine the presence of HIV by looking at a person; you can't tell by questioning unless the person has been tested recently, is HIV negative, and is giving an honest answer. So what should you do?

Of course, the simplest answer is abstinence. If you don't exchange body fluids, you won't get the disease.

As a second line of defense, if you decide to be intimate, the next best option is to use a condom. However, in spite of all the educational campaigns, surveys consistently indicate that most college students throw caution to the wind if they think they "know" someone—and they have unprotected sex.

Recognize the risk factors, and remember, if you do not engage in activities that are known to spread the virus, your chances of becoming infected are extremely small. The following activities are high-risk behaviors.

Exchange of Body Fluids The greatest risk factor is the exchange of HIV-infected body fluids during vaginal or anal intercourse. Substantial research indicates that blood, semen, and vaginal secretions are the major fluids of concern. However, even though these risks are well documented, millions of Americans report inconsistent safer sex practices, particularly when drugs or alcohol affect rational thinking.

Although the virus was found in one person's saliva (out of 71 people in a study population), most health officials state that saliva is a less significant risk than other shared body fluids (see the Reality Check box on page 398 on tattooing and piercing for additional risks). The fact that the virus has been found in saliva does provide a good rationale for caution when engaging in deep, wet kissing.

Initially, public health officials included breast milk in the list of high-risk fluids because a few infants apparently contracted HIV while breastfeeding. Subsequent research has indicated that HIV could have been transmitted by bleeding nipples as well as by actual consumption of breast milk and other fluids. Infection through contact with feces and urine is believed to be highly unlikely though technically possible.

Injecting Drugs A significant percentage of AIDS cases in the United States result from sharing or using HIV-contaminated needles and syringes. Though users of illegal drugs are commonly considered the only members of this category, others may also share needles—for example, people with diabetes who inject insulin or athletes who inject steroids. People who share needles and also engage in sexual activities with members of high-risk groups, such as those who exchange sex for drugs, increase their risks dramatically.

Receiving a Blood Transfusion Prior to 1985 A small group of people became infected after receiving blood transfusions. In 1985, the Red Cross and other blood donation programs implemented a stringent testing program for all donated blood. Today, because of these massive screening efforts, the risk of receiving HIV-infected blood is almost nonexistent.

Mother-to-Infant (Perinatal) Transmission

Approximately one in three of children with AIDS received the virus from their infected mothers

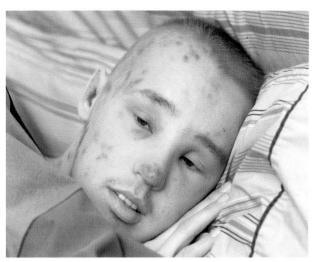

The effects of HIV/AIDS can be seen here in the form of Kaposi's sarcoma and wasting syndrome.

while in the womb or while passing through the vaginal tract during delivery.

Symptoms of HIV Disease

A person may go for months or years after infection by HIV before any significant symptoms appear. The incubation time varies greatly from person to person. For adults who receive no medical treatment, it takes an average of eight to ten years for the virus to cause the slow, degenerative changes in the immune system that are characteristic of AIDS. During this time, the person may experience *opportunistic infections* (infections that gain a foothold when the immune system is not functioning effectively). Colds, sore throats, fever, tiredness, nausea, night sweats, and other generally non–life-threatening conditions commonly appear and are described as pre-AIDS symptoms.

Testing for HIV Antibodies

Once antibodies have formed in reaction to HIV, a blood test known as the **ELISA** (enzyme-linked immunosorbent assay) may detect their presence. If sufficient antibodies are present, the test will be positive. When a person who previously tested *negative* (no HIV antibodies present) has a subsequent test that is *positive,* seroconversion is said to have occurred. In such a situation, the person would typically take another ELISA test, followed by a more precise test known as the **Western blot,** to confirm the presence of HIV antibodies.

ELISA Blood test that detects presence of antibodies to HIV virus.

Western blot A test more accurate than the ELISA to confirm presence of HIV antibodies.

A look around any college campus reveals many examples of the widespread trend of body piercing and tattooing, also referred to as "body art." Many view the trend as a desire for self-expression. Whatever the reason, there is a booming business in both tattooing and body piercing.

However, health professionals cite several health concerns. The most common health-related problems associated with tattoos and body piercing include skin reactions, infections, and scarring. The average healing times for piercings depend on the size of the insert, location, and the person's overall health. Facial and tongue piercings tend to heal more quickly than areas not commonly exposed to open air or light and which are often teeming with bacteria, such as the genitals. (Tongue piercings are now being cited as a significant cause of damage to teeth.) Because the hands are great germ transmitters, touching pierced areas poses a significant risk for infection.

Of even greater concern is the potential transmission of dangerous pathogens that any puncture of the human body exacerbates. The use of unsterile needles—which can cause serious infections and can transmit HIV, hepatitis B and C, tetanus, and a host of other diseases—poses a very real risk. (Consider actress Pamela Anderson, who claims to have con-

tracted hepatitis C from sharing a tattoo needle with her ex-husband Tommy Lee.) Laws and policies regulating body piercing and tattooing vary greatly by state. While some states don't allow tattoo and body-piercing parlors, others may regulate them carefully, and still others provide few regulations and standards by which parlors have to abide. Standards for safety usually include minimum age of use, standards of sanitation, use of aseptic techniques, sterilization of equipment, informed risks, instructions for skin care, record keeping, and recommendations for dealing with adverse reactions. Because of the lack of standards regulating this business and the potential for transmission of dangerous pathogens, anyone who receives a tattoo, body piercing, or permanent makeup tattoo cannot donate blood for one year.

If you opt for tattooing or body piercing, remember the following points:

✓ Look for clean, well-lit work areas, and ask about sterilization procedures.

✓ Immediately before piercing or tattooing, the body area should be carefully sterilized. The artist should put on new latex gloves and touch nothing else while working.

✓ Packaged, sterilized needles should be used only once and then discarded. A piercing gun should not be

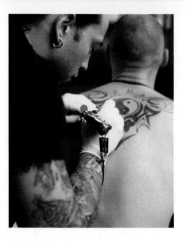

used because it cannot be sterilized properly.

✓ Leftover tattoo ink should be discarded after each procedure. Do not allow the artist to reuse ink that has been used for other customers.

✓ Only jewelry made of noncorrosive metal, such as surgical stainless steel, niobium, or solid 14-karat gold, is safe for new piercing.

✓ If any signs of pus, swelling, redness, or discoloration persist, remove the piercing object and contact a physician.

Sources: Center for Food Safety and Applied Nutrition, "Tattoos and Permanent Makeup," *Office of Cosmetics Fact Sheet*, 2004, www.cfsan.fda .gov/~dms/cos-204.html; M. L. Armstrong and K. P. Murphy, "Adolescent Tattooing and Body Piercing," *The Prevention Researcher* 5 (Eugene, OR: Integrated Research Services, 1998):5.

It should be noted that these tests are not AIDS tests per se. Rather, they detect antibodies for the disease, indicating the presence of HIV in the person's system. Whether the person will develop AIDS depends to some extent on the strength of the immune system. Although we have made remarkable progress in prolonging the relatively symptom-free period between infection, HIV-positive status, and progression to symptomatic AIDS, it is important to note that a cure does not yet exist. The vast majority of all infected people eventually develop some form of the disease.

As testing for HIV antibodies has improved, scientists have explored various ways of making it easier for individuals to be tested. Health officials distinguish between *reported* and *actual* cases of HIV infection because it is believed that many HIV-positive people avoid being tested. One reason is fear of knowing the truth. Another is the fear of recrimination from employers, insurance companies, and medical staff. However, early detection and reporting are important, because immediate treatment for someone in the early stages of HIV disease is critical.

New Hope and Treatments

New drugs have slowed the progression from HIV to AIDS and have prolonged life expectancies for most AIDS patients. While these new therapies offer the promise of extended life for many, they may have inadvertently led to an increase in risky behaviors and a noteworthy rise in cases in 2002. Advocates for AIDS patients believe medications still cost too much money and cause too many side effects. The cost of multidrug treatment for one person now exceeds $15,000 per year.[35]

Current treatments combine selected drugs, especially protease inhibitors and reverse transcriptase inhibitors. *Protease inhibitors* (for example, amprenavir, ritonavir, and saquinavir) act to prevent the production of the virus in chronically infected cells that HIV has already invaded. Other drugs, such as AZT, ddI, ddC, d4T, and 3TC, inhibit the HIV enzyme *reverse transcriptase* before the virus has invaded the cell so prevent the virus from infecting new cells.

All of the protease drugs seem to work best in combination with other therapies. These combination treatments are still quite experimental, and no combination has proven to be absolute for all people. As with other antiviral treatments, resistance to the drugs can develop. Individuals who already show resistance to AZT may not be able to use a protease-AZT combination. This can pose a problem for many people who have been taking the common drugs and then find their options for combination therapy limited.

Although these drugs provide new hope and longer survival rates for people living with HIV, it is important to maintain caution. New drugs that held much promise are becoming less effective as HIV develops resistance to them. Costs of taking multiple drugs are becoming prohibitive and side effects common. Apathy and carelessness may abound if too much confidence is placed in these treatments. Indeed, the number of people becoming HIV-infected each year has stabilized and even increased in some communities. While AIDS death rates in America have dropped, we are now seeing increases in rates of HIV infection rise again in certain populations.[36] We are still a long way from beating this disease.

Preventing HIV Infection

Although scientists have been working on a variety of HIV vaccine trials, none are currently available.[37] The only way to prevent HIV infection is to avoid risky behaviors. HIV infection and AIDS are not uncontrollable conditions. You can reduce your risk by the choices you make in sexual behaviors and by taking responsibility for your own health and the health of your loved ones. The Skills for Behavior Change box on page 400 presents ways to reduce your risk for contracting HIV and other STIs.

Where to Go for Help If you are concerned about your own risk or the risk of a close friend, arrange a confidential meeting with the health educator or other health professional at your college health service. He or she will provide you with the information that you need to decide whether you should be tested for HIV antibodies. If the student health service is not an option for you, seek assistance through your local public health department or community STI clinic. Local physicians, counselors, professors, and other responsible people can help you discover the answers you are looking for.

NONINFECTIOUS DISEASES: MODERN MALADIES

Typically, when we think of major noninfectious ailments, we think of "killer" diseases such as cancer and heart disease. Clearly, these diseases make up the major portion of life-threatening diseases—accounting for nearly two-thirds of all deaths (see Chapters 12 and 13). Although these diseases capture much media attention, other chronic conditions can also cause pain, suffering, and disability. Fortunately, most of them can be prevented or their symptoms relieved.

Generally, noninfectious diseases are not transmitted by a pathogen or by any form of personal contact. Lifestyle and personal health habits are often implicated as underlying causes. Healthy changes in lifestyle and public health efforts aimed at research, prevention, and control can minimize the effects of these diseases.

CHRONIC LUNG DISEASE

Chronic lung diseases pose a serious and significant threat to Americans today. Collectively, they have become the fourth leading cause of death, with most sufferers living with a condition known as chronic **dyspnea,** or chronic breathlessness. Depending on

Dyspnea Chronic breathlessness.

HIV transmission depends on specific behaviors; this is true of other STIs as well. The following will help you protect yourself and reduce your risk.

■ Avoid casual sexual partners. Ideally, have sex only if you are in a long-term, mutually monogamous relationship with someone who is equally committed to the relationship and whose HIV status is negative.

■ Avoid unprotected sexual activity involving the exchange of blood, semen, or vaginal secretions with people whose present or past behaviors put them at risk for infection. Postpone sexual involvement until you are assured that he or she is not infected.

■ Practice safer sex by using latex condoms. Remember, however, that condoms still do not provide 100 percent safety.

■ Never share any devices through which the exchange of blood could occur, including needles, razors, tattoo instruments, body-piercing instruments, and any other sharp objects.

■ Avoid injury to body tissue during sexual activity. HIV can enter the bloodstream through microscopic tears in anal or vaginal tissues.

■ Avoid unprotected oral sex or any sexual activity in which semen, blood, or vaginal secretions could penetrate mucous membranes through breaks in the membrane. Always use a condom or a dental dam during oral sex.

■ Avoid using drugs (including alcohol) that may dull your senses and affect your ability to take responsible precautions with potential sex partners.

■ Although total abstinence is the only absolute means of preventing the sexual transmission of HIV, abstinence can be a difficult choice to make. Consider other means of intimacy. Try massage, dry kissing, hugging, holding and touching, and masturbation (alone or with a partner).

■ Be sure medical professionals take appropriate precautions to prevent potential transmission, including washing their hands and wearing gloves and masks. All equipment used for treatment should be properly sterilized.

■ If you are worried about your own HIV status, have yourself tested. Don't risk infecting others.

■ If you are a woman and HIV positive, you should take the steps necessary to ensure that you do not become pregnant.

■ If you suspect that you may be infected or if you test positive for HIV antibodies, do not donate blood, semen, or body organs.

At no time in your life is it more important to communicate openly than when you are considering an intimate relationship. Remember that you can't tell if someone has an STI. The following will help you to communicate about potential risks.

■ Remember that you have a responsibility to your partner to disclose your own status. You also have a responsibility to yourself to stay healthy. Ask about your partner's HIV status. Suggest going through the testing together as a means of sharing something important.

■ Be direct, honest, and determined in talking about sex before you become involved. Do not act silly or evasive. Get to the point, ask clear questions, and do not be put off in receiving a response. A person who does not care enough to talk about sex probably does not care enough to take responsibility for his or her actions.

■ Discuss the issues without sounding defensive or accusatory. Develop a personal comfort level with the subject prior to raising the issue with your partner. Be prepared with

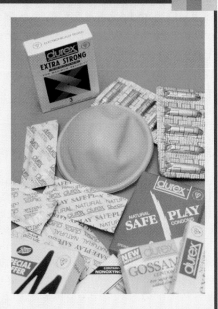

complete information, and articulate your feelings clearly. Reassure your partner that your reasons for desiring abstinence or safer sex arise from respect and not distrust.

■ Encourage your partner to be honest and to share feelings. This will not happen overnight. If you have never had a serious conversation with this person before you get into an intimate situation, you cannot expect honesty and openness when the lights go out.

■ Analyze your own beliefs and values ahead of time. Know where you will draw the line on certain actions, and be very clear with your partner about what you expect. If you believe that using a condom is necessary, make sure you communicate this.

■ Decide what you will do if your partner does not agree with you. Anticipate potential objections or excuses, and prepare your responses accordingly.

■ Discuss the significance of monogamy in your partner's relationships. Decide early how important this relationship is to you and how much you are willing to work at arriving at an acceptable compromise on lifestyle.

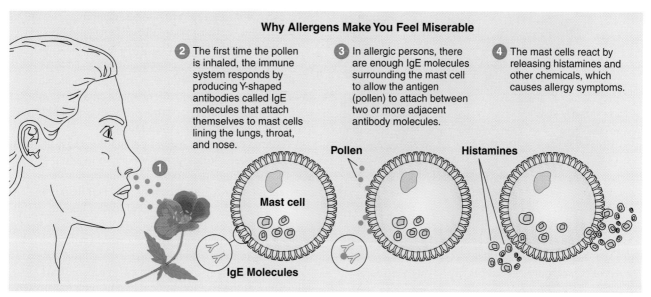

Figure 14.5 ■ Stages of an Allergic Response

the situation, dyspnea may limit the ability to climb stairs, walk unassisted, or even sleep. Chronic lung disease can result in major disability and lack of function as the lungs fill with mucous, become susceptible to bacterial or viral infections, or cause acute stress on the heart as they struggle to get valuable oxygen. Chronic cough, excessive phlegm, wheezing, or coughing up blood are frequent symptoms. Over time, many of these underlying conditions lead to hospitalization and possible death.

Among the more deadly chronic lung diseases are the **chronic obstructive pulmonary diseases (COPDs):** asthma, emphysema, and chronic bronchitis. Other chronic lung diseases also cause significant health risks, the most common of which are allergy-induced problems and hay fever. Each of these may exacerbate or contribute to the development of COPD.

Allergy-Induced Respiratory Problems

An **allergy** occurs as a part of the body's attempt to defend itself against a specific *antigen* (or *allergen* in this case) by producing specific *antibodies*. When foreign pathogens such as bacteria or viruses invade the body, the body responds by producing antibodies to destroy these invading antigens. Under normal conditions, the production of antibodies is a positive element in the body's defense system. However, for unknown reasons, in some people the body overreacts by developing an overly elaborate protective mechanism against relatively harmless substances. The resultant *hypersensitivity reaction* to specific antigens in the environment is fairly common, as anyone who has awakened with a runny nose or itchy eyes will testify. Most commonly, these hypersensitivity, or allergic, responses occur as a reaction to environmental antigens such as molds, animal

dander (hair and dead skin), pollen, ragweed, or dust. Once excessive antibodies to these antigens are produced, they trigger the release of **histamines,** chemical substances that dilate blood vessels, increase mucous secretions, cause tissues to swell, and produce other allergy-like symptoms, particularly in the respiratory system (Figure 14.5).

Over 60 million Americans have asthma or allergies.[38] Although many people think of allergies as childhood diseases, in reality allergies tend to become progressively worse with time and with increased exposure to allergens. Many people take allergy shots to reduce the severity of their symptoms, with some success. In most cases, once the offending antigen has disappeared, allergy-prone people suffer few symptoms.

Hay Fever

Perhaps the best example of a chronic respiratory disease is **hay fever.** Usually considered a seasonally related disease (caused by pollen exposure and most

---

Chronic obstructive pulmonary diseases (COPDs)
A collection of chronic lung diseases including asthma, emphysema, and chronic bronchitis.

Allergy Hypersensitive reaction to a specific antigen or allergen in the environment in which the body produces excessive antibodies to that antigen or allergen.

Histamines Chemical substances that dilate blood vessels, increase mucous secretions, and produce other symptoms of allergies.

Hay fever A chronic respiratory disorder that is triggered by pollen.

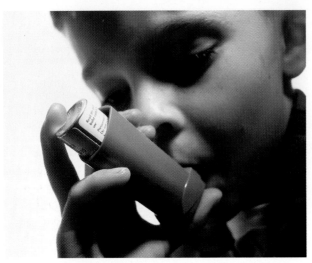

The marked increase of asthma cases among young children worries health officials.

prevalent when ragweed and flowers are blooming), hay fever is common throughout the world. Hay fever attacks, which are characterized by sneezing and itchy, watery eyes and nose, make countless people miserable. The disorder appears to run in families, and research indicates that lifestyle is not as great a factor in developing hay fever as it is in other chronic diseases. Instead, an overzealous immune system and exposure to environmental allergens including pet dander, dust, pollen from various plants, and other substances appear to be the critical factors that determine vulnerability. For those people who are unable to get away from the cause of their hay fever response, medical assistance in the form of injections or antihistamines may provide the only relief.

Asthma

Unfortunately, for many persons who suffer from allergies such as hay fever, their condition often becomes complicated by the development of one of the major COPDs: asthma, emphysema, or bronchitis. **Asthma** is a long-term, chronic inflammatory disorder that blocks air flow in and out of the lungs. Asthma causes tiny airways in the lung to overreact with spasms in response to certain triggers. Symptoms include wheezing, difficulty breathing, shortness of breath, and coughing spasms. Although most asthma attacks are mild and non–life-threatening, they can trigger *bronchospasms* (contractions of the bronchial tubes in the lungs) that are so

severe that without rapid treatment, death may occur. Between attacks, most people have few symptoms.

A number of things can trigger an asthma attack, including air pollutants; particulate matter, such as wood dust; indoor air pollutants, such as secondhand smoke from tobacco; and allergens, such as dust mites, cockroach saliva, and pet dander. Stress is also believed to trigger attacks in some individuals.[39]

Asthma can occur at any age, but it is most likely in children between infancy and age 5 and in adults before age 40. In childhood, asthma strikes more boys than girls; in adulthood, it strikes more women than men. Also, the asthma rate is 50 percent higher among African Americans than whites, and four times as many African Americans die of asthma than do whites. Midwesterners appear to be more prone to asthma than people from other areas of the country. In recent years, concern over the rise in incidence of asthma has grown considerably.

People with asthma fall into one of two distinctly different types. *Intrinsic asthma* may be triggered by any unpleasant event or stimulant, including allergies. The most common form, known as *extrinsic* (or *slow onset*) *asthma,* is typically associated with allergic triggers; it tends to run in families and develop in childhood. Often, by adulthood, a person has few episodes or the disorder completely goes away. A common form of extrinsic asthma is *exercise-induced asthma (EIA),* which may or may not have an allergic connection. Some athletes have no allergies yet live with asthma. Cold, dry air is believed to exacerbate EIA; thus, keeping the lungs moist and warming up prior to working out may help. The warm, moist air around a swimming pool is one of the best environments for people with asthma.

Relaxation techniques appear to help some asthma sufferers. Drugs may be necessary for serious cases. Determining whether a specific allergen provokes asthma attacks, taking steps to reduce exposure, avoiding triggers such as certain types of exercise or stress, and finding the most effective medications are big steps in asthma prevention and control. Numerous new drugs are available that cause fewer side effects than older medications.

Try it ►NOW

Eliminate dust to control allergies or asthma. **If you, or someone you live with has allergies, take these steps today to control dust. Keep pillows, cushions, and mattresses in zippered covers. Wash bedding weekly in hot water, and wipe surfaces with a damp rag weekly to keep dust to a minimum.**

Asthma   A chronic respiratory disease characterized by attacks of wheezing, shortness of breath, and coughing spasms.

Emphysema

Emphysema involves the gradual destruction of the **alveoli** (tiny air sacs) of the lungs. As the alveoli are destroyed, the affected person finds it more and more difficult to exhale. The victim typically struggles to take in a fresh supply of air before the air held in the lungs has been expended. The chest cavity gradually begins to expand, thus producing the barrel-shaped chest characteristic of the chronic emphysema victim. (For more on emphysema and smoking, see Chapter 8.)

Bronchitis

Bronchitis refers to an inflammation of the lining of the bronchial tubes. These tubes, the bronchi, connect the windpipe with the lungs. When the bronchi become inflamed or infected, less air is able to flow from the lungs, and heavy mucus begins to form. *Acute bronchitis* is the most common of the bronchial diseases and results in millions of visits to the doctor every year at a cost of more than $300 million per year.[40] More than 95 percent of these acute cases are caused by viruses; however, they are often misdiagnosed and treated with antibiotics, even though little evidence supports this treatment. Typically, misdiagnosis occurs when a cluster of symptoms is labeled as bronchitis, despite the fact that there is no true laboratory diagnosis. (See Chapter 8 for information on chronic bronchitis.)

Sleep Apnea

Sleep apnea is believed to affect more than 18 million Americans. This condition is characterized by periodic episodes when breathing stops almost completely for ten seconds or longer. Each time it occurs, the sleeper awakens and breathing resumes, but the pattern causes a restless night's sleep. Sleep apnea can lead to high blood pressure, irregular heartbeats, heart attack, and stroke.[41] Reducing alcohol use, losing weight, changing sleeping position, and other medical interventions are common treatments.

What Do You Think?
Which of the respiratory diseases described in this section do you, your family, or friends have problems with? ■ What difficulties do they have in controlling their diseases? ■ Why do you think the incidence of COPDs is increasing? ■ What actions can you take to reduce risks and problems from these diseases?

NEUROLOGICAL DISORDERS

Headaches

Almost all of us have experienced at least one major headache. In fact, more than 80 percent of women and 65 percent of men experience headaches on a regular basis.[42] Common types of headaches and their treatments are described in this section.

Tension Headaches Tension headaches, also referred to as muscular contraction headaches, are generally caused by muscle contractions or tension in the neck or head. This tension may be caused by actual strain placed on neck or head muscles due to overuse, static positions held for long periods of time, or tension triggered by stress. Other possible triggers include red wine, lack of sleep, fasting, menstruation, among others. Relaxation, hot water treatment, and massage are holistic treatments, while aspirin, Tylenol, Aleve, and Advil remain the old standby forms of pain relief.

Migraine Headaches More than 28 million Americans—three times more women than men—suffer from **migraines,** a type of headache that often has severe, debilitating symptoms.[43] Usually migraine incidence peaks in young adulthood, the prime years for college students (ages 20–45).[44] Migraines are often hereditary. If both parents have them, there is a 75 percent chance their children will have them; if only one parent has them, there is a 50 percent chance their children will have them. If your relatives have them, there is 20 percent risk for you.[45]

Symptoms vary greatly by individual and attacks typically last anywhere from 4 to 72 hours, with distinct phases of symptoms. In about 15 percent of cases, migraines are preceded by a sensory warning sign known as an *aura,* such as flashes of light, flickering vision, blind spots or tingling in arms or legs, or sensation of odor or taste. Sometimes, nausea, vomiting, and extreme sensitivity to light and sound are present.[46] Symptoms of migraine include excruciating pain behind or around one eye and usually on the same side of

---

Emphysema   A respiratory disease in which the alveoli become distended or ruptured and are no longer functional.

Alveoli   Tiny air sacs of the lungs where all gas exchange must occur.

Bronchitis   An inflammation of the lining of the bronchial tubes.

Sleep apnea   Disorder in which a person has numerous episodes of breathing stoppage during a night's sleep.

Migraine   A condition characterized by localized headaches that possibly result from alternating dilation and constriction of blood vessels.

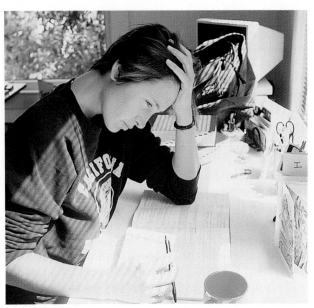

Tension headaches are triggered by many factors, including lack of sleep, stress, and strain on head and neck muscles.

the head. In some people, there is sinus pain, neck pain, or an aura without headache.

Migraines may occur when blood vessels dilate in the membrane that surrounds the brain. Historically, treatments have centered on reversing or preventing this dilation, with the most common treatment derived from the rye fungus *ergot*. Today, fast-acting ergot compounds are available by nasal spray, vastly increasing the speed of relief. However, ergot drugs have many side effects, the least of which may be that they are habit forming.[47]

Critics of the blood vessel dilation theory question why only blood vessels of the head dilate in these situations. Furthermore, why aren't people who take hot baths or those who exercise more prone to migraine attacks? They suggest that migraines originate in the cortex of the brain, where certain pain sensors are stimulated.[48] Other researchers believe that migraines are started by disturbances that keep the pain-regulating chemical serotonin from doing its job, which would explain why drugs that interact with serotonin reduce headaches.[49]

When true migraines occur, relaxation is only minimally effective as a treatment. Imitrex, a drug tailor-made for migraines, works for about 80 percent of those who try it. However, Imitrex is expensive, and its side effects make it inappropriate for anyone with uncontrolled high blood pressure or heart disease. Recently,

---

Epilepsy A neurological disorder caused by abnormal electrical brain activity; can be accompanied by altered consciousness or convulsions.

---

treatment with lidocaine has shown promising results, and newer drugs called triptans, such as Zomig, Amerge, and Maxalt, are now available. All triptans, however, are cleared from the body in a few hours, and the migraine sometimes returns.[50]

Secondary Headaches Secondary headaches arise as a result of some other underlying condition. Hypertension, blocked sinuses, allergies, low blood sugar, diseases of the spine, the common cold, poorly fitted dentures, problems with eyesight, and other problems can trigger this condition. Relaxation and pain relievers are of little help in treating secondary headaches. Rather, medications or other therapies designed to relieve the underlying organic cause of the headache must be included in the treatment regimen.

Seizure Disorders

The word **epilepsy** derives from the Greek *epilepsia,* meaning "seizure." Approximately 2 million people in the United States suffer from some form of seizure-related disorder and between 5 and 10 percent of the population will experience at least one seizure in their lives.[51] These disorders are generally caused by abnormal electrical activity in the brain and are characterized by loss of control of muscular activity and unconsciousness. Symptoms vary widely and can range from temporary confusion to major motor seizing. Not all types of seizures involve convulsions.

Typically seizures fall into one of two categories. When they seem related to abnormal activity in just one region of the brain, they are classified as *partial*. When they involve all or most parts of the brain, they are *generalized*. About half of all cases of seizure disorder are of unknown origin. Possible causes include stroke, head injury, congenital abnormalities, injury or illness resulting in inflammation of the brain or spinal column, drug or chemical poisoning, tumors, nutritional deficiency, and heredity.

In most cases, people afflicted with seizure disorders can lead normal, seizure-free lives when under medical supervision. Public ignorance about these disorders is one of the most serious obstacles confronting them. Improvements in medication and surgical interventions to reduce some causes of seizures are among the most promising treatments today.

What Do You Think? Do you suffer from recurrent headaches or other neurological problems? ■ What might cause your problems? ■ What actions could you take to reduce your risks and symptoms?

Parkinson's Disease

Over 1.5 million Americans—including actor Michael J. Fox—have **Parkinson's disease,** a chronic, slowly progressive neurological condition. Rates of Parkinson's have quadrupled in the past 30 years and may increase even more dramatically as more baby boomers pass age 60. Nearly 60,000 new cases are diagnosed each year. Fifteen percent of the people diagnosed are under age 50.[52]

The hallmark of Parkinson's disease is a tremor or "shaking palsy." Other symptoms are rigid or stiff muscles, slow movement, poor balance, shuffling steps, and slurred speech. The most common theories concerning its causes include familial predisposition, acceleration of age-related changes, and exposure to environmental toxins. Although Parkinson's is progressive and incurable, new drug therapies can keep symptoms under control, possibly for years. Surgical options such as brain tissue transplants and the use of fetal tissue or genetically engineered cell transplants have also provided promising results.

Multiple Sclerosis

Multiple sclerosis (MS) is a degenerative disease in which myelin, a fatty material that serves as an insulator and conduit for transmission of nerve impulses, breaks down and causes nerve malfunction. Multiple sclerosis typically appears between ages 15 and 50 and is characterized by a periods of relapse (when symptoms flare up) and remissions (when symptoms are not present). Symptoms can range in severity from fatigue and episodic numbness to severe weakness. Most MS patients have few flare-ups and can lead fairly normal lives. The cause of MS is unknown.

GENDER-RELATED DISORDERS

Menstrual Problems

Premenstrual syndrome (PMS) comprises the mood changes and physical symptoms that occur in some women a week to ten days preceding the menstrual period. Symptoms may include depression, irritability, headaches, tender breasts, bloating, backache, abdominal cramps, acne, diarrhea, and fatigue. About 80 percent of all women have some negative symptoms associated with their menstrual cycle; about 3 to 5 percent have more severe symptoms, which are known collectively as **premenstrual dysphoric disorder (PMDD).** Unlike PMS, PMDD symptoms are severe and difficult to manage. They include severe mood disturbances in addition to the physical symptoms associated with PMS.

Strategies for managing PMS include decreasing caffeine and salt intake, increasing intake of complex carbohydrates, practicing stress reduction techniques, and getting exercise. These strategies can also help PMDD. The use of selective serotonin reuptake inhibitors (SSRI antidepressants) has shown significant promise in the treatment of the mood disturbances associated with PMDD.

Endometriosis Whether the incidence of **endometriosis** is on the rise in the United States or whether the disorder is simply attracting more attention is difficult to determine. Victims of endometriosis tend to be women between the ages of 20 and 40. Symptoms include severe cramping during and between menstrual cycles, irregular periods, unusually heavy or light menstrual flow, abdominal bloating, fatigue, painful bowel movements with periods, painful intercourse, constipation, diarrhea, menstrual pain, infertility, and low back pain. (For more on endometriosis, see Chapter 6.)

DIGESTION-RELATED DISORDERS

Diabetes: Disabling, Deadly, and on the Rise

Diabetes is a serious, widespread, and costly chronic disease, affecting not just the 18 million Americans who must live with it, but their families and communities. Between 1980 and 2002, diagnosed diabetes increased over 50 percent among U.S. adults, giving it the dubious distinction of being the fastest growing chronic disease in American history.[53] Diabetes is increasing even more dramatically among younger adults—it is up by almost 70 percent among those in their thirties.[54] Over 2,200 people are diagnosed with diabetes each day in America, and over 200,000 die each year of related

---

Parkinson's disease A chronic, progressive neurological condition that causes tremors and other symptoms.

Multiple sclerosis (MS) A degenerative neurological disease in which myelin, an insulator of nerves, breaks down.

Premenstrual syndrome (PMS) The mood changes and physical symptoms that occur in many women prior to menstruation.

Premenstrual dysphoric disorder (PMDD) A group of symptoms similar to but more severe than PMS; especially involves mood disturbances.

Endometriosis Abnormal development of endometrial tissue outside the uterus; results in serious side effects.

complications—making it the sixth leading cause of death in America today.[55]

What causes this serious disease? In healthy people, the *pancreas*, a powerful enzyme-producing organ, produces the hormone **insulin** in sufficient quantities to allow the body to use or store glucose (blood sugar). When the pancreas fails to produce enough insulin to regulate sugar metabolism or when the body fails to use insulin effectively, a disease known as **diabetes mellitus** occurs. Diabetics exhibit **hyperglycemia,** or elevated blood sugar levels, and high glucose levels in their urine. Other symptoms include excessive thirst, frequent urination, hunger, tendency to tire easily, wounds that heal slowly, numbness or tingling in the extremities, changes in vision, skin eruptions, and, in women, a tendency toward vaginal yeast infections.

The most serious form, *type 1 diabetes* (insulin-dependent diabetes), is an autoimmune disease in which the immune system destroys the insulin-making beta cells and most often appears during childhood or adolescence.[56] Type 1 diabetics must depend on insulin injections or oral medications for the rest of their lives because their bodies lack insulin.

In *type 2 diabetes* (noninsulin-dependent diabetes), the body resists or is unable to utilize available insulin. Type 2 diabetes accounts for 90 to 95 percent of all diabetes cases and most often appears after age 40.[57] However, type 2 diabetes is now being diagnosed at younger ages, even among children and teens. This form of diabetes is typically linked to obesity and physical inactivity. If people with type 2 diabetes change their lifestyle, they may be able to avoid oral medications or insulin indefinitely.

A third type, *gestational diabetes*, can develop in a woman during pregnancy and affects 2 to 5 percent of all pregnant women. The condition usually disappears after childbirth, but it does leave the woman at greater risk of developing type 2 diabetes in the future.

Understanding Risk Factors Diabetes tends to run in families. Being overweight, coupled with inactivity, dramatically increases the risk of type 2

What can I do to reduce my risk for diabetes?

diabetes. Older persons and mothers of babies weighing over 9 pounds also run an increased risk. Approximately 80 percent of all type 2 patients are overweight at the time of diagnosis. Weight loss, better nutrition, control of blood glucose levels, and regular exercise can lower blood sugar and improve the efficiency of cellular use of insulin. These improvements can help to prevent overwork of the pancreas and the development of diabetes. In fact, modest, consistent physical activity and a healthy diet can cut a person's risk of type 2 diabetes by nearly 60 percent.[58] For unknown reasons, African Americans, Hispanics, and Americans Indians have the highest rates of type 2 diabetes in the world—much higher than that of whites.[59]

Controlling Diabetes Most physicians attempt to control type 1 diabetes and later stages of type 2 with a variety of insulin-related drugs. Most of these drugs are taken orally, although self-administered hypodermic injections are prescribed when other treatments are inadequate. Recent breakthroughs in individual monitoring and implantable insulin monitors and insulin infusion pumps have provided many people with diabetes the opportunity to lead normal lives. Newer forms of insulin that last longer in the body and have fewer side effects are now available. An insulin inhaler is being tested for possible widespread use.

Lactose Intolerance

As many as 50 million Americans are unable to eat dairy products such as milk, cheese, ice cream, and other foods that the rest of us take for granted. These people suffer from **lactose intolerance,** which means that they have lost the ability to produce the digestive enzyme (lactase) that is necessary for the body to convert milk sugar (lactose) into glucose. That glass of milk becomes a source of stomach cramping, diarrhea, nausea, gas, and related symptoms. Once diagnosed, however, lactose intolerance can be treated by introducing low-lactose or lactose-free foods into the diet. Through trial and error, people usually find that they can tolerate one type of low-lactose food better than others. Someone who is lactose intolerant may need to experiment before settling into a diet that works.

Colitis and Irritable Bowel Syndrome

Ulcerative colitis is a disease of the large intestine in which the mucous membranes of the intestinal walls become inflamed. Those with severe cases may have as many as 20 bouts of bloody diarrhea a day. Colitis can

---

Insulin A hormone produced by the pancreas; required by the body for the metabolism of carbohydrates.

Diabetes mellitus A disease in which the pancreas fails to produce enough insulin or the body fails to use insulin effectively.

Hyperglycemia Elevated blood sugar levels.

Lactose intolerance The inability to produce lactase, an enzyme needed to convert milk sugar into glucose.

Ulcerative colitis An inflammatory disorder that affects the mucous membranes of the large intestine, producing bloody diarrhea.

---

also produce severe stomach cramps, weight loss, nausea, sweating, and fever. Although some experts believe that colitis occurs more frequently in people with high stress levels, this theory is controversial. Hypersensitivity reactions to certain foods have also been considered as a possible cause. It is difficult to determine the cause of colitis because the disease goes into unexplained remission and then recurs without apparent reason. This pattern often continues over periods of years and may be related to the later development of colorectal cancer. Treatment focuses on relieving the symptoms. Increasing fiber intake and taking anti-inflammatory drugs, steroids, and other medications to reduce inflammation and soothe irritated intestinal walls can relieve symptoms.

Irritable bowel syndrome (IBS), characterized by nausea, pain, gas, diarrhea, or cramps after eating certain foods or during unusual stress, commonly begins in early adulthood. Symptoms may vary from week to week and can fade for long periods of time, only to return.

The cause is unknown, but researchers suspect that people with IBS have digestive systems that are overly sensitive to what they eat and drink, to stress, and to certain hormonal changes. Stress management, relaxation techniques, regular activity, and diet can control IBS in the vast majority of cases. Problems with diarrhea can be reduced by cutting down on fat and avoiding caffeine and excessive amounts of sorbitol, a sweetener found in dietetic foods and chewing gum. Constipation can be relieved by a gradual increase in fiber. Some sufferers benefit from anticholinergic drugs, which relax the intestinal muscle, or from antidepressant drugs and psychological counseling. Medical advice should be sought whenever such conditions persist.

Peptic Ulcers

An ulcer is a lesion or wound that forms in body tissue as a result of some irritant. A **peptic ulcer** is a chronic ulcer that occurs in the lining of the stomach or the section of the small intestine known as the *duodenum*. The lining of these organs becomes irritated, the protective covering of mucus is reduced, and the gastric acid begins to digest the dying tissue, just as it would a piece of food. Typically, this irritation causes pain that disappears when the person eats, but it returns about an hour later.

Research indicates that most peptic ulcers result from infection by a common bacterium, *Helicobacter pylori*. The disorder, which affects more than 4 million Americans every year, generally responds to antibiotics. Peptic ulcers caused by excess stomach acid or overuse of stomach-irritating drugs such as aspirin and ibuprofen can be treated with acid-reducing medications.

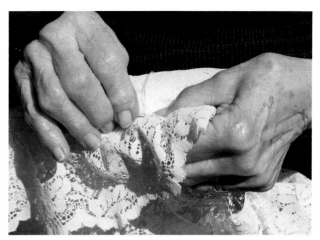

Arthritis can make simple tasks both painful and difficult to accomplish.

What Do You Think? What role can a healthy diet play in reducing risks for and symptoms of the diseases discussed here? ■ Are you or any of your family members at risk for these problems? ■ What actions can you take today that will cut your risk?

MUSCULOSKELETAL DISEASES

Arthritis

Called "the nation's primary crippler," **arthritis** strikes one in seven Americans, or over 38 million people. Symptoms range from the occasional tendinitis in the weekend athlete to the horrific pain of rheumatoid arthritis. There are over 100 types of arthritis diagnosed today, accounting for over 30 million lost workdays annually. The cost to the U.S. economy is over $65 billion per year in lost wages and productivity and untold amounts in hospital and nursing home services, prescriptions, and over-the-counter pain relief.[60]

Osteoarthritis (OA), also known as degenerative joint disease, is a progressive deterioration of bones and joints that has been associated with the "wear and tear" theory of aging. Bones rub directly against each other,

---

Irritable bowel syndrome (IBS) Nausea, pain, gas, or diarrhea caused by certain foods or stress.

Peptic ulcer Damage to the stomach or intestinal lining, usually caused by digestive juices.

Arthritis Painful inflammatory disease of the joints.

Osteoarthritis (OA) A progressive deterioration of bones and joints that has been associated with the "wear and tear" theory of aging.

---

causing the pain, swelling, and limited movement characteristic of arthritis. Obesity, joint trauma, and repetitive joint usage all increase the risk and thus are important targets for prevention.

Over 80 percent of those with OA report an activity limitation. Joint replacement and bone fusion are common surgical repair techniques. Anti-inflammatory drugs and pain relievers, applications of heat, mild exercise, and massage may relieve the pain.

Rheumatoid arthritis is an autoimmune disease involving chronic inflammation that most commonly appears between ages 20 and 45 and affects over 2.1 million Americans. Symptoms include stiffness, pain, redness, and swelling of multiple joints (often including the hands and wrists) and can be gradually progressive or sporadic, with occasional unexplained remissions.

Treatment of rheumatoid arthritis is similar to that for osteoarthritis, emphasizing pain relief and improved functional mobility. Immunosuppressant drugs can reduce the inflammatory response.

Systemic Lupus Erythematosus

Systemic lupus erythematosus (SLE), or **lupus,** is an autoimmune disease in which antibodies destroy or injure organs such as the kidneys, brain, and heart. The symptoms vary from mild to severe and may disappear for periods of time. A butterfly-shaped rash covering the bridge of the nose and both cheeks is common. Nearly all lupus sufferers have aching joints and muscles, and 60 percent of them develop redness and swelling that move from joint to joint. The disease is two to three times more prevalent among people of color, including African Americans, Asians, Native Americans, and Hispanics; 90 percent of all victims are female.[61] Extensive research has not yet found a cure for this sometimes fatal disease.

Lower Back Pain

Approximately 80 percent of all Americans will experience lower back pain (LBP) at some point. Some LBP

---

episodes result from muscular damage and may be short-lived and acute. Other episodes may involve dislocations, fractures, or other problems with spinal vertebrae or discs, thus resulting in chronic pain or requiring surgery.

Almost 90 percent of all back problems occur in the lumbar spine (lower back). You can avoid many problems by consciously maintaining good posture. Other preventive hints include:

- Purchase a supportive mattress, and avoid sleeping on your stomach.
- Avoid high-heeled shoes, which tilt the pelvis forward.
- Control your weight.
- Lift objects with your legs, not your back.
- Buy a good chair for doing your work, preferably one with lumbar support.
- Move your car seat forward so your knees are elevated slightly.
- Warm up before exercising.
- Engage in regular exercise, particularly exercises that strengthen the abdominal muscles and stretch the back muscles.

OTHER MALADIES

During the past 20 years, several afflictions have surfaced that seem to be products of our time. Some of these health problems relate to specific groups of people, some are due to technological advances, and others have not been explained.

Chronic Fatigue Syndrome

The diagnosis of **chronic fatigue syndrome (CFS)** depends on two major criteria and eight or more minor criteria. The major criteria are debilitating fatigue that persists for at least six months and the absence of other illnesses that could cause the symptoms. Minor criteria include headaches, fever, sore throat, painful lymph nodes, weakness, fatigue after exercise, sleep problems, and rapid onset of these symptoms. Treatment focuses on improved nutrition, rest, counseling for depression, judicious exercise, and development of a strong support network.

Despite extensive testing, no viral cause has been found. In the absence of a known pathogen, many researchers believe that the illness may have strong psychosocial roots.

Fibromyalgia

Persons with **fibromyalgia** experience an array of symptoms, including headaches, dizziness, numbness and tingling, itching, fluid retention, chronic joint pain, abdominal or pelvic pain, and even occasional diarrhea. Suspected causes include sleep disturbances, stress,

---

Rheumatoid arthritis A serious inflammatory joint disease.

Lupus A disease in which the immune system attacks the body and produces antibodies that destroy or injure organs such as the kidneys, brain, and heart.

Chronic fatigue syndrome (CFS) A debilitating fatigue that lasts for at least 6 months and the absence of another illness that could be causing the symptoms.

Fibromyalgia A chronic rheumatoid-like disorder that can be highly painful and difficult to diagnose.

emotional distress, viruses, and autoimmune disorders; however, none has been proved in clinical trials. Because of fibromyalgia's multiple symptoms, it is usually diagnosed only after myriad tests have ruled out other disorders.

Many people with fibromyalgia also become depressed and report chronic fatigue–like symptoms. Treatment varies based on the severity of symptoms. Typically, adequate rest, stress management, relaxation techniques, dietary supplements and selected herbal remedies, and pain medications are prescribed.

Repetitive Stress Injuries

The Bureau of Labor Statistics estimates that 25 percent of all injuries in the labor force that result in lost work time are due to a **repetitive stress injury (RSI).** These are injuries to nerves, soft tissue, or joints that result from the physical stress of repeated motions. They are estimated to cost employers up to $120 billion a year.[62]

One of the most common RSIs is **carpal tunnel syndrome.** Hours spent typing at the computer, flipping groceries through computerized scanners, or other jobs made simpler by technology can irritate the median nerve in the wrist, thus causing numbness, tingling, and pain in the fingers and hands. Although carpal tunnel syndrome risk can be reduced by proper placement of the keyboard, mouse, wrist pads, and other techniques, RSIs are often overlooked until significant damage has been done. Better education and ergonomic workplace designs can eliminate many injuries of this nature.

> **Repetitive stress injury (RSI)** An injury to nerves, soft tissue, or joints due to the physical stress of repeated motions.
>
> **Carpal tunnel syndrome** A common occupational injury in which the median nerve in the wrist becomes irritated, thus causing numbness, tingling, and pain in the fingers and hands.

Taking Charge

Summary

- The major uncontrollable risk factors for contracting infectious diseases are heredity, age, environmental conditions, and organism resistance. The major controllable risk factors are stress, nutrition, fitness level, sleep, hygiene, avoidance of high-risk behaviors, and drug use.

- The major pathogens are bacteria, viruses, fungi, protozoa, prions, and parasitic worms. Bacterial infections include staphylococcal infections, streptococcal infections, pneumonia, and tuberculosis. Major viruses include the common cold, influenza, mononucleosis, hepatitis, and measles.

- Your body uses a number of defense systems to keep pathogens from invading. The skin is the body's major protection, helped by enzymes. The immune system creates antibodies to destroy antigens. Fever and pain play a role in defending the body. Vaccines bolster the body's immune system against specific diseases.

- Emerging and resurgent diseases pose significant threats for future generations. Many factors contribute to these risks. Possible solutions focus on a public health approach to prevention.

- Sexually transmitted infections (STIs) are spread through intercourse, oral sex, anal sex, hand–genital contact, and sometimes through mouth-to-mouth contact. Major STIs include chlamydia, pelvic inflammatory disease (PID), gonorrhea, syphilis, pubic lice, genital warts, candidiasis, trichomoniasis, and herpes. Sexual transmission may also be involved in some general urinary tract infections.

- Acquired immunodeficiency syndrome (AIDS) is caused by the human immunodeficiency virus (HIV). Globally, HIV/AIDS has become a major threat to the world's population. Anyone can get HIV by engaging in high-risk sexual activities that include exchange of body fluids, by having received a blood transfusion before 1985, and by injecting drugs (or having sex with someone who does). Women appear to be particularly susceptible to infection. You can cut your risk for AIDS by deciding not to engage in risky sexual activities.

- Chronic lung diseases include allergies, hay fever, asthma, emphysema, and chronic bronchitis. Allergies are part of the body's natural defense system. Chronic obstructive pulmonary diseases are the fourth leading cause of death in the United States.

- Neurological conditions include headaches, seizure disorders, Parkinson's disease, and multiple sclerosis. Headaches may be caused by a variety of factors, the most common of which are tension, dilation and/or rapid contraction of blood vessels in the brain, chemical influences on muscles and vessels that cause inflammation and pain, and underlying physiological and psychological disorders.

- Premenstrual syndrome (PMS) and premenstrual dysphoric disorder (PMDD) are conditions related to the menstrual cycle. Endometriosis is the buildup of endometrial tissue in regions of the body other than the uterus.

■ Diabetes occurs when the pancreas fails to produce enough insulin to regulate sugar metabolism or the body's receptors for insulin no longer function. Other conditions, such as colitis, irritable bowel syndrome (IBS), and peptic ulcers, result from functional problems in various digestion-related organs or systems.

■ Musculoskeletal diseases such as arthritis, lower back pain, repetitive stress injuries, and other problems cause significant pain and disability in millions of people. Chronic fatigue syndrome (CFS) and repetitive stress injuries (RSIs, such as carpal tunnel syndrome) have emerged as major chronic maladies. CFS is associated with depression. Repetitive stress injuries are preventable by proper equipment placement and usage.

Chapter Review

1. What inherited blood disease primarily affects African Americans and results in organ damage and premature death?
   a. AIDS
   b. sickle cell anemia
   c. diabetes
   d. muscular dystrophy

2. The smallest of the pathogens are
   a. prions.
   b. viruses.
   c. protozoa.
   d. bacteria.

3. What is the single greatest factor influencing your longevity?
   a. gender
   b. socioeconomic status
   c. parents' longevity
   d. marital status

4. Which of the following is a *viral* disorder?
   a. measles
   b. pneumonia
   c. tuberculosis
   d. streptococcal infections

5. Acne, boils, and styes are a type of
   a. virus.
   b. fungi.
   c. staphylococcal infection.
   d. streptococcal infection.

6. The Epstein-Barr virus causes
   a. hepatitis.
   b. measles.
   c. pneumonia.
   d. infectious mononucleosis.

7. During what stage of syphilis does a chancre develop?
   a. primary syphilis
   b. secondary syphilis
   c. latent syphilis
   d. late syphilis

8. Many researchers believe that the world is due for a flu pandemic, causing much anxiety over an emerging virulent flu strain called
   a. avian influenza.
   b. E. coli O157:H7.
   c. ebola hemorrhagic fever.
   d. severe acute respiratory syndrome.

9. The Western blot is a test used to detect the presence of
   a. hepatitis.
   b. syphilis.
   c. chlamydia.
   d. HIV antibodies.

10. What degenerative disease involves the breakdown of myelin?
    a. epilepsy
    b. multiple sclerosis
    c. cerebral palsy
    d. Parkinson's disease

Answers to these questions can be found on page A-1.

Questions for Discussion and Reflection

1. What are the major controllable risk factors for contracting infectious diseases? Using this knowledge, how would you change your current lifestyle to prevent such infection?

2. What is a pathogen? What are the similarities and differences between pathogens and antigens? Discuss uncontrollable and controllable risk factors that can threaten your health.

3. What are the six types of pathogens? What are the various means by which they can be transmitted? How have social conditions among the poor and homeless increased the risks for certain diseases, such as tuberculosis, influenza, and hepatitis? Why are these conditions a challenge to the efforts of public health officials?

4. Identify possible reasons for the spread of emerging and resurgent diseases. Indicate public policies and programs that might reduce this trend.

5. Identify five STIs and their symptoms. How do they develop? What are their potential long-term effects?

6. Should Americans be concerned about soaring HIV/AIDS rates elsewhere in the world? Explain your answer.

7. What are some of the major noninfectious chronic diseases affecting Americans today? Do you think there is a pattern in the types of diseases that we get? What are the common risk factors?

8. List common respiratory diseases affecting Americans. Which of these diseases has a genetic basis? An environmental basis? An individual basis? What, if anything, is being done to prevent, treat, and control each of these conditions?

9. Describe the symptoms and treatment of diabetes. What is the difference between type 1 diabetes and type 2 diabetes?

10. What are the major disorders of the musculoskeletal system? Why do you think there aren't any cures? Describe the difference between osteoarthritis and rheumatoid arthritis.

Accessing Your Health on the Internet

The following websites explore further topics and issues related to personal health. For links to the websites below, visit the Companion Website for *Health: The Basics*, Seventh Edition at www.aw-bc.com/donatelle.

1. *American Academy of Allergy, Asthma, and Immunology.* Provides an overview of asthma and allergies. Offers interactive quizzes to test your knowledge and an ask-an-expert section.

2. *American Diabetes Association.* Excellent resource for diabetes information.

3. *Centers for Disease Control and Prevention (CDC).* Home page for the government agency dedicated to disease intervention and prevention, with links to all the latest data and publications put out by the CDC, including the *Morbidity and Mortality Weekly Report, HIV/AIDS Surveillance Report*, and the *Journal of Emerging Infectious Diseases*, and access to the CDC research database, Wonder.

4. *National Center for Chronic Disease Prevention and Health Promotion (NCCDPHP).* Provides access to a wide range of information from this CDC-affiliated organization dedicated to chronic diseases and health promotion.

5. *World Health Organization (WHO).* Provides access to the latest information on world health issues, including infectious disease; direct access to publications and fact sheets, with keywords to help users find topics of interest.

Further Reading

Champeau, D. and R. Donatelle. *AIDS and STIs: A Global Perspective.* Englewood Cliffs, NJ: Prentice Hall, 2002.

An overview of issues, trends, and ethics surrounding the global pandemic of HIV/AIDS and STIs.

Chin, J., ed. *Control of Communicable Diseases Manual*, 17th ed. Washington, DC: American Public Health Association, 2003.

Outstanding pocket reference for information on infectious diseases. Updated every three to five years to cover emerging diseases.

National Center for Health Statistics. *Monthly Vital Statistics Report and Advance Data from Vital and Health Statistics.* Hyattsville, MD: Public Health Service.

Detailed government reports, usually published monthly, concerning mortality and morbidity data for the United States. Includes changes occurring in the rates of particular diseases and in health practices so patterns and trends can be analyzed.

References

1. K. Nelson, C. Williams, and N. Graham, *Infectious Disease Epidemiology: Theory and Practice* (Gaithersburg, MD: Aspen, 2001), 17–39.

2. University of Michigan Health System, "Toxic Shock Syndrome," 2004, www.med.umich.edu/1libr/aha/aha_toxic_crs.htm.

3. Ibid.

4. American Lung Association, "Pneumonia Fact Sheet," June 2005, www.lungusa.org/site/paasp?c=duluk900E&b=35692.

5. National Center for HIV, STD, and TB Prevention, "Surveillance Report: Reported Tuberculosis in the United States, 2004," 2005, www.cdc.gov/nchstp/tb/surv/surv2003/default.htm.

6. World Health Organization (WHO), "Tuberculosis Facts and Figures," March 2005, www.wpo.wha.int/media_centre?fact_sheets/fs_20050324.htm.

7. Ibid.

8. A. Evans and R. Kaslow, *Viral Infections in Humans: Epidemiology and Control*, 4th ed. (New York: Plenum, 1997), 6–11.

9. Centers for Disease Control and Prevention (CDC), *Preventing the Flu: Key Facts about Influenza Vaccine* (Atlanta: CDC, 2005), www.cdc.gov/flu/protect/keyfacts.htm.

10. World Health Organization (WHO), "Immunization, Vaccines and Biologicals: Hepatitis A Vaccine," www.who.int/vaccines/en/hepatitisa.shtml.

11. K. W. Link and J. T. Kirchner, "Hepatitis B," *American Family Physician* 69:75–82.

12. Centers for Disease Control and Prevention (CDC), *Viral Hepatitis C Fact Sheet* (Atlanta, GA: CDC, 2005), www.cdc.gov/ncidod/diseases/hepatitis/c/fact.htm.

13. Ibid.

14. Seattle Biomedical Research Institute, "Global Connections, Infectious Diseases Hinder Environment," 2003, www.sbri.org.news/GC%20summer03.pdf.

15. K. Nelson, C. Williams, and N. Graham, *Infectious Disease Epidemiology*, 17–39.

16. National Center for Infectious Diseases, "BSE and CJD Information and Resources," 2005, www.cdc.gov/ncidod/diseases/cjdcjd.htm.

17. Centers for Disease Control and Prevention (CDC), *Fact Sheet: Basics Information about SARS* (Atlanta: CDC, 2005), www.cdc.gov/ncidod/sars/factsheet.htm.

18. Centers for Disease Control and Prevention (CDC), "Diseases—Ebola Hemorrhagic Fever," 2005, www.cdc.gov/ncidod/dvrd/spb/mnpages/dispages/ebola.htm.

19. Ibid.

20. K. Nelson, C. Williams, and N. Graham, *Infectious Disease Epidemiology*, 325.

21. R. Fenner, *The History of Smallpox and Its Spread around the World* (Geneva, Switzerland: World Health Organization, 1988).

22. National Center for HIV, STD, and TB Prevention, "STD Surveillance 2004," 2005, www.cdc.gov/std/stats/toc2002.htm.

23. Ibid.
24. National Center for HIV, STD, and TB Prevention, "Chlamydia Fact Sheet," 2004, www.cdc.gov/std/Chlamydia/STDFact-Chlamydia.htm.
25. Ibid.
26. National Center for HIV, STD, and TB Prevention, "Gonorrhea Fact Sheet," 2004, www.cdc.gov/std/Gonorrhea/STDFact-Gonorrhea.htm.
27. National Institute of Allergy and Infectious Diseases, "Gonorrhea" www.niaid.nih.gov/factsheets/stdgon.htm.
28. National Center for HIV, STD, and TB Prevention, "Genital Herpes Fact Sheet," 2005, www.cdc.gov/std/herpes/STDFact-Herpes.htm.
29. Ibid.
30. Ibid.
31. The CARE Exchange, "HIV/ADIS Statistics, 2005," www.caree.org/aids.htm.
32. Centers for Disease Control and Prevention (CDC), "HIV/AIDS Surveillance," 2005, www.cdc.gov/programs/hiv06.htm.
33. Ibid.
34. National Institute of Allergy and Infectious Diseases, "HIV Infection and IADS: An Overview," 2005, www.niaid.nih.gov/factsheets/hivinf.htm.
35. AVERT, "Providing Drug Treatment for Millions," www.avert.org/drugtreatment.htm.
36. AVERT, "AIDS in America," www.avert.org/aids-america.htm.
37. Ibid.
38. Asthma and Allergy Foundation of America, "Asthma Facts and Figures, " 2005, www.aafa.org.
39. American Academy of Allergy, Asthma, and Immunology, *Tips to Remember: Asthma Triggers and Management,* (Milwaukee, WI: Author) www.aaaai.org/patients/publicedmat/tips/asthmatriggersandmgmt.stm.
40. MayoClinic,com, "Bronchitis," 2005, www.mayoclinic.com/invoke.cfm?id-DS00031.
41. Canadian Lung Association, "Symptoms of Sleep Apnea," www.sleepapnea.ab.ca/symptoms.htm.
42. National Headache Foundation (NFH), "NFH Headache Fact Sheet," 2004, www.headaches.org.
43. Ibid.
44. Ibid.
45. Ibid.
46. MayoClinic.com, "Migraine," 2005, www.mayoclinic.com/invoke.cfm?id=DS00120.
47. McKinley Health Center, "Migraine Headaches," www.mckinley.uiuc.edu/health-info/dis-cond/headache/migr-hea.htm.
48. Condell Health Network, "Coping with Migraine Pain," www.condell.org/health-information/migraines.php.
49. Ibid.
50. Ibid.
51. MayoClinic.com, "Epilepsy," 2005, www.mayoclinic.com/invoke.cfm?id=DS00342.
52. National Parkinson Foundation, "Parkinson Primer," 2004, www.parkinson.org.
53. J. Gerberding, "Diabetes: Disabling, Deadly, and on the Rise. At A Glance 2004," 2004, www.cdc.gov/nccdphp/aag/aag_ddt.htm; Centers for Disease Control and Prevention, "Diabetes Surveillance System," 2005, www.cdc.gov/diabetes/statistics.
54. Ibid.
55. Ibid.
56. Ibid.
57. Ibid.
58. Ibid.
59. J. Adler and C. Kalb, "An American Epidemic: Diabetes," *Newsweek,* September 4, 2000, 40–48; Centers for Disease Control and Prevention (CDC), "Diabetes Surveillance System."
60. Arthritis Foundation, "Disease Center," 2005, www.arthritis.org/conditions/DiseaseCenter/oa.asp.
61. Lupus Foundation of America, "Statistics About Lupus," 2005. www.lupus.org/education/stats.html
62. Commission Behavioral and Social Sciences and Education, *Work Related Musculo Skeletal Disorders: Report, 1999.* Washington D.C.: National Academies Press.

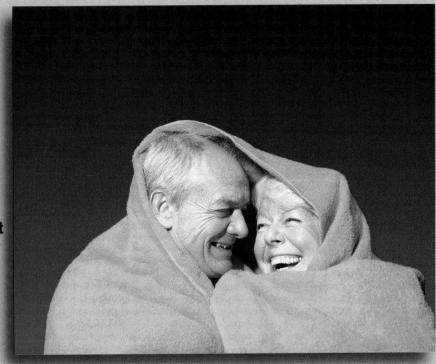

■ Is it really possible to "age gracefully"?

■ Why should I create a living will?

■ What types of physical changes can I expect as I grow older?

■ What makes stem cells different from other types of cells?

15 Life's Transitions
The Aging Process

Objectives

- **Define** aging, and explain the related concepts of biological, psychological, social, legal, and functional age.
- **Discuss** the unique health challenges faced by older adults.
- **Discuss** strategies for healthy aging that can begin during young adulthood.
- **Explain** death, the stages of the grieving process, and strategies for coping with death.

- **Describe** the ethical concerns that arise from the concepts of the right to die and rational suicide.
- **Review** the decisions that need to be made when someone is dying or has died, including hospice care, funeral arrangements, wills, and organ donations.

Grow old along with me!
The best is yet to be,
The last of life, for which the first was made . . .

Robert Browning, *Rabbi Ben Ezra*

In a society that seems to worship youth, researchers have begun to offer good—even revolutionary—news about the aging process. Growing old doesn't have to mean a slow slide to declining physical and mental health. Health promotion, disease prevention, and wellness-oriented activities can prolong vigor and productivity, even among those who haven't always led model lifestyles or made healthful habits a priority. In fact, getting older can mean getting better in many ways—particularly socially, psychologically, and intellectually.

The manner in which you view aging (either as a natural part of living or an inevitable decline toward disease and death) is a crucial factor in how successfully you will adapt to life's transitions. If you view these transitions as periods of growth in your development as a human being, your journey through even the most difficult times will be easier. Explore your own notions about aging in the Assess Yourself box on page 416.

Aging has traditionally been described as the patterns of life changes that occur in members of all species as they grow older. Some people believe that aging begins at the moment of conception. Others contend that it starts at birth. Still others believe that true aging does not begin until we reach our forties. Typically, experts and laypersons alike have used chronological age to assign a person to a particular life-cycle stage.

REDEFINING AGING

The study of individual and collective aging processes, known as **gerontology**, explores the reasons for aging and the ways in which people cope with and adapt to this process. Gerontologists have identified several age-related characteristics that define where a person is in terms of biological, psychological, social, legal, and functional life-stage development:[1]

- *Biological age* refers to the relative age or condition of the person's organs and body systems. There are 70-year-old runners who have the cardiovascular system of a 40-year-old, and 40-year-olds who have less energy than their parents do. Arthritis and other chronic conditions can accelerate the aging process.

Aging The patterns of life changes that occur in members of all species as they grow older.

Gerontology The study of individual and collective aging processes.

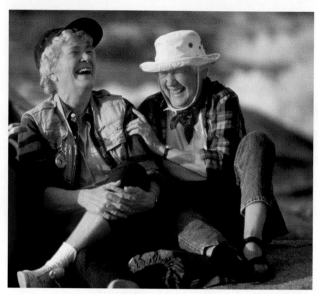

For many, the secret to aging well is to stay active and enjoy the company of good friends.

- *Psychological age* refers to a person's adaptive capacities, such as coping abilities and intelligence, and to the person's awareness of his or her individual capabilities, self-efficacy, and general ability to adapt to situations. Research documents that people who maintain a positive attitude and stay mentally active are more likely to age well and be happy.[2] Although chronic illness may render people physically handicapped, they may possess tremendous psychological reserves and remain alert and fully capable of making decisions.

- *Social age* refers to a person's habits and roles relative to society's expectations. People in a particular life stage usually share similar tastes in music, television shows, and politics.

- *Legal age* is probably the most common definition of age in the United States. Based on chronological years, legal age is used as a factor in determining voting rights, driving privileges, drinking age, eligibility for Social Security payments, and a host of other rights and obligations.

- *Functional age* refers to the ways—heart rate, hearing, etc.—in which people compare to others of a similar age. It is difficult to separate functional aging from other types of aging, particularly chronological and biological aging.

What Is Successful Aging?

Many of today's older individuals lead active, productive lives. For instance, 49,000 Americans age 65 and older are currently enrolled in college, and 14 percent are employed. In the last presidential election, 72 percent of U.S. citizens aged 65 to 74 voted—a higher percentage than any other age group.[3]

Typically, people who have aged successfully have the following characteristics:

- They have managed to avoid serious, debilitating diseases and disability.
- They maintain a high level of physical functioning, live independently, and engage in most normal activities of daily living.
- They have maintained cognitive functioning and are actively engaged in mentally challenging and stimulating activities.
- They are actively engaged in social and productive activities.
- They are resilient and able to cope reasonably well with physical, social, and emotional changes.

Though the process of aging has often been viewed with dread because of the inevitable physical changes, only in the past decade have we begun to fully appreciate the gains and positive aspects of normal adult development throughout the lifespan. According to gerontologist Dr. Karen Hooker, older adults as a population display much more differentiation in personalities, coping styles, and "possible selves" than any other age group. She states that "successful aging and development as individuals can be viewed as dynamic processes of adaptation between the self and the environment."[4]

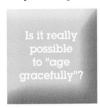

Is it really possible to "age gracefully"?

Aging is not a static process, but one in which we change and become someone uniquely fashioned by our life's story. Gerontologists have devised several categories for specific age-related characteristics. People aged 65 to 74 are viewed as the **young-old;** those aged 75 to 84 are the **middle-old** group; those 85 and over are classified as **old-old.**

However, chronological age is not the only issue to be considered. *Quality-of-life* (discussed in Chapter 1), combined with the chronological process, appears to be the best indicator of the phenomenon of "aging gracefully." Most experts agree that the best way to experience a productive, full, and satisfying old age is to lead a productive, full, and satisfying life prior to old age.

Older Adults: A Growing Population

There are almost 36 million people aged 65 or older in the United States—over 12 percent of the total population—and almost 4.2 million people aged 85 or older (Figure 15.1). This statistic represents more than a tenfold increase since 1900, when there were only 3 million residents in the 65-or-older category and only 100,000 people aged 85 or more. The number of those 65 and over is projected to hit 71.5 million by 2030,

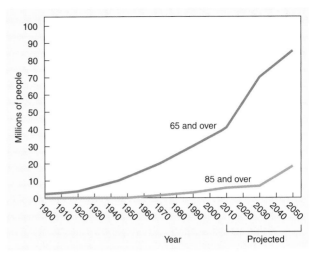

Figure 15.1 ■ Number of Americans 65 and Older (in Millions), Years 1900–2000, and Projected 2010–2050

Note: Data from 2010–2050 are projections of the population.

Source: Federal Interagency Forum on Aging-Related Statistics, "Indicator 1: Number of Older Americans," *Older Americans 2004: Key Indicators of Well-Being* (Hyattsville, MD: Federal Interagency Forum on Aging-Related Statistics, 2005).

almost 20 percent of the U.S. population.[5] Some researchers predict that this will have as big an impact on our society as immigration did at the turn of the last century.[6]

HEALTH ISSUES FOR AN AGING SOCIETY
Health Care Costs

Older Americans average $3,741 per year in out-of-pocket medical expenses, an increase of 45 percent since 1992.[7] As people live longer, the chances of developing a costly chronic disease increase; and, as technology improves, chronic illnesses that once were quickly fatal may now be treated successfully for years. Projected future costs from these two trends are staggering.

If Social Security goes bankrupt, large numbers of Americans will no longer have Medicare coverage. Even if they could afford to buy their own health insurance, most older individuals would face high out-of-pocket expenses and limited choices in treatments. Major questions loom: Will working Americans be willing to pay an increased share of the health care costs for people on fixed incomes who cannot pay for themselves? If not, what will become of older Americans? Perhaps most important, who will ultimately pay?

Young-old   People aged 65 to 74.

Middle-old   People aged 75 to 84.

Old-old   People aged 85 and over.

Where Do You Want to Be?

my health lab

Fill out this assessment online at
www.aw-bc.com/MyHealthLab or www.aw-bc.com/donatelle.

When we are young, aging is the furthest thing from our minds. However, thinking about aging and what we expect from life are important elements of a satisfying adult devel-opment process. Take a few minutes to answer the follow-ing questions. Your answers may tell you a great deal about yourself.

1. At this point in your life, what do you value most?
2. What do you think will be most important to you when you reach your forties? Fifties? Sixties? What similari-ties and differences do you notice, and what causes these similarities and differences?
3. Do you think your parents are happy with the way their lives have turned out? If they could change anything, what do you think they might do differently?
4. What about your own direction thus far in life is similar to that of your parents? What have you done differ-ently? Are the similarities and differences good? Why or why not?
5. What do you think are the keys to a happy and satisfying life?
6. What do you want to accomplish by the time you are 40? By the time you are 50? By the time you are 60?
7. Have you ever thought of retirement? Describe your retirement.
8. Describe the "you" that you would like to be at the age of 70. How is that person similar to or different from the "you" of today? What actions will you need to take to be that person in the future?

Make It Happen!

Assessment: The Assess Yourself activity encouraged you to consider some of the deepest questions in life: What are your values? How do you want your life to compare with that of your parents? How would you like to be described at age 70? Now that you have considered your answers, per-haps there are actions you can take that will help you create the life that you want.

Making a Change: In order to change your behavior, you need to develop a plan. Follow these steps below and com-plete your Behavior Change Contract to take action.

1. Evaluate your behavior, and identify patterns and spe-cific things you are doing. What can you change now? What can you change in the near future?
2. Select one pattern of behavior that you want to change.
3. Fill out the Behavior Change Contract found at the front of your book. It should include your long-term goal for change, your short-term goals, the rewards you'll give yourself for reaching these goals, potential obstacles along the way, and strategies for overcoming these obstacles. For each goal, list the small steps and spe-cific actions that you will take.

4. Chart your progress in a journal. At the end of a week, consider how successful you were in following your plan. What helped you be successful? What made change more difficult? What will you do differently next week?
5. Revise your plan as needed: Are the short-term goals attainable? Are the rewards satisfying?

Example: When Eric answered the Assess Yourself ques-tions, he realized he had not thought deeply about where he wanted to be at various stages in his life. In particular, he wanted to take more time to look at his parents' lives and careers, as well as those of older adults around him in the community. He set a goal of asking his parents and grand-parents some of these same questions about their goals and lives to see where he might agree and disagree with them and how he might develop his own values and priori-ties. As he began thinking more seriously about the types of careers that might be fulfilling, he arranged to meet with people who had gone into professions that he was consid-ering. He also decided to take a philosophy class as one of his electives in the next year, so he could actually get school credit for thinking about these big questions.

Housing and Living Arrangements

Contrary to popular opinion, most older people (more than 95 percent) never live in a nursing home. Community living, assisted living, skilled nursing care, and other options are new possibilities for those who have financial means or who have purchased some form of long-term care insurance. However, housing problems for low-income individuals remain. Who will provide the necessary social services, and who will pay the bill? Will the family of the future be forced to coexist with several generations under one roof?

Ethical and Moral Considerations

Difficult ethical questions arise when we consider the implications for an already overburdened health care system. Given the shortage of donor organs, will we be forced to decide whether a 50-year-old should receive a heart transplant instead of a 75-year-old? Questions have already surfaced regarding the efficacy of hooking up a terminally ill older person to costly machines that prolong life for a few weeks or months but overtax health care resources. Is the prolongation of life at all costs a moral imperative, or will future generations be forced to devise a set of criteria for deciding who will be helped and who will not? Understanding the process of aging and knowing what actions you can take to prolong your own healthy years are part of our collective responsibility.

What Do You Think? Do you currently have health insurance? If not, why not? ■ What do you think people over 65 would do if they suddenly didn't have Medicare? ■ Should older Americans be left out of the health insurance industry because they are at high risk for illness and disability? ■ Why are the aging of the population and the impending difficulties with health care costs and access important to all of us?

THEORIES OF AGING
Biological Theories

Explanations for the biological causes of aging include:

■ The *wear-and-tear theory* states that, like everything else in the universe, the human body wears out. Inherent in this theory is the idea that the more you abuse your body, the faster it will wear out. Fortunately, today's older adults have a variety of resources and opportunities to keep their bodies strong and healthy.

Walking, gardening, and other activities allow even the most out of shape to improve.

■ The *cellular theory* states that at birth we have only a certain number of usable cells, which are genetically programmed to divide or reproduce a limited number of times. Once these cells reach the end of their reproductive cycle, they die, and the organs they make up begin to deteriorate. The rate of deterioration varies from person to person, and its impact depends on the system involved.

■ The *autoimmune theory* attributes aging to the decline of the body's immunological system. Studies indicate that as we age, our immune systems become less effective in fighting disease. Eventually, bodies that are subjected to too much stress, lack of sleep, and so on, show signs of disease and infirmity, especially if these factors are coupled with poor nutrition. Although autoimmune disorders occur in all age groups, some gerontologists believe that they increase in frequency and severity with age.

■ The *genetic mutation theory* proposes that the number of cells exhibiting unusual or different characteristics increases with age. Proponents of this theory believe that aging is related to the amount of mutational damage within the genes. The more mutation, the greater the chance that cells will not function properly, which leads to eventual dysfunction of body organs and systems.

Psychosocial Impacts on Aging

Numerous psychological and sociological factors also influence the manner in which people age. Psychologists Erik Erikson and Robert Peck have formulated theories of personality development that emphasize adaptation and adjustment. In his developmental model, Erikson states that people must progress through eight critical stages during a lifetime. If a person does not receive the proper stimulus or develop effective methods of coping with life's turmoil from infancy onward, problems are likely to develop later in life. According to this theory, maladjustments in old age are often a result of problems encountered in earlier stages of life.

Peck argues that during middle age and old age, people face a series of increasingly stressful tasks. Those who are poorly adjusted psychologically or who have not developed appropriate coping skills are likely to undergo a painful aging process.

Both Erikson and Peck suggest that a combination of psychosocial and biological factors and environmental trigger mechanisms causes each of us to age in a unique manner. But what is normal and what is unique in aging? How much change is inevitable, and how much can we avoid?

CHANGES IN THE BODY AND MIND

Typical Physical Changes

> **What types of physical changes can I expect as I grow older?**

Although the physiological consequences of aging can differ in severity and timing, certain standard changes occur as a result of the aging process.

The Skin As a normal consequence of aging, the skin becomes thinner and loses elasticity, particularly in the outer surfaces. Fat deposits, which add to the soft lines and shape of the skin, diminish. Starting at about age 30, lines develop on the forehead as a result of smiling, squinting, and other facial expressions. These lines become more pronounced, with added "crow's feet" around the eyes, during the forties. During a person's fifties and sixties, the skin begins to sag and lose color, which leads to pallor in the seventies. Body fat in underlying layers of skin continues to be redistributed away from the limbs and extremities into the trunk region of the body. Age spots become more numerous because of excessive pigment accumulation under the skin, particularly in areas of the skin exposed to heavy sun.

Bones and Joints Throughout the life span, bones are continually changing because of the accumulation and loss of minerals. By the third or fourth decade of life, mineral loss from bones becomes more prevalent than does mineral accumulation, which results in a weakening and porosity (diminishing density) of bony tissue. This loss of minerals (particularly calcium) occurs in both sexes, although it is more common in females. Loss of calcium can contribute to **osteoporosis,** a disease characterized by low bone density and structural deterioration of bone tissue. These porous, fragile bones are susceptible to fracture.

However, osteoporosis can occur at any age and develops over the course of many years.[8] There are several risk factors for osteoporosis, some of which cannot be controlled (gender, age, body size, ethnicity, and family history). However, there are factors that can be controlled starting from adolescence. Young women should receive adequate nutrients, particularly calcium and vitamin D, to reduce risk. All young adults, both female and male, should avoid cigarette smoking and should achieve adequate levels of exercise. Weight-bearing exercise such

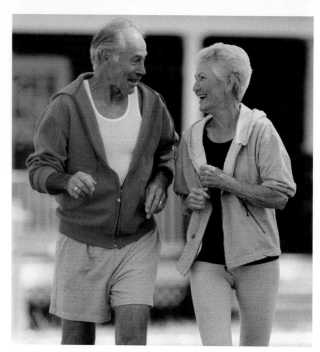

Regular weight-bearing exercises, such as vigorous walking, are an excellent way to strengthen bones.

as walking, jogging, weight training, and tennis all strengthen bone and improve bone density.[9]

Another bone condition that afflicts almost 21 million Americans is *osteoarthritis,* a progressive breakdown of joint cartilage that becomes more common with age and is the leading cause of disability in the United States.[10] (For information on osteoarthritis and other forms of arthritis, see Chapter 14.)

The Head With age, features of the head enlarge and become more noticeable. Increased cartilage and fatty tissue cause the nose to grow a half-inch wider and another half-inch longer. Earlobes get fatter and grow longer. As the skull becomes thicker with age, the overall head circumference increases one-quarter of an inch per decade, even though the brain itself shrinks.

The Urinary Tract At age 70, the kidneys can filter waste from the blood only half as fast as they could at age 30. The need to urinate more frequently occurs because the bladder's capacity declines from 2 cups of urine at age 30 to 1 cup at age 70.

One problem often associated with aging is **urinary incontinence,** which ranges from passing a few drops of urine while laughing or sneezing to having no control over urination. Approximately 35 percent of older women and 22 percent of older men have some degree of urinary incontinence.[11]

Incontinence can pose major social, physical, and emotional problems. Embarrassment and fear of wetting oneself may cause an older person to become isolated and avoid social functions. Caregivers may

---

Osteoporosis A degenerative bone disorder characterized by increasingly porous bones.

Urinary incontinence The inability to control urination.

become frustrated with incontinent patients. Prolonged wetness and the inability to properly care for oneself can lead to irritation, infections, and other problems.

However, incontinence is not an inevitable part of aging. Most cases are caused by medications, highly treatable neurological problems that affect the central nervous system, infections of the pelvic muscles, weakness in the pelvic wall, or other problems. When the problem is treated, the incontinence usually vanishes.[12]

The Heart and Lungs Resting heart rate stays about the same over the course of a person's life, but the stroke volume (the amount of blood the muscle pushes out per beat) diminishes as heart muscles deteriorate. Vital capacity, or the amount of air that moves when you inhale and exhale at maximum effort, also declines with age. Exercise can do a great deal to preserve heart and lung function.

Eyesight By age 30, the lens of the eye begins to harden, which causes problems by the early forties. The lens begins to yellow and loses transparency, while the pupil of the eye shrinks, which allows less light to penetrate. Activities such as reading become more difficult, particularly in dim light. By age 60, depth perception declines, and farsightedness often develops. A need for glasses usually develops in the forties, and this often evolves into a need for bifocals in the fifties and trifocals in the sixties. **Cataracts** (clouding of the lens) and **glaucoma** (elevated pressure within the eyeball) become more likely. Eventually, a tendency toward color blindness may develop, especially for shades of blue and green. **Macular degeneration** is the breakdown of the light-sensitive part of the retina responsible for the sharp, direct vision needed to read or drive. Its effects can be devastating to independent older adults; the causes are still being investigated.

Hearing The ability to hear high-frequency consonants (for example, s, t, and z) diminishes with age. Much of the actual hearing loss lies in the inability to distinguish extreme ranges of sound rather than in the inability to distinguish normal conversational tones.

Sexual Changes As people age, they experience noticeable changes in sexual function. While the degree and rate of change vary greatly from person to person, the following changes generally occur in men:

- Diminished ability to obtain and maintain an erection
- Longer refractory period between orgasms
- Shortened duration of orgasm

Women also experience several changes:

- Menopause usually occurs between the ages of 45 and 55. Women may experience a variety of symptoms (see Chapter 5).

- The walls of the vagina become less elastic and the epithelium thins, which may make intercourse painful.
- Vaginal secretions, particularly during sexual activity, diminish.
- The breasts become less firm. Loss of fat in various areas leads to fewer curves, with a decrease in the soft lines of the body contours.

While these physiological changes may sound somewhat discouraging, the fact is that many people remain sexually active all their lives.[13] Indeed, a landmark study by the National Council on Aging refuted long-held beliefs that sexual desire decreases as we age. Results indicated that nearly half of Americans over age 60 engage in sexual activity at least once a month and four out of ten would like to have sex more frequently than they currently do.[14] With the advent of drugs designed to treat sexual dysfunction, such as Viagra, many older adults may get their wish.

Body Comfort Because of the loss of body fat, thinning of the epithelium, and diminished glandular activity, older people experience greater difficulty in regulating body temperature. This limits their ability to withstand extreme cold or heat, which increases the risks of hypothermia, heatstroke, and heat exhaustion.

Try it ►NOW_____

Protect your ears now to spare you hearing later. **Turn down the volume on your headset a notch, and purchase some earplugs to have on hand for music concerts, mowing the lawn, or any other activity that causes your ears to ring, a telltale sign they've had enough!**

Typical Mental Changes

Intelligence Recent research demonstrates that many of our previous beliefs about intelligence later in life were based on inappropriate testing procedures.

Cataracts Clouding of the lens that interrupts the focusing of light on the retina, which results in blurred vision or eventual blindness. This condition is correctable with surgery.

Glaucoma Elevation of pressure within the eyeball, which leads to hardening of the eyeball, impaired vision, and possible blindness.

Macular degeneration Disease that breaks down the macula, the light-sensitive part of the retina responsible for sharp, direct vision.

Given an appropriate length of time, older people learn and develop skills in a similar manner to younger people. Researchers have also determined that what many older adults lack in speed of learning they make up for in practical knowledge—that is, they have the wisdom of age.

Memory Have you ever wondered why your grandfather seems unable to remember what he did last weekend even though he can graphically describe an event that occurred 40 years ago? This phenomenon is not unusual. Although short-term memory may fluctuate on a daily basis, the ability to remember events from past decades seems to remain largely unchanged.

Adaptability Having lived through a multitude of experiences and faced diverse joys, sorrows, and obstacles, the typical older person has developed unique methods of coping with life. These unique adaptive variations make for interesting differences in how we confront the many changes brought on by the aging process. As a group, older adults are extremely heterogeneous. They adapt and "make do" in ways that younger adults may not be able to duplicate.

Depression Most adults continue to lead healthy, fulfilling lives. However, some older people do suffer from mental and emotional disturbances. Some research indicates that depression may be the most common psychological problem facing older adults. However, the rate of major depression is actually lower among older people than among younger adults.

Regardless of age, people who have a poor perception of their health, have multiple chronic illnesses, take a lot of medications, abuse alcohol or other drugs, lack social support, and do not exercise face more challenges that may require emotional strength. Strong coping skills and support systems can lessen the duration and severity of the depression.

Senility: Getting Rid of Ageist Attitudes

Discrimination against people based on age is known as **ageism.** When directed against the elderly, this discrimination carries with it social ostracism and negative portrayals of older people. Over the years, older adults have often suffered from ageist attitudes. People who were chronologically old were often labeled **senile** whenever they displayed memory failure, errors in judgment, disorientation, or erratic behaviors. Today scientists recognize that these same symptoms can occur at any age and for various reasons, including disease or the use of over-the-counter and prescription drugs. When the underlying problems are corrected, the memory loss and disorientation also improve.

Alzheimer's Disease **Dementias** are progressive brain impairments that interfere with memory and normal intellectual functioning. Although there are many types of dementia, one of the most common forms is **Alzheimer's disease (AD).** Currently, AD afflicts an estimated 1 in 10 Americans over the age of 65 and nearly half of people over age 85, and it costs society over $100 billion a year. With the U.S. population gradually aging, the number of people afflicted and the economic burden are certain to increase.[15] Patients with AD live for an average of 8 years after diagnosis, though the disease can last for up to 20 years.[16] Although most people associate the disease with the aged, AD has been diagnosed in people in their late forties. In fact, about 5 percent of all cases occur before age 65.

Alzheimer's is a degenerative brain disease in which nerve cells stop communicating with one another. Ordinarily, brain cells communicate by releasing chemicals that allow the cells to receive and transmit messages for various types of behavior. In AD patients, the brain doesn't produce enough of these chemicals, cells can't communicate, and eventually the cells die. Degeneration occurs in the sections of the brain that affect memory, speech, and personality, leaving the areas that control other bodily functions, such as heartbeat and breathing, functioning at near normal levels. Thus, the mind begins to go as the body lives on. Alzheimer's is generally detected first by families, who note changes, particularly memory lapses and personality changes, in their loved ones. Medical tests rule out underlying causes, and certain neurological tests help confirm the diagnosis.

Researchers are investigating possible causes of the disease, including genetic predisposition, malfunction of the immune system, a slow-acting virus, chromosomal or genetic defects, chronic inflammation, and neurotransmitter imbalance. Preliminary research indicates that a defect in the chromosomes may be the most likely cause, partly because virtually everyone with Down's syndrome eventually develops AD. A recent study indicates that being overweight or obese may predispose individuals to AD.[17] While the link is not clear, obesity increases the incidence of high blood pressure, high cholesterol, and high blood sugar, all of which have been implicated as risk factors.

Ageism   Discrimination based on age.

Senile   A term associated with loss of memory and judgment and orientation problems occurring in a small percentage of the elderly.

Dementias   Progressive brain impairments that interfere with memory and normal intellectual functioning.

Alzheimer's disease (AD)   A chronic condition involving changes in nerve fibers of the brain that results in mental deterioration.

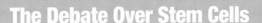
Stem cells are unique—and controversial. Stem cells are body cells with two important characteristics: (1) they are unspecialized (meaning their specific function is yet to be determined) and capable of renewing themselves by dividing repeatedly, and (2) they can be induced to become specialized cells that perform specific functions, such as muscle cells that make the heart beat or nerve cells that enable the brain to function.

What makes stem cells different from other types of cells?

These qualities have led many scientists to believe that stem cells have the potential to cure debilitating health problems such as Alzheimer's, heart disease, diabetes, Parkinson's, and glaucoma. These conditions all involve the destruction of certain crucial cells—in the case of type 1 diabetes, for example, the pancreatic cells that secrete insulin. In the laboratory, researchers are working to coax stem cells to develop into these pancreatic cells. The plan is to transplant the new cells into diabetic patients, where they could replace the patients' damaged cells and produce insulin. If successful, this approach could prevent the destructive complications of the disease and free diabetics from the painful burden of injecting insulin for the rest of their lives. Other therapies under investigation involve growing new cells to replace those ravaged by spinal injuries, heart attacks, muscular dystrophy, and vision and hearing loss.

The controversy over stem cells arises from their origins. Generally stem cells are derived from eggs that were fertilized in vitro. Typically these are "extra" embryos created during fertility treatments at clinics but not used for implantation. Only four to five days old, embryonic stem cells are *pluripotent* (capable of developing into many different cell types).

Embryonic stem cell research has provoked fierce debate. Opponents believe that an embryo is a human being and we have no right to create life and then destroy it, even for humanitarian purposes. Advocates counter that the eggs from which these embryos developed were given freely by donors and would otherwise be discarded.

Are adult stem cells a solution to this ethical dilemma? An adult stem cell is an undifferentiated cell found in body tissues and which can specialize to replace certain types of cells. For example, human bone marrow contains at least two kinds of adult stem cells. One kind gives rise to the various types of blood cells, while the other can differentiate into bone, cartilage, fat, or fibrous connective tissue. Other tissues that may contain adult stem cells include the brain, liver, skeletal muscles, and blood vessels. While research indicates that adult stem cells may be more versatile than previously thought, many scientists believe that embryonic stem cells, with their unlimited potential, are far more promising medically.

In the United States, embryonic stem cell research is limited by law. Federal funding—a major source of support for universities and labs—is restricted to experiments on only 71 stem cell lines (a stem cell line refers to a set of pluripotent, embryonic stem cells that have grown in the laboratory for at least six months). Some scientists worry that this pool is too small to develop valid medical therapies. Opponents believe that even this compromise allows unethical practices to continue. California has established a research initiative that would ban human reproductive cloning but permit embryonic stem cell research for therapeutic purposes.

As debate rages in the United States, embryonic stem cell research is moving forward in other countries. For example, the United Kingdom has licensed a British university to clone stem cells for diabetes research, and South Korean scientists have developed better laboratory techniques for deriving new stem cell lines.

Do you feel that embryonic stem cell research is ethical? Explain your answer. Would you feel differently if you or a loved one suffered from a disease that might respond to stem cell therapy?

Sources: F. Yates et al., "New Breakthrough in Nuclear Transfer," International Society for Stem Cell Research, June 9, 2005, http://www.isscr.org/public/breakthrough.htm; National Institutes of Health, Stem Cell Information, "Stem Cell Basics," revised August 12, 2005, http://stemcells.nih.gov/info/basics/; M. Waldholz and A. Regalado, "Biggest Struggles in Stem-Cell Fight May Be in the Lab," *The Wall Street Journal,* August 12, 2004, pp. A1, A6; International Society for Stem Cell Research, "The Ethics of Embryonic Stem Cell Research," updated February 2, 2005, http://www.isscr.org/public/ethics.htm; Associated Press, "U.K. Grants First Cloning License to Develop Research Stem Cells," *The Wall Street Journal,* August 12, 2004, p. D3.

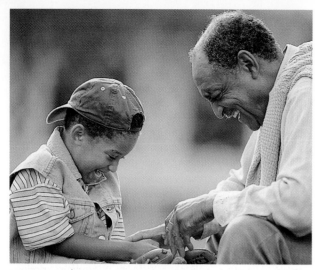
Learning to cope with challenges and changes early in life develops attitudes and skills that contribute to a full and satisfying old age.

AD treatment focuses on several prescription drugs. Some physicians also prescribe vitamin E supplements because the vitamin may help protect brain cells against damage from free radicals. Some researchers are looking at anti-inflammatory drugs, theorizing that AD may develop in response to an inflammatory ailment. Others are focusing on stimulating the brains of AD-prone individuals, believing that as people learn, more connections between cells are formed that may offset those that are lost.

HEALTH CHALLENGES OF OLDER ADULTS

Some health problems common in the elderly are brought on by failing health, others by society or a perceived loss of control over life's events. Developing life skills and a network of social support during earlier years can reduce problems in old age significantly.

Alcohol Use and Abuse

A person who is prone to alcoholism during the younger and middle years is more likely to continue during later years. The older alcoholic is probably no more common in American society than the young alcoholic, despite the stereotype of the old, lost soul hiding his or her sorrows in a bottle. Often, when people think they see a drunken older person, they are really seeing a confused individual who has taken too many different prescription medications and is experiencing a form of drug interaction.

Alcohol abuse is five times more common among older men than among older women. Yet as many as half of all older men and an even higher proportion of older women don't drink at all. Those who do drink do so less than younger persons, consuming only five to six drinks weekly.

Prescription Drug Use

It is extremely rare for older people to use illicit drugs, but some do overuse and grow dependent on prescription drugs. Some take four to six prescription drugs a day. Anyone who combines different drugs runs the risk of dangerous drug interactions. The risks of adverse effects are even greater for people with impaired circulation and declining kidney and liver function. To avoid drug interactions and other problems, older adults should use the same pharmacy consistently, ask questions about medicines and dosages, and read the directions carefully.

Over-the-Counter Remedies

A substantial segment of the over-60 population avoids orthodox medical treatment and views it as a last resort. This is becoming increasingly true as Medicare coverage becomes less adequate and older adults are forced to pay larger medical bills out of their own resources. The poor are particularly prone to turn to folk medicine and over-the-counter preparations as cheaper, less intimidating alternatives.

STRATEGIES FOR HEALTHY AGING

As you know from reading this book, you can do many things to prolong and improve the quality of your life. Some of these preventive measures are especially important. To provide for healthy older years, make each of the following part of your younger years.

Develop and Maintain Healthy Relationships

Social bonds lend vigor and energy to life. Be willing to give to others, and seek variety in your relationships rather than befriending only people who agree with you. By experiencing diverse people and interacting with different points of view, we gain a new perspective on life.

Enrich the Spiritual Side of Life

Although we often take this for granted, cultivating a relationship with nature, the environment, a higher being, and yourself is a key factor in personal growth and development. Take time for thought and quiet contemplation, and enjoy the sunsets, sounds, and energy of life. These moments spent in time prioritized for you will leave you invigorated and fresh—better able to cope with the ups and downs of life. If you don't take time for yourself now, it may be that you won't have time in the later years.

Improve Fitness

If you're basically sedentary, just about any moderate-intensity exercise that gets your heart beating faster and increases strength and/or flexibility will maximize your physical health and functional years. One of the inevitable physical changes that the body undergoes is **sarcopenia,** age-associated loss of muscle mass. The less muscle you have, the less energy you will burn even while resting. The lower your metabolic rate, the more likely you will gain weight. With regular strength training, you can increase your muscle mass, boost your metabolism, strengthen your bones, prevent osteoporosis, and, in general, feel better and function more efficiently.

Eat for Health

Although other chapters in this text provide detailed information about nutrition and weight control, certain nutrients are especially essential to healthy aging:

- *Calcium.* Bone loss tends to increase in women, particularly in the hip region, shortly before menopause. During perimenopause and menopause, this bone loss accelerates rapidly, with an average of about 3 percent skeletal mass lost per year over a five-year period. The result is an increased risk for fracture and disability. Few women actually consume the 1,000 milligrams of calcium recommended during the younger years or the 1,500 milligrams recommended during and after menopause.
- *Vitamin D.* Vitamin D is necessary for adequate calcium absorption, yet as people age, particularly in their fifties and sixties, they do not absorb vitamin D from foods as readily as they did in their younger years. If vitamin D is unavailable, calcium levels are also likely to be lower.
- *Protein.* As older adults become more concerned about cholesterol and fatty foods, and as their budgets shrink, one nutrient that often is cut back is protein. It costs more, takes longer to cook, and has that "fat" stigma associated with animal products. Many older people cut back on protein to a point that is below the recommended daily amount. Because protein is necessary for muscle mass, protein insufficiencies can spell trouble.

 Other nutrients, including vitamin E, folic acid (folate), iron, potassium, and vitamin B_{12}, are important to the aging process, and most of these are readily available in any diet that follows USDA dietary guideline recommendations (see Chapter 9).

CARING FOR OLDER ADULTS

Elderly women far outnumber elderly men in American society, and the discrepancy increases with age. Because women live seven years longer than men do on average, older women are more likely to live alone. Further, they are more likely to experience poverty and multiple chronic health problems, a situation referred to as **comorbidity.** Consequently, more women than men are likely to need assistance from children, other relatives, friends, and neighbors.

 Women usually have been the primary caregivers for older Americans, often for their ailing husbands. Research also indicates that women spend more hours than men do (38 hours versus 27 hours per week) in caregiving activities and perform a wider range of services. Regardless of the time spent, caregiving is a difficult and stressful experience for both women and men. **Respite care,** or care that is given by someone who relieves the primary caregiver, should be available to ease the burden. As the population ages and more older adults require care, it will become even more important to support caregivers' health and well-being.

What Do You Think? Why are women often the primary caregivers for aging spouses and other family members? ■ What problems can such caregiving cause? ■ How can caregivers learn to cope with the stresses and strains of their situation?

UNDERSTANDING DEATH

Death eventually comes to everyone, but if you live life to the fullest and learn as much about end-of-life issues as you can, you will be better able to accept the inevitable. To cope effectively with dying, we must address the needs of those facing life's final transition. Let's begin by investigating what death means, at least in medical terms.

Sarcopenia Age-related loss of muscle mass.

Comorbidity The presence of a number of diseases at the same time.

Respite care The care provided by substitute caregivers to relieve the principal caregiver from his or her continuous responsibility.

Defining Death

Dying is the process of decline in body functions that results in the death of an organism. **Death** can be defined as the "final cessation of the vital functions" and also refers to a state in which these functions are "incapable of being restored."[18] This definition has become more significant as medical advances make it increasingly possible to postpone death.

Legal and ethical issues led to the Uniform Determination of Death Act in 1981, which has been endorsed by the American Medical Association, the American Bar Association, and the National Conference for Commissioners on Uniform State Laws. This act, which has been adopted by several states, reads as follows: "An individual who has sustained either (1) irreversible cessation of circulatory and respiratory functions, or (2) irreversible cessation of all functions of the entire brain, including the brain stem, is dead. A determination of death must be made in accordance with accepted medical standards."[19]

The concept of **brain death,** defined as the irreversible cessation of all functions of the entire brain stem, has gained increasing credence. As defined by the Ad Hoc Committee of the Harvard Medical School, brain death occurs when the following criteria are met:[20]

- Unreceptivity and unresponsiveness—that is, no response even to painful stimuli

- No movement for a continuous hour after observation by a physician and no breathing after three minutes off a respirator

- No reflexes, including brain stem reflexes; fixed and dilated pupils

- A "flat" electroencephalogram (EEG, which monitors electrical activity of the brain) for at least ten minutes

- All of these tests repeated at least 24 hours later with no change

- Certainty that hypothermia (extreme loss of body heat) and depression of the central nervous system caused by use of drugs such as barbiturates are not responsible for these conditions

The Harvard report provides useful guidelines; however, the definition of *death* and all its ramifications continue to concern us.

Dying   The process of decline in body functions, resulting in the death of an organism.

Death   The permanent ending of all vital functions.

Brain death   The irreversible cessation of all functions of the entire brain stem.

What Do You Think?   Why is there so much concern over the definition of death? ■ How does modern technology complicate the understanding of when death occurs?

Denying Death

Attitudes toward death tend to fall on a continuum. At one end of the continuum, death is viewed as the mortal enemy of humankind. Both medical science and certain religions have promoted this idea. At the other end of the continuum, death is accepted and even welcomed by some religious groups and segments of the population. For people whose attitudes fall at this end, death is a passage to a better state of being. But most of us perceive ourselves to be in the middle of this continuum. From this perspective, death is a bewildering mystery that elicits fear and apprehension while profoundly influencing beliefs and actions throughout life.

In the United States, a high level of discomfort is associated with death and dying. We may avoid speaking about death to limit our own discomfort. Those who deny death tend to:

- Avoid people who are grieving after the death of a loved one so they won't have to talk about it

- Fail to validate a dying person's frightening situation by talking to the person as if nothing were wrong

- Substitute euphemisms for the word death (for example, "passing away," "kicking the bucket," "no longer with us," "going to heaven," or "going to a better place")

- Give false reassurances to dying people by saying things like "everything is going to be okay"

- Shut off conversation about death by silencing people who are trying to talk about it

- Avoid touching people who are dying

Recent years have shown a greater effort on the part of the American public to mourn openly, as is indicated by roadside memorials placed at the sites of violent or unexpected deaths. Although these are fairly new additions to the American landscape, these memorials have long been popular in other parts of the world, particularly in predominantly Catholic countries.[21]

THE PROCESS OF DYING

Dying is a complex process that includes physical, intellectual, social, spiritual, and emotional dimensions. Now that we have examined the physical indicators of death, we must consider the emotional aspects of dying and "social death."

Coping Emotionally with Death

Science and medicine have enabled us to understand many changes throughout the life span, but they have not fully explained the nature of death. This may explain why the transition from life to death evokes so much mystery and emotion. Although emotional reactions to dying vary, many people share similar experiences during this process. Terms such as *tasks, stages,* and *phases* have been used in models that have been developed to understand the process of dying.

Kübler-Ross and the Stages of Dying

Much of our knowledge about reactions to dying stems from the work of Elisabeth Kübler-Ross, a pioneer in **thanatology**, the study of death and dying. In 1969, Kübler-Ross published *On Death and Dying,* a sensitive analysis of the reactions of terminally ill patients. This pioneering work encouraged the development of death education as a discipline and prompted efforts to improve the care of dying patients. Kübler-Ross identified five psychological stages that those coping with death often experience:

1. *Denial.* ("Not me, there must be a mistake.") A person intellectually accepts the impending death but rejects it emotionally and feels a sense of shock and disbelief. The patient is too confused and stunned to comprehend "not being" and thus rejects the idea.

2. *Anger.* ("Why me?") The person becomes angry at having to face death when others, including loved ones, are healthy and not threatened. The dying person perceives the situation as unfair or senseless and may be hostile to friends, family, physicians, or the world in general.

3. *Bargaining.* ("If I'm allowed to live, I promise . . .") This stage generally occurs at about the middle of the progression. The dying person may resolve to be a better person in return for an extension of life or may secretly pray for a short reprieve from death in order to experience a special event, such as a family wedding or birth.

4. *Depression.* ("It's really going to happen to me, and I can't do anything about it.") Depression eventually sets in as vitality diminishes and the person begins to experience symptoms with increasing frequency. The person's deteriorating condition becomes impossible for him or her to deny. Common feelings experienced in this stage include doom, loss, worthlessness, and guilt over the emotional suffering of loved ones and the arduous but seemingly futile efforts of caregivers.

5. *Acceptance.* ("I'm ready.") This is often the final stage. The patient stops battling with emotions and becomes tired and weak. With acceptance, the person does not give up and become sullen or resent-

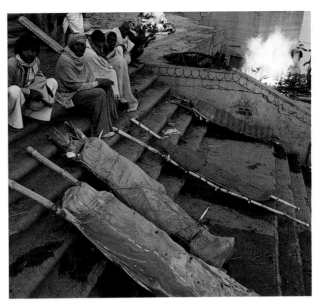

There is no single way to mourn. Each culture has its own unique ways of saying goodbye to the deceased.

fully resigned to death but rather becomes passive. According to one dying person, the acceptance stage is "almost void of feelings . . . as if the pain had gone, the struggle is over, and there comes a time for the final rest before the long journey."[22] Death usually occurs quietly and painlessly while the victim is unconscious.

Some of Kübler-Ross's contemporaries consider her stage theory too neat and orderly. Subsequent research has indicated that the experiences of dying people do not fit easily into specific stages, and patterns vary from person to person. Some people may never go through this process and instead remain emotionally calm; others may pass back and forth between the stages. Even if it is not accurate in all its particulars, however, Kübler-Ross's theory offers valuable insights for those seeking to understand or deal with the process of dying.

Corr's Coping Approach Others have developed alternative models for understanding the ways in which we cope with death and significant losses. Charles Corr believes that there are unique challenges and responses for the dying person and those who love them.[23] He suggests four dimensions of coping with loss: *physical*—doing everything possible to make ourselves comfortable and minimize pain; *psychological*—living to the fullest, focusing on life accomplishments, and seeking satisfaction in daily activities; *social*—nurturing relationships, keeping loved ones involved and sharing emotions; and *spiritual*—identifying what matters in life and reaffirming meaningful experiences.

Thanatology   The study of death and dying.

Social Death

The need for recognition and appreciation within a social group is nearly universal. Although the size and nature of the social group may vary widely, the need to belong exists in all of us. Loss of being valued or appreciated by others can lead to **social death,** a seemingly irreversible situation in which a person is not treated like an active member of society. Dramatic examples of social death include the exile of nonconformists from their native countries or the excommunication of dissident members of religious groups. More often, however, social death is inflicted by denying a person normal social interaction. Numerous studies indicate that people are treated differently when they are dying. The following common behaviors contribute to the social death that often isolates people who are terminally ill:[24]

- The dying person is referred to as if he or she were already dead.

- The dying person may be inadvertently excluded from conversations.

- Dying patients often are moved to terminal wards and given minimal care.

- Bereaved family members are avoided, often for extended periods, because friends and neighbors feel uncomfortable in the presence of grief.

- Medical personnel may make degrading comments about patients in their presence.[25]

This decrease in meaningful social interaction often strips dying and bereaved people of their identity as valued members of society at a time when belonging is critical. Some dying people choose not to speak of their inevitable fate in an attempt to make others feel more comfortable and thus preserve vital relationships.

Coping with Loss

The losses resulting from the death of a loved one are extremely difficult to cope with. The dying person, as well as close family and friends, frequently suffers emotionally and physically from the impending loss of critical relationships and roles.

Bereavement generally is defined as the loss or deprivation experienced by a survivor when a loved one dies. Because relationships vary in type and intensity, reactions to loss also vary. In the lives of the bereaved or of close survivors, the loss of loved ones leaves "holes." We can think of bereavement as the awareness of these holes. Time and courage are necessary to fill these spaces.

A special case of bereavement occurs in old age. Loss is an intrinsic part of growing old. The longer we live, the more losses we are likely to experience. They include physical, social, and emotional losses as our bodies deteriorate and more and more of our loved ones die. The theory of *bereavement overload* has been proposed to explain the effects of multiple losses and the accumulation of sorrow in the lives of some older people. This theory suggests that the gloomy outlook, disturbing behavior patterns, and apparent apathy that characterize these people may be related more to bereavement overload than to intrinsic physiological degeneration in old age.[26]

Grief is a state of mental distress that occurs in reaction to significant loss, including one's own impending death, the death of a loved one, or a quasi-death experience (a loss, such as the end of a relationship or job, that resembles death because it involves separation, grief, or change in personal identity). Grief reactions include any adjustments needed for one to make it through the day and may include changes in patterns of eating, sleeping, working, and even thinking.

When a person experiences a loss that cannot be openly acknowledged, publicly mourned, or socially supported, coping may be much more difficult. This type of grief is referred to as **disenfranchised grief.**[27] It may occur among those who miscarry, are developmentally disabled, or are close friends rather than blood relatives of the deceased. It may also include those relationships that are not socially approved, such as those between extramarital lovers or homosexual couples. When society does not assign significance to a high-grief death, grieving becomes more difficult.

The term **mourning** is often incorrectly equated with the term *grief.* As we have noted, *grief* refers to a wide variety of feelings and actions that occur in response to bereavement. *Mourning,* in contrast, refers to culturally

---

Social death   A seemingly irreversible situation in which a person is not treated like an active member of society.

Bereavement   The loss or deprivation experienced by a survivor when a loved one dies.

Grief   The state of mental distress that occurs in reaction to significant loss, including one's own impending death, the death of a loved one, or a quasi-death experience.

Disenfranchised grief   Grief concerning a loss that cannot be openly acknowledged, publicly mourned, or socially supported.

Mourning   The culturally prescribed behavior patterns for the expression of grief.

prescribed and accepted time periods and behavior patterns for the expression of grief. In Judaism, for example, *sitting shiva* is a designated mourning period of seven days that involves prescribed rituals and prayers. Depending on a person's relationship with the deceased, various other rituals may continue for up to a year.

Symptoms of grief vary in severity and duration, depending on the situation and the individual. However, the bereaved person can benefit from emotional and social support from family, friends, clergy, employers, and the traditional support organizations, including the medical community and the funeral industry. The larger and stronger the support system, the easier readjustment is likely to be.

What Is "Normal" Grief?

Grief responses vary widely from person to person but frequently include the following symptoms:

- Periodic waves of physical distress lasting from 20 minutes to an hour
- A feeling of tightness in the throat
- Choking and shortness of breath
- A frequent need to sigh
- Feelings of emptiness and muscular weakness
- Intense anxiety that is described as actually painful

Other common symptoms of grief include insomnia, memory lapse, loss of appetite, difficulty concentrating, a tendency to engage in repetitive or purposeless behavior, an "observer" sensation or feeling of unreality, difficulty in making decisions, lack of organization, excessive speech, social withdrawal or hostility, guilt feelings, and preoccupation with the image of the deceased. Susceptibility to disease increases with grief and may even be life threatening in severe and enduring cases.

Coping with Grief

A bereaved person may suffer emotional pain and exhibit a variety of grief responses for many months after the death. The rate of the healing process depends on the amount and quality of grief work that a person does. **Grief work** is the process of integrating the reality of the loss into everyday life and learning to feel better. Often, the bereaved person must deliberately and systematically work at reducing denial and coping with the pain that results from memories of the deceased. This process takes time and requires emotional effort.

Worden's Model of Grieving Tasks

William Worden, a researcher into the death process, developed an active grieving model which suggests four developmental tasks to complete in the grief work process (see Figure 15.2):[28]

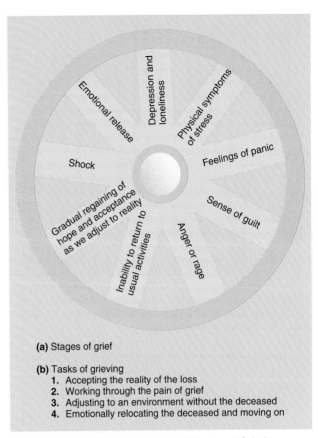

(a) Stages of grief

(b) Tasks of grieving
1. Accepting the reality of the loss
2. Working through the pain of grief
3. Adjusting to an environment without the deceased
4. Emotionally relocating the deceased and moving on

Figure 15.2 ■ **The Stages and Tasks of Grief**
(a) People react differently to losses, but most eventually adjust. Generally, the stronger the social support system, the smoother the progression through the stages of grief. (b) Worden's developmental tasks associated with grief are another way to understand the grieving process.

1. *Accept the reality of the loss.* This task requires acknowledging and realizing that the person is dead. Traditional rituals, such as the funeral, help many bereaved people move toward acceptance.

2. *Work through to the pain of grief.* It is necessary to acknowledge and work through the pain associated with loss or it will manifest itself through other symptoms or behaviors.

3. *Adjust to an environment in which the deceased is missing.* The bereaved may feel lonely and uncertain about a new identity without the person who has died. This loss confronts them with the challenge of adjusting to their own sense of self.

4. *Emotionally relocate the deceased and move on with life.* Individuals never lose memories of a significant relationship. They may need help in letting

Grief work The process of accepting the reality of a person's death and coping with memories of the deceased.

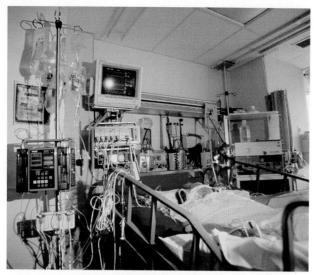

Sophisticated life-support technology allows a patient's life to be prolonged even in cases of terminal illness or mortal injury. It has also raised legal and moral questions for patients, their families, and health care professionals.

go of the emotional energy that used to be invested in the person who has died, finding an appropriate place for the deceased in their emotional lives.

Models of the grief process can be viewed as "generalized maps"—each theory is an attempt by an investigator to understand and guide grieving people through their pain. However, each individual will travel through grief at his/her own speed using an appropriate route.

What Do You Think? If you have experienced death among your family or friends, how did you grieve? ■ Did you accomplish Worden's tasks? ■ Does the model match your experience?

LIFE-AND-DEATH DECISION MAKING

Many complex—and often expensive—life-and-death decisions must be made during a highly distressing period in people's lives. We will not attempt to present definitive answers to moral and philosophical questions about death; instead, we offer these topics for your consideration. We hope that this discussion of the needs of the dying person and the bereaved will help you negotiate these difficult decisions in the future.

The Right to Die

Few people would object to a proposal for the right to a dignified death. Going beyond that concept, however, many people today believe that they should be allowed to die if their condition is terminal and their existence depends on mechanical life support devices or artificial feeding or hydration systems. Artificial life support techniques that may be legally refused by competent patients in some states include:

■ Electrical or mechanical heart resuscitation
■ Mechanical respiration by machine
■ Nasogastric tube feedings
■ Intravenous nutrition
■ Gastrostomy (tube feeding directly into the stomach)
■ Medications to treat life-threatening infections

As long as a person is conscious and competent, he or she has the legal right to refuse treatment, even if this decision will hasten death. However, when a person is in a coma or otherwise incapable of speaking on his or her own behalf, medical personnel, family members, and administrative policy will dictate treatment. This issue has evolved into a battle involving personal freedom, legal rulings, health care administration policy, and physician responsibility. The living will was developed to assist in solving these conflicts.

Why should I create a living will?

Even young, apparently healthy people need a living will. Consider Terri Schiavo, who collapsed at age 26 from heart failure that led to irreversible brain damage. Schiavo, unable to survive without life support, never left any written guidelines about her wishes should she become incapacitated. After a 15-year legal battle between her parents, who wanted her to be kept alive, and her husband, who felt she should be allowed to die, the courts sided with her husband, and she was removed from life support.

In other instances, the wishes of people who had signed a living will (or advance directive) indicating their desire not to receive artificial life support were not honored by their physician or medical institution. Many legal experts suggest that you take the following steps to ensure that your wishes are carried out:

1. *Be specific.* Complete an advanced directive that permits you to make very specific choices about a variety of procedures, including cardiopulmonary resuscitation (CPR); being placed on a ventilator; being given food, water, or medication through tubes; being given pain medication; and organ donation. It is also essential to attach that document to a completed copy of the standard advance directive for your state.

2. *Get an agent.* You may want to also appoint a family member or friend to act as your agent, or *proxy,* by making out a form known as either a *durable power of attorney for health care* or a *health care proxy.*

3. *Discuss your wishes.* Discuss your preferences in detail with your proxy and your doctor. Going over

the situations described in the form will give them a clear idea of just how much you are willing to endure to preserve your life.

4. *Deliver the directive.* Distribute several copies, not only to your doctor and your agent but also to your lawyer and to immediate family members or a close friend. Make sure *someone* knows to bring a copy to the hospital in the event you are hospitalized.[29]

Rational Suicide

Although exact numbers are not known, medical ethicists and specialists in forensic medicine (the study of legal issues in medicine) estimate that thousands of terminally ill people every year decide to kill themselves rather than endure constant pain and slow decay. This alternative to the extended dying process is known as **rational suicide.** To these people, the prospect of an undignified death is unacceptable. This issue has been complicated by advances in death prevention techniques that allow terminally ill patients to exist in an irreversible disease state for extended periods of time. Medical personnel, clergy, lawyers, and patients all must struggle with this ethical dilemma.

Euthanasia is often referred to as "mercy killing." The term **active euthanasia** refers to ending the life of a person (or animal) who is suffering greatly and has no chance of recovery. An example might be a physician-prescribed lethal injection. **Passive euthanasia** refers to the intentional withholding of treatment that would prolong life. Deciding not to place a person with massive brain trauma on life support is an example of passive euthanasia.

Dr. Jack Kevorkian, a physician in Michigan, started a one-person campaign to force the medical profession to change its position regarding physician-assisted death. Kevorkian has assisted many terminally ill patients in dying and, until recently, had escaped conviction despite being taken into court several times for his actions. Kevorkian believes that the present situation in our society demands a shift in the practice of medicine and the acceptance of euthanasia, specifically in the practice of physician-assisted death. In 1998, Kevorkian took his argument to prime time, as the CBS News program *60 Minutes* broadcast his latest case of assisting a terminally ill patient with ending his life. This time, however, the courts determined that Kevorkian had gone too far. He was convicted of murder and sentenced to prison, where he remains.

Kevorkian's actions have focused attention on the issue, causing many to discuss the merits of physician-assisted suicide. Roughly six in ten Americans say they think people have a right to end their own life only if they have an incurable disease.[30] Currently, 38 states have enacted statues explicitly prohibiting assisted suicide, 4 states are undecided (meaning there are no statutes or case law specifically prohibiting assisted

suicide), and only 1 state, Oregon, allows physician-assisted suicide under certain circumstances.[31]

Try it ➤NOW

Complete an advanced directive. Right now, go to www.uslivingwillregistry.com/forms.shtm, select the state you live in, and print out your state's advanced directive for health care form. Read through the form, and think about the health care decisions you would make to complete the form.

MAKING FINAL ARRANGEMENTS

Caring for dying people and dealing with the practical and legal questions surrounding death can be difficult and painful. The problems of the dying person and the bereaved loved ones involve a wide variety of psychological, legal, social, spiritual, economic, and interpersonal issues.

Hospice Care: Positive Alternatives

Since the mid-1970s, **hospice** programs have grown from a mere handful to more than 2,500 and are available in nearly every community. Improving quality of care at the end of life is a top priority of the American Medical Association.

The primary goals of hospice programs are to relieve the dying person's pain; offer emotional support to the dying person and loved ones; and restore a sense of control to the dying person, family, and friends. Although home care with maximum involvement by loved ones is emphasized, hospice programs are directed by cooperating physicians; coordinated by specially trained nurses; and fortified with the skills of counselors, clergy, and trained volunteers. Hospital inpatient beds are available if necessary. Hospice programs usually include the following characteristics.

Rational suicide   The decision to kill oneself rather than endure constant pain and slow decay.

Active euthanasia   "Mercy killing" in which a person or organization knowingly acts to hasten the death of a terminally ill person.

Passive euthanasia   The intentional withholding of treatment that would prolong life.

Hospice   A concept of care for terminally ill patients designed to maximize quality of life.

Whether we have months to prepare for death or it comes suddenly, most people have difficulty knowing what to do. We push death from our consciousness, which leads to problems before and after the moment of death comes for loved ones. Although you can never be fully prepared for the loss of a loved one, you can learn skills that will help you through the trauma of loss. The following suggestions will help, particularly if you have time to prepare.

1. *Follow the wishes of the patient.* Make sure that a copy of his or her advance directive is available and accepted as the wishes of the patient. Most people, particularly in hospice, want a natural death. Think of comfort, not cure. Whenever possible, talk to the patient and allow choices to be made about the dying process. For example, if the patient wants to stay at home but being in a hospital bed would be easier for caregivers, talk this out with the patient.

2. *Help with comfort and rest.* Don't be afraid to ask for medications to help the patient deal with pain, sleeplessness, or anxiety.

3. *Prepare a list of people to call near the time of death, including family, friends, and religious support.* Talk about who the patient wants present, if anyone. Make a list of people to notify once death occurs. Keep a list of home health nurses, hospice staff, and physicians nearby so they can be contacted quickly.

4. *Call for professional help if any of the following occur:*
   - The patient experiences extreme pain or discomfort.
   - The patient has difficulty breathing. Oxygen can calm the person and make the last hours more comfortable.
   - The patient has trouble urinating or passing stool. Usually the urine will be dark and in small quantity. Medications can help ease discomfort.
   - Your emotions are getting the best of you. Thoughts of impending loss can prevent you from being supportive.

5. *Touch is often comforting for the dying person.* Give back, hand, or foot rubs; apply skin lotion. Do not stand back and avoid contact. Help the patient adjust his or her position in bed if at all possible. Usually an extra sheet placed under the patient and the help of a second person will make this easier.

6. *Make the person as physically comfortable as possible.* Moisten the eyes and lips with warm, damp cloths. Apply warm or cool compresses if the person wants them.

7. *Know what to expect.* Be ready to say goodbye. Talk to the person. In some cases soft, relaxing music may be comforting. During the last moments of life, the body begins to slow down, breathing rates slow, sometimes there are long pauses between breaths. Sometimes the person will appear to wake up but will be unable to speak or recognize you. Usually this means patients are in or near coma state, and they may progress to longer and longer periods of sleep. The skin may be cool, especially around the feet and hands, and may become blue- or gray-tinged. In the last stages as death nears, the person may become incontinent or lose bowel control. Finally, the chest will stop rising, the eyes may appear glassy, and there is no more pulse.

8. *Prepare for the activities that will occur after death.* You may choose to assist with preparing the body for transport to the funeral home or other facility, or you may prefer to let others take over. Try to think about this in advance and make decisions based on your own wishes and needs.

1. The patient and family constitute the unit of care, because the physical, psychological, social, and spiritual problems of dying confront the family as well as the patient.

2. Emphasis is placed on symptom control, primarily the alleviation of pain. Curative treatments are curtailed as requested by the patient, but sound judgment must be applied to avoid a feeling of abandonment.

3. There is overall medical direction of the program, with all health care being provided under the direction of a qualified physician.

4. Services are provided by an interdisciplinary team because no one person can provide all the needed care.

5. Coverage is provided 24 hours a day, seven days a week, with emphasis on the availability of medical and nursing skills.

6. Carefully selected and extensively trained volunteers who augment but do not replace staff service are an integral part of the health care team.

7. Care of the family extends through the bereavement period.

8. Patients are accepted on the basis of their health needs, not on their ability to pay.

Despite the growing number of people considering the hospice option, many people prefer to go to a hospital to die. Others choose to die at home, without the intervention of medical staff or life-prolonging equipment. Each dying person and his or her family should decide as early as possible what type of terminal care is most desirable and feasible. This will allow time for necessary emotional, physical, and financial preparations. Hospice care also may help survivors cope better with the death experience. See the Skills for Behavior Change box for things you can do to prepare for the death of a loved one.

Making Funeral Arrangements

Anthropological evidence indicates that all cultures throughout history have developed some sort of funeral ritual. For this reason, social scientists agree that funerals assist survivors of the deceased in coping with their loss.

In the United States, with its diversity of religious, regional, and ethnic customs, funeral patterns vary. In some faiths, the deceased may be displayed to formalize last respects and increase social support for the bereaved. This part of the funeral ritual is referred to as a *wake* or *viewing*. The funeral service may be held in a church, in a funeral chapel, or at the burial site. Some people choose to replace the funeral service with a simple memorial service held within a few days of the burial. Social interaction associated with funeral and memorial services is valuable in helping survivors cope with their loss.

Common methods of body disposal include burial in the ground, entombment above ground in a mausoleum, cremation, and anatomical donation. Expenses vary according to the method chosen and the available options. It should be noted that if burial is selected, an additional charge may be assessed for a burial vault. Burial vaults—concrete or metal containers that hold the casket—are required by most cemeteries to limit settling of the gravesite as the casket disintegrates and collapses. The actual container for the remains is only one of many tasks that must be dealt with when a person dies.

Pressures on Survivors

There are many other decisions concerning the funeral ritual that can be burdensome for survivors. Many have to be made within 24 hours. These decisions relate to the method and details of body disposal, the type of memorial service, display of the body, the site of burial or body disposition, the cost of funeral options, organ donation, ordering floral displays, contacting friends and relatives, planning for guests, choosing markers, gathering and submitting obituary information to newspapers, printing memorial folders, and many other details. In our society, people who make their own funeral arrangements can save their loved ones from having to deal with unnecessary problems. Even making the

National Kidney Foundation
Please detach and give this portion of the card to my family

This is to inform you that, should the occasion ever arise, I would like to be an organ and tissue donor. Please see that my wishes are carried out by informing the attending medical personnel that I have indicated my wishes to become a donor.
Thank you.

Signature _____ Date _____

For further information write or call:
National Kidney Foundation
30 East 33rd Street, New York, NY 10016
(800) 622-9010

- -

Uniform Donor Card

Of _____
(print or type name of donor)

In the hope that I may help others, I hereby make this anatomical gift, if medically acceptable, to take effect upon my death. The words and marks below indicate my wishes.

I give: ☐ any needed organs or parts
☐ only the following organs or parts

_____
(specify the organ(s), tissue(s) or part(s))

for the purposes of transplantation, therapy, medical research or education;
☐ my body for anatomical study if needed.

Limitations or special wishes, if any: _____

Figure 15.3 ■ Organ Donor Card

Source: Reprinted with permission from "Uniform Donor Card." Copyright National Kidney Foundation.

decision regarding the method of body disposal can reduce the stress on survivors greatly.

Organ Donation

Another decision concerns organ donation. Organ transplant techniques have become so refined, and the demand for transplant tissues and organs is so great, that many people are being encouraged to donate these gifts of life upon death. Uniform donor cards are available through the National Kidney Foundation (Figure 15.3); donor information is printed on the backs of drivers' licenses; and many hospitals include the opportunity for organ donor registration in their admission procedures. Although some people are opposed to organ transplants and tissue donation, others experience personal fulfillment from knowing that their organs may extend and improve someone else's life after their own deaths.

Wills

The issue of inheritance is controversial in some families and should be resolved before the person dies to reduce conflict and needless expense. Unfortunately, many people are so intimidated by the thought of making a will that they never do so and die **intestate** (without a will). This is tragic, especially because the procedure for establishing a legal will is relatively simple and inexpensive. In addition, if you don't make a will before you die, the courts (as directed by state laws) will make a will for you. Legal issues, rather than your wishes,

will preside. Furthermore, it usually takes longer to settle an estate when the person dies intestate. Clearly, we all need wills that are updated regularly.

In some cases, other types of wills may substitute for the traditional legal will. One alternative is the **holographic will,** which is written in the handwriting of the **testator** (person who leaves a will) and unwitnessed. However, be very cautious concerning any alternatives to legally written and witnessed wills because they are not honored in all states. For example, holographic wills are contestable in court. Think of the parents who never approved of the fact that their child lived with someone outside marriage; they could challenge the holographic will in court successfully.

Intestate   Not having made a will.

Holographic will   A will written in the testator's own handwriting and unwitnessed.

Testator   A person who leaves a will or testament at death.

What Do You Think? What can you do to ensure that your wishes will be carried out at the time of your death?

■ Taking Charge

Summary

- Aging can be defined in terms of biological age (a person's physical condition); psychological age (a person's coping abilities and intelligence); social age (a person's habits and roles relative to society's expectations); legal age (based on chronological years); or functional age (relative to how other people function at varied ages).

- The growing numbers of older adults (people aged 65 and older) will have a growing impact on society in terms of economy, health care, housing, and ethical considerations.

- Two broad groups of theories—biological and psychosocial—purport to explain the physiological and psychological changes that occur with aging. Biological explanations include the wear-and-tear theory, the cellular theory, the autoimmune theory, and the genetic mutation theory. Psychosocial theories center on adaptation and adjustments related to self-development.

- Aging changes the body and mind in many ways. Physical changes occur in the skin, bones and joints, head, urinary tract, heart and lungs, senses, sexual function, and temperature regulation. Major physical concerns are osteoporosis and urinary incontinence. Most older people maintain a high level of intelligence and memory. Potential mental problems include depression and Alzheimer's disease.

- Special challenges for older adults include alcohol abuse, prescription and over-the-counter drug interactions, questions about vitamin and mineral supplementation, and issues regarding caregiving.

- Lifestyle choices we make today will affect health status later in life. Choosing to exercise, eat a healthy diet, and foster lasting relationships will contribute to healthy aging. Decisions about caring for older adults and stresses related to caregiving are ongoing concerns as the United States population ages.

- Death can be defined biologically in terms of brain death and/or the final cessation of vital functions. Denial of death results in limited communication about death, which can lead to further denial.

- Death is a multifaceted process, and individuals may experience emotional stages of dying such as denial, anger, bargaining, depression, and acceptance. Social death results when a person is no longer treated as living. Grief is the state of distress felt after loss.

- The right to die by rational suicide involves ethical, moral, and legal issues.

- Choices of care for the terminally ill include hospice care. After death, funeral arrangements must be made almost immediately, which adds to pressures on survivors. Decisions should be made in advance of death through wills and organ donation cards.

Chapter Review

1. Your habits and roles relative to society's expectations define your
   a. functional age.
   b. psychological age.
   c. legal age.
   d. social age.

2. People who are classified as "young-old" are
   a. 55–64 years of age.
   b. 65–74 years of age.
   c. 75–84 years of age.
   d. 85 years of age and older.

3. According to the genetic mutation theory, aging is caused by
   a. the human body wearing out.
   b. the body's cells have reached the end of their reproductive cycle.
   c. the decline of the body's immunological system.
   d. an increased number of cells exhibiting unusual or different characteristics with increased age.

4. Menopause usually occurs between the ages of
   a. 35 and 45.
   b. 40 and 50.
   c. 45 and 55.
   d. 50 and 60.

5. Walt's ophthalmologist tells him that there is an elevation of pressure within his eyeball. What is this condition?
   a. cataracts
   b. glaucoma
   c. far-sightedness
   d. near-sightedness

6. What is the most common form of dementia in older adults?
   a. Alzheimer's disease
   b. incontinence
   c. depression
   d. psychosis

7. The first psychological state that terminally ill patients often experience as they approach death is
   a. anger.
   b. denial.
   c. depression.
   d. bargaining.

8. The study of death and dying is called
   a. thanatology.
   b. gerontology.
   c. ageism.
   d. senescence.

9. Grief work is
   a. the process of integrating the reality of the loss with everyday life and learning to feel better.
   b. the total acceptance that a loved one has died.
   c. assigning feelings to the loss of a loved one.
   d. completing the cultural rituals that are required to express one's grief.

10. Kerri's elderly grandmother is terminally ill and wants to die without receiving medical intervention. Her family has agreed to withhold treatment that may prolong her life. This is called
    a. rational suicide.
    b. self-deliverance.
    c. passive euthanasia.
    d. active euthanasia.

Answers for these questions can be found on page A-1.

Questions for Discussion and Reflection

1. Discuss the various definitions of aging. At what age would you place your parents for each category?

2. As the older population grows, how will it affect your life? Would you be willing to pay higher taxes to support government social programs for the elderly? For example, do you believe that Social Security should continue its yearly increases in payments, which are pegged to inflation? Why or why not?

3. Which of the biological theories of aging do you think is most correct? Why?

4. List the major physiological changes that occur with aging. Which of these, if any, can you change?

5. Explain the major health challenges that older adults may face. What advice would you give to your grandparents before they took a prescription or over-the-counter drug?

6. Discuss actions you can start taking now to ensure a healthier aging process.

7. Discuss why so many of us deny death. How could death become a more acceptable topic to discuss?

8. Debate whether rational suicide should be legalized for the terminally ill. What restrictions would you include in a law?

9. Compare and contrast the hospital experience with hospice care. What must one consider before arranging for hospice care?

10. Discuss the legal matters surrounding death, including wills, physician directives, organ donations, and funeral arrangements.

Accessing Your Health on the Internet

The following websites explore further topics and issues related to personal health. For links to the websites below, visit the Companion Website for *Health: The Basics,* Seventh Edition at www.aw-bc.com/donatelle.

1. *Administration on Aging.* A link to the U.S. Department of Health and Human Services, dedicated to addressing the health needs of older adults.

2. *Alzheimer's Association.* Includes media releases, position statements, fact sheets, and research on Alzheimer's disease.

3. *Funerals: A Consumer Guide.* Guides the consumer through the thinking process of planning for a funeral, including preplanning, types of funerals, costs, choosing a casket, burial, and many other aspects of funeral preparation.

4. *Hospice Web.* Includes information and links about hospice, including frequently asked questions.

5. *Loss, Grief, and Bereavement.* This site from the National Cancer Institute covers a variety of topics related to loss, grief, and bereavement. Includes a summary written by cancer experts.

6. *SeniorCom.* Home page links to numerous resources for senior citizens, including chatrooms, databases, and services dedicated to assisting the aging.

7. *Social Security Online.* Provides information about Social Security benefits and entitlements. Also offers links to related sites.

8. *Terminal Illness and Hospice.* Addresses all aspects of dealing with terminal illness, including loss, ALS (amyotrophic lateral sclerosis or Lou Gehrig's disease), Alzheimer's disease, legal issues, and funeral planning.

Further Reading

The Johns Hopkins Medical Letter—Health After 50. www.hopkinsafter50.com.

> *Monthly newsletter providing comprehensive, accurate overviews of health topics relevant to older adults.*

Jacobs Altman, L. *Death: An Introduction to Medical–Ethical Dilemmas.* Berkeley Heights, NJ: Enslow, 2000.

> *A multifaceted exploration of death that gives the reader much to consider.*

Muth, A. S., ed. *Death and Dying Sourcebook: Basic Consumer Health Information for the Layperson About End-of-Life Care and Related Ethical and Legal Issues.* Detroit, MI: Omnigraphics, 2000.

> *Provides up-to-date information on the issues of nursing care, living wills, pain management, and counseling.*

References

1. J. Kavenaugh, *Adult Development and Aging* (Pacific Grove, CA: Brooks/Cole/ITP, 1996), 45.
2. National Institute on Aging, "Life Extension: Science Fact or Science Fiction?" *Age Page,* September 2002, www.niapublications.org/engagepages/lifeext.asp.
3. Illinois Department on Aging, "Facts on Aging," June 1, 2002, www.state.il.us/aging/1news_pubs/onage53.htm.
4. W. Madar, "Life Stories as Well as Theory Needed to Understand Aging," *Center for the Humanities Newsletter* (Consortium of Humanities Centers and Institutes, Oregon State University, Spring 2000), 8.
5. Federal Interagency Forum on Aging-Related Statistics, "Indicator 1: Number of Older Americans," *Older Americans 2004: Key Indicators of Well-Being* (Hyattsville, MD: Author, 2005), http://agingstats.gov/chartbook2004/population.html.
6. U.S. Department of Health and Human Services, Administration on Aging, "A Profile of Older Americans 2003: Future Growth," March 8, 2004, www.aoa.gov/prof/Statistics/profile/2003/4.asp.
7. U.S. Department of Health and Human Services, "A Profile of Older Americans 2004: Health and Health Care," Updated May 20, 2005, www.aoa.gov/prof/Statistics/profile/2004/2.asp.
8. Osteoporosis and Related Bone Diseases National Resource Center, "Osteoporosis Overview," Revised June 2005, www.osteo.org/newfile.asp?doc=r106i&doctitle=Osteoporosis+Overview+%2D+HTML+Version&doctype=HTML+Fact+SheetT.
9. Ibid.
10. Mayo Clinic staff, "Osteoarthritis: Overview," *Mayoclinic.com,* April 8, 2005, www.mayoclinic.com/invoke.cfm?objectid=2B275878-8417-41E5-AB4FA4B6646DD7F6.
11. National Kidney and Urologic Diseases Information Clearinghouse, "Kidney and Urologic Diseases Statistics for the United States," (NIH Publication No. 04-3895), February 2004, www.kidney.niddk.nih.gov/kudiseases/pubs/kustats/index.htm.
12. Ibid.
13. Philadelphia Corporation for Aging, *Health Matters,* no. 14, August 2004, www.pcaphl.org/healthmatters/agingsexuality.pdf.
14. National Council on Aging, "Half of Older Americans Report They Are Sexually Active, 4 in 10 Want More Sex, Says New Survey," September 28, 1998, http://ncoa.org/mews/archives.sexsurvey.htm.
15. Alzheimer's Association, "Fact Sheet," April 5, 2004, www.alz.org/Resources/FactSheets/FSAlzheimerStats.pdf.
16. Ibid.
17. Alzheimer's Association, "Data Suggest Benefits to Shedding the Spare Tire," 2004, www.alz.org/Perspective/shedding.asp.
18. *Oxford English Dictionary* (Oxford, UK: Oxford University Press, 1969), 72, 334, 735.
19. President's Commission for the Study of Ethical Problems in Medicine and Biomedical and Behavioral Research, *Deciding to Forgo Life-Sustaining Treatment* (New York: Concern for Dying, 1983), 9.
20. Ad Hoc Committee of the Harvard Medical School to Examine the Definition of Brain Death, "A Definition of Irreversible Coma," *Journal of the American Medical Association* 205 (1968): 377.
21. *Civilization* 6, no. 6 (2000): 30, 33–34.
22. E. Kübler-Ross, *On Death and Dying* (New York: Macmillan, 1969), 113.
23. C. Corr, C. Nabe, and D. Corr, *Death and Dying: Life and Living,* 4th ed. (Belmont, CA: Wadsworth, 2003).
24. R. J. Kastenbaum, *Death, Society, and Human Experience,* 8th ed. (Boston: Allyn & Bacon, 2003).
25. Ibid.
26. Ibid.
27. K. J. Doka, ed., *Disenfranchised Grief: Recognizing Hidden Sorrow* (Lexington, MA: Lexington Books, 1989).
28. J. W. Worden, *Grief Counseling and Grief Therapy: A Handbook for the Mental Health Practitioner,* 3rd ed. (New York: Springer, 2001).
29. National Cancer Institute, "Advance Directives, Cancer Facts 8.12," 2000, http://cis.nci.nih.gov/fact/8_12.htm.
30. Public Agenda, "Right-to-Die," 2004, www.publicagenda.org.
31. Oregon Department of Human Services, "Oregon's Death with Dignity Act," 2004, www.dhs.state.or.us/publichealth/chs/pas/pas.cfm.

What has our government done to prevent destruction of the ozone layer?

Can talking on my cell phone cause cancer?

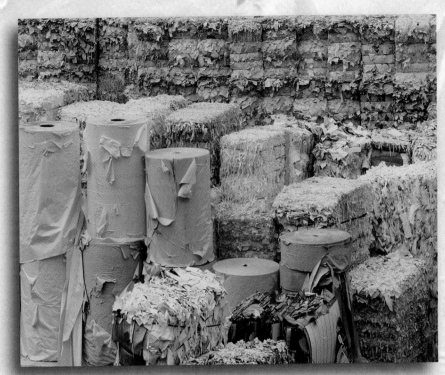

What is a Superfund site?

What are some benefits of using nuclear power?

16 Environmental Health
Thinking Globally, Acting Locally

Objectives

- *Explain* problems and ethical issues associated with current levels of global population growth.
- *Discuss* major causes of air pollution and the global consequences of the accumulation of greenhouse gases and of ozone depletion.
- *Identify* sources of water pollution and the chemical contaminants often found in water.
- *Describe* the physiological consequences of noise pollution.
- *Distinguish* between municipal solid waste and hazardous waste.
- *Discuss* the health concerns associated with ionizing and nonionizing radiation.

Human health and the survival of all living things depend on the health and integrity of the planet on which we live. Today the natural world is under siege from a burgeoning population that consumes massive amounts of natural resources to survive. Consequently, many citizens are interested in the human health effects of such environmental concerns as global warming; depletion of the ozone layer; air, water, and solid waste pollution; deforestation; endangered species; human population control; and dwindling natural resources.

In response to public and political concerns, there has been a surge in federal and state regulations along with a multibillion-dollar national infrastructure—but doubt remains about the effectiveness of that infrastructure in reducing environmental health risks.[1] While the federal government has decided not to participate in several international policy and planning groups designed to protect the global environment, environmental problems continue to escalate. International groups continue to promote an agenda based on sustainable development, or efforts to ensure that the level of productivity and activity that are undertaken in one generation do not compromise the environmental integrity or needed resources of the next generation.[2] In such a period of environmental pressures, an informed citizenry with a strong commitment to be responsible for the planet is essential to the survival of Earth and all living things. This chapter reviews major global environmental issues that affect us today and will continue to affect us in generations to come. What can *you* do to preserve the environment? See the Assess Yourself box on page 438 to find out.

OVERPOPULATION

Anthropologist Margaret Mead wrote, "Every human society is faced with not one population problem but two: how to beget and rear enough children and how not to beget and rear too many."[3] The United Nations projects that the world population will grow from its present total of 6.5 billion to 9.4 billion by 2050 and to 11.5 billion by 2150.[4] Though our population is expanding, the Earth's resources are not. Population experts believe that many areas of the world are already struggling to sustain increasing consumption and the most critical environmental challenge today is to slow the population growth of the world.[5]

The global population explosion is not distributed equally. Nearly 99 percent of all population increases take place in poor countries, while population size is static or declining in wealthy countries. Overpopulation threats are most evident in Latin America, Africa, and parts of Asia. The country projected to have the largest increase in population is India, which could add another 600 million people by the year 2050 and surpass China as the most populous country in the world. Put into

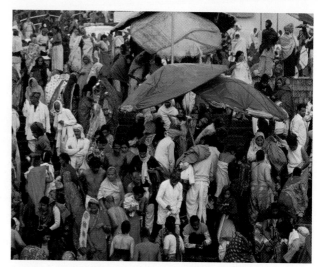

As population levels increase, countries' resources are overloaded. In many parts of the world, governments struggle to meet the needs of the increasing numbers of citizens.

perspective, the U.S. population had not yet reached 300 million by the end of 2004.[6]

As the global population expands, so does competition for the Earth's resources. There is already heavy pressure on the capacity of natural resources to support human life and world health.[7] Many argue that at the current rate we are already exceeding our capacity to provide food and clean water and to dispose of human waste. Every week, the population of the world's urban centers grows by more than 1 million.[8]

Recognizing that population control will be essential in the decades ahead, many countries have enacted strict population control measures or encouraged their citizens to limit the size of their families. Proponents of *zero population growth (ZPG)* believe that each couple should produce only two offspring. When the parents die, these two children are their replacements, allowing the population to stabilize. By 2000, Italy, Spain, Portugal, Greece and Sweden were among the first to achieve ZPG.[9] Germany, Russia, Ukraine, Hungary, and Bulgaria have actually achieved negative population growth.[10] Ironically, while other nations, many of which consume far fewer natural resources and contribute far less to environmental decline, have worked hard to achieve zero or negative population growth, the United States is the only major industrialized nation to continue to have significant population growth. In 2005, the rate of U.S. growth is estimated to be nearly 1 percent, far greater than that of Canada, England, or other world leaders.[11] Unless the United States takes action to reduce population growth at home and diminish our heavy consumption patterns, we will continue to be part of the problem instead of part of the solution.

We can also do our part by recognizing that the United States consumes far more energy and raw materials per person than another other nation on Earth. Although the United States makes up only 5 percent of the world's population, it is responsible for nearly 30 percent of total global consumption.[12] Many of these resources come from other countries, and our consumption is depleting the resource balance of those countries. (Table 16.1 shows a comparison of U.S. oil consumption with that of selected other countries.)

The continued preference for large families in many developing nations is related to several factors: high infant mortality rates; the traditional view of children as "social security" (working from a young age to assist families in daily survival and supporting parents when they grow too old to work); the low educational and economic status of women, which often leaves women with few reproductive choices; and the traditional desire for sons, which keeps parents of daughters reproducing until they have male offspring.

Education may be the single biggest contributor to zero population growth. As education levels of women increase and women achieve equality in pay and job status, fertility rates decline. However, U.S. funding for this kind of education and family planning has declined dramatically in the last four years as highly controversial "abstinence only" messages have been promoted as the only allowable interventions in many regions of the world. In countries such as the United States, policies that encourage zero-population rates or provide incentives to young parents through tax breaks for reduced family size may be a viable option.

AIR POLLUTION

The daily impact of a growing population makes clean air more difficult to find. Concern about air quality prompted Congress to pass the Clean Air Act in 1970 and to amend it in 1977 and again in 1990. The object was to develop standards for six of the most widespread air pollutants that seriously affect health: sulfur dioxide, particulates, carbon monoxide, ozone, nitrogen dioxide, and lead.

Sources of Air Pollution

Sulfur Dioxide A yellowish brown gas, **sulfur dioxide** is a by-product of burning fossil fuels. Electricity-generating stations, smelters, refineries, and industrial boilers are the main source points. In humans, sulfur dioxide aggravates symptoms of heart and lung disease; obstructs breathing passages; and increases the incidence of respiratory diseases such as colds, asthma, bronchitis, and emphysema. Sulfur dioxide is toxic to plants, destroys some paint pigments, corrodes metals, impairs visibility, and is a precursor to acid deposition, which we discuss later in this chapter.

Particulates **Particulates** are tiny solid particles or liquid droplets that are suspended in the air. Cigarette smoke, for example, releases particulates. They are also

Table 16.1

Oil Consumption in Selected Countries (millions of barrels per day)

	1995	2004
United States	17,700	20,700
China	3,360	6,500
Japan	5,680	5,400
Germany	2,880	2,600
Russia	2,980	2,600
India	1,570	2,300
Brazil	1,790	2,200
Canada	1,820	2,300
France	1,920	2,000
Mexico	1,820	2,000

Source: U.S. Energy Information Administration, "Top World Oil Consumers, 2004"; U.S. Energy Information Administration, "World Petroleum Consumption," 1995, www.eia.doe.gov.

by-products of industrial processes and the internal combustion engine. Particulates irritate the lungs and can carry heavy metals and carcinogenic agents deep into the lungs. When combined with sulfur dioxide, they exacerbate respiratory diseases. Particulates also can corrode metals and obscure visibility. Numerous scientific studies have found significant links between adverse health effects (including premature death) and exposure to air particulate concentrations at or below current standards.[13] A recent study in Montana showed significant improvements in employee health after workplace smoking bans were implemented.[14]

Carbon Monoxide An odorless, colorless gas, **carbon monoxide** originates primarily from motor vehicle emissions. Carbon monoxide interferes with the blood's ability to absorb and carry oxygen and can impair thinking, slow reflexes, and cause drowsiness, unconsciousness, and death. Many people have purchased home monitors to test for carbon monoxide.

Ozone Ground-level **ozone** is a form of oxygen that is produced when nitrogen dioxide reacts with sunlight and oxygen molecules. In the lower atmosphere, ozone irritates the mucous membranes of the respiratory system, which causes coughing and choking. It can impair

---

Sulfur dioxide A yellowish brown gaseous by-product of the burning of fossil fuels.

Particulates Nongaseous air pollutants.

Carbon monoxide An odorless, colorless gas that originates primarily from motor vehicle emissions.

Ozone A gas formed when nitrogen dioxide interacts with hydrogen chloride.

What Can I Do to Preserve the Environment?

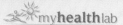

Fill out this assessment online at
www.aw-bc.com/MyHealthLab or www.aw-bc.com/donatelle.

Environmental problems often seem too big for one person to make a difference. Each day, though, there are things you can do that contribute to the health of the planet.

Making a Difference

For each statement, indicate how commonly you follow the described behavior.

	Always	Usually	Sometimes	Never
1. Whenever I can, I try to walk or ride my bicycle rather than take a car.	1	2	3	4
2. I try to carpool with others to school or work.	1	2	3	4
3. I have my car tuned up and inspected every year.	1	2	3	4
4. When I have the oil in my car changed, I make sure the oil goes into a recycling bin, not on the ground or into a floor drain.	1	2	3	4
5. I try to save fuel by not using the air conditioner except in extreme conditions.	1	2	3	4
6. I turn off the lights when a room is not being used.	1	2	3	4
7. I take a shower rather than a bath most of the time.	1	2	3	4
8. I have water-saving devices installed on my shower, toilet, and sinks.	1	2	3	4
9. I make sure faucets and toilets do not leak.	1	2	3	4
10. I use my bath towels more than once before putting them in the wash.	1	2	3	4
11. I wear my clothes more than once between washings when possible.	1	2	3	4
12. I make sure that the washing machine is full before I wash a load of clothes.	1	2	3	4
13. I try to purchase biodegradable soaps and detergents.	1	2	3	4
14. I try to use biodegradable trash bags.	1	2	3	4
15. At home, I use dishes and silverware rather than Styrofoam or plastic.	1	2	3	4
16. When I buy pre-packaged foods, I choose the ones with the least packaging.	1	2	3	4
17. I try not to subscribe to newspapers and magazines when I can view them online.	1	2	3	4
18. I try not to use a hair dryer.	1	2	3	4
19. I recycle plastic bags that I get when I bring something home from the store.	1	2	3	4
20. I don't run water continuously when washing the dishes, shaving, or brushing my teeth.	1	2	3	4
21. I prefer to use unbleached or recycled paper.	1	2	3	4
22. I use both sides of printer paper and other paper when possible.	1	2	3	4

	Always	Usually	Sometimes	Never
23. If I have items I do not want to use anymore, I donate them to charity so someone else can use them.	1	2	3	4
24. I try not to buy drinks in cans with plastic rings attached to them.	1	2	3	4
25. I try not to buy bottled water in small plastic containers.	1	2	3	4
26. I clean up after myself while enjoying the outdoors (picnicking, camping, etc.).	1	2	3	4
27. I volunteer for clean-up days in the community in which I live.	1	2	3	4
28. I consider candidates' positions on environmental issues before casting my vote.	1	2	3	4

For Further Thought

Review your scores. Are your responses mostly 1s and 2s? If not, what actions can you take to become more environmentally responsible? Are there ways to help the environment on the list that you had not thought of before? Are there behaviors not on the list that you are already doing?

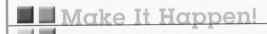

Make It Happen!

Assessment: The Assess Yourself activity gave you the chance to look at your behavior and consider ways of saving water, reducing waste, and protecting the planet in other ways. Now that you have considered these results, you can begin to take steps to become more environmentally responsible.

Making a Change: In order to change your behavior, you need to develop a plan. Follow these steps below and complete your Behavior Change Contract to take action.

1. Evaluate your behavior, and identify patterns and specific things you are doing. What can you change now? What can you change in the near future?
2. Select one pattern of behavior that you want to change.
3. Fill out the Behavior Change Contract found at the front of your book. It should include your long-term goal for change, your short-term goals, the rewards you'll give yourself for reaching these goals, potential obstacles along the way, and strategies for overcoming these obstacles. For each goal, list the small steps and specific actions that you will take.
4. Chart your progress in a journal. At the end of a week, consider how successful you were in following your plan.

What helped you be successful? What made change more difficult? What will you do differently next week?

5. Revise your plan as needed. Are the short-term goals attainable? Are the rewards satisfying?

Example: Marta saw that she was already doing several of the items recommended in the self-assessment. However, she had not considered several of the ideas regarding excess packaging of her food, drinks, and so on, although she knew that extra plastic wraps and other excess packaging contribute to the need for more landfills and other environmental problems. She decided that for a week she would try to pay more attention to the packaging of her favorite foods and to buy large sizes whenever possible instead of individually packed products. This meant spending more time in the grocery store to be sure she found items with the least packaging (although she also didn't have to make as many trips to the store that week). The next week, Marta looked at how many plastic bottles she used for her water each day. She bought a durable, dishwasher-safe plastic bottle and started filling it with water each day before she left the house. After a week she was happy to discover that her garbage was not full of plastic water bottles, and she had actually saved herself some money.

lung functioning; reduce resistance to colds and pneumonia; and aggravate heart disease, asthma, bronchitis, and pneumonia. Ozone corrodes rubber and paint and can kill vegetation. The natural ozone found in the upper atmosphere (sometimes called "good" ozone), however, serves as a protective shield against heat and radiation from the sun. We will discuss atmospheric ozone later in the chapter.

Nitrogen Dioxide Coal-powered electrical utility boilers and motor vehicles emit **nitrogen dioxide,** an amber-colored gas. High concentrations can be fatal. Lower concentrations increase susceptibility to colds and flu, bronchitis, and pneumonia. Nitrogen dioxide is also toxic to plant life and causes a brown discoloration of the atmosphere. It is a precursor of ozone and, along with sulfur dioxide, of acid deposition.

Lead **Lead** is a metal pollutant found in paint, batteries, drinking water, pipes, dishes with lead-glazed bases, dirt, soldered cans, and some candies made in Mexico. It affects the circulatory, reproductive, urinary, and nervous systems and can accumulate in bone and other tissues. Lead is particularly detrimental to children and fetuses. It can cause birth defects, behavioral abnormalities, and decreased learning abilities.[15]

The elimination of lead from gasoline and vehicle exhaust in the 1970s was one of the great public health accomplishments of all time. However, although stricter standards prevail, an estimated 300,000 children in the United States still have unsafe blood lead levels.[16]

Hydrocarbons Although not listed as one of the six major air pollutants in the Clean Air Act, hydrocarbons encompass a wide variety of pollutants in the air and play a major part in the formation of smog. Sometimes known as volatile organic compounds,

hydrocarbons are chemical compounds containing different combinations of carbon and hydrogen. Most automobile engines emit hundreds of different hydrocarbon compounds. By themselves, hydrocarbons seem to cause few problems, but when they combine with sunlight and other pollutants, they form such poisons as formaldehyde, ketones, and peroxyacetyl nitrate, all of which are respiratory irritants. Hydrocarbon combinations such as benzene and benzo[a]pyrene are carcinogenic.

What Do You Think? Why do you think American auto manufacturers have not pursued low-emission and hybrid automobiles more aggressively?

■ As a motorist, how can you help eliminate carbon monoxide emissions?

Photochemical Smog

When oxygen-containing compounds of nitrogen and hydrocarbons react in the presence of sunlight, **photochemical smog,** a brown, hazy mix of particulates and gases, forms. It is sometimes called *ozone pollution* because ozone is created when nitrogen dioxide from vehicle exhaust reacts with sunlight. In most cases, smog forms in areas that experience a **temperature inversion,** a weather condition in which a cool layer of air is trapped under a layer of warmer air, which prevents the air from circulating. When gases such as hydrocarbons and nitrogen oxides are released into the cool air layer, they remain suspended until winds move away the warmer air layer. Sunlight filtering through the air causes chemical changes in the hydrocarbons and nitrogen oxides, which results in smog. Smog is more likely to be produced in valley regions blocked by hills or mountains—for example, Tokyo, Los Angeles, and Mexico City.

The most noticeable adverse effects of exposure to smog are difficulty breathing, burning eyes, headaches, and nausea. Long-term exposure poses serious health risks, particularly for children, older adults, pregnant women, and people with chronic respiratory disorders such as asthma and emphysema.

Acid Deposition and Acid Rain

Acid deposition is a term used to describe the acidification process that occurs when rain, sleet, snow, clouds, and fog hold acid particles. In many scientific circles, it is replacing the term *acid rain*. Acid deposition refers to precipitation that has fallen through acidic air pollutants, particularly those containing sulfur dioxides and nitrogen dioxides.

Nitrogen dioxide An amber colored gas found in smog; can cause eye and respiratory irritations.

Lead A metal found in the exhaust of motor vehicles powered by fuel containing lead and in emissions from lead smelters and processing plants.

Hydrocarbons Chemical compounds that contain carbon and hydrogen.

Photochemical smog The brownish-yellow haze resulting from the combination of hydrocarbons and nitrogen oxides.

Temperature inversion A weather condition occurring when a layer of cool air is trapped under a layer of warmer air.

Acid deposition The acidification process that occurs when pollutants are deposited by precipitation, directly on the land or by clouds.

Acidic pollutants can be deposited in three ways:[17]

- *Wet deposition.* Pollutants are deposited in rain and snow (what has been termed *acid rain*). This is the major acid deposition found in most of the Northern hemisphere.
- *Dry deposition.* Gases and particles are deposited directly onto the land. This is the most common form of acid deposition in much of Europe.
- *Cloud deposition.* Clouds can provide a significant input of acidic pollutants over high ground.

Sources of Acid Deposition More than 95 percent of acid deposition originates in human actions, chiefly burning of fossil fuels. The greatest sources of acid deposition in the United States are coal-fired power plants, ore smelters, oil refineries, and steel mills. When these and other industries burn fuels, the sulfur and nitrogen in the emissions combine with oxygen and sunlight in the air to become sulfur dioxide and nitrogen oxides (precursors of sulfuric acid and nitric acids, respectively). Small acid particles are carried by the wind and combine with moisture to produce acidic rain or snow.

Effects of Acid Deposition When introduced into lakes and ponds, this precipitation gradually acidifies the water. When the acid content of the water reaches a certain level, plant and animal life cannot survive. Ironically, acidified lakes and ponds become a crystal-clear deep blue, giving the illusion of beauty and health. Every year acid deposition destroys millions of trees in Europe and North America. Scientists have concluded that much of Europe's forestlands are experiencing damaging levels of sulfur deposition.[18]

Doctors believe that acid deposition aggravates and may even cause bronchitis, asthma, and other respiratory problems. People with emphysema or heart disease may also suffer from exposure, and it may be hazardous to a pregnant woman's unborn child.

Acidic precipitation can cause metals such as aluminum, cadmium, lead, and mercury to **leach** (dissolve and filter) out of the soil. If these metals make their way into water or food supplies (particularly fish), they can cause cancer in humans who consume them. Acid deposition also damages crops; laboratory experiments show that it can reduce seed yield by up to 23 percent. Actual crop losses are being reported with increasing frequency. A final consequence is the destruction of public monuments and structures, with billions of dollars in building damage each year.[19]

Indoor Air Pollution

In the last several years, a growing body of scientific evidence indicates that the air within homes and other buildings can be 10 to 40 times more hazardous than

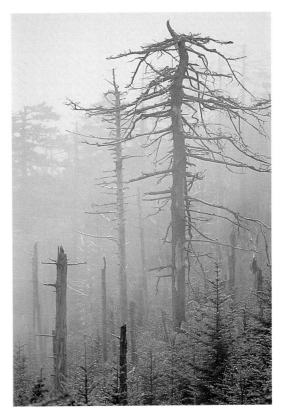

Acid rain has many harmful effects on the environment. Because its toxins seep into groundwater and enter the food chain, it also poses health hazards to humans.

outdoor air in even the most industrialized cities. Research also indicates that some of the most vulnerable people, particularly the young, older adults, and chronically ill, often spend over 90 percent of their time indoors.[20]

There are 20 to 100 potentially dangerous chemical compounds in the average American home. Most indoor air pollution comes from sources that release gases or particles into the air. Inadequate ventilation, particularly in heavily insulated buildings with airtight windows, may increase pollution by not allowing in outside air. Some sources, such as building materials, furnishings, and household products such as air fresheners, release pollutants continuously. Others release pollutants intermittently. Several factors affect risk, including age, pre-existing medical conditions, individual sensitivity, room temperature and humidity, and functioning of the liver, immune, and respiratory systems.[21]

Prevention should focus on three main areas: source control (eliminating or reducing individual contaminants), ventilation improvements (increasing the amount of outdoor air coming indoors), and air cleaners (removing particulates from the air).[22] Indoor pollution comes primarily from woodstoves, furnaces, passive

---

Leach To dissolve and filter through soil.

---

cigarette exposure, asbestos, formaldehyde, radon, and household chemicals. Mold may also be a significant source.

Home Heating

Woodstoves emit significant levels of particulates and carbon monoxide in addition to other pollutants, such as sulfur dioxide. If you rely on wood for heating, make sure that your stove is properly installed, vented, and maintained. Burning properly seasoned wood reduces particulates.

People who rely on oil- or gas-fired furnaces also need to make sure that these appliances are properly installed, ventilated, and maintained. Inadequate cleaning and maintenance can allow deadly carbon monoxide to build up in the home.

Asbestos

Asbestos is a mineral that was commonly used in insulating materials in buildings constructed before 1970. When bonded to other materials, asbestos is relatively harmless, but if its tiny fibers become loosened and airborne, they can embed themselves in the lungs. Their presence leads to cancer of the lungs, stomach, and chest lining, and a fatal lung disease called mesothelioma.

Formaldehyde

Formaldehyde is a colorless, strong-smelling gas present in some carpets, draperies, furniture, particle board, plywood, wood paneling, countertops, and many adhesives. It is released into the air in a process called *outgassing*. Outgassing is highest in new products, but the process can continue for many years. Exposure to formaldehyde can cause respiratory problems, dizziness, fatigue, nausea, and rashes. Long-term exposure can lead to central nervous system disorders and cancer. If you experience symptoms of formaldehyde exposure, have your home tested by a city, county, or state health agency.

Radon

Radon, an odorless, colorless gas, is the natural by-product of the decay of uranium and radium in the soil. Radon penetrates homes through cracks, pipes, sump pits, and other openings in the foundation. The EPA estimates that 1 in 15 American homes has an elevated radon level.[23] An estimated 15,000 to 22,000 lung cancer deaths per year have been attributed to radon, making it second only to smoking as a cause of lung cancer.[24] You can evaluate your own home with a home-testing kit.

Indoor air pollution is also a concern in the classroom and workplace. Studies show that one in five U.S. schools has indoor air quality problems, and one in four has ventilation problems.[25] Poor air quality can lead to drowsiness and headaches and may affect physical growth and development. Children with asthma are particularly at risk. Many people who work indoors complain of maladies that lessen or vanish when they leave the building. **Sick building syndrome (SBS)** is said to exist when 80 percent of a building's occupants report problems. Poor ventilation is a primary cause of sick building syndrome. Other causes include faulty furnaces that emit carbon monoxide, nitrogen dioxide, and sulfur dioxide; biological air pollutants such as dander, molds, and dust; volatile organic compounds from products such as hairspray, cleaners, and adhesives; and heavy metals such as lead, particularly in older buildings. Symptoms include eye irritation, sore throat, queasiness, and worsened asthma.[26]

Ozone Layer Depletion

What has our government done to prevent destruction of the ozone layer?

As mentioned earlier, the ozone layer forms a protective layer in the Earth's stratosphere—the highest level of our atmosphere, located 12 to 30 miles above the Earth's surface. The ozone layer in the stratosphere protects our planet and its inhabitants from ultraviolet B (UVB) radiation, a primary cause of skin cancer. Such radiation damages DNA and weakens immune systems in both humans and animals.

In the 1970s, scientists began to warn of a breakdown in the ozone layer. Instruments developed to test atmospheric contents indicated that chemicals used on Earth, especially **chlorofluorocarbons (CFCs),** were contributing to its rapid depletion.

At first believed to be miracle chemicals, chlorofluorocarbons were used as refrigerants (Freon), aerosol propellants in hairsprays and deodorants, and cleaning solvents and in medical sterilizers, rigid foam insulation, and Styrofoam. But, along with halons (found in many fire extinguishers), methyl chloroform, and carbon tetrachloride (cleaning solvents), CFCs were eventually found to be a major cause of ozone depletion. When released into the air through spraying or outgassing, CFCs migrate upward toward the ozone layer,

---

Asbestos A mineral that separates into stringy fibers and lodges in the lungs, where it can cause various diseases.

Formaldehyde A colorless, strong-smelling gas released through outgassing; causes respiratory and other health problems.

Radon A naturally occurring radioactive gas resulting from the decay of certain radioactive elements.

Sick building syndrome (SBS) Problem that exists when 80 percent of a building's occupants report maladies that tend to lessen or vanish when they leave the building.

Chlorofluorocarbons (CFCs) Chemicals that contribute to the depletion of the ozone layer.

where they decompose and release chlorine atoms. These atoms cause ozone molecules to break apart (Figure 16.1).

The U.S. government banned the use of aerosol sprays containing CFCs in the 1970s. The discovery of an ozone "hole" over Antarctica led to the 1987 Montreal Protocol treaty, whereby the United States and other nations agreed to further reduce the use of CFCs and other ozone-depleting chemicals. The treaty was amended in 1995 to ban CFC production in developed countries. Today, over 160 countries have signed the treaty, as the international community strives to preserve the ozone layer.[27]

Although the ban on CFCs is believed to be responsible for slowing the depletion of the ozone layer, CFC replacements (including two greenhouse gases, hydrofluorocarbons and perfluorocarbons) appear to be equally damaging. A United Nations treaty signed in Kyoto in 1997 attempted to control these newer greenhouse gases. Unfortunately, the United States has so far refused to sign the treaty, amid much controversy. As the greatest producer of greenhouse gases, the United States would have been required to reduce emissions by 33 percent.

Global Warming

More than 100 years ago, scientists theorized that carbon dioxide emissions from fossil-fuel burning would create a buildup of *greenhouse gases* in the Earth's atmosphere that could have a warming effect on the Earth's surface. The century-old predictions now seem to be coming true, with alarming results. According to the National Academy of Sciences, the Earth's surface temperature has risen 1 degree Fahrenheit in the past century, with accelerated warming in the past two decades, and there is new evidence that most of the warming over the last 50 years is due to human activities.[28]

With average global temperatures higher today than at any time since first recorded, the change in atmospheric temperature may be taking a heavy toll on humans and crops. In 1975, climate researchers predicted that the buildup of greenhouse gases would produce life-threatening natural phenomena, including drought in the Midwestern United States, more frequent and severe forest fires, flooding in India and Bangladesh, extended heat waves over large areas of the Earth, and massive hurricanes (like Hurricane Katrina) in the southeastern United States. Recently, the planet has experienced all of these phenomena, although whether they are connected to global warming remains a matter of debate.

Greenhouse gases include carbon dioxide, CFCs, ground-level ozone, nitrous oxide, and methane. They become part of a gaseous layer that encircles the earth, allowing solar heat to pass through and then trapping it

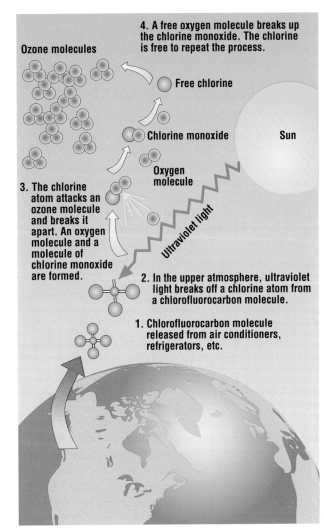

Figure 16.1 ■ How the Ozone Layer Is Being Depleted

close to the earth's surface. The most predominant is carbon dioxide, which accounts for 49 percent of all greenhouse gases, and Eastern Europe and North America are responsible for approximately half of all carbon dioxide emissions. Since the late nineteenth century, carbon dioxide concentrations in the atmosphere have increased by 30 percent, with half of this increase occurring since the 1950s. Carbon emissions from the burning of fossil fuels, oil, coal, and gas continue to climb. The United States is the greatest producer of greenhouse gases, and this output is expected to increase by 43 percent by 2025.[29]

Rapid deforestation of the tropical rain forests of Central and South America, Africa, and Southeast Asia also contributes to the rapid rise in greenhouse gases. Trees take in carbon dioxide, transform it, store the

> **Greenhouse gases**   Gases that contribute to global warming by trapping heat near the Earth's surface.

carbon for food, and release oxygen into the air. As we lose forests, at the rate of hundreds of acres per hour, we lose the capacity to dissipate carbon dioxide.

Reducing Air Pollution

Air pollution problems are rooted in our energy, transportation, industrial practices, and our own lack of resolve to make the necessary changes now to improve the air for future generations. We must develop comprehensive national strategies that encourage the use of renewable resources such as solar, wind, and water power. Most experts agree that shifting away from fossil fuel–burning automobiles as the primary source of transportation is the only way to reduce air pollution significantly. Many cities have taken steps in this direction by setting high parking fees and road-usage tolls and imposing bans on city driving. Local governments should be encouraged to provide convenient, inexpensive public transportation.

Although stricter laws on carbon emissions from cars and trucks and new hybrid cars that operate on electricity and gas are promising, we have a long way to go to reduce fossil fuel consumption. Hybrid cars, capable of significantly lower emissions and less reliance on fossil fuels, have gained popularity in the United States and abroad. Tax incentives and other initiatives have made them a realistic alternative to traditional cars in some areas. Another promising initiative is "bicycle power," with bicycles gaining popularity worldwide. In Germany, bicycle use has increased by 50 percent, and England has a plan to quadruple bicycle use by the year 2012.[30] Currently, China leads the world in bicycle use, followed by India; however, as the economies of these countries continue to flourish, increased use of automobiles is expected.

Try it → NOW

Put your computer to bed! Nearly $1 billion a year is wasted on electricity for computer monitors that remain on when not in use. Resolve to turn off your monitor (if not your entire computer) whenever you aren't using it for more than an hour, or activate your computer's sleep setting so it will go into an energy saving low-power mode automatically.

WATER POLLUTION

Seventy-five percent of the Earth is covered with water in the form of oceans, seas, lakes, rivers, streams, and wetlands. Beneath the landmass are reservoirs of groundwater. We draw our drinking water from either

Table 16.2		
Daily per Capita Water Use (in Gallons) in Single-Family Homes		
Type of Use	With Water-Conserving Devices	Without Water-Conserving Devices
Showers	10.0	12.6
Washing machines	10.6	15.1
Toilets	9.3	20.1
Dishwashers	1.0	1.0
Baths	1.2	1.2
Leaks	5.0	10.0
Faucets	10.8	11.1
Other domestic use	1.5	1.5
Total	**49.4**	**72.6**
Total savings: 23.3 gallons per day		

Source: Adapted from "1999 Residential Water Use Summary," by permission. Copyright © 2002, American Water Works Association.

this underground source or from surface freshwater. The status of our water supply reflects the pollution level of our communities and, ultimately, of the entire Earth.

According to a 2004 World Health Organization/UNICEF report, the world faces a silent emergency of a shortage of clean water for almost half the world's population. Table 16.2 illustrates how much water might be saved daily through simple conservation methods. More than 2.6 billion people, about 40 percent of those on the planet, have no access to basic sanitation or adequate toilet facilities. More than 1 billion have no access to clean water, and over 4,000 children die every day from illnesses caused by their lack of safe water and sanitation.[31]

Water Contamination

Any substance that gets into the soil can potentially enter the water supply. Industrial pollutants, acidic precipitation, and pesticides eventually work their way into the soil, then into groundwater. The potential health hazards of mixing these thousands of chemicals together can barely be imagined.[32]

In a recent survey carried out by a group of U.S. Geological Survey researchers, the presence of low levels of many chemical compounds, including prescription and nonprescription drugs, hormones, and other wastewater compounds was discovered in a network of 139 targeted streams across the United States. Steroids, nonprescription drugs, and insect repellent were among the most frequently detected groups of chemicals.[33]

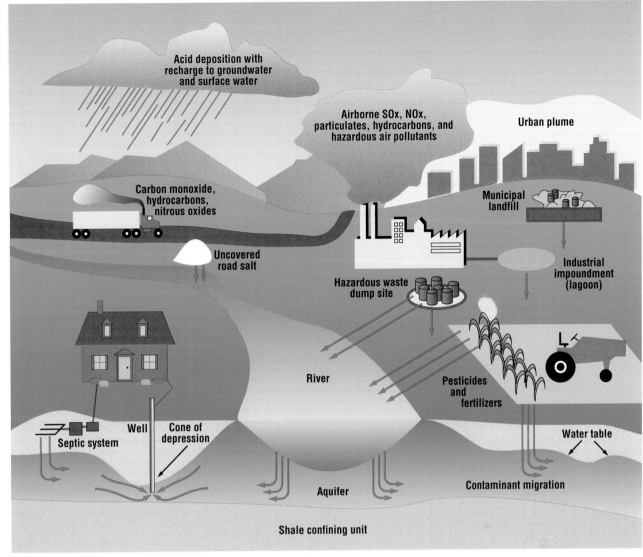

Figure 16.2 ■ Sources of Groundwater Contamination

Sources of Water Contamination

Congress has coined two terms, *point source* and *nonpoint source,* to describe the two general sources of water pollution. **Point source pollutants** enter a waterway at a specific location through a pipe, ditch, culvert, or other conduit. The two major sources of point source pollution are sewage treatment plants and industrial facilities.

Nonpoint source pollutants—commonly known as *runoff* and *sedimentation*—run off or seep into waterways from broad areas of land rather than through a discrete conduit. Nonpoint pollution results from a variety of human land use practices. It includes soil erosion and sedimentation, construction wastes, pesticide and fertilizer runoff, urban street runoff, acid mine drainage, wastes from engineering projects, leakage from septic tanks, and sewage sludge.[34] Figure 16.2 shows various sources of water contamination.

Gasoline and Petroleum Products There are more than 2 million underground storage tanks for gasoline and petroleum products in the United States, most of which are located at gasoline filling stations. One-quarter of them are thought to be leaking.[35]

Most of these tanks were installed 25 to 30 years ago and are made of fabricated steel that was unprotected from corrosion. Over time, pinpoint holes develop in the steel, and the petroleum products leak into groundwater. The most common way to detect the presence of petroleum products in water is to test for benzene, a component of oil and gasoline. Benzene is highly toxic and associated with the development of cancer.

> **Point source pollutants** Pollutants that enter waterways at a specific point.
>
> **Nonpoint source pollutants** Pollutants that run off or seep into waterways from broad areas of land.

Chemical Contaminants *Organic solvents* are chemicals designed to dissolve grease and oil. These extremely toxic substances, such as carbon tetrachloride, tetrachloroethylene, and trichloroethylene, are used to clean clothing, painting equipment, plastics, and metal parts. Many household products (such as stain and spot removers, degreasers, drain cleaners, septic system cleaners, and paint removers) also contain these toxic chemicals.

Organic solvents work their way into the water supply in different ways. Consumers often dump leftover products into the toilet or into street drains. Industries pour leftovers into large barrels, which are then buried. After a while, the chemicals eat through the barrels and leach into the groundwater system.

PCBs Fire resistant and stable at high temperatures, **polychlorinated biphenyls (PCBs)** were used for many years as insulating materials in high-voltage electrical equipment such as transformers. They bind to dust particles in the air, are deposited on plants, and end up in the food supply.[36] The human body does not excrete PCBs but rather stores them (they *bioaccumulate*) in fatty tissues and the liver. Exposure to PCBs are associated with birth defects and is known to cause cancer. The manufacture of PCBs was discontinued in the United States in 1977, but approximately 500 million pounds of them have been dumped into landfills and waterways, where they continue to pose an environmental threat.[37] Western European countries phased out the use of many of these chemicals in the 1970s, but elevated levels can still be detected at the mouths of major rivers, and some countries continue to produce them.

Dioxins **Dioxins** are chlorinated hydrocarbons found in herbicides (chemicals that are used to kill vegetation) and produced during certain industrial processes. Dioxins have the ability to bioaccumulate and are much more toxic than PCBs. Long-term effects include possible damage to the immune system and increased risk of infections and cancer. Exposure to high concentrations of PCBs or dioxins for a short period of time can also have severe consequences, including nausea, vomiting, diarrhea, painful rashes and sores, and chloracne, an ailment in which the skin develops hard, black, painful pimples that may never go away.

Polychlorinated biphenyls (PCBs) Toxic chemicals that were once used as insulating materials in high-voltage electrical equipment.

Dioxins Highly toxic chlorinated hydrocarbons contained in herbicides and produced during certain industrial processes.

Pesticides Chemicals that kill pests.

Noise Levels of Various Activities (in Decibels)

Decibels (db) measure the volume of sounds. Here are the decibel levels of some common sounds.

Type of Sound	Noise Level (db)
Jet takeoff from 200 feet	140
Rock concert	120 (painful)
Auto horn (3 feet)	110 (extremely loud)
Motorcycle	100
Garbage truck	100
Pneumatic drill	90
Lawnmower	90
Heavy traffic	80
Alarm clock	80
Shouting, arguing	80 (very loud)
Vacuum cleaner	75 (loud)
Normal conversation	60
Light auto traffic	50 (moderate)
Soft whisper	30 (faint)

Pesticides **Pesticides** are chemicals that are designed to kill insects, rodents, plants, and fungi. Americans use more than 1.2 billion pounds of pesticides each year, but only 10 percent actually reach the targeted organisms. The remaining 1.1 billion pounds of pesticides settle on the land and in our air and water. Many pesticides, such as DDT, whose uses are banned in the United States are shipped abroad. Mexico, a major crop producer for the American market, continues to use DDT.[38]

Pesticides are volatile and evaporate readily, often being dispersed by winds over a large area or carried to the sea. This is particularly true in tropical regions, where many farmers use pesticides heavily and the climate promotes their rapid release into the atmosphere. In Nigeria, for example, 98 percent of the DDT applied to a cowpea crop evaporated within four years.[39]

Pesticide residues cling to fresh fruits and vegetables and can accumulate in the body when people eat these items. One study found a correlation between breast cancer and dieldrin, a popular pesticide used until the 1970s.[40] Women who had the highest traces of dieldrin in their blood were twice as likely as women with the lowest levels to develop breast cancer. Other potential hazards associated with exposure to pesticides include birth defects, liver and kidney damage, and nervous system disorders.[41]

Lead The U.S. Environmental Protection Agency (EPA) has issued new standards to reduce dramatically the levels of lead in drinking water. The new rules stipulate that tap water lead values must not exceed 15 parts per billion (the previous standard allowed an average lead level of 50 parts per billion).

If lead does exist in your home's water, you can reduce your risk by running tap water for several minutes before taking a drink or cooking with it. This flushes out water that has been standing overnight in lead-contaminated lines. Although leaded paints and ceramic glazes used to pose health risks, particularly for small children who put painted toys in their mouths, the use of lead in such products has effectively been reduced in recent years.

NOISE POLLUTION

Our bodies have definite physiological responses to noise, and it can become a source of physical or mental distress. Short-term exposure to loud noise reduces productivity and concentration and may affect mental and emotional health. Symptoms of noise-related distress include disturbed sleep patterns, headaches, and tension.

Sounds are measured in decibels. A decibel level of 110 is 10 times higher than 100 decibels. A jet take-off from 200 feet has a noise level of approximately 140 decibels, while voice in normal conversation has a level of about 60 decibels (Table 16.3). Hearing can be damaged by varying lengths of exposure to sound. If the duration of allowable daily exposure to different decibel levels is exceeded, hearing loss will result.

Unfortunately, despite increasing awareness that noise pollution is more than just a nuisance, noise control programs have received low budgetary priority in the United States According to the National Institute for Occupational Safety and Health, 30 million Americans are exposed to hazardous noise at work, and 10 million suffer from permanent hearing loss.[42] Clearly, to protect your hearing, you must take it upon yourself to avoid voluntary and involuntary exposure to excessive noise.

LAND POLLUTION
Solid Waste

Each day, every person in the United States generates more than four pounds of **municipal solid waste**—containers and packaging, discarded food, yard debris, and refuse from residential, commercial, institutional, and industrial sources. Approximately 73 percent of this waste is buried in landfills. Cities throughout the country are in danger of exhausting their landfill space.

As communities run out of landfill space, it is becoming more common to haul garbage out to sea to dump it or ship it to landfills in developing countries. Although experts believe that up to 90 percent of our trash is recyclable, only about 30 percent of it is currently recycled (Figure 16.3). In today's throwaway society, we need to become aware of the amount of waste we generate every day and to look for ways to recycle, reuse, and—most desirable of all—reduce what we use.

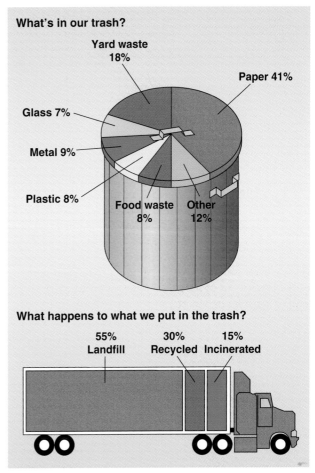

What's in our trash?

Yard waste 18%
Paper 41%
Glass 7%
Metal 9%
Plastic 8%
Food waste 8%
Other 12%

What happens to what we put in the trash?

55% Landfill   30% Recycled   15% Incinerated

Figure 16.3 ■ The Composition and Disposal of Trash

Source: Energy Information Administration, "What We Do with Our Trash" www.eia.doe.gov/kids/energyfacts; 2005.

Try it ▸ NOW

Put a stop to junk mail! Tired of all those credit card offers and unwanted catalogs flooding your mailbox? Take a second to contact Mail Preference Service, Direct Marketing Association, PO Box 643, Carmel, NY 15012-0643. Include your complete name, address, zip code and a request to "activate the preference service." You can also telephone 1-888-5 OPT OUT to put an end to unwanted mail.

Municipal solid waste Solid wastes such as durable goods, nondurable goods, containers and packaging, food wastes, yard wastes, and miscellaneous wastes from residential, commercial, institutional, and industrial sources.

Here are several ways to help preserve and protect the environment:

- Listen carefully to what political candidates say about the environment. Vote for those who prioritize environmental issues and actively promote preservation, protection, and sustainable development.

- Consider state and federal initiatives on issues such as logging, fishing industries, preservation of parks, oil and natural gas drilling, protection of the food supply, restrictions on industrial polluters, solid waste disposal, and water quality.

- Become an environmentally oriented consumer. Buy products with less packaging, foods that are produced with minimal or sustainable energy, and foods with fewer chemicals and pesticides. Buy organic whenever possible.

- Do not use caustic cleansers, chemicals that remove film in your shower, or dyes and fragrances in your laundry products. Use soap or baking soda and water to clean surfaces, not disposable cleaning cloths and spray-on shower cleaners. All these chemicals are flushed down the drain and into the local water supply.

- Let your legislators know how you feel about environmental issues and that you will vote according to their record on the issues. When writing to any public official, keep the letter simple and to the point; avoid inflammatory statements and attacks; state the facts, cite reputable sources, and indicate what you want changed; and say it in one page or less. Proofread the letter for accuracy.

- If you buy a product with excessive packaging, call the toll free number on the package and let the manufacturer know about your concerns.

- Educate yourself and others. Organize a discussion group of friends to read books and articles or discuss speakers focused on environmental issues. Request environmental speakers in your class or at campus events.

- Stop buying plastic bottles of water and other beverages. Plastics are among the fastest growing sources of pollution in America. Purchase a hard plastic, wide-mouth water bottle and fill it from a filtered source. Reuse the bottle, and wash it frequently.

- Get active in community groups that deal with environmental issues. Volunteer for commissions, boards, and other groups involved in decision-making. Participate in clean-up days and recycling drives. Parks, land use, animal control, zoning, public transit, street cleanup, and trash collection are a few of the many issues that have environmental components.

- Run for student government. Help your school become more involved in environmental issues. Seek practicum or internship credits working for environmental causes. Take coursework in environmental health or science.

Hazardous Waste

Hazardous waste is defined as waste with properties that make it capable of harming human health or the environment.[43] In the United States, the EPA sets the criteria for what constitutes a hazardous waste product.

The community of Love Canal, New York, has come to symbolize hazardous waste dump sites. Used by the Hooker Chemical Company as a chemical dump site for nearly 30 years, starting in the 1920s, the area was later filled in by land developers and built up with homes and schools. In 1976, homeowners began noticing strange seepage in their basements and strong chemical odors. Babies were born with birth defects, and the rate of cancer and miscarriages was far above normal. The New York State Department of Health investigation found high concentrations of PCBs in the storm sewers near the old canal. Eventually, more than 900 families were evacuated and the expensive process of cleaning up the waste dump began. Many lawsuits for damages are still being litigated.

What is a Superfund site?

In 1980, the Comprehensive Environmental Response Compensation and Liability Act **(Superfund)** was enacted to provide funds for cleaning up chemical dump sites that endanger public health and land, as well as liability compensation to those affected. This fund is financed through taxes on the chemical and petroleum

> **Hazardous waste** Solid waste that, because of its toxic properties, poses a hazard to humans or to the environment.
>
> **Superfund** Fund established under the Comprehensive Environmental Response Compensation and Liability Act to be used for cleaning up toxic waste dumps.

industries (87 percent) and through general federal tax revenues (13 percent). Cost estimates for cleanup covering the years 1990 through 2020 range from $106 to $500 billion. Billions continue to be spent annually.[44]

To date, 32,500 potentially hazardous waste sites have been identified across the nation. After investigation, 17,800 of these sites were determined to require no further action. However, 1,498 sites were listed on the National Priorities List (NPL), and 46 percent of the sites assessed from 1992 through 1996 were a hazard to human health.[45] As of the end of 2004, clean-up work had been completed at 926 of the sites. Funding has been scaled back due to competing economic priorities.

The large number of hazardous waste dump sites in the United States indicates the severity of our toxic chemical problem. American manufacturers generate more than 1 ton of chemical waste per person per year (approximately 275 million tons). The EPA and individual states have undertaken an aggressive program to manage hazardous wastes by monitoring their generation, transportation, storage, treatment, and final disposal.[46]

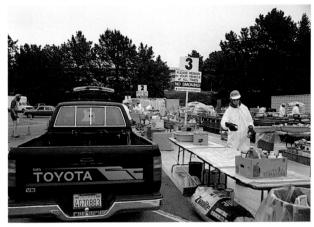

Many communities now provide special programs where their residents can drop off any kind of hazardous waste for safe disposal.

What Do You Think? What items do you currently recycle? ■ What are some of the reasons you do not recycle? ■ What might encourage you to recycle more than you do? ■ What concerns would you have about living near a landfill or hazardous waste disposal site?

RADIATION

A substance is said to be *radioactive* when it emits high-energy particles from the nuclei of its atoms. There are three types of radiation: alpha particles, beta particles, and gamma rays. *Alpha particles* are relatively massive and are not capable of penetrating human skin. They pose health hazards only when inhaled or ingested. *Beta particles* can penetrate the skin slightly and are harmful if ingested or inhaled. *Gamma rays* are the most dangerous because they can pass straight through the skin, which causes serious damage to organs and other vital structures.

Ionizing Radiation

Exposure to ionizing radiation is an inescapable part of life on this planet. **Ionizing radiation** is caused by the release of particles and electromagnetic rays from atomic nuclei during the normal process of disintegration. Some naturally occurring elements, such as uranium, emit radiation. Radiation can wreak havoc on human cells, which leads to mutations, cancer, miscarriages, and other problems.

Reactions to radiation differ from person to person. Exposure is measured in **radiation absorbed doses,** or **rads** (also called roentgens). Recommended maximum "safe" dosages range from 0.5 to 5 rads per year. Approximately 50 percent of the radiation to which we are exposed comes from natural sources, such as building materials. Another 45 percent comes from medical and dental X rays. The remaining 5 percent comes from computer display screens, microwave ovens, television sets, luminous watch dials, and radar screens and waves. Most of us are exposed to far less radiation than the safe maximum dosage per year.

Radiation can cause damage at dosages as low as 100 to 200 rads. At this level, signs of radiation sickness include nausea, diarrhea, fatigue, anemia, sore throat, and hair loss, but death is unlikely. At 350 to 500 rads, these symptoms become more severe, and death may result because the radiation hinders bone marrow production of the white blood cells we need to protect us from disease. Dosages above 600 to 700 rads are invariably fatal. The effects of long-term exposure to relatively low levels of radiation are unknown. Some scientists believe that such exposure can cause lung cancer, leukemia, skin cancer, bone cancer, and skeletal deformities. Researchers are also investigating the effects of exposure to the radio frequency waves generated by cell phones (see the Consumer Health box).

Ionizing radiation Radiation produced by photons having energy high enough to ionize atoms.

Radiation absorbed doses (rads) Units that measure exposure to radioactivity.

In less than a decade, cell phones have become a household staple, with the number of subscribers skyrocketing from 16 million in 1994 to over 110 million today and still rising by 1 million per month.

Although cell phones have become commonplace, their use continues to spur controversy, particularly regarding questions of potential health risk. While the cell phone industry assures consumers that phones are safe, a former industry research director, Dr. George Carlo, argues that past studies have not provided conclusive evidence of safety and we do not know the effects of cell phone usage on future generations. He observed, "This is the first generation that has put relatively high-powered transmitters against the head, hour after hour, day after day."

> **Can talking on my cell phone cause cancer?**

Are increases in the prevalence of brain tumors and other neurological conditions in the last decade related to cell phone use? At high power levels, radiofrequency energy (the energy used in cell phones) can rapidly heat biological tissue and cause damage, such as burns. However, cell phones operate at power levels well below the level at which such heating occurs. Many countries, including the United States and most of Europe, follow standards set by the Federal Communications Commission (FCC) for radiofrequency energy based on research by several scientific groups. These groups identified a whole-body *specific absorption rate (SAR)* value for exposure to radiofrequency energy. Four watts per kilogram was identified as a threshold level of exposure at which harmful biological effects may occur. The FCC requires wireless phones to comply with a safety limit of 1.6 watts per kilogram. To find the SAR for your phone, see this website: www.fda.gov/cellphones/qa.html.

The U.S. Food and Drug Administration (FDA), the World Health Organization, and other major health agencies agree that the research to date has not shown radiofrequency energy emitted from cell phones to be harmful. However, they also point to the need for more research and caution that, because cell phones have only been widely used for less than a decade and no long-term studies have been done, there is not enough information to say they are risk-free. Three large, case-control studies and one large cohort study have compared cell phone use among brain cancer patients and individuals free of brain cancer. Key findings from these studies indicate that:

■ Brain cancer patients did not report more cell phone use overall than controls. In fact, for unclear reasons, most of the studies showed a lower risk of brain cancer among cell phone users.

■ None of the studies showed a clear link between the side of the head on which the cancer occurred and the side on which the phone was used.

■ There was no correlation between brain tumor risk and dose of exposure, as assessed by duration of use, date since first subscription, age at first subscription, or type of cell phone used.

However, these studies are not conclusive, and preliminary results from smaller, well-designed studies have continued to raise questions. A recent Swedish study found higher risk of a benign brain tumor among adults who had used analog cell phones (which produce higher exposure levels than their digital counterparts) for at least

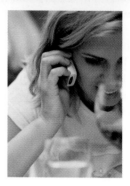

ten years. At the moment, the biggest risk from cell phones appears to come from using them while driving, with a corresponding increase in vehicle crashes. However, if you prefer to err on the side of caution, follow these hints to lower your risk:

■ Use lighter- or dash-mounted phones or headphones/ear buds when driving. This not only keeps your hands free, but, if subsequent studies indicate a health risk, you will have minimized your exposure to radiofrequency energy. Exposure levels drop dramatically with distance.

■ Limit cell phone usage. Use land-based phones whenever possible.

■ Check the SAR level of your phone. Purchase one with a lower level if yours is near the FCC limit.

Sources: S. Grund, "Cell Phones: Do They Cause Cancer?" *Medline Plus,* 2004 update, www.nlm.nih.gov/medlineplus/ency/article/007151.htm; S. Lönn et al., "Mobile Phone Use and the Risk of Acoustic Neuroma," *Epidemiology* 15, no. 6 (2004): 653–659; H. Frumkin and M. Thun, "Environmental Carcinogens—Cellular Phones and Risk of Brain Tumors," *California Cancer Journal for Clinicians* 51 (2001): 137–141; R. Westerman and B. Hocking, "Diseases of Modern Living: Neurological Changes Associated with Mobile Phones and Radiofrequency Radiation in Humans," *Neuroscience Letters* 361, no. 1–3 (2004): 13–16; U.S. Food and Drug Administration, "Cell Phone Facts: Consumer Information on Wireless Phones," 2004, www.fda.gov/cellphones/qa.html.

Electromagnetic Fields: Emerging Risks?

If you believe what you hear on TV, electromagnetic fields (EMFs) generated by electric power delivery systems are responsible for risks for cancer (particularly among children), reproductive dysfunction, birth defects, neurological disorders, Alzheimer's disease, and other ailments. Does research support these claims about EMFs? Though many believe that the threat is legitimate, others point to major discrepancies and inconsistencies in the research. In spite of many questions, fears have increased, and there is probably more potential for exploitation of consumers than real hazard to health from this nonionizing form of exposure.

Nuclear Power Plants

What are some benefits to using nuclear power?

Nuclear power plants account for less than 1 percent of the total radiation to which we are exposed. Other producers of radioactive waste include medical centers that use radioactive materials as treatment and diagnostic tools and nuclear weapons production facilities.

Proponents of nuclear energy believe that it is a safe and efficient way to generate electricity. Initial costs of building nuclear power plants are high, but actual power generation is relatively inexpensive. A 1,000-megawatt reactor produces enough energy for 650,000 homes and saves 420 million gallons of fossil fuels each year. In some areas where nuclear power plants were decommissioned, electricity bills tripled when power companies turned to hydroelectric or fossil fuel sources to generate electricity.

Nuclear reactors discharge fewer carbon oxides into the air than fossil fuel–powered generators. Advocates believe that conversion to nuclear power could help slow the global warming trend. Over the past 15 years, carbon emissions were reduced by 298 million tons, or 5 percent.

All these advantages of nuclear energy must be weighed against the disadvantages. Currently, disposal of nuclear waste is extremely problematic. In addition, a reactor core meltdown could pose serious threats to a plant's immediate environment and to the world in general.

A **nuclear meltdown** occurs when the temperature in the core of a nuclear reactor increases enough to melt both the nuclear fuel and the containment vessel that holds it. Most modern facilities seal their reactors and containment vessels in concrete buildings with pools of cold water on the bottom. If a meltdown occurs, the building and the pool are supposed to prevent the escape of radioactivity.

Human error and mechanical failure were the reported causes of the 1986 reactor core fire and explosion at the Chernobyl nuclear power plant in Russia. In just 4.5 seconds, the temperature in the reactor rose to 120 times normal, causing an explosion. Eighteen people were killed immediately, 30 workers died later from radiation sickness, and 200 other workers were hospitalized for severe radiation sickness. Officials evacuated towns and villages near the plant. Some medical workers estimate that the eventual death toll from radiation-induced cancers related to the Chernobyl incident topped 100,000. Direct costs of the disaster totaled more than $13 billion, including lost agricultural output and the cost of replacing the power plant. Nuclear accidents continue to pose risks to human health, even in well-controlled settings.

> **Nuclear meltdown** An accident that results when the temperature in the core of a nuclear reactor increases enough to melt the nuclear fuel and the containment vessel housing it.

▧ Taking Charge

Summary

- Population growth is the single largest factor affecting the demands on the environment. Demand for more food, products, and energy—as well as places to dispose of waste, particularly in the industrialized world—places great strain on the Earth's resources.

- The primary constituents of air pollution are sulfur dioxide, particulate matter, carbon monoxide, nitrogen dioxide, ozone, lead, and hydrocarbons. Air pollution includes photochemical smog and acid deposition, among others. Indoor air pollution is caused primarily by woodstove smoke, furnace emissions, asbestos, passive smoke, formaldehyde, radon, and household chemicals. Pollution is depleting the Earth's protective ozone layer, which causes global warming.

- Water pollution can be caused by either point (direct entry through a pipeline, ditch, etc.) or nonpoint (runoff or seepage from a broad area of land) sources. Major contributors to water pollution include dioxins, pesticides, and lead.

- Noise pollution affects our hearing and produces other symptoms such as decreased productivity, reduced concentration, headaches, and tension.

- Solid waste pollution includes household trash, plastics, glass, metal products, and paper. Limited landfill space creates problems. Hazardous waste is toxic; improper disposal creates health hazards for those in surrounding communities.

- Ionizing radiation results from the natural erosion of atomic nuclei. Nonionizing radiation is caused by the electric and magnetic fields around power lines and household appliances, among other sources. The disposal and storage of radioactive waste from nuclear power and weapons production plants pose serious potential problems for public health.

Chapter Review

1. The only major industrialized country that has significant population growth is
   a. Spain.
   b. Sweden.
   c. Germany.
   d. the United States.

2. Even though the United States makes up only 5 percent of the world's population, it is responsible for what percent of total global consumption?
   a. 10 percent
   b. 30 percent
   c. 50 percent
   d. 68 percent

3. Jason and Elaine believe in the concept of zero population growth, so they decide to limit their offspring to
   a. 0.
   b. 1.
   c. 2.
   d. 3.

4. Soon after Sandra and Dean moved into their new house, they began experiencing respiratory problems, dizziness, fatigue, nausea, and rashes. One possible source of their problem is a colorless, strong-smelling gas present in some carpets called
   a. lead.
   b. asbestos.
   c. radon.
   d. formaldehyde.

5. The single biggest contributor to zero population growth is
   a. income.
   b. gender.
   c. education.
   d. ethnicity.

6. Cigarette smoke releases what air pollutant?
   a. particulates
   b. sulfur dioxide
   c. nitrogen dioxide
   d. hydrocarbons

7. What substance separates into stringy fibers, embeds itself in lungs, and causes mesothelioma?
   a. asbestos
   b. particulate matter
   c. radon
   d. formaldehyde

8. The terms *point source* and *nonpoint source* are used to describe the two general sources of
   a. water pollution.
   b. air pollution.
   c. noise pollution.
   d. ozone depletion.

9. The air pollutant that originates primarily from motor vehicle emissions is
   a. particulates.
   b. nitrogen dioxide.
   c. sulfur dioxide.
   d. carbon monoxide.

10. Ed's job involves the use of herbicides. Ed is now experiencing nausea, vomiting, diarrhea, and painful sores. Ed may be suffering from the long-term effects of accumulating toxic substances in the herbicides called
    a. THMs.
    b. PCPs.
    c. dioxins.
    d. leachates.

Answers for these questions can be found on page A-1.

Questions for Discussion and Reflection

1. How are the rapidly increasing global population and consumption of resources related? Is population control the best solution? Why or why not?

2. What are the primary sources of air pollution? What can be done to reduce air pollution?

3. What causes poor indoor air quality? How does indoor air pollution affect schoolchildren?

4. What are the causes and consequences of global warming?

5. What are point and nonpoint sources of water pollution? What can be done to reduce or prevent water pollution?

6. What are the physiological consequences of noise pollution? What can you do to lessen your exposure to it?

7. Why do you think so little recycling occurs in the United States?

8. Would you feel comfortable living near a nuclear power plant? Do you think nuclear power is an important source of energy in the future? Why or why not?

Accessing Your Health on the Internet

The following websites explore further topics and issues related to personal health. For links to the websites below, visit the Companion Website for *Health: The Basics,* Seventh Edition at www.aw-bc.com/donatelle.

1. *Environmental Protection Agency (EPA).* Government agency responsible for overseeing environmental regulation and protection issues in the United States.

2. *National Center for Environmental Health (NCEH).* A section of the Centers for Disease Control and Prevention website, this site provides information on a wide variety of environmental health issues, including a series of helpful fact sheets.

3. *National Environmental Health Association (NEHA).* This organization provides educational resources and opportunities for environmental health professionals. The NEHA website lists conferences, trainings, and publications and offers informational position papers.

Further Reading

Cayne, B. and J. Tesar. *Food and Water: Threats, Shortages, and Solutions.* New York: Facts on File, 2002.

A basic introduction that discusses the vital importance of an adequate supply of food and water and the need for alternative water storage and agricultural strategies.

Kennedy, R. F. *Crimes against Nature: How George W. Bush and His Corporate Pals Are Plundering the Country and Hijacking Our Democracy.* New York: HarperCollins, 2004.

Michaels, P. *Meltdown: The Predictable Distortion of Global Warming by Scientists, Politicians, and the Media.* Washington, DC: Cato Institute, 2004.

The two books offer sharply contrasting perspectives on the environment and public policy and will provoke debate and discussion. The factual basis of the assertions made in both books should be compared to commentary and statistics available from objective sources in the scientific community.

Speth, J. G. *Red Sky at Morning: America and the Crisis of the Global Environment.* New Haven, CT: Yale University Press, 2004.

Overview of major environmental threats to health and projections for the future.

References

1. G. Moore, *Living with the Earth,* 2nd ed. (Boca Raton, FL: Lewis Publisher/CRC Press, 2002), 519–542.
2. A. Yassi et al., *Basic Environmental Health* (New York: Oxford University Press, 2001), 14.
3. Moore, *Living with the Earth,* 60.
4. U.S. Census Bureau, "World Clock Projections," 2005, www.census/gov/ipc.wwa.popclockworld.html.
5. A. Nadakavukaren, *Our Global Environment* (Long Grove, IL: Waveland Press, 2000), 45–80.
6. U.S. Census Bureau, "World Clock Projections."
7. Moore, *Living with the Earth,* 62.
8. Population Reference Bureau, "2005 World Population Data Sheet," www.prb.org.
9. Nadakavukaren, *Our Global Environment,* 76.
10. Ibid.
11. Population Reference Bureau, "2005 World Population Data Sheet."
12. H. Franklin, *Environmental Health: From Global to Local* (San Francisco: Jossey-Bass, 2005), 25.
13. J. Schwartz, "Health Effects of Particulate Air Pollution," *The Center for Environmental Health Newsletter* (University of Connecticut, College of Agriculture and Natural Resources) 7 (1998).
14. R. Sargent, R. Shepard, and S. Glantz, "Reduced Incidence of Admissions for Myocardial Infarction Associated with Public Smoking Ban: Before and After Study," *British Medical Journal* 328 (2004): 977–980.
15. K. Koller et al., "Recent Developments in Low-Level Lead Exposure and Intellectual Impairment in Children," *Environmental Health Perspectives* 112 (2004): 987–994.
16. Children's Health Environmental Coalition, "Children's Blood-Lead Levels Declining, But Studies Show Exposure Causes Long-Term Risks," *Chec's Healthehouse,* January 12, 2003, www.Checnet.Org/Healthehouse/Education/Articles-Detail.Asp?Main_Id=527.
17. Environment Agency, "Acid Rain," 2005, www.environment-agency.gov.uk/yourenv/eff/pollution/acid_rain.
18. L. Brown, "A New Era Unfolds," in: *State of the World, 1993,* ed. L. Brown (New York: W. W. Norton Co., 1993), 107.
19. U.S. Environmental Protection Agency, "Effects of Acid Rain," 2005, www.epa.gov/acidrain.
20. U.S. Environmental Protection Agency, "The Inside Story: A Guide to Indoor Air Quality" (EPA Document #402-K-93-007), January 2002, http://epa.gov/iaq/pubs/insidest.html.
21. Ibid.
22. Ibid.
23. Ibid.
24. National Cancer Institute, "Radon and Cancer: Questions and Answers," 2005, http://cis.nci.nih.gov/fact3_52.htm.
25. U.S. Environmental Protection Agency, "Air—Indoor Air Quality," 2004, www.epa.gov/iaq.
26. N. Carpenter, " 'Sick' Buildings Can Be Root of Work-Related Maladies," *Boston Business Journal* 20 (2000): 36–37.
27. U.S. Environmental Protection Agency, *Questions and Answers on Ozone Depletion* (Washington, DC: Stratospheric Protection Division, 1998).
28. U.S. Environmental Protection Agency, "Global Warming—Climate," 2002, http://yosemite.epa.gov/oar/globalwarming.nsf/content/climate.html.
29. United States General Accounting Office, *Climate Change: Trends in Greenhouse Gas Emissions and Emissions Intensity in the United States and Other High-Emitting Nations,* GAQ04.146R, 2003.
30. J. Abramovitz, *Taking a Stand: Cultivating a New Relationship with the World's Forests* (Washington, DC: Worldwatch Institute, 1998).
31. World Health Organization, "Meeting the Millennium Development Goals Drinking Water and Sanitation Target—A Mid-Term Assessment of Progress," 2004, www.who.int/water_sanitation_health/monitoring/jmp2004.

32. P. Hamilton, T. Miller, and D. Meyers, "Water Quality in the Nations Streams and Aquifers—Overview of Selected Findings," *U.S. Geological Survey Circular* 1265 (2004): 20.

33. D. Kolpin et al., "Pharmaceuticals, Hormones, and Other Organic Wastewater Contaminants in U.S. Streams, 1999–2000: A National Reconnaissance," *Environmental Science & Technology* 36, no. 6 (2002): 1202–1211.

34. Ibid.

35. Moore, *Living with the Earth,* 203.

36. Ibid.

37. Ibid.

38. Ibid., 248.

39. Global Programme of Action for the Protection of the Marine Environment from Land-Based Activities, "Inputs of POPs in Coastal and Marine Environment," 2001, http://pops.gpa.unep.org/031marin.htm.

40. A. Hoyer, "Organochlorine Exposure and Risk of Breast Cancer," *The Lancet* 352 (1998): 1816–1831.

41. D. Barr et al., "Concentrations of Dialkyl Phosphate Metabolites of Organophosphorus Pesticides in the U.S. Population," *Population and Environmental Health Perspectives* 112, no. 2 (2004): 186–200.

42. Ibid.

43. Ibid.

44. U.S. Environmental Protection Agency "Superfund National Accomplishments Summary Fiscal Year 2004," 2004, www.epa.gov/superfund/action/process/numbers04.htm.

45. Ibid.

46. Ibid.

Answers to Chapter Review Questions

Chapter 1
1. d; 2. b; 3. c; 4. c; 5. d;
6. b; 7. a; 8. a; 9. a; 10. c

Chapter 2
1. d; 2. b; 3. b; 4. d; 5. a;
6. c; 7. b; 8. b; 9. c; 10. b

Chapter 3
1. c; 2. c; 3. d; 4. d; 5. b;
6. b; 7. c; 8. d; 9. c; 10. b

Chapter 4
1. b; 2. a; 3. a; 4. c; 5. d;
6. d; 7. c; 8. a; 9. a; 10. a

Chapter 5
1. b; 2. b; 3. d; 4. c; 5. c;
6. d; 7. c; 8. a; 9. d; 10. b

Chapter 6
1. c; 2. d; 3. a; 4. a; 5. a;
6. b; 7. c; 8. d; 9. d; 10. a

Chapter 7
1. a; 2. b; 3. a; 4. c; 5. d;
6. c; 7. d; 8. c; 9. a; 10. b

Chapter 8
1. c; 2. c; 3. c; 4. c; 5. b;
6. d; 7. a; 8. c; 9. d; 10. d

Chapter 9
1. c; 2. c; 3. a; 4. b; 5. d;
6. c; 7. d; 8. b; 9. d; 10. a

Chapter 10
1.b; 2.c; 3. b; 4.c; 5. c;
6. c; 7. a; 8. d; 9. a; 10. b

Chapter 11
1. c; 2. c; 3. c; 4. a; 5. a;
6. d; 7. b; 8. d; 9. b; 10. c

Chapter 12
1. d; 2. c; 3. a; 4. c; 5. b;
6. d; 7. c; 8. a; 9. d; 10.a

Chapter 13
1. b; 2. a; 3. c; 4. b; 5. d;
6. a; 7. d; 8. c; 9. c; 10. c

Chapter 14
1. b; 2. b; 3. c; 4. a; 5. c;
6. d; 7. a; 8. a; 9. d; 10. b

Chapter 15
1. d; 2. b; 3. c; 4. c; 5. b;
6. a; 7. b; 8. a; 9. a; 10. c

Chapter 16
1. d; 2. b; 3. c; 4. d; 5. c;
6. a; 7. a; 8. a; 9. d; 10. c

Chapter 17
1. b; 2. b; 3. a; 4. c; 5. d;
6. a; 7. b; 8. b; 9. a; 10. b

Chapter 18
1. d; 2. c; 3. b; 4. b; 5. a;
6. d; 7. a; 8. c; 9. c; 10. b

Health Resources

Injury Prevention and Emergency Care

Injury Prevention

Unintentional injuries are one of the major public health problems facing the United States today. On an average day, more than a million people will suffer a nonfatal injury; almost 100,000 people die each year as a result of unintentional injuries. Unintentional injuries are the leading cause of death for Americans under the age of 44. In the United States, they are the fifth leading cause of death, after heart disease, cancer, stroke, and lung disease.

Vehicle Safety

The risk of dying in an automobile crash is related to age. Young drivers (aged 16 to 24) have the highest death rate, which is attributable to their inexperience and immaturity. Each year about 40,000 Americans die in automobile crashes, and another 1.9 million are disabled—140,000 permanently. Most of these were avoidable. The best way to prevent crashes is to practice risk-management driving and accident-avoidance techniques and to be aware of safety technology when purchasing a car.

Risk-Management Driving Risk-management driving techniques, which help reduce chances of being involved in a collision, include the following:

- *Surround your car with a bubble space.* The rear bumper of the car ahead of you should be three seconds away. To measure your safety bubble, choose a roadside landmark such as a signpost or light pole as a reference point. When the car in front of you passes this point, count "one-one-thousand, two-one-thousand." Make sure you are not passing the reference point before you've finished saying "three-one-thousand."
- Scan the road ahead of you and to both sides.
- *Drive with your low-beam headlights on.* Being seen is an important safety factor. Driving with your low-beam headlights on, *day and night,* makes you more visible to other drivers.

Other important techniques include anticipating other drivers' actions, avoiding driving when tired or stressed, driving sober, obeying all traffic laws, and using safety belts.

Accident-Avoidance Techniques Sometimes when driving, you need to react instantly to a situation. To avoid a more severe accident, you may need to steer into another, less severe collision. The point of accident avoidance is to save lives. Here are the Automobile Association of America's (AAA) rules for avoidance:

- Generally, veer to the right.
- Steer, don't skid, off the road. (It is easy to roll a vehicle over if you swerve suddenly off the edge of the road.)
- If you have to hit a vehicle, hit one moving in the same direction as your own.
- If you have to hit a stationary object, try to hit a soft one (bushes, small trees) rather than a hard one (boulders, brick walls, giant trees).
- If you have to hit a hard object, hit it with a glancing blow.
- Avoid hitting pedestrians, motorcyclists, and bicyclists at all costs.

Safety Technology The last line of defense against a collision is the car itself. How a car is equipped can mean the difference between life and death. When purchasing a car, the Insurance Institute for Highway Safety recommends that you look for the following features:

- Does the car have airbags? Remember, airbags do not eliminate the need for everyone to wear safety belts and could cause injury to small adults and children.
- Does the car have antilock brakes? Antilock brakes rapidly pump the brakes to prevent them from locking up and, hence, prevent the car from skidding.
- Does the car have impact-absorbing crumple zones?
- Are there strengthened passenger compartment side walls?
- Is there a strong roof support? (The center door post on four-door models gives you an extra roof pillar that helps protect passengers if a vehicle rolls over.)

In Case of Mechanical Breakdown

- Try to get off the road as far as possible.
- Turn on your car's emergency flashers, and raise the hood. Set out flares or reflective triangles.

- Stay in the car until a law enforcement officer arrives. If others stop to help, roll down your window only an inch or so and ask them to contact the police, sheriff's office, or the state patrol.
- If you must leave your car, leave a note with the car explaining the problem (as best you can), the time and date, your name, the direction in which you are walking, and what you are wearing. This information will help anyone who needs to look for you.
- Remove all valuables from the car if you must leave it.

Safe Refueling Gasoline is a flammable substance. Follow these guidelines from the Petroleum Equipment Institute any time you are filling up a car, truck, or motorcycle:

- Turn off the engine while refueling.
- Do not reenter your vehicle during refueling. In the unlikely event of a static-caused fire, leave the nozzle in the tank and back away from the vehicle. Notify the attendant immediately.
- Avoid prolonged breathing of gasoline vapors. Keep gasoline away from your eyes and skin; it can cause irritation. Never use it to wash your hands or as a cleaning solvent.
- If you are dispensing gasoline into a container or storing it, be sure the container is approved for such a use.
- Never siphon gasoline by mouth; it can be harmful or fatal if swallowed.

Pedestrian Safety

Each year approximately 13 percent of all motor vehicle deaths involve pedestrians, and another 82,000 pedestrians are injured each year. The highest death rates involving pedestrians occur among the very young and older populations. Pedestrian injuries occur most frequently after dark, in urban settings, and primarily in intersections where pedestrians may walk or dart into traffic. It is not uncommon for alcohol to play a role in the death or injury of a pedestrian. How can you protect yourself from being injured or becoming a fatality? AAA has the following suggestions for joggers and walkers:

- Carry or wear reflective material or lights at night to help drivers see you.
- Cross only at crosswalks. Keep to the right in crosswalks.
- Before crossing, look both ways. Be sure the way is clear before you cross.
- Cross only on the proper signal.

- Watch for turning cars.
- Never enter the roadway from between parked cars.
- Where there is no sidewalk and it is necessary to walk in a roadway, walk on the left side, facing traffic.
- Don't wear headphones for a radio or CD player. These may interfere with your ability to hear sounds of motor vehicles.

Cycling Safety

Currently over 63 million Americans of all ages ride bicycles for transportation, recreation, and fitness. The Consumer Product Safety Commission reports about 800 deaths per year from cycling accidents. The biggest risk factors are failure to wear a helmet, being male, and riding after dark.

Children aged 10 to 14 also are at higher risk for injury. Approximately 87 percent of fatal collisions were due to cyclists' errors, usually failure to yield at intersections. Alcohol also plays a significant role in bicycle deaths and injuries. The following are suggestions cyclists should consider to reduce risk of injury or death.

- Wear a helmet that is ANSI or Snell approved. This can reduce head injuries by 85 percent.
- Don't drink and ride.
- Respect traffic and ride with the flow of traffic.
- Stop at stop signs and traffic lights.
- Wear light reflective clothing that is easily seen at night and during the day.
- Avoid riding after dark.
- Know and use proper hand signals.
- Keep your bicycle in good working condition.
- Use bike paths whenever possible.

Water Safety

Drowning is the third most common cause of accidental death in the United States, according to the National Safety Council. About 85 percent of drowning victims are teenage males. Many drowned swimmers are actually strong swimmers. Alcohol plays a significant role in many drowning cases. Most drownings occur in unorganized or unsupervised facilities, such as ponds or pools with no lifeguards present. Swimmers should take the following precautions:

- Don't drink alcohol before or while swimming.
- Don't enter the water unless you can swim at least 50 feet unassisted.
- Know your limitations; get out of the water as soon as you start to feel even slightly fatigued.

- Never swim alone, even if you are a skilled swimmer. You never know what might happen.
- Never leave a child unattended, even in extremely shallow water or wading pools.
- Before entering the water, check the depth. Most neck and back injuries result from diving into water that is too shallow.
- Never swim in muddy or dirty water that obstructs your view of the bottom.
- Never swim in a river with currents too swift for easy, relaxed swimming.

Emergency Care

In certain situations, it may be necessary to administer first aid. Ideally, first aid procedures should be performed by someone who has received formal training from the American Red Cross or some other reputable institution. If you do not have such training, contact a physician or call your local emergency medical service (EMS) by dialing 911 or your local emergency number. In life-threatening situations, however, you may not have time to call for outside assistance. In cases of serious injury or sudden illness, you may need to begin first aid immediately and continue until help arrives. This section contains basic information and general steps to follow for various emergency situations. Simply reading these directions, however, may not prepare you fully to handle these situations. For this reason, you may want to enroll in a first aid course.

Calling for Emergency Assistance

When calling for emergency assistance, be prepared to give exact details. Be clear and thorough, and do not panic. Never hang up until the dispatcher has informed you that he or she has all the information needed and that it is alright to do so. Be ready to answer the following questions:

1. Where are you and the victim located? This is the most important information the EMS will need.
2. What is your phone number and name?
3. What has happened? Was there an accident, or is the victim ill?
4. How many people need help?
5. What is the nature of the emergency? What is the victim's apparent condition?

6. Are there any life-threatening situations that the EMS should know about (for example, fires, explosions, or fallen electrical lines)?
7. Is the victim wearing a medic-alert tag (a tag indicating a specific medical condition such as diabetes)?

Are You Liable?

According to the laws in most states, you are not required to administer first aid unless you have a special obligation to the victim. For example, parents must provide first aid for their children, and a lifeguard must provide aid to a swimmer.

Before administering first aid, you should obtain the victim's consent. If the victim refuses aid, you must respect that person's rights. However, you should make every reasonable effort to persuade the victim to accept your help. In emergency situations, consent is *implied* if the victim is unconscious. Once you begin to administer first aid, you are required by law to continue. You must remain with the victim until someone of equal or greater competence takes over.

Can you be held liable if you fail to provide adequate care or if the victim is further injured? To help protect people who render first aid, most states have Good Samaritan laws, which grant immunity (protection from civil liability) if you act in good faith to provide care to the best of your ability and in accordance with your certified level of training. Because these laws vary from state to state, you should become familiar with the Good Samaritan laws in your state.

When Someone Stops Breathing

If someone has stopped breathing, you should perform mouth-to-mouth resuscitation. This involves the following steps:

1. Check for responsiveness by gently tapping or shaking the victim. Ask loudly, "Are you OK?"
2. Call the local EMS for help (usually 911).
3. Gently roll the victim onto his or her back.
4. Open the airway by tilting the victim's head back, placing your hand nearest the victim's head on the victim's forehead, and applying backward pressure to tilt the head back and lift the chin.
5. Check for breathing (3 to 5 seconds): look, listen, and feel for breathing.
6. Give two slow breaths.
   - Keep the victim's head tilted back.
   - Pinch the victim's nose shut.

- Seal your lips tightly around the victim's mouth.
- Give two slow breaths, each lasting 1½ to 2 seconds.

7. Check for pulse at side of neck; feel for pulse for 5 to 10 seconds.

8. Begin rescue breathing.
   - Keep the victim's head tilted back.
   - Pinch the victim's nose shut.
   - Give one breath every 5 to 6 seconds.
   - Look, listen, and feel for breathing between breaths.

9. Recheck pulse every minute.
   - Keep the victim's head tilted back.
   - Feel for pulse for 5 to 10 seconds.
   - If the victim has a pulse but is not breathing, continue rescue breathing. If there is no pulse, begin CPR.

There are some variations when performing this procedure on infants and children. For children aged one to eight, at step 8, give one slow breath every 4 seconds. For infants, seal your lips tightly around the infant's nose and mouth instead of pinching the nostrils shut and at step 8, you should give one slow breath every 3 seconds.

In cases in which the victim has no pulse, cardiopulmonary resuscitation (CPR) should be performed. This technique involves a combination of artificial respiration and chest compressions. You should not perform CPR unless you have received up-to-date certification to perform it. You cannot learn CPR simply by reading directions; and, without training, you could cause further injury to the victim. The American Red Cross offers courses in mouth-to-mouth resuscitation and CPR, as well as general first aid. If you have taken a CPR course in the past, you should be aware that certain changes have been made in the procedure. Consider taking a refresher course.

When Someone Is Choking

Choking occurs when an object obstructs the trachea (windpipe), thus preventing normal breathing. Failure to expel the object and restore breathing can lead to death within 6 minutes. The universal signal of distress related to choking is the clasping of the throat with one or both hands. Other signs of choking include not being able to talk and/or noisy and difficult breathing. If a victim can cough or speak, do not interfere. The most effective method for assisting choking victims is the Heimlich maneuver, which involves the application of pressure to the victim's abdominal area to expel the foreign object. The Heimlich maneuver involves the following steps.

If the Victim Is Standing or Seated

1. Recognize that the victim is choking. Ask if they want assistance.

2. Wrap your arms around the victim's waist, making a fist with one hand.

3. Place the thumb side of one fist on the middle of the victim's abdomen, just above the navel and well below the tip of the sternum.

4. Cover your fist with your other hand.

5. Press fist into victim's abdomen, using up to five quick upward thrusts.

6. After every five abdominal thrusts, check the victim and your technique.

7. If the victim becomes unconscious, gently lower him or her to the ground.

8. Look to see if you can find the obstruction in the person's throat. Try to clear the airway by using your finger to sweep the object from the victim's mouth or throat.

9. Give two rescue breaths. If the passage is still blocked and air will not go in, proceed with the Heimlich maneuver.

If the Victim Is Lying Down

1. Facing the person, kneel with your legs astride the victim's hips. Place the heel of one hand against the abdomen, slightly above the navel and well below the tip of the sternum. Put the other hand on top of the first hand.

2. Press inward and upward using both hands with up to five quick abdominal thrusts.

3. Repeat the following steps in this sequence until the airway becomes clear or the EMS arrives:
   a. Finger sweep.
   b. Give two rescue breaths.
   c. Do up to five abdominal thrusts.

Alcohol Poisoning Alcohol overdose is considered a medical emergency when an irregular heartbeat or coma occur. The two immediate causes of death in such cases are cardiac arrhythmia and respiratory depression. If a person is seriously uncoordinated and has possibly also taken a depressant, the risk of respiratory failure is serious enough that a physician should be contacted. When dealing with someone who is drunk, remember these points:

1. Stay calm. Assess the situation.

2. Keep the person still and comfortable.

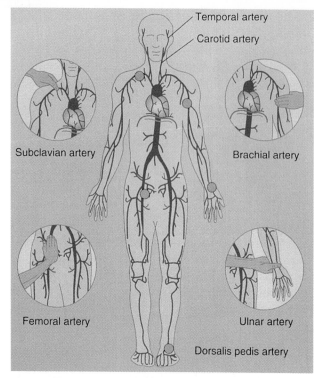

Figure H.1 ■ **Pressure Points**
Pressure can be applied to these points to stop bleeding.
However, unless absolutely necessary, avoid applying pressure
to the carotid arteries, which supply blood to the brain. Never
apply pressure to both carotid arteries at the same time.

The image is labeled with: Temporal artery, Carotid artery, Subclavian artery, Brachial artery, Femoral artery, Ulnar artery, Dorsalis pedis artery.

3. Stay with the person if he or she is vomiting. When helping him or her to lie down, turn the head to the side to help keep the person from choking on vomit.

4. Monitor the person's breathing.

5. Keep your distance. Before approaching or touching the person, explain what you intend to do.

6. Speak in a clear, firm, reassuring manner.

When Someone Is Bleeding

External Bleeding Control of external bleeding is an important part of emergency care. Survival is threatened by the loss of one quart of blood or more. There are three major procedures for the control of external bleeding.

1. *Direct pressure.* The best method is to apply firm pressure by covering the wound with a sterile dressing, bandage, or clean cloth. Wearing disposable latex gloves or an equally protective barrier, apply pressure for 5 to 10 minutes to stop bleeding.

2. *Elevation.* Elevate the wounded section of the body to slow the bleeding. For example, a wounded arm or leg should be raised above the level of the victim's heart.

3. *Pressure points.* Pressure points are sites where an artery that is close to the body's surface lies directly over a bone. Pressing the artery against the bone can limit the flow of blood to the injury. This technique should be used only as a last resort when direct pressure and elevation have failed to stop bleeding.

Knowing where to apply pressure to stop bleeding is critical (see Figure H.1). For serious wounds, seek medical attention immediately.

Internal Bleeding Although internal bleeding may not be immediately obvious, you should be aware of the following signs and symptoms:

1. Symptoms of shock (discussed on page H-7)

2. Coughing up or vomiting blood

3. Bruises or contusions of the skin

4. Bruises on chest or fractured ribs

5. Black, tarlike stools

6. Abdominal discomfort or pain (rigidity or spasms)

In some cases, a person who has suffered an injury (such as a blow to the head, chest, or abdomen) that does not cause external bleeding may experience internal bleeding. If you suspect that someone is suffering from internal bleeding, follow these steps:

1. Have the person lie on his or her back on a flat surface with knees bent.

2. Treat for shock. Keep the victim warm. Cover the person with a blanket, if possible.

3. Expect vomiting. If vomiting occurs, keep the victim on his or her side for drainage, to prevent inhalation of vomit, and to prevent expulsion of vomit from the stomach.

4. Do *not* give the victim any medications or fluids.

5. Send someone to call for emergency medical help immediately.

Nosebleeds To control a nosebleed, follow these steps:

1. Have the victim sit down and lean slightly forward to prevent blood from running into the throat. If you do not suspect a fracture, pinch the person's nose firmly closed using the thumb and forefinger and pressing just below the bony bridge of the nose

to compress the blood vessels. Keep the nose pinched for at least 5 minutes.

2. While the nose is pinched, apply a cold compress to the surrounding area.

3. If pinching does not work, gently pack the nostril with gauze or a clean strip of cloth. Do not use absorbent cotton, which will stick. Be sure that the ends of the gauze or cloth hang out so that it can be easily removed later. Once the nose is packed with gauze, pinch it closed again for another 5 minutes.

4. If the bleeding persists, seek medical attention.

Treatment for Burns

Minor Burns For minor burns caused by fire or scalding water, apply running cold water or cold compresses for 20 to 30 minutes. Never put butter, grease, salt water, aloe vera, or topical burn ointments or sprays on burned skin. If the burned area is dirty, gently wash it with soap and water, and blot it dry with a sterile dressing.

Major Burns For major burn injuries, call for help immediately. Wrap the victim in a clean, dry sheet. Do not clean the burns or try to remove any clothing attached to burned skin. Remove jewelry near the burned skin immediately, if possible. Keep the victim lying down and calm.

Chemical Burns Remove clothing surrounding the burn. Wash skin that has been burned by chemicals by flushing with water for at least 20 minutes. Seek medical assistance as soon as possible.

Shock

Shock is a condition in which the cardiovascular system fails to provide sufficient blood circulation to all parts of the body. Victims of shock display the following symptoms:

- Dilated pupils
- Cool, moist skin
- Weak, rapid pulse
- Vomiting
- Delayed or unrelated responses to questions

All injuries result in some degree of shock. Therefore, treatment for shock should be given after every major injury. The following are basic steps for treating shock:

1. Have the victim lie flat with his or her feet elevated approximately 8 to 12 inches. (If there is no sign of spinal injury, and there is a chest injury, difficulty breathing, or severe pain, the victim's head should be slightly elevated.)

2. Keep the victim warm. If possible, wrap him or her in blankets or other material. Keep the victim calm and reassured.

3. Seek medical help.

Electrical Shock

Do not touch a victim of electrical shock until the power source has been turned off. Approach the scene carefully, avoiding any live wires or electrical power lines. Pay attention to the following:

1. If the victim is holding onto the live electrical wire, do not remove it unless the power has been shut off at the plug, circuit breaker, or fuse box.

2. Check the victim's breathing and pulse. Electrical current can paralyze the nerves and muscles that control breathing and heartbeat. If necessary, give mouth-to-mouth resuscitation. If there is no pulse, CPR might be necessary. (Remember that only trained people should perform CPR.)

3. Keep the victim warm and treat for shock. Once the person is breathing and stable, seek medical help or send someone else for help.

Poisoning Of the 1 million cases of poisoning reported in the United States each year, about 75 percent occur in children under age five, and the majority are caused by household products. Most cases of poisoning involving adults are attempted suicides or attempted murders.

You should keep emergency telephone numbers for the Poison Control center and the local EMS close at hand. Many people keep these numbers on labels on their telephones. Check the front of your telephone book for these numbers. The National Safety Council recommends that you be prepared to give the following information when calling for help:

- What was ingested? Have the container of the product and the remaining contents ready so you can describe it. You should also bring the container to the emergency room with you.
- When was the substance taken?
- How much was taken?
- Has vomiting occurred? If the person has vomited, save a sample to take to the hospital.
- Are there any other symptoms?
- How long will it take to get to the nearest emergency room?

When caring for a person who has ingested a poison, keep these basic principles in mind:

1. Maintain an open airway. Make sure the person is breathing.

2. Call the local poison control center. Follow their advice for neutralizing the poison.

3. If the poison control center or another medical authority advises you to induce vomiting, then do so.

4. If a corrosive or caustic (that is, acid or alkali) substance was swallowed, immediately dilute it by having the victim drink at least one or two 8-ounce glasses of cold water or milk.

5. Place the victim on his or her left side. This position will delay advancement of the poison into the small intestine, where absorption into the victim's circulatory system is faster.

Injuries of Joints, Muscles, and Bones

Sprains Sprains result when ligaments and other tissues around a joint are stretched or torn. The following steps should be taken to treat sprains:

1. Elevate the injured joint to a comfortable position.

2. Apply an ice pack or cold compress to reduce pain and swelling.

3. Wrap the joint firmly with a roller bandage.

4. Check the fingers or toes periodically to ensure that blood circulation has not been obstructed. If the bandage is too tight, loosen it.

5. Keep the injured area elevated, and continue ice treatment for 24 hours.

6. Apply heat to the injury after 48 hours if there is no further swelling.

7. If pain and swelling continue or if a fracture is suspected, seek medical attention.

Fractures Any deformity of an injured body part usually indicates a fracture. A fracture is any break in a bone, including chips, cracks, splinters, and complete breaks. Minor fractures (such as hairline cracks) might be difficult to detect and might be confused with sprains. If there is doubt, treat the injury as a fracture until X rays have been taken.

Do not move the victim if a fracture of the neck or back is suspected because this could result in a spinal cord injury. If the victim must be moved, splints should be applied to immobilize the fracture in order to prevent further damage and to decrease pain. The following are

some basic steps for treating fractures and applying splints to broken limbs:

1. If the person is bleeding, apply direct pressure above (*not* on) the site of the wound.

2. If a broken bone is exposed, do not try to move it back into the wound. This can cause contamination and further injury.

3. Do not try to straighten out a broken limb. Splint the limb as it lies.

4. The following materials are needed for splinting:
   - *Splint:* wooden board, pillow, or rolled up magazines and newspapers.
   - *Padding:* towels, blankets, socks, or cloth.
   - *Ties:* cloth, rope, or tape.

5. Place splints and padding above and below the joint. Never put padding directly over the break. Padding should protect bony areas and the soft tissue of the limb.

6. Tie splints and padding into place.

7. Check the tightness of the splints periodically. Pay attention to the skin color, temperature, and pulse below the fracture to make sure the blood flow is adequate.

8. Elevate the fracture and apply ice packs to prevent swelling and reduce pain.

Head Injuries

A head injury can result from an auto accident, a fall, an assault, or a blow from a blunt object. All head injuries can potentially lead to brain damage, which may result in a cessation of breathing and pulse.

For Minor Head Injuries

1. For a minor bump on the head resulting in a bruise without bleeding, apply ice to decrease the swelling.

2. If there is bleeding, apply even, moderate pressure. Because there is always the danger that the skull may be fractured, excessive pressure should not be used.

3. Observe the victim for a change in consciousness. Observe the size of pupils, including whether both pupils are dilated to the same degree, and note signs of inability to think clearly. Check for any signs of numbness or paralysis. Allow the victim to sleep, but wake him or her periodically to check for awareness.

For Severe Head Injuries

1. If the victim is unconscious, check the airway for breathing. If necessary, perform mouth-to-mouth resuscitation.

2. If the victim is breathing, check the pulse. If it is less than 55 or more than 125 beats per minute, the victim may be in danger.

3. Check for bleeding. If fluid is flowing from the ears or nose, do not stop it.

4. Do not remove any objects embedded in the victim's skull.

5. Cover the victim with blankets to maintain body temperature, but guard against overheating.

6. Seek medical help as soon as possible.

Temperature-Related Emergencies

Frostbite Frostbite is damage to body tissues caused by intense cold. Frostbite generally occurs at temperatures below 32°F. The body parts most likely to suffer frostbite are the toes, ears, fingers, nose, and cheeks. When skin is exposed to the cold, ice crystals form beneath the skin. Avoid rubbing frostbitten tissue because the ice crystals can scrape and break blood vessels. To treat frostbite, follow these steps:

1. Bring the victim to a health facility as soon as possible.

2. Cover and protect the frostbitten area. If possible, apply a steady source of external warmth, such as a warm compress. The victim should avoid walking if the feet are frostbitten.

3. If the victim cannot be transported, you must rewarm the body part by immersing it in warm water (100°F to 105°F). Continue to rewarm until the frostbitten area is warm to the touch when removed from the bath. Do not allow the body part to touch the sides or bottom of the water container. After rewarming, gently dry and wrap the body part in bandages to protect from refreezing.

Hypothermia Hypothermia is a condition of generalized cooling of the body, resulting from exposure to cold temperatures or immersion in cold water. It can occur at any temperature below 65°F and can be made more severe by wind chill and moisture. The following are key symptoms of hypothermia:

- Shivering
- Vague, slow, slurred speech
- Poor judgment
- A cool abdomen
- Lethargy or extreme exhaustion

- Slowed breathing and heartbeat
- Numbness and loss of feeling in extremities

After contacting the EMS, you should take the following steps to provide first aid to a victim of hypothermia:

1. Get the victim out of the cold.

2. Keep the victim in a flat position. Do not raise the legs.

3. Squeeze as much water as possible from wet clothing, and layer dry clothing over wet clothing. Removal of clothing may jostle victim and lead to other problems.

4. Give the victim warm drinks only if he or she is able to swallow. Do not give the victim alcohol or caffeinated beverages, and do not allow the victim to smoke.

5. Do not allow the victim to exercise.

Heatstroke Heatstroke, the most serious heat-related disorder, results from the failure of the brain's heat-regulating mechanism (the hypothalamus) to cool the body. The following are signs and symptoms of heatstroke:

- Rapid pulse
- Hot, dry, flushed skin (absence of sweating)
- Disorientation leading to unconsciousness
- High body temperature

As soon as these symptoms are noticed, the body temperature should be reduced as quickly as possible. The victim should be immersed in a cool bath, lake, or stream. If there is no water nearby, loosen clothing and use a fan to help lower the victim's body temperature.

Heat Exhaustion Heat exhaustion results from excessive loss of salt and water. The onset is gradual, with the following symptoms:

- Fatigue and weakness
- Anxiety
- Nausea
- Profuse sweating
- Clammy skin
- Normal body temperature

To treat heat exhaustion, move the victim to a cool place. Have the victim lie down flat, with feet elevated 8 to 12 inches. Replace lost fluids slowly and steadily. Sponge or fan victim.

Heat Cramps Heat cramps result from excessive sweating, resulting in an excessive loss of salt and water. Although heat cramps are the least serious heat-related emergency, they are the most painful. The symptoms include muscle cramps, usually starting in the arms and legs. To relieve symptoms, the victim should drink electrolyte-rich beverages or a light saltwater solution or eat salty foods.

First Aid Supplies

Every home, car, or boat should be supplied with a basic first aid kit. In order to respond effectively to emergencies, you must have the basic equipment. This kit should be stored in a convenient place, but it should be kept out of the reach of children. Following is a list of supplies that should be included:

- Bandages, including triangular bandages (36 inches by 6 inches), butterfly bandages, a roller bandage, rolled white gauze bandages (2- and 3-inch widths), adhesive bandages

- Sterile gauze pads and absorbent pads

- Adhesive tape (2- and 3-inch widths)
- Cotton-tip applicators
- Scissors
- Thermometer
- Antibiotic ointment
- Aspirin
- Calamine lotion
- Antiseptic cream or petroleum jelly
- Safety pins
- Tweezers
- Latex gloves
- Flashlight
- Paper cups
- Blanket

You cannot be prepared for every medical emergency. Yet these essential tools and a knowledge of basic first aid will help you cope with many emergency situations.

Behavior Change Contract

Complete the Assess Yourself questionnaire, and read the Skills for Behavior Change box describing the stages of change. After reviewing your results and considering the various factors that influence your decisions, choose a health behavior that you would like to change, starting this quarter or semester (see other side for a sample filled-in contract.) Sign the contract at the bottom to affirm your commitment to making a healthy change, and ask a friend to witness it.

My behavior change will be:
_____

My long-term goal for this behavior change is:
_____

These are three obstacles to change (things that I am currently doing or situations that contribute to this behavior or make it harder to change):

1. _____
2. _____
3. _____

The strategies I will use to overcome these obstacles are:

1. _____
2. _____
3. _____

Resources I will use to help me change this behavior include:

a friend/partner/relative: _____

a school-based resource: _____

a community-based resource: _____

a book or reputable website: _____

In order to make my goal more attainable, I have devised these short-term goals:

short-term goal _____   target date _____   reward _____

short-term goal _____   target date _____   reward _____

short-term goal _____   target date _____   reward _____

When I make the long-term behavior change described above, my reward will be:

_____   target date _____

I intend to make the behavior change described above. I will use the strategies and rewards to achieve the goals that will contribute to a healthy behavior change.

Signed: _____   Witness: _____

Sample Behavior Change Contract

Complete the Assess Yourself questionnaire, and read the Skills for Behavior Change box describing the stages of change. After reviewing your results and considering the various factors that influence your decisions, choose a health behavior that you would like to change, starting this quarter or semester (see other side for a sample filled-in contract.) Sign the contract at the bottom to affirm your commitment to making a healthy change, and ask a friend to witness it.

My behavior change will be:

To snack less on junk food and more on healthy foods

My long-term goal for this behavior change is:

Eat junk food snacks no more than once a week

These are three obstacles to change (things that I am currently doing or situations that contribute to this behavior or make it harder to change):

1. *The grocery store is closed by the time I come home from school*
2. *I get hungry between classes, and the vending machines only carry candy bars*
3. *It's easier to order pizza or other snacks than to make a snack at home*

The strategies I will use to overcome these obstacles are:

1. *I'll leave early for school once a week so I can stock up on healthy snacks in the morning*
2. *I'll bring a piece of fruit or other healthy snack to eat between classes*
3. *I'll learn some easy recipes for snacks to make at home*

Resources I will use to help me change this behavior include:

a friend/partner/relative: *my roommates—I'll ask them to buy snacks insteads of chips when they do the shopping*

a school-based resource: *the dining hall—I'll ask for healthy foods we can take to eat between classes*

a community-based resource: *the library—I'll check out some cookbooks to find easy snack ideas*

a book or reputable website: *the USDA nutrient database at www.nal.usda.gov/fnic—I'll use this site to make sure the foods I select are healthy choices*

In order to make my goal more attainable, I have devised these short-term goals:

short-term goal *Eat a healthy snack 3X per week*   target date *September 15*   reward *new CD*

short-term goal *Learn to make a healthy snack*   target date *October 15*   reward *concert ticket*

short-term goal *Eat a healthy snack 5X per week*   target date *November 15*   reward *new shoes*

When I make the long-term behavior change described above, my reward will be:

Ski lift tickets for winter break   target date *December 15*

I intend to make the behavior change described above. I will use the strategies and rewards to achieve the goals that will contribute to a healthy behavior change.

Signed: *Elizabeth King*   Witness: *Susan Bauer*

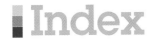

Index

Page references followed by *p* indicates a photograph; followed by *fig* indicates an illustrated figure.

Gender-related disorders, 405
Gender roles, 130
Gender-role stereotypes, 130
Gender selection science, 175
General urinary tract infections (UTIs), 395
Generic drugs, 185
Genetic history
    alcohol abuse/alcoholism and, 218–219
    bipolar disorder and, 48
    BRCA1/BRCA2 genes, 362
    cancer risk and, 357–358
    CVD risk and, 342
    depression risk and, 46
    migraine headaches and, 403–404
    as obesity risk factor, 282
    ovarian cancer and, 368
    prostate cancer risk and, 365
    sickle cell disease, 376
    See also Families
Genetic mutation theory, 417
Genital herpes, 393–394
Genital warts (human papillomavirus), 394–395
German Commission E, 487–488
Gerontology, 414
Gestational diabetes, 406
GHB (gamma-hydroxybutyrate), 105, 142, 200, 202
GIFT (gamete intrafallopina transfer), 174
Ginkgo biloba, 482
Ginseng, 485
Glaucoma, 419
Global health issues
    avian influenza, 382
    bioterrorism/terrorism, 95–96, 388
    challenges of, 15p
    factors contributing to cancer, 357fig
    overpopulation, 436–437
    pollution, 358, 437, 440–451
Global warming, 443–444
Globesity, 281
GLP-1 (ghrelin), 284
Glucose, 247
Glycemic index, 296–297
Glycogen, 248
GnRH (gonadotropin-releasing hormone), 129, 133
Goals
    establishing realistic weight loss, 280, 294
    identifying fitness, 317–318
    self-esteem and setting realistic expectations, 42
    setting realistic health behavior change, 27
    stress of inconsistent behaviors and, 66–67
Gonadatropins, 129, 133
Gonads, 128
Gonorrhea, 392
Graded exercise test, 309
GRAE (Generally Recognized as Effective), 186
GRAS (Generally Recognized as Safe), 186
Gratuitous violence, 92–95
Greenhouse gases, 443
Green tea, 483
Grief
    coping with, 427–428
    definition of, 426–427
    "normal," 427
Grief work, 427
Grieving tasks model, 427–428

Group A cancer-causing agent, 230
Group sex, 140
Gurin, J., 284

H

H5N1 (avian influenza), 382
Hallucinogens (psychedelics), 198–200
Hantavirus, 388
Happiness
    physical health and, 43–44
    satisfaction with life scale, 44fig
    SWB (subjective well-being) and, 43
Harrison Act (1914), 196
Hashish, 195
Hassles, 66
Hate/bias crimes, 93–94, 95
Hate Crime Statistics Report (FBI), 93
Hay fever, 401–402
Hazardous waste, 448–449
Hazing, 104
HBM (Health Belief Model), 19
HBP (high blood pressure), 341
HBV (hepatitis B), cancer risk and, 360
hCG (human chorionic gonadotropin), 134, 166–167
HCV (hepatitis C), 360
HDLs (high-density lipoproteins), 250, 339
Headaches, 403–404p
Health
    challenges of gender differences in, 15–16
    challenges of older adults, 422
    definition of, 3
    dental, 195p, 300
    dimensions of, 4–5fig
    evolution toward wellness as part of, 4–5fig
    impact of stress on, 63
    new directions for, 5–6
    physical fitness to improve, 308
    preparing for better 21st century, 1416
    reducing disparities of, 6
    self-assessment of your, 8–13
    yesterday and today's perspective of, 3–4
    See also Wellness
Health behavior intentions, 19–20
Health care costs, 415
Health information
    CAM consumer protection, 487
    CAM resources on the Internet, 489
    locating reliable Internet, 22
Health insurance
    CAM treatment coverage by, 488
    ethnic/racial minorities and, 356p
Health Professional Follow-Up Study, 347
Health promotion
    definition of, 7
    new focus on, 6–7
Health status, 16–17fig
Health status report, 12–14
Healthy behavior change
    choosing behavior-change technique for, 23–25
    health influenced by, 17
    improving health through, 2p–3
    preparing for, 17–22
    process of, 25–27
Healthy behavior change preparation
    beliefs and attitudes, 19
    identifying factors that influence behavior change, 17–19
    intentions to change, 19–20
    motivation and readiness, 19
    significant others as change agents, 20–22

Healthy behavior change process
    analyzing personal behavior, 26
    decision making: choices for change, 26–27
    finding reliable information on the Internet, 22
    overcoming barriers, 26fig
    self-assessment: antecedents and consequences, 25
    setting realistic goals, 27
    staging for, 20–22
Healthy behavior change techniques
    changing self-talk, 24–25
    controlling the situation, 23–24
    modeling, 23
    problem solving: art of self-instruction, 25
    reinforcement, 24
    shaping, 23
    visualization, 23
Healthy life expectancy, 14
Healthy People 2010, 5–6
Hearing loss, 419
Heart
    aging impact on the, 419
    anatomy of the, 329–330fig
    fibrillation, 336–337
    function of, 330–331
Heart attack (MI), 335, 336, 385
Heart disease. *See* CVD (cardiovascular disease)
Heart murmurs, 337
Heat cramps, 322
Heat exhaustion, 322
Heat stroke, 322–323
Hemochromatosis, 257
Hepatitis A (HAV), 381–382
Hepatitis B (HBV), 360, 382–383
Hepatitis C (HCV), 360, 383
Herbal preparations, 180
Herbal remedies, 481–483
Heroin, 197
Herpes, 393–394
Herpes simplex viruses (HSV), 393–394
Heterosexual orientation, 130–131
High-risk sexual behavior, 396–397
Histamines, 401
HIV disease
    symptoms of, 397
    testing for antibodies, 397–398
HIV (human immunodeficiency virus)
    definition of, 395
    new hope and treatments for, 399
    preventing infection due to, 399
    as shifting epidemic, 395–396
    transmission of, 396–397
    See also AIDS (acquired immunodeficiency syndrome)
Holistic approach, 5
Holmes, T., 65, 66
Holographic will, 432
Home heating pollution, 442
Homeopathy, 447
Homeostasis, 61
Homicide
    gratuitous violence of, 93
    United States as international capital of, 91
    YPLL (years of potential life lost) due to, 94
Homocysteine, 335
Homophobia, 131
Homosexual orientation, 130–131
Hope, 38
Hormonal methods, 148

Paternal health, 163
Pathogens
    body defenses against, 383–386fig
    body's defenses against, 377fig
    definition of, 376
    types/routes of transmission, 377–383
    See also Immune system
Pathogen types
    animal-borne, 377–378
    bacterial, 378–379
    fungi, protozoa, parasitic worms, 383
    prions, 383, 387
    viruses, 379–383
PCBs (polychlorinated biphenyls), 446, 448
PCP (phencyclidine), 199
PEA (phenylethylamine), 119
Peck, R., 417
Pedophilia, 140
Penis, 135fig–136
Peptic ulcer, 407
Perfect failure rate, 148
Perineum, 132
Periods of communicability, 389
Personal behavior assessment, 26
Personal control, 40
Personality
    characteristics of, 40
    resiliency (protective factors) part of, 41
    Type A, 63, 69, 73
    Type B, 63, 69
Pesticides water contamination, 446
PET scan (positron emission tomography
    scan), 345
Peyote cactus, 199
Pheromones, 120
Phobias, 51
Photochemical smog, 440
Physical activity
    benefits of, 306–309
    cardiorespiratory fitness and, 306–307,
        309–310, 312–313
    definition of, 306
    improving flexibility, 315–317, 318fig
    levels of, 311fig
    prostate cancer risk and, 365
    resistance exercise, 310–315, 423
    See also Exercise
Physical fitness
    body composition component of, 317
    cardiorespiratory fitness component of,
        306–307, 309–310, 312–313, 319
    components of, 307
    creating your own program for, 317–324
    definition of, 306
    flexibility component of, 315–317
    health aging and, 423
    muscular strength/endurance component
        of, 310–315fig, 423
Physical fitness program
    appropriate footwear for, 320–321
    avoiding injuries, 319, 321–322
    components of, 318–319
    dealing with heat or cold conditions,
        322–323
    designing your, 318
    identifying fitness goals, 317–318
    preventing cramps, 323–324
    starting exercise routine, 323
    workout machines/equipment for, 320
Physical health
    as dimension of health, 4, 5fig
    happiness and, 43–44
    psychosocial health and maintaining, 42
Physiological (physical) dependence, 182

PID (pelvic inflammatory disease), 153, 173,
    392
Pilates, 316p, 317
Pilates, J., 317
PIN (prostatic intraephithelial neoplasia), 365
Pituitary gland, 62, 129
Placenta, 168
Plantar fasciitis, 321
Plaque (arteries), 250, 331, 334p
Plateau (weight loss), 284
Platelet adhesiveness, 228
PMDD (premenstrual dysphoric disorder),
    53, 405
PMS (premenstrual syndrome), 46, 52–53, 405
Pneumonia, 379
PNF (proprioceptive neuromuscular facilita-
    tion), 316
PNI (psychoneuroimmunology), 64, 481
Point source pollutants, 445
Pollution
    air, 437, 440–444
    land, 447–449
    noise, 447
    radiation, 358, 449–451
    water, 444–447
Polydrug use, 187
Polysaccharides, 248
"Portion Distortion" quiz, 283
Portion distortion (serving sizes), 260, 263,
    283
Positive reinforcement, 24
Postpartum depression, 171
Potentiation (synergism), 187–188
Preconception care, 163
Predisposing factors, 18
Preeclampsia, 172
Pregnancy
    caffeine consumption during, 235
    complications of, 172–173
    ectopic, 173
    factors involved in planning, 163–164
    FAS (fetal alcohol syndrome), 165–166p,
        215–216
    fertilization resulting in, 167fig
    gender selection science and, 175
    genital herpes and, 394
    gestational diabetes developed during,
        406
    prenatal care, 164–166
    prenatal testing and screening, 168–169fig
    process of, 167–168p
    testing for, 166–167
    trimesters of, 167–168, 169fig
    woman's reproductive years and, 166
    See also Abortion; Childbirth; Women
Preimplantation genetic diagnosis, 175
Prejudice, 37, 94
Premature ejaculation, 141
Prenatal care, 164–166
Prenatal testing/screening, 168–169fig
Prescription drugs
    costs of, 185
    described, 183
    generic, 185
    improving safety of, 184
    interactions of, 187–188
    older adults and use of, 422
    switched to being OTC products, 185
    types of, 183–185
Pressure
    downshifting to control, 75
    stressful impact of, 66

Prevalence reduction, 12
Primary aggression, 92
Primary prevention
    definition of, 7
    to reduce incidence and prevalence, 12
Prions, 383, 387
Probiotics, 264
Problem solving
    art of self-instruction for, 25
    examining problems/seeking help if nec-
        essary, 42
    See also Decision making
Progesterone, 133, 134
Progestin-only pills (minipills), 153
Progressive muscle relaxation, 83
Prostaglandin inhibitors, 186
Prostate cancer, 364, 365
Prostate gland, 136
Protease inhibitors, 399
Proteins
    CRP (C-reactive protein), 335
    nutrition and, 243, 246
    older adults and need for, 423
    RDA (Recommended Dietary
        Allowance), 247fig
Protooncogenes, 356
Protozoa, 383
Prozac, 48
PSA (prostate-specific antigen) test, 365
Psilocybin, 199
Psychedelics (hallucinogens), 198–200
Psychiatric nurse specialist, 55
Psychiatrist, 54
Psychoactive drugs, 180
Psychoeducation, 128
Psychological aging, 414
Psychological factors
    cancer risks and, 358–359
    hardiness, 73
Psychological stress, 73
Psychologist, 55
Psychoneuroimmunology (PNI), 64, 481
Psychosocial factors
    aging and, 417
    CFS (chronic fatigue syndrome), 408
    obesity and, 285
Psychosocial health
    assessing your, 34–36
    characteristics of, 32fig–33fig
    definition of, 32
    deterioration of, 45–53
    emotional health as part of, 36–37
    factors influencing, 39–41
    mental health as part of, 36
    seeking professional help with, 54–55
    social health as part of, 37
    spiritual health as part of, 37–39
    strategies to enhance, 41–45
    suicide, 53–54
    tips for building self-esteem and, 41
Psychosocial health deterioration
    anxiety disorders, 49–52
    depression, 45–48
    gender issues in, 52–53
    overview of, 45
    SAD (seasonal affective disorder), 52
    schizophrenia, 52
    seeking professional help, 54–55
    suicide and, 53–54
PTSD (post-traumatic stress disorder), 76–77
Puberty
    definition of, 129
    menstrual cycle and onset of, 133–134

∎ Credits

Chapter 1, p. 1: Randy Faris/CORBIS; p. 2: Digital Stock/CORBIS; p. 7: Scott Barbour/Allsport; p. 14: Richard Price/Getty Images; p. 15: Kirsty Wigglesworth/Associated Press, PAMPC PA; p. 20: Randy M. Ury/CORBIS; p. 24: Tom Prettyman/PhotoEdit; Chapter 2, p. 31: SuperStock; p. 37: Timothy Shonnard/Getty Images; p. 45: Randy Faris/CORBIS; p. 46: Lawrence Manning/CORBIS; p. 49: Andrew Errington/Getty Images; p. 51: CORBIS;Chapter 3, p. 59: Spike Mafford/Photodisc; p. 60: DanielGarcia/AFP/Getty Images; p. 64: CORBIS; p. 69: Leland Bobbe/Getty Images; p. 73: Ulrike Welsch/ PhotoEdit; p. 77: Reuters/CORBIS; p. 78: Chuck Savage/CORBIS; p. 82: CORBIS; p. 84: Jason Homa/Getty Images; Chapter 4, p. 89: Mary-Arthur Johnson/Taxi; p. 95: AP Wide World Photos; p. 97: Bill Aron/PhotoEdit; p. 102: AP Wide World Photos; p. 107: William Thomas Cain/Getty Images; p. 108: James Lauritz/Getty Images; Chapter 5, p. 113: Stockbyte; p. 114: Charles Gupton/CORBIS; p. 115: Jose Luis Pelaez, Inc./CORBIS; p. 123: AP Wide World Photos; p. 126: Ellen Senisi/The Image Works; p. 130: Michael Pole/CORBIS; p. 141:The Image Bank; p. 142:Bill Stanton/Rainbow; Chapter 6, p. 147: Michelangelo Gratton/Digital Vision; p. 151: Dorling Kindersley; p. 152: Jules Selmes and Debi Treloar/Dorling Kindersley; p. 154: Joel Gordon/Joel Gordon Photography; p. 162: AP Wide World Photos; p. 165: Michael Newman/PhotoEdit; p. 166: Ann P. Streigssgoth/ Fetal Alcohol & Drug Unit (FAS); p. 168: Claude Edelman/Photo Researchers; p. 168: Petit Format-Nestle/Photo Researchers; p. 168: Petit Format-Nestle/Photo Researchers; p. 172: Photodisc; Chapter 7, p. 179: Stockbyte; p. 183: Bonnie Kamin/PhotoEdit; p. 190: Garry Watson/Photo Researchers; p. 190: Bill Aron/PhotoEdit, Inc.; p. 190: Michael Newman/PhotoEdit, Inc.; p. 191: SPL/Photo Researchers; p. 195: Charles Tatlock; p. 196: Gary Retherford/Photo Researchers; p. 201: Luc Beziat/Getty Images; p. 202: Reuters/CORBIS; Chapter 8, p. 207: Ryan McVay/Photodisc; p. 208: Chuck Savage/CORBIS; p. 214: Mark Peterson/CORBIS; p. 216: Yva Momatiuk & John Eastcott/Stock Boston; p. 221: Jon Feingersh/CORBIS; p. 226: Oral Health America; Chapter 9, p. 239: Peter Cade/The Image Bank; p. 240: Michael Keller/CORBIS; p. 248: VCL/Taxi/Getty Images; p. 253: Peter Nicholson/Getty Images; p. 260: Photolibrary.com/Index Stock Imagery, Inc.; p. 262: Brian Hagiwara/Foodpix; p. 265: Reg Charity/ CORBIS; Chapter 10, p. 275: Comstock/CORBIS; p. 278: Guang Niu/CORBIS; p. 283: C Squared Studios/Photodisc; p. 283: James Noble/CORBIS; p. 285: Ariel Skelley/CORBIS; p. 290: Table Mesa Prod/IndexStock; p. 295: APF/LIU Jin/CORBIS; p. 296: Chris Hondros/Getty Images; p. 298: Tammie Arroyo/AP Photo; Chapter 11, p. 305: Photodisc; p. 308: David Stoecklein/CORBIS; p. 310: David Young-Wolff/PhotoEdit; p. 310: Esbin-Anderson/The Image Works; p. 316: PhotoEdit Inc.; p. 322: Bob Daemmrick/The Image Works; p. 323: Jim Cummins/Getty Images; Chapter 12, p. 327: Steve Allen/ Digital Vision; p. 328: Mike Fiala/CORBIS; p. 334: Visuals Unlimited; p. 334: Visuals Unlimited; p. 340: Chris Fotoman Smith/Alamy; p. 344: Thinkstock; p. 345: Richard T. Nowitz/Photo Researchers; Chapter 13, p. 351: David Becker/Stone; p. 356: Mark Richards/PhotoEdit Inc.; p. 358: Jonathan A. Meyers/Photo Researchers; p. 362: Charles Gupton/Stock Boston; p. 366: James Stevenson/SPL/Photo Researchers; p. 366: Dr. P. Marazzi/SPL/Photo Researchers; p. 366: Dr. P. Marazzi/SPL/Photo Researchers; p. 367: Anthony Redpath/ CORBIS; p. 368: Joel Saget/AFP Photo; p. 372: Bill Greenplatt/ Newsmakers / Liaison; Chapter 14, p. 375: Arthur Tilley/Taxi; p. 379: Jeff Greenberg/AGE Fotostock; p. 382: Marius Nemes/Pool/Reuters/ CORBIS; p. 388: PETER PARKS/AFP/Getty Images; p. 393: Steve Mercer/Getty Images; p. 397: A. Ramy/Stock Boston; p. 398: Stonehill/ zefa/CORBIS; p. 400: Francoise Sauze/Photo Researchers; p. 402: John Millar/Stone; p. 404: Elena Dorfman/Offshoot Inc.; p. 407: Bonnie Kamin; Chapter 15, p. 413: Jim Naughten/Taxi; p. 414: John Henley/ CORBIS; p. 418: Ariel Skelley/CORBIS; p. 422: Dan Bosler/Stone Allstock / Getty Images; p. 425: Arvind Garg/Photo Researchers; p. 428: Mark Richards/PhotoEdit Inc.; Chapter 16, p. 435: Comstock; p. 436: Richard L'Anson/Lonelyplanet Images/Getty Images; p. 441: Will & Demi McIntyre/Photo Researchers; p. 449: Bonnie Kamin/ PhotoEdit; p. 450: Jenns Lucking/Getty Images; Chapter 17, p. 455: Stockbyte; p. 457: Jim Sulley/The Image Works; p. 461: SuperStock, Inc.; p. 464: Paul Conklin/PhotoEdit; p. 468: David Young-Wolff/ PhotoEdit Inc.; p. 469: A. Ramey/PhotoEdit Inc.; Chapter 18, p. 473: Mel Yates/Photodisc; p. 480: Novastock/The Stock Connection; p. 481: Willie Hill, Jr./The Image Works; p. 482: Michael Newman/PhotoEdit; p. 487: Richard Levine/Alamy